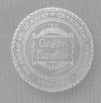 American Academy of Orthopaedic Surgeons

# OKU
## Orthopaedic Knowledge Update:

# Spine

# 3

Edited by
Jeffrey M. Spivak, MD
Patrick J. Connolly, MD

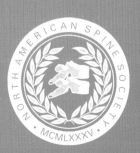

Developed by

North American
Spine Society

Published 2006
by the American Academy of Orthopaedic Surgeons
6300 North River Road
Rosemont, IL 60018
1-800-626-6726

The material presented in *Orthopaedic Knowledge Update: Spine 3* has been made available by the American Academy of Orthopaedic Surgeons for educational purposes only. This material is not intended to present the only, or necessarily best, methods or procedures for the medical situations discussed, but rather is intended to represent an approach, view, statement, or opinion of the author(s) or producer(s), which may be helpful to others who face similar situations.

Some drugs or medical devices demonstrated in Academy courses or described in Academy print or electronic publications have not been cleared by the Food and Drug Administration (FDA) or have been cleared for specific uses only. The FDA has stated that it is the responsibility of the physician to determine the FDA clearance status of each drug or device he or she wishes to use in clinical practice.

Furthermore, any statements about commercial products are solely the opinion(s) of the author(s) and do not represent an Academy endorsement or evaluation of these products. These statements may not be used in advertising or for any commercial purpose.

Some of the authors or the departments with which they are affiliated have received something of value from a commercial or other party related directly or indirectly to the subject of their chapter.

Third Edition
Copyright ©2006 by the
American Academy of Orthopaedic Surgeons

ISBN 10: 0-89203-354-1
ISBN 13: 978-0-89203-354-6
Printed in the USA

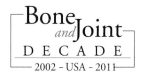

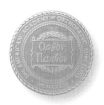

*American Academy of Orthopaedic Surgeons*

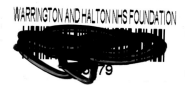

# Orthopaedic Knowledge Update:

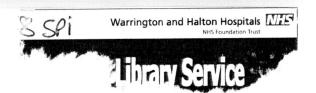

# Spine

# Acknowledgments

## Editorial Board, OKU: Spine 3

Jeffrey M. Spivak, MD
Director, New York University Hospital
   for Joint Diseases Spine Center
Department of Orthopaedic Surgery
New York University Hospital for Joint Diseases
New York, New York

Patrick J. Connolly, MD
Chief, Division of Spinal Surgery
University of Massachusetts
Department of Orthopaedic Surgery
University of Massachusetts
Worcester, Massachusetts

Denis S. Drummond, MD
Professor Emeritus
Department of Orthopaedic Surgery
Children's Hospital of Philadelphia
Philadelphia, Pennsylvania

Sanford E. Emery, MD, MBA
Professor and Chairman
Department of Orthopaedics
West Virginia University
Morgantown, West Virginia

Alexander Ghanayem, MD
Associate Professor
Chief, Division of Spine Surgery
Department of Orthopaedic Surgery and Rehabilitation
Loyola University Medical Center
Maywood, Illinois

Joel M. Press, MD
Medical Director
Spinal Sports Rehabilitation Center
Rehabilitation Institute of Chicago
Chicago, Illinois

Henry Claude Sagi, MD
Orhopaedic Trauma Service
Florida Orthopaedic Institute
Tampa General Hospital
Tampa, Florida

Jeffrey C. Wang, MD
Chief, Spine Service
Associate Professor of Orthopaedics and Neurosurgery
UCLA Department of Orthopaedic Surgery
UCLA School of Medicine
Los Angeles, California

## North American Spine Society

*Board of Directors, 2006*

Joel Press, MD
   *President*
Richard D. Guyer, MD
   *1st Vice President*
Hallet Mathews, MD
   *Secretary*
Robert J. Gatchel, PhD
   *Treasurer*
Tom Faciszewski, MD
   *2nd Vice President*
Jean-Jacques Abitbol, MD
   *Past President*
Ray Baker, MD
   *Education Council Co-Director*
J. Kenneth Burkus, MD
   *Education Council Co-Director*
Michael Heggeness, MD
   *Research Council Director*
Jerome Schofferman, MD
   *Clinical Care Council Director*
Greg Przybylski, MD
   *Socio-Economic Affairs Council Director*
Charles Mick, MD
   *Socio-Economic Affairs Council Co-Director*
Stuart Weinstein, MD
   *Member Services Council Director*
Marjorie Eskay-Auerbach, MD, JD
   *Public Education Council Director*
Eric J. Muehlbauer, MJ, CAE
   *Executive Director*

# Contributors

Behrooz A. Akbarnia, MD
Clinical Professor
Department of Orthopaedics
University of California, San Diego
San Diego Center for Spinal Disorders
La Jolla, California

Todd J. Albert, MD
Professor and Vice Chairman
Department of Orthopaedic Surgery
Thomas Jefferson University Hospital
Rothman Institute
Philadelphia, Pennsylvania

D. Greg Anderson, MD
Associate Professor
Department of Orthopaedic Surgery
Rothman Institute
Thomas Jefferson University Hospital
Philadelphia, Pennsylvania

Paul A. Anderson, MD
Associate Professor of Orthopedic
    Surgery and Rehabilitation
University of Wisconsin
Madison, Wisconsin

Gunnar B. J. Andersson, MD, PhD
Professor and Chairman
Department of Orthopedic Surgery
Rush University Medical Center
Chicago, Illinois

Joshua D. Auerbach, MD
Department of Orthopaedic Surgery
The University of Pennsylvania
Philadelphia, Pennsylvania

John N. Awad, MD
Department of Orthopaedics,
    Spine Division
Hospital for Joint Disease
New York University
New York, New York

Vaibhav Bagaria, MD
Fellow
Department of Orthopaedic Surgery
Medical College of Wisconsin
Milwaukee, Wisconsin

Aleksander Beric, MD, DSC
Professor of Neurophysiology
New York University School of
    Medicine
Department of Clinical Neurology
Hospital for Joint Diseases
New York, New York

John A. Bendo, MD
Department of Orthopaedics,
    Spine Division
Hospital for Joint Disease
New York University
New York, New York

James B. Billys, MD
Department of Orthopaedics
Florida Orthopaedic Institute
Tampa, Florida

Michael J. Bolesta, MD
Associate Professor
Orthopaedic Surgery
University of Texas Southwestern
    Medical School
Dallas, Texas

Christopher M. Bono, MD
Assistant Professor
Director, Spine Surgery
Department of Orthopaedic Surgery
Boston University School of Medicine
Boston, Massachusetts

Darrel S. Brodke, MD
Associate Professor
Department of Orthopaedic Surgery
University of Utah
Salt Lake City, Utah

Robert J. Campbell, MD
Assistant Instructor in Orthopaedic
    Surgery
Brown University School of Medicine
Chief Resident in Orthopaedic Surgery
Rhode Island Hospital
Department of Orthopaedics
Providence, Rhode Island

Elliot Carlisle, MD
Orthopaedic Spine Surgeon
Orthopaedic Consultants Medical
    Group
Encino-Tarzana Medical Center
Encino, California

George E. Charuk, DO
Medical Director, Outpatient
    Rehabilitation
Department of Orthopaedic Surgery
    and Rehabilitation
Loyola University Medical Center
Maywood, Illinois

David Chen, MD
Director, Spinal Cord Injury Program
Rehabilitation Institute of Chicago
Chicago, Illinois

Jack Chen, MD
Spine Surgeon
Orthopaedic Specialty Institute
Orange, California

Kingsley R. Chin, MD
Chief, Division of Spine Surgery
Assistant Professor of Orthopaedic
    Surgery
Department of Orthopaedic Surgery
University of Pennsylvania Medical
    School
Philadelphia, Pennsylvania

Geoffrey A. Cronen, MD
Chief Resident
Department of Orthopaedics
West Virginia University
Morgantown, West Virginia

Kirk W. Dabney, MD
Department of Orthopaedics
A.I. duPont Hospital for Children
Wilmington, Delaware

Hargovind DeWal, MD
Fellow, Spinal Surgery
Cleveland Clinic Spine Institute
Cleveland Clinic Foundation
Cleveland, Ohio

Rob D. Dickerman, DO, PhD
Neurosurgeon
North Texas Neurosurgical Associates
Department of Neurosurgery
Plano Presbyterian Hospital
Plano, Texas

Daniel M. Doleys, PhD
Director
Pain and Rehabilitation Institute
Birmingham, Alabama

John P. Dormans, MD
Chief of Orthopaedic Surgery
Children's Hospital of Philadelphia
Professor of Orthopaedic Surgery
University of Pennsylvania School
    of Medicine
Philadelphia, Pennsylvania

Denis S. Drummond, MD
Professor Emeritus
Department of Orthopaedic Surgery
Children's Hospital of Philadelphia
Philadelphia, Pennsylvania

Jason C. Eck, DO, MS
Resident
Department of Orthopaedic Surgery
Memorial Hospital
York, Pennsylvania

Frank Eismont, MD
Co-Chairman
Department of Orthopaedic Surgery
Orthopaedic Surgeon
University of Miami
Miami, Florida

Sanford E. Emery, MD, MBA
Professor and Chairman
Department of Orthopaedics
West Virginia University
Morgantown, West Virginia

Tom Faciszewski, MD
Department of Orthopaedic Spine
    Surgery
Marshfield Clinic
Marshfield, Wisconsin

Daniel R. Fassett, MD
Neurosurgical Resident
Department of Neurosurgery
University of Utah
Salt Lake City, Utah

Jeffrey S. Fischgrund, MD
Spine Surgeon
Department of Orthopaedic Surgery
William Beaumont Hospital
Royal Oak, Michigan

John M. Flynn, MD
Associate Professor
University of Pennsylvania
Attending Surgeon
Division of Orthopaedic Surgery
The Children's Hospital of Philadelphia
Philadelphia, Pennsylvania

John C. France, MD
Associate Professor
Department of Orthopaedics
West Virginia University
Morgantown, West Virginia

Christopher G. Furey, MD
Assistant Professor
Department of Orthopaedic Surgery
Case Western Reserve University
Cleveland, Ohio

Ioannis N. Gaitanis, MD
Research Fellow
Department of Orthopaedic Surgery
    and Rehabilitation
Loyola University, Chicago
Maywood, Illinois

Timothy A. Garvey, MD
Associate Professor
Twin Cities Spine Center
Minneapolis, Minnesota

Robert J. Gatchel, PhD, ABPP
Professor and Chairman
Department of Psychology
College of Science
University of Texas
Arlington, Texas

Lars G. Gilbertson, PhD
Associate Professor
Department of Orthopaedic Surgery
University of Pittsburgh
Pittsburgh, Pennsylvania

Kevin Gill, MD
Professor
Department of Orthopaedic Surgery
University of Texas Southwestern
    Medical School
Dallas, Texas

Bernard H. Guiot, MD, FRCSC
Director of Spine
Department of Neurosurgery
University of South Florida
Tampa, Florida

Michael H. Haak, MD
Assistant Professor of Orthopaedic
    Surgery
The Feinberg School of Medicine
Northwestern University
Chicago, Illinois

Martin J. Herman, MD
Assistant Professor of Orthopedic
    Surgery
Drexel College of Medicine
Orthopedic Center for Children
St. Christopher's Hospital for Children
Philadelphia, Pennsylvania

Alan S. Hilibrand, MD
Associate Professor of Orthopaedic
    Surgery and Neurosurgery
Director of Medical Education
The Rothman Institute
Jefferson Medical College
Philadelphia, Pennsylvania

Harish S. Hosalkar, MD, MBMS (Orth),
    D (Orth), FCPS (Orth), DNB (Orth)
Department of Orthopaedic Surgery
Children's Hospital of Philadelphia
Philadelphia, Pennsylvania

Joji Inamasu, MD, PhD
Spine Fellow
Department of Neurosurgery
University of South Florida
Tampa, Florida

Louis G. Jenis, MD
Clinical Assistant Professor,
    Orthopaedic Surgery
Tufts University School of Medicine
New England Baptist Hospital
Department of Orthopaedic Surgery
Boston, Massachusetts

James D. Kang, MD
Vice Chairman, Orthopaedic Surgery
Associate Professor
Orthopaedic Surgery and Division
    of Neurological Spinal Surgery
University of Pittsburgh Medical Center
Pittsburgh, Pennsylvania

Reilly Keffer, DO
Spine Fellow
Spine Center
Department of Physical Medicine
    and Rehabilitation
New England Baptist Hospital
Boston, Massachusetts

Natasha J. Kim, DC
Chiropractor
Spine and Sports Rehabilitation
Rehabilitation Institute of Chicago
Chicago, Illinois

John S. Kirkpatrick, MD
Associate Professor
Division of Orthopaedic Surgery
University of Alabama, Birmingham
Birmingham, Alabama

Nancy D. Kishino, OTR, CVE
Director/Owner
West Coast Spine Restoration Center
Riverside, California

James W. Larson III, MD
Resident Physician
Department of Orthopaedic Surgery
University of Pittsburgh Medical Center
Pittsburgh, Pennsylvania

Eric A. Levicoff, MD
Orthopaedic Surgery Research Resident
Department of Orthopaedic Surgery
University of Pittsburgh Medical Center
Pittsburgh, Pennsylvania

Richard E. McCarthy, MD
Clinical Professor
Arkansas Spine Center
Department of Orthopaedics
University of Arkansas for Medical
    Sciences
Little Rock, Arkansas

Fergus E. McKiernan, MD
Center for Bone Disease
Marshfield Clinic
Marshfield, Wisconsin

Robert F. McLain, MD
Professor
Lerner College of Medicine
Director, Spine Surgery Fellowship
    Program
The Cleveland Clinic Spine Institute
Department of Orthopaedic Surgery
The Cleveland Clinic Foundation
Cleveland, Ohio

Freeman Miller, MD
Department of Orthopaedics
A.I. duPont Hospital for Children
Wilmington, Delaware

Leslie Moroz
Clinical Research Coordinator
Division of Orthopaedic Surgery
Children's Hospital of Philadelphia
Philadelphia, Pennsylvania

Elisha Ofiram, MD
Department of Spine Surgery
Twin Cities Spine Center
Minneapolis, Minnesota

Mark Palumbo, MD
Associate Professor of Orthopaedic
    Surgery
Department of Orthopaedic Surgery
Brown Medical School
Rhode Island Hospital
Providence, Rhode Island

Nilesh M. Patel, MD
Orthopedic Spine Surgeon
Michigan Orthopedic Specialists
Oakwood Hospital and Medical Center
Dearborn, Michigan

Ajit V. Patwardhan, MD, MS
Clinical Spine Fellow
Orthopedics
Yale New Haven Hospital
Yale University
New Haven, Connecticut

Avinash G. Patwardhan, PhD
Professor and Director
Musculoskeletal Biomechanics
    Laboratory
Department of Orthopaedic Surgery
    and Rehabilitation
Loyola University, Chicago
Maywood, Illinois

Bernard A. Pfeifer, MD
Assistant Clinical Professor of
    Orthopaedic Surgery
Boston University School of Medicine
Department of Orthopaedic Surgery
Lahey Clinic
Burlington, Massachusetts

Amy H. Phelan, MD
Physical Medicine and Rehabilitation/
    Pain Medicine
Magnolia Diagnostics
New Orleans, Louisiana

Peter D. Pizzutillo, MD
Director, Orthopaedic Surgery
Department of Surgery
St. Christopher's Hospital for Children
Philadelphia, Pennsylvania

John B. Pracyk, MD, PhD
Neurological Surgeon
Iowa Spine and Brain Institute
Covenant Health System
Waterloo, Iowa

Joel M. Press, MD
Medical Director
Spinal Sports Rehabilitation Center
Rehabilitation Institute of Chicago
Chicago, Illinois

James Rainville, MD
Assistant Clinical Professor
Department of Physical Medicine and
    Rehabilitation
Harvard Medical School
Boston, Massachusetts

Raj Rao, MD
Associate Professor
Director of Spine Surgery
Department of Orthopaedic Surgery
Medical College of Wisconsin
Milwaukee, Wisconsin

John M. Rhee, MD
Assistant Professor
Department of Orthopaedic Surgery
Emory Spine Center
Emory University School of Medicine
Atlanta, Georgia

K. Daniel Riew, MD
Professor
Chief, Cervical Spine Surgery
Department of Orthopaedic Surgery
Washington University School of
    Medicine
St. Louis, Missouri

Marie D. Rinaldi, BA
New Jersey Medical School
Newark, New Jersey

Anthony Rinella, MD
Assistant Professor
Department of Orthopaedic Surgery
    and Rehabilitation
Loyola University Medical School
Maywood, Illinois

Henry Claude Sagi, MD
Orhopaedic Trauma Service
Florida Orthopaedic Institute
Tampa General Hospital
Tampa, Florida

Lee S. Segal, MD
Associate Professor of Orthopaedic
    Surgery
Department or Orthopaedics and
    Rehabilitation
The Pennsylvania State University
    College of Medicine
The Milton S. Hershey Medical Center
Hershey, Pennsylvania

Arya Nick Shamie, MD
Assistant Professor of Orthopaedic
    Surgery and Neurosurgery
Chief, Wadsworth VA Spine Service
UCLA Department of Orthopaedic
    Surgery
UCLA School of Medicine
Los Angeles, California

Brad Sorosky, MD
Physiatrist
Department of Physical Medicine and
    Rehabilitation
Desert Pain Institute
Mesa, Arizona

Susan C. Sorosky, MD
Physiatrist
Department of Physical Medicine and
    Rehabilitation
Desert Pain Institute
Mesa, Arizona

David A. Spiegel, MD
Department of Orthopaedic Surgery
Children's Hospital of Philadelphia
Philadelphia, Pennsylvania

Steven Stanos, DO
Medical Director, Chronic Pain Care
    Center
Rehabilitation Institute of Chicago
Department of Physical Medicine and
    Rehabilitation
Northwestern University Medical
    School
Feinberg School of Medicine
Chicago, Illinois

Michael P. Steinmetz, MD
Spine Fellow
Neurosurgery
University of Wisconsin
Madison, Wisconsin

Alan M. Strezak, MD
Associate Clinical Professor of
    Orthopaedic Surgery
Department of Orthopaedic Surgery
University of California, Irvine
Orange, California

Chadi Tannoury, MD
Research Assistant in Orthopaedic
    Surgery
Department of Spine Surgery
Thomas Jefferson University Hospital
Rothman Institute
Philadelphia, Pennsylvania

John J. Triano, DC, PhD, FCCSC
Texas Back Institute
Research Professor
University of Texas
Biomedical Engineering Program
Arlington, Texas

Vincent C. Traynelis, MD
Professor
Department of Neurosurgery
The University of Iowa
Iowa City, Iowa

Leonard I. Voronov, MD, PhD
Research Associate
Adjunct Instructor
Department of Orthopaedic Surgery
    and Rehabilitation
Loyola University, Chicago
Maywood, Illinois

Jeffrey C. Wang, MD
Chief, Spine Service
Associate Professor of Orthopaedics
    and Neurosurgery
UCLA Department of Orthopaedic
    Surgery
UCLA School of Medicine
Los Angeles, California

Andrew P. White, MD
Clinical Instructor and Chief Resident
Department of Orthopaedics and
    Rehabilitation
Yale Medical School
New Haven, Connecticut

Susan Lai Williams, MD
Department of Orthopaedic Surgery
George Washington University
Washington, DC

Warren D. Yu, MD
Assistant Professor
Department of Orthopaedic Surgery
George Washington School of Medicine
Washington, DC

James J. Yue, MD
Assistant Professor of Orthopaedic
    Surgery
Yale School of Medicine
Department of Orthopaedic Surgery
Yale University
New Haven, Connecticut

Jack E. Zigler, MD
Clinical Associate Professor of
    Orthopaedic Surgery
University of Texas Southwestern
    Medical School
Co-Director, Fellowship Training
    Program
Texas Back Institute
Plano, Texas

# Preface

When asked by the North American Spine Society to be editors of the third edition of Orthopaedic Knowledge Update: Spine, we realized we were taking on an extensive project. The care of spinal disorders is truly a multidisciplinary field, encompassing a large number of health care subspecialties. It involves not only orthopaedic surgeons, but also colleagues in the fields of physical medicine and rehabilitation, anesthesia, radiology, neurology, neurosurgery, rheumatology, and internal medicine. We felt strongly that it was important to approach this project keeping this aspect in mind, and draw from the varied expertise of many nonorthopaedic subspecialists.

The challenges of spine care have led to a recent explosion of new technologies, improving our ability to treat many spinal disorders. Physicians must be able to incorporate these new technologies into patient care where appropriate, and be able to review and critically evaluate the literature in order to practice proper evidence-based medicine. Some of these new technologies represent a natural progression toward making surgical procedures more efficient and less destructive to normal surrounding tissues; examples of these would include thoracoscopic diskectomies and minimally invasive posterior lumbar fusions. Other technologies may represent a significant change in traditional thinking and care; examples of these would include motion-sparing stabilization procedures (including total disk replacement) and gene therapy for intervertebral disk repair. As physicians caring for our patients, we must act as advocates for them, and seek the truth within the usual "hype" of these new and different procedures. We must also act responsibly in order to avoid depleting our health care resources on unnecessary tests and ineffective interventions. In order to provide the reader with the latest information in all of the varied fields regarding spinal disorder diagnosis and treatment, we have assembled a group of contributors who are not only experts regarding their assigned topics but who also actively participate in clinical patient care.

This text is divided into five main sections. Section one is devoted to the basics of spine care and includes chapters on anatomy, physical examination, diagnostic testing, and outcomes assessment. Section two focuses on management of acute and chronic spine-related pain, including medical and interventional management and rehabilitation. Section three addresses the evaluation and treatment of specific adult disorders including degenerative disease, adult deformity, and spinal trauma. Section four is dedicated to the pediatric spine. Section five provides the reader with the latest update (at the time of printing) on new and future trends in osteobiologics and device technology, all aimed at improving and expanding the treatment of spinal disorders. Expanding on the previous OKU Spine editions, each chapter in this edition highlights updates since the previous edition, but also reviews and emphasizes the basic concepts of the various spinal disorders and their treatment. In this manner, the current edition can act as more of a review text than prior editions. The authors have incorporated radiographs, photographs, illustrations, and tables into the chapters to highlight significant points. The annotated bibliography of recent articles and the classic article listings in each chapter provide an excellent resource for further in-depth learning on specific topics.

Practicing medicine in this day and age requires more time spent on non- patient care, practice-related activities than ever before, constantly pulling on our family and personal time. The time spent by all of the contributors creating these chapters represents a special type of volunteerism that often goes unrecognized. We would like to acknowledge and thank all of the contributors to OKU Spine 3, for taking the extra time out of their already busy schedules to help make this volume a strong learning tool.

The scope of this text, with more than 50 chapters and 75 individual contributors, requires the assistance of a team of section editors, who are true experts in their fields of specialization and act as the 'first-line' reviewers of the chapter submissions. We are indebted to Alex Ghanayem, Joel Press, Sandy Emery, Claude Sagi, Denis Drummond, and Jeff Wang for all of their time and effort.

The strength of any edited manuscript with many contributors, including the AAOS OKU series, requires a tremendous effort and incredible attention to detail on the part of the administrative staff. The AAOS Department of Publications headed by Marilyn Fox, PhD, director, and Lisa Claxton Moore, managing editor, Kathy Anderson, medical editor, are truly the unsung heroes of this project. We cannot thank them enough for all of their hard work.

*Patrick J. Connolly, MD*
*Jeffrey M. Spivak, MD*
*Editors*

# Table of Contents

## Section 1: Basic Concepts
**Section Editor:       Alexander Ghanayem, MD**

## Section 2: Pain Treatments and Rehabilitation
**Section Editor:     Joel M. Press, MD**

## Section 3: Adult Topics
**Section Editors:**   **Sanford E. Emery, MD**
                       **Henry Claude Sagi, MD**

## Section 4: Pediatric Topics

**Section Editor:    Denis S. Drummond, MD**

# Section 1

# Basic Concepts

Section Editor:
Alexander Ghanayem, MD

# Chapter 1

# Human Embryology Emphasizing Spinal and Neural Development

Anthony Rinella, MD

## General Concepts

It takes 266 days for the human zygote, the initial sperm/egg pair, to develop into a neonate. This process requires a complex yet coordinated interaction of events. The initial cells are pluripotent, meaning that individual cells can follow more than one developmental pathway. Cells acquire special features through a process called differentiation. Morphogenesis is the organization of differentiated cells into tissues and organs. As the cells become more specialized, they lose their pluripotential ability.

The development of any specific structure, such as a vertebra, begins with the creation of a critical cell mass called an anlage—the earliest discernible indication of an organ or part. The anlage is then subjected or exposed to inductive biochemical and biophysical factors that promote further cell differentiation into modified or additional anlagen followed by an intermediate structure, and then the final structure. These genetic and microenvironmental factors include biochemical gradients, morphogen concentrations, mechanical forces, and cellular migrations and adhesions. Within certain cell lines, a system known as determination may encourage, for example, ectodermal tissue to become neural tissue as opposed to other ectodermal pathways. The precise timing and order of specific protein synthesis at the molecular level is critical for proper embryologic development.

Questions arise as to how an initial group of homogeneous cells can differentiate into specific structures such as a vertebra or foot. Homeotic genes may provide the answer in their function in coordinating the process of differentiation. A group of homeotic genes called *HOX* genes are important in positioning cell types along the AP axis.

From a clinical perspective, pathologic development can occur because of errors that occur in three time periods: prefertilization (errors in gametogenesis); gestation (errors in embryo and/or fetal development); and the postnatal period (errors after birth). Pathologic development that occurs after birth is not within the scope of this chapter.

## Prefertilization

Gametogenesis is the production of gametes (spermatozoa and oocytes). Most cells in the human body are diploid (having 46 chromosomes: 44 autosomes and 2 sex chromosomes, X and Y). During mitosis, diploid cells are duplicated into two identical diploid daughter cells. Meiosis is a special process in which diploid cells are converted into haploid gametes (23 chromosomes). One DNA replication cycle is followed by two cell divisions resulting in haploid cells: either four spermatozoa, or one oocyte and two polar bodies. Mitosis takes 30 to 60 minutes in mammals, whereas meiosis can take 3 weeks in males or years in females. After fertilization, the two gametes combine their nuclear material to form the first embryonic diploid cell—the human zygote. Errors in this phase of development can lead to atypical numbers of chromosomes (for example, various monosomies or trisomies) that may lead to abnormal development. Meiosis is important because it maintains a constant chromosome number, allows a random assortment of maternal and paternal chromosomes, and allows "shuffling" of genes.

In theory, the male spermatozoa and female oocyte form through similar processes; however, the timing and results of each meiotic division are very different.

### Spermatogenesis

During spermatogenesis, immature spermatogonia are transformed into mature spermatozoa. Immature spermatogonia remain dormant until puberty. During the first meiotic division, diploid primary spermatocytes are converted into two equal haploid secondary spermatocytes. Each secondary spermatocyte then divides into two spermatids during the second meiotic division. Therefore, each primary spermatocyte results in four spermatids after two meiotic divisions. Spermatids mature into spermatozoa through a process called spermiogenesis.

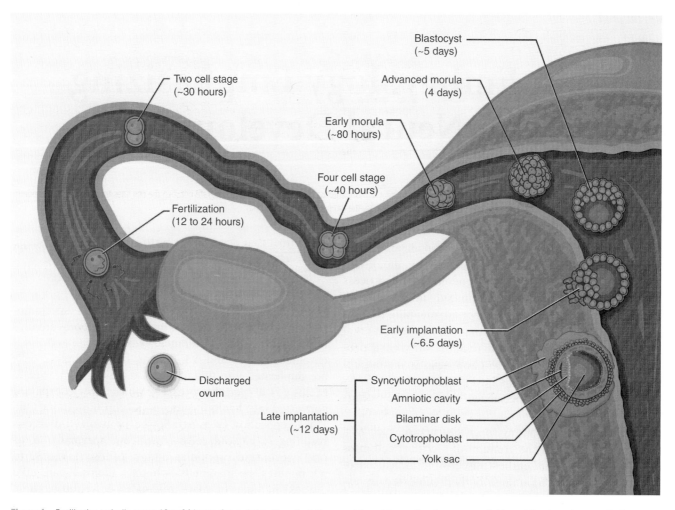

**Figure 1** Fertilization typically occurs 12 to 24 hours after ovulation. The cells divide several times (cleavage) as they are propelled toward the uterus; however, the fetus stays approximately the same size. Before implantation, the morula develops a fluid-filled cavity forming the blastocyst. Trophoblasts assist the embryo during implantation into the uterine wall. Late in implantation, an amniotic cavity forms a separating layer, the bilaminar disk, that is two cells thick.

### Oogenesis

Oogonia mature into primary oocytes during the fetal period and initiate the first meiotic division. The process is suspended in prophase until adolescence. After birth, no primary oocytes form, in contrast to continuous production of primary spermatocytes in males. The first meiotic division is completed just before ovulation. The primary oocyte divides into a single secondary oocyte and a small nonfunctional polar body. At ovulation, the second meiotic division begins, but is suspended in metaphase until fertilization occurs.

### Errors in Gametogenesis

The long duration of the first meiotic division in females (up to 45 years) may account for the relatively high rate of meiotic errors. The primary oocytes suspended in prophase are vulnerable to environmental agents. Chromosome pairs may fail to separate during the first meiotic division, leading to nondysjunction. As a result, some gametes may have 24 chromosomes whereas oth-

ers have 22 chromosomes. Nondysjunction may lead to trisomy (three chromosomes) in some cells and monosomy (one chromosome) in other cells instead of two equal pairs.

## Gestation

Gestation is typically divided into an embryonic period (fertilization to the eighth week of gestation) and fetal period (the remainder of gestation). By the end of the embryonic period, all major organ systems are complete. The embryonic period is divided into five stages: fertilization, cleavage, gastrulation, neurulation, and organogenesis.

### Fertilization

Fertilization is the process by which the male and female gametes fuse (Figure 1); haploid sperm and oocyte pronuclei combine to form the diploid zygote (46 chromosomes). Of the 200 to 300 million spermatozoa that enter the female genital tract, 1% will enter the cervix, and

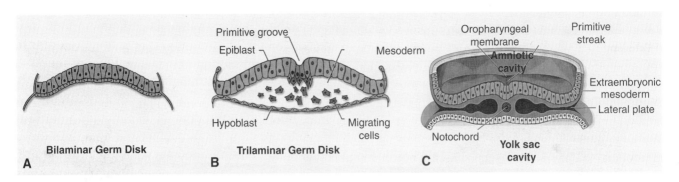

**Figure 2** Gastrulation. **A,** Early gastrulation: two germ cell lines are present. **B,** Formation of trilaminar disk: epiblasts migrate between the cell lines to establish the mesoderm layer. **C,** Late gastrulation: A three-dimensional view of the trilaminar disk showing the three layers and notochord.

only 300 to 500 will reach the site of fertilization. The sperm must undergo activation processes called capacitation (in the uterine tube) and acrosome reaction (near the oocyte) to fuse to and enter the oocyte. Once conditioned, the spermatozoa must penetrate the corona radiata and zona pellucida of the egg. A single sperm will penetrate the zona pellucida triggering a zona reaction that prevents other sperms from entering. Soon after, the corona radiata disappears. The sperm leaves its plasma membrane behind, but maintains its head and tail as it enters the oocyte cytoplasm. This process causes completion of the second meiotic division within the oocyte forming the mature female pronucleus and the second polar body. The tail of the sperm degenerates and the sperm head enlarges forming the male pronucleus. The pronuclei fuse forming the diploid zygote. Fertilization takes place in the uterine tube, and the zygote is propelled toward the uterus by ciliary action.

## Cleavage

Approximately 30 hours after fertilization, the large zygote divides into blastomeres (mitotic divisions 1 through 3), and later the morula (Latin, Mulberry) composed of 16 cells after 4 mitotic divisions (Figure 1). Through a process called blastogenesis, uterine fluid enters the dense morula creating the blastocyst. The blastomeres separate into an inner cell mass (embryoblast, which later becomes the embryo) and outer trophoblasts (which become the embryonic portion of the placenta). Implantation into the uterus begins approximately at day 6 or day 7 after fertilization. The trophoblasts proliferate and invade the uterine epithelium. The trophoblasts differentiate into cytotrophoblasts (a single mononuclear layer that surrounds the blastocyst) and syncytiotrophoblasts (a multinucleated mass that invades the uterine wall). By the 10th day, the embryo is completely embedded within the uterine lining. During implantation, amniotic fluid enters the embryoblast separating the bilaminar embryonic disk from the trophoblasts. The outer trophoblasts proliferate very quickly relative to the bilaminar disk.

Problems that occur during this phase of gestation can lead to abnormal implantation (such as uterine tube or mesenteric implantation), spontaneous abortion (failure to implant), or proliferation of the trophoblasts without embryonic growth (hydatidiform mole). If the blastocyst divides, monozygotic twins will develop. If two eggs are fertilized, dizygotic twins occur.

## Gastrulation

Gastrulation is the beginning of morphogenesis (Figure 2). During the third week, the embryo develops a planar structure just before the development of the central nervous system. During gastrulation, a thickened linear band of epiblasts called the primitive streak begins at the caudal end of the bilaminar disk and moves cranially establishing the three-dimensional axis of the embryo. The primitive streak deepens to form the primitive groove. As the groove deepens, cells migrate between the bilaminar layers, causing formation of the mesodermal layer and thus the trilaminar disk. The trilaminar disk is composed of three primary tissue layers: the inner endoderm, middle mesoderm, and outer ectoderm (Table 1). Some of the mesenchymal cells migrate cranially to form the notochordal process.

The embryo is highly sensitive to teratogens at this point in development. Gastrulation can be disrupted, leading to insufficient mesoderm in the caudal regions of the embryo. This situation may lead to formational abnormalities in the lower extremities (hypoplasia or fusion of limbs), urogenital (renal agenesis, imperforate anus), or lumbosacral abnormalities. Remnants of the primitive streak may persist, which can lead to sacrococcygeal teratomas.

## Neurulation

The midsagittal groove deepens within the ectoderm and begins to fold onto itself, creating the neural tube (Figure 3). As it closes, the neural crest forms dorsal to the neural tube, whereas the notochord remains ventral. The neural tube will form the spinal cord, the neural crest will form the peripheral nervous system, and the

| **Table 1** \| **Structures Originating From Various Germ Layers** | | |
|---|---|---|
| **Ectoderm** | **Mesoderm** | **Endoderm** |
| Surface ectoderm | Notochord | Gastrointestinal tract |
|   Skin |   Nucleus pulposus |   Thyroid gland |
|   Lens of eye |   Induces neurulation |   Bronchial tree |
|   Inner ear | | |
|   Anterior pituitary | | |
| Neural tube | Somites | Pharyngeal pouches |
|   Central nervous system |   Skeletal muscle |   Middle ear |
|   Presynaptic autonomic neurons |   Bone |   Thymus |
|   Retina/optic nerves |   Connective tissue |   Parathyroids |
|   Posterior pituitary | | |
| Neural crest | Other | |
|   Peripheral sensory neurons |   Kidneys and ureters | |
|   Postsynaptic autonomic neurons |   Reproductive system | |
| All ganglia |   Heart | |
| Adrenal medulla | | |
| Melanocytes | | |
| Bone, muscle, and connective tissue in head and heart | | |

notochord will form the anterior vertebral bodies. The neural tube initially closes in the middle of the embryo and progresses both cranially and caudally in a zipper-like fashion. As it closes, the open ends are called the cranial and caudal neuropores. Somite pairs form adjacent to the closed neural tube, whereas the neural crest forms superficial to the neural tube. Over time, the level of the somites will correspond to individual vertebral levels and innervations.

Failure of the cranial neuropore to close can cause anencephaly, whereas failure to close the caudal neuropore may lead to spina bifida occulta, meningocele, myelomeningocele, or myeloschisis (Figure 4).

### Organogenesis

Undifferentiated mesenchymal cells called somites divide into the sclerotome, myotome, and dermatome (Figure 5). These divisions differentiate into the axial skeleton, head and trunk musculature, and associated dermis, respectively. All major organ systems develop concurrently. During the fetal period, the arms and legs begin to move, primitive reflexes appear, and the fetus grows rapidly as it refines its organ structure.

## Overview of Abnormal Development

Alterations in the normal molecular processes may lead to structural abnormalities in the spine and surrounding soft tissues. These defects may occur prenatally or postnatally. The most common patterns of abnormal development during gestation include malformation, disrup-

tion, and deformation. Malformation is a failure of embryologic differentiation, development, or both, leading to the absence of or the improper formation of structures before the fetal period begins. Examples of malformation include hemivertebra and vertebral bars. Disruption is structural deviation of a part that otherwise is forming normally during the embryonic period. Examples include amniotic band syndrome or autoamputation. Deformation is an alteration to the normal shape of a part during the fetal or postnatal periods (such as scoliosis). Deformations can be caused by intrinsic forces (inability to move away from normal imposed forces because of neuromuscular problems) or extrinsic forces (cause by space limitations in utero). The prognosis for deformations depends on the amount of time the deforming forces are present, and the age of the fetus or child when the forces are applied.

## Overview of Bone Formation

Bones are formed through a process called osteogenesis. The two major types of osteogenesis are intramembranous and endochondral ossification. Depending on the mechanism, bone either replaces fibrous mesenchyme or cartilaginous tissue. Overall, the first bones to ossify are the clavicle and mandible. In both instances, ossification begins early in the seventh week by intramembranous ossification (direct transformation of fibrous mesenchyme). The scapula and humerus follow. These bones form through endochondral ossification (cartilaginous precursor). The clavicle is the only bone in the appendicular skeleton to form by intramembranous ossifica-

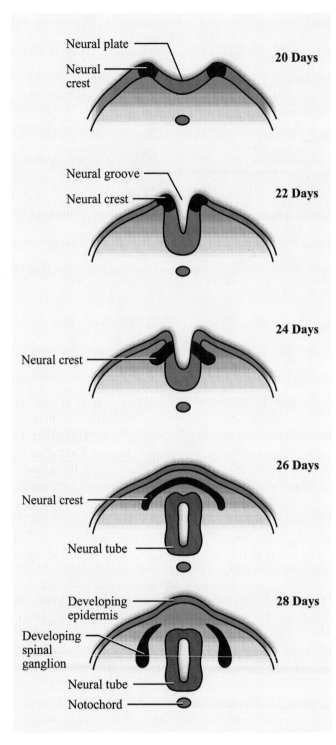

**Figure 3** Neurulation. The midsagittal groove deepens within the ectoderm and begins to fold onto itself, creating the neural tube.

tion. All bones use both endochondral and intramembranous mechanisms for future remodeling.

### Intramembranous Bone Formation
Intramembranous bones form from a fibrous mesenchymal analogue that is structurally similar to the eventual bone. At the site of primary ossification, cells differentiate into osteoblasts to calcify and form osteoid. The ossification centers expand outward to form the cranial bones, facial bones, and the clavicle. This process does not normally form the spine, although occipitocervical developmental deformities may include the spine. The outer surface of the skull hardens quickly after birth, but the inner tables may remain soft during the process of remodeling and growth. For this reason, children younger than 10 years are particularly sensitive to inner table penetration when halo pins are placed.

### Endochondral Ossification
Endochondral ossification is the process by which condensed scleroblastema divide and differentiate into chondroblasts in the central portion of the limb bud. The chondroblasts mature into chondrocytes and synthesize the extracellular matrix of the cartilaginous anlagen. The chondrocytes undergo a series of cellular changes before ossification. Eventually, bone completely replaces the cartilage model.

## Spine and Limb Development
### Vertebral Column, Ribs, and Disks
The notochord and somites are the prominent features in the development of the vertebral column. Vertebrae develop from cells induced from the somites to surround the notochord and the neural tube. The notochord extends from the oropharyngeal membrane (cranially) to the caudal neuropore. Somites initially appear at 3.5 weeks gestation; approximately 30 pairs are present at 4.5 weeks gestation. The full complement of somites is approximately 38 to 39 pairs (4 occipital, 8 cervical, 12 thoracic, 5 lumbar, 5 sacral, and 4 to 5 coccygeal). Somites initially differentiate into sclerotomes (later forming the vertebrae and ribs) and dermatomyotomes (later forming muscle and skin) (Figure 5). One theory of spinal development is known as resegmentation. During a process called metameric shift (resegmentation), the superior portion of each sclerotome divides and combines with the caudal portion of the sclerotome above (Figure 6). The combined regions develop into vertebra, whereas the intervertebral disk develops where the sclerotomes divided. Some authors adhere to a broader definition of resegmentation, believing that metameric shift probably does not occur in mammals.

It is believed that all vertebrae are composed of three portions: centrum (anterior vertebral body), neural arch (posterior elements, pedicles, and a small portion of the anterior vertebra), and costal element (the anterior part of the lateral mass or transverse process in the cervical and lumbar spines, respectively, and the ribs in the thoracic spine). Each area is a primary ossification center. At birth, most vertebrae present three ossific areas: one for the centrum, and one for each half of

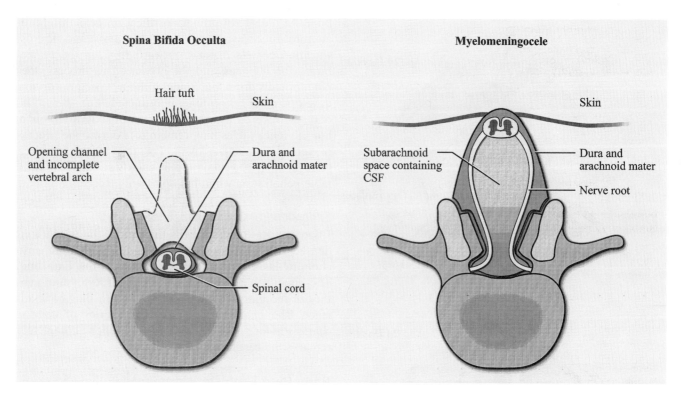

**Figure 4** Failure of the caudal neuropore to close may lead to spina bifida occulta or myelomeningocele. CSF = cerebrospinal fluid.

the neural arch. During spinal development, the neural processes extend dorsally on each side of the neural tube. They unite during the fetal period completing the neural arch (Figure 5). Cells between the surface ectoderm and neural tube interact, leading to the formation of the spinous process.

The occiput, atlas, and axis are formed by a separate mechanism than the other vertebral bodies. Four sclerotomes are involved in the formation of the occiput. Some authors believe that the portion of the skull that develops around the notochord is comparable to one or more vertebrae. The resegmentation theory postulates that part of the first cervical (C1) sclerotome and the cranial portion of the C2 sclerotome contribute cells to the odontoid process and arch of C1. A failure of craniocaudal resegmentation at this level causes the dens to remain attached to C2. The remainder of the postaxial cervical vertebrae develops in a manner similar to the rest of the spine. The eight cervical somites develop into seven cervical vertebrae and eight cervical nerves. The superior portion of the first cervical somite contributes to the occiput, and the caudal portion of the eighth cervical somite contributes to T1.

The nucleus pulposus develops from cells of the notochord, whereas the anulus fibrosus originates from sclerotomal cells associated with resegmentation. During this resegmentation process, the spinal nerves can pass between the precartilaginous vertebrae to innervate the segmental myotomes and dermatomes (Figure 6).

Occasionally, notochordal cells will remain at the cranial and caudal regions of the spine, leading to chordomas in the occipitocranial or lumbosacral regions.

The ribs develop from the sclerotomes and are contiguous with the future neural arches and intervertebral disks. *PAX3* gene expression is important for normal rib development. The costal elements are probably present at all levels of the spine. Chondrification begins at about 6 weeks gestation, and a well-formed cartilaginous thoracic rib cage is present at the end of the embryonic period. The ribs ossify by endochondral ossification from a primary ossification center near the angle of the rib. Secondary centers appear at puberty.

Costal anomalies include bifid ribs and supernumerary ribs. Cervical ribs are more important clinically than lumbar ribs because they may cause neurovascular compression on the lower trunk of the brachial plexus and on the subclavian artery. Ribs may fuse in association with other vertebral anomalies.

Kyphosis of the thoracic spine and sacrum are considered primary processes and appear before birth. Cervical and lumbar lordosis occurs after birth. Some authors believe that, at the least, cervical lordosis appears early in fetal life.

### Vertebral Variations and Anomalies

Variations in the number, shape, and position of vertebrae are common. In the lumbar spine, sacralization of the last lumbar vertebra or lumbarization of S1 is com-

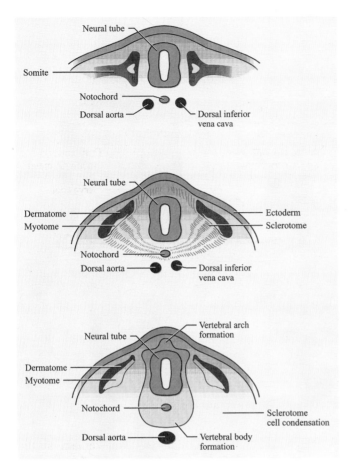

**Figure 5** Somite differentiation. Undifferentiated mesenchymal cells divide into the sclerotome, myotome, and dermatome.

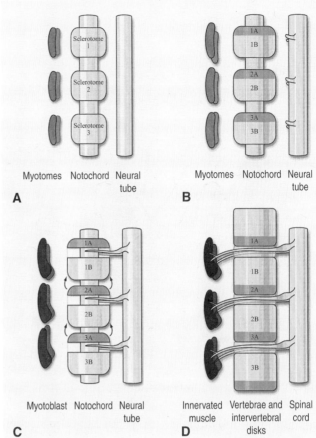

**Figure 6** Vertebral development. **A,** Somite differentiation: The somites differentiate into sclerotomes overlying the notochord and dermomyoblasts. **B,** Metameric shift: The sclerotomes begin to divide into two components. **C,** Each sclerotome divides forming an intervertebral disk between the two segments. **D,** Formation of vertebral bodies and innervation of the dermatomes and myotomes.

mon. Vertebral anomalies can typically be classified as either "failure of formation" or "failure of segmentation" of the vertebrae. Failure of formation can lead to the development of hemivertebra, whereas failure of segmentation can lead to unsegmented bars or block vertebrae. A hemivertebra is a wedged vertebra situated between two other vertebrae causing congenital scoliosis. The embryologic origin of hemivertebra remains unclear. Possible etiologies include absence of one of the bilateral chondrific centers and lateral deviation of the notochord. Vertebral bars may be situated laterally (causing scoliosis), anteriorly (leading to kyphosis), or at any location in between (causing kyphoscoliosis). Block vertebrae essentially have a normal shape, but have failed to separate. This variation may be the result of complete chondrification of the mesenchymal zone that normally would have formed the intervertebral disk. Other variations include sagittal cleft (butterfly vertebra) or coronal cleft vertebra, which may result from the failure of fusion of bilateral chondrific centers or premature degeneration of the notochord. Another defect caused by failure of segmentation is congenital brevicollis (Klippel-Feil sequence). This condition occurs in 1 in 42,000 births; 65% of those affected are fe-

male. The embryologic anomaly is nonsegmentation of two or more cervical vertebra. As described earlier, spina bifida is caused in part by a failure of formation of the posterior elements of the spine.

Split notochord syndrome may result from notochordal derangement leading to vertebral and neural malformations. Many variations exist, including diastematomyelia (a partial longitudinal split of the spinal cord caused by a fibrocartilaginous or bony spur in the vertebral canal), diplomyelia (duplication of the entire spinal cord), or anterior/posterior spina bifida. Diastematomyelia is believed to be caused by the persistence of the neurenteric canal, which is a temporary communication between the amniotic cavity and umbilical vesicle normally present between 3 and 4 weeks of gestation. Other variations include extrusion of the intestine on the back, diaphragmatic hernia, and dorsal enteric fistula.

## Limb Development

Appendicular bones develop from the mesenchymal cells that arise from the mesoderm. The development of

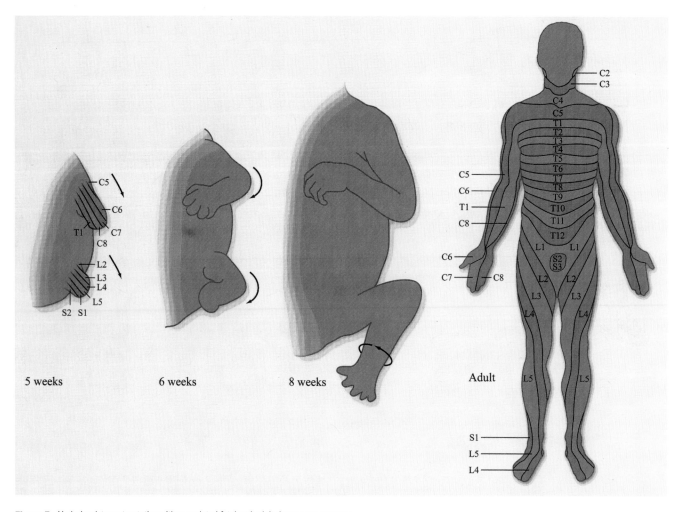

**Figure 7** Limb development: rotation with speculated fetal and adult dermatome patterns.

the upper extremities begins in the third week with an embryonic epidermal swelling that progresses into a limb bud during the fourth postovulatory week. By 7 weeks, a clear longitudinal axis is present with the thumb and big toe lying on the preaxial border of the hand and foot plates, respectively. The development of the lower extremities lags behind the upper extremities by a few days. The limbs develop in a proximodistal sequence. Thus, the arm and forearm appear before the palm and fingers. Chondrification of the bones also occurs in a proximodistal order. Ossification begins in the clavicle (by intramembranous ossification), followed by the humerus, radius, femur, tibia, and ulna (by endochondral ossification). At the time of birth, most primary ossific centers for the limbs are present.

The upper extremity limb bud occurs at the base of the neck next to somites C5-T1. The limb buds grow perpendicular to the trunk, allowing somite innervations to remain parallel (perpendicular to the long axis of the embryo) (Figure 7). Angioblasts derived from somites invade the limb buds early establishing the vascular supply to the limbs. Skeletal bone and muscle development

precede the ingrowth of nerves. By 5 weeks after fertilization, the ventral rami of several spinal nerves have united to form the brachial plexus (C5-T1) and lumbosacral plexus (L1-S2). Cutaneous innervation also is present. By 7 weeks, major named nerves appear in a similar pattern to the adult.

Approximately 4 days after the upper extremity limb buds occur, the lower extremity limb buds form adjacent to the L2-S2 somites. In general, there is a cranial-caudal, proximal-to-distal sequence to limb development. The lower extremities are initially externally rotated and supinated (the plantar aspect of the foot pointing at the torso). During the sixth week, the lower extremities internally rotate almost 90° to a neutral position, explaining the wrapping nature of the mature dermatomal distributions (Figure 7).

### Nervous System Development

The central nervous system consists of the brain and spinal cord, whereas the peripheral nervous system consists of cranial and spinal nerves. As described previously, neurulation is the process by which the neural tube and

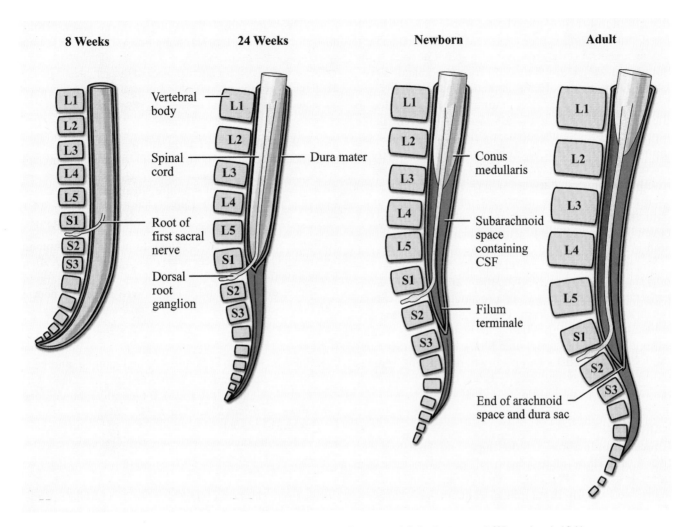

**Figure 8**  The spinal cord changes position relative to the vertebral bodies with growth. The conus medullaris migrates upward. CSF = cerebrospinal fluid.

plate form. Primary neurulation continues until closure of the cranial and caudal neuropores, which takes approximately 10 days. Secondary neurulation takes place after the rostral neuropore closes. At the opposite end of the embryo, neuromeres, morphologically distinct transverse subdivisions, develop perpendicular to the long axis. The neuromeres form the various regions of the brain.

Dorsal to the neural tube, the neural crest develops from neural ectoderm. The cells quickly migrate in a rostrocaudal sequence to many regions of the body. In the brain, some cells differentiate into ganglia and cranial nerves and others form parts of the pharyngeal arches. At the level of the spinal cord, cells form the pia mater and spinal ganglia, and then the sympathetic trunk and ganglia. Cells also encircle the dorsal and ventral roots of the spinal nerves.

The spinal cord and spinal nerves develop during primary and secondary neurulation. As the neural tube closes, the dorsal cells (alar laminae) develop into cells/roots that are primarily afferent (sensory) in function,

whereas the ventral cells (basal laminae) develop into cells/roots that are primarily efferent (motor) in function (the Bell-Magendie law). The sulcus limitans divides the two halves of the neural tube over the entire length of the spinal cord.

The spinal cord changes position relative to the vertebral bodies with growth (Figure 8). At the end of the first trimester, the spinal cord extends the entire length of the vertebral column. The embryonic trunk, vertebrae, and dura grow at a faster rate than the spinal cord, causing the conus medullaris to move in a cranial direction. At birth, the conus lies at the level of the third lumbar vertebra and moves to the L1-2 level at skeletal maturity. The disproportionate growth between the vertebral column and spinal cord leads to progressive obliquity of the spinal nerves distal to the cervical spine.

The peripheral nervous system connects the central nervous system with the periphery via afferent and efferent nerves. Spinal nerves develop as follows: (1) spinal ganglion cells (derived from the neural crest) send processes centrally and peripherally constituting the dorsal (afferent) root of the spinal nerve; (2) cells in the basal lamina of the neural tube send processes peripherally as a ventral (efferent) root of a spinal nerve; (3) the dorsal and ventral roots unite to form the spinal nerves, which then divide almost immediately to supply the body wall and limbs; (4) autonomic fibers are added to the roots and rami for the afferent and efferent nerve supply to the visceral structures. Cranial nerves have additional types of nerve fibers in addition to the afferent/ efferent visceral and somatic nerves.

The autonomic nervous system is divided into the sympathetic and parasympathetic components. The sympathetic division arises from preganglionic neurons between T1 and L2. The postganglionic neurons are situated in the sympathetic trunk (paravertebral ganglia) or in collateral ganglia found on arteries. Neural crest cells migrate to the future sympathetic trunk. The parasympathetic division arises from preganglionic neurons in the brain stem or sacrum. Postganglionic neurons are situated in terminal ganglia of the head or in ganglia in various viscera. Postganglionic fibers in the parasympathetic system tend to be short, whereas in the sympathetic system they are long because of the position of the ganglia.

## Summary

Critical coordination, relationships, and signaling between cells allow each specific cell line to mature in a normal manner. Pathologic interactions can lead to many well-known developmental anomalies and syndromes.

## Annotated Bibliography
### General Concepts

O'Rahilly R, Müller F: *Human Embryology and Teratology*, ed 3. New York, NY, Wiley-Liss Publishers, 2001.
  This book is a detailed reference of all aspects of embryology with annotated bibliographies at the end of each chapter.

### Spine and Limb Development

Dasen JS, Tice BC, Brenner-Morton S, Jessell TM: A Hox regulator network establishes motor neuron pool identity and target-muscle connectivity. *Cell* 2005;123: 363-365.
  This article describes important findings leading to how Hox genes regulate motor neurons connections to specific myotomes.

Kasemeier-Kulesa JC, Kulesa PM, Lefcort F: Imaging neural crest cell dynamics during formation of dorsal root ganglia and sympathetic ganglia. *Development* 2005;132:235-245.
  Time-lapse microscopy is used to follow fluorescently labeled trunk neural crest cells and their interactions with neighboring cells.

Liu A, Niswander LA: Signalling in development: Bone morphogenetic protein signaling and vertebrate nervous system development. *Nat Rev Neurosci* 2005; 6:945-954.
  A review of protein interactions and their influence on the development of the peripheral and central nervous systems is presented.

Muller F, O'Rahilly R: The primitive streak, the caudal eminence and related structures in staged human embryos. *Cells Tissues Organs* 2004;177:2-20.
  A thorough review of primitive streak and somite development in human embryos is presented.

Muller F, O'Rahilly R: Segmentation in staged human embryos: The occipitocervical region revisited. *J Anat* 2003;203:297-315.
  Critical distinctions are made between chick and human occipitocervical development, and a review of the development of this region is presented.

O'Rahilly R, Muller F: Somites, spinal ganglia, and centra: Enumeration and interrelationships in staged human embryos, and implications for neural tube defects. *Cells Tissues Organs* 2003; 173: 5-92.
  This article presents a thorough review of somite relationships with centra, neural crest, and ganglia cells and their involvement in neural tube defects.

Tsirikos AI, McMaster MJ: Congenital anomalies of the ribs and chest wall associated with congenital deformities of the spine. *J Bone Joint Surg Am* 2005;87:2523-2536.
  A review of the relationship between thorax malformations and congenital scoliosis is presented.

## Classic Bibliography

Dalgleish AE: A study of the development of thoracic vertebrae in the mouse assisted by autoradiography. *Acta Anat (Basel)* 1985;122:91-98.

Gamble JG: Development and maturation of the neuromusculoskeletal system, in Morrisey RT, Weinstein SL (eds): *Lovell & Winter's Pediatric Orthopaedics*, ed 4. Philadelphia, PA, Lippincott-Raven Publishers, 1996.

Kelly RO, Fallon JF, Kelly RE: Vertebrate limb morphogenesis. *Issues Rev Terato* 1984;2:219-265.

Lemire RJ, Loeser JD, Leech RW, et al: *Normal and Abnormal Development of the Human Nervous System.* Hagerstown, MD, Harper & Row, 1975.

Müller F, O'Rahilly R: Occipitocervical segmentation in staged human embryos. *J Anat* 1994;185:251-258.

Peacock A: Observations on the prenatal development of the intervertebral disc in man. *J Anat* 1951;85:260-274.

Shinohara H, Naora H, Hashimoto R, Hatta T, Tanaka O: Development of the innervation pattern in the upper limb of staged human embryos. *Acta Anat (Basel)* 1990; 138:265-269.

Vettivel S: Vertebral level of the termination of the spinal cord in human fetuses. *J Anat* 1991;179:149-161.

Wilting J, Kurz H, Brand-Saberi B, et al: Kinetics and differentiation of somite cells forming the vertebral column: Studies on human and chick embryos. *Anat Embryol (Berl)* 1994;190:573-581.

# Chapter 2

# Anatomy

Kingsley R. Chin, MD

## Alignment of the Spine

The osseous spinal column is composed of 7 cervical, 12 thoracic, 5 lumbar, 5 sacral, and 4 to 5 coccygeal vertebral segments. From a frontal view the spine tends to be straight although it may curve to the right in some individuals, possibly as a result of the position of the aorta and right-hand dominance. On lateral plain radiographs, the mean occipitocervical angles between McRae's line (a line intersecting the basion and the opisthion) and the C3 superior end plate are approximately 24.2° in flexion, 44.0° in neutral, and 57.2° in extension. The mean occipitocervical distance, which is measured as the shortest distance from the superiormost aspect of the C2 spinous process to the occipital protuberance, is 21.5 mm in neutral, 28.0 mm in flexion, and 14.8 mm in extension. The McGregor line is the most reliable and reproducible method for measuring the occipitocervical angle (Figure 1).

Normal thoracic kyphosis averages 35° (range, 20° to 50°) whereas normal lumbar lordosis averages 60° (range, 20° to 80°). Up to 75% of the lumbar lordosis occurs between L4 and S1, and up to 47% occurs between L5 and S1. Lumbar lordosis varies widely; however, there is limited evidence that women and patients with a higher body mass index tend to have more prominent lordosis. Men with low back pain tend to have reduced lumbar lordosis. Asymptomatic patients older than 70 years tend to have increased thoracic kyphosis (range, 29° to 79°), decreased lumbar lordosis (mean, –57°; range, –96° to –20°) and an anteriorly displaced C7 sagittal plumb line (on average 40 mm anterior to the posterosuperior margin of the S1 end plate). Visual assessment of cervical and lumbar lordosis is not reliable.

## Osseous Anatomy for Anterior Cervical Fixation

From C2 to C6, the depth and width of the vertebral surfaces average 15 mm and 17 mm respectively and increases to a depth of approximately 17 mm and a width of approximately 20 mm at C7. The midsagittal height of the posterior wall of the vertebral body ranges from

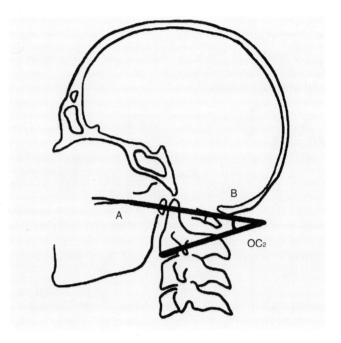

**Figure 1** The McGregor line is depicted to measure the occipitocervical angle. A = the posterosuperior aspect of the hard palate; B = the most caudal aspect point on the midline occipital curve. OC2 is the occipitocervical angle and is measured between McGregor's line and the inferior end plate of C2. (*Reproduced with permission from Shoda N, Takeshita K, Seichi A, et al: Measurement of occipitocervical angle. Spine 2004;29(10):E204-E208.*)

11 mm to 13 mm. The sagittal diameters of the canal are 17 mm to 18 mm at C3 to C6, and 15 mm at C7. On average, males have larger vertebral dimensions of approximately 1 mm in all measurements and therefore have longer screw paths. Males and females have similar sagittal canal diameter and therefore males have a smaller Torg (canal/body) ratio, which may explain the preponderance of cervical myelopathy in males. For anterior cervical plating, the mean length of the sagittal, parasagittal, and convergent screw paths for men and women is 16 mm. The mean length of the safe divergent screw path is 15 mm. The central portions of the end plates are thinner than the peripheral parts; this difference is more pronounced in the superior versus the inferior end plates. Anteriorly, the distance between the vertebral arteries

decreases caudad to cephalad, similar to the distance between the lateral border of the uncinate process and the medial border of the transverse foramen. The transverse processes become smaller and the intertransverse space and the amount of vertebral artery exposed become larger proceeding from caudal to rostral. The vertebral artery courses closer to the lateral aspect of the vertebral body than to the medial border of the anterior tubercle of the transverse process. The lower half of the anterior root of the transverse process tends to have defects or thinning from C3-C5, possibly caused by the erosive effects of the vertebral artery. Anterior transarticular screws may be placed in the inferior facet of C1 and the body of C2 for atlantoaxial instability via a prevascular retropharyngeal approach. The AP diameter of the inferior C1 facet articular surface ranges from 16.2 mm (± 1.6 mm) to 17.1 mm (± 1.8 mm). The AP diameter of the C2 vertebral body ranges from 9.3 mm (± 1 mm) to 16.2 mm (± 1.8 mm).

## Osseous Anatomy for Posterior Cervical Fixation

Lateral mass and transpedicular pedicle screws are being used more often for posterior spine fixation. The diameter of the pedicle in the transverse plane, the angles of insertion into the vertebral bodies, and the dimensions of the lateral mass and C2 isthmus/pedicle are essential determinants of successful screw placement. The vertebral artery is at risk for injury with posterior instrumentation and dissection around the posterior arch of C1. From midline, the artery is at risk with lateral dissection at C1 beyond 12 mm (range, 12 to 23 mm) on the dorsal surface, and 8 mm (range, 8 to 13 mm) on the cephalad surface. Between the C1 and C2 laminas and lateral masses there is a large venous plexus. The internal carotid artery and hypoglossal nerves are at risk for injury anteriorly with bicortical C1 fixation. The hypoglossal nerve lies approximately 2 to 3 mm lateral to the middle of the anterior aspect of the C1 lateral mass. The internal carotid artery lies within 1 mm of the ideal exit point of a bicortical C1-2 transarticular screw or a C1 lateral mass screw (Figure 2). Cervical rotation does not have a predictable effect on the internal carotid artery but medial angulation of C1 lateral mass screws increases the margin of safety. The C1 lateral mass varies on average between 9 to 15 mm in width, 17 to 19 mm in thickness, and 10 to 15 mm in height.

There is a mean angulation of 6° medially from the midpoint of the C3-C5 lateral mass to the lateral aspect of the vertebral foramen, and 6° laterally at C6. The lateral border of the vertebral artery with respect to the middle of the C7 lateral mass is 14.1° (± 6.1°). Lateral mass screws angled 30° lateral and 15° cephalad are ideal for use from C3 to C6 and will avoid the vertebral artery, whereas pedicle screws are preferred for use at C7.

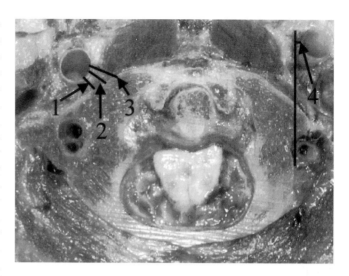

**Figure 2** Axial section of the C1 vertebra showing measurements made directly from the cadaveric specimen and from comparable CT images. 1, Shortest distance from C1 to the internal carotid artery; 2, Shortest distance from the anterior cortex of the center of the lateral mass of C1 to the internal carotid artery; 3, Shortest distance from a point on the anterior cortex of the C1 lateral mass where a screw tip would exit with the screw directed 15° medially through the lateral mass; 4, Distance between the internal carotid artery and a line drawn in the sagittal plane at the medial border of the C1 vertebral foramen. This line represents the most lateral screw position possible (with neutral angulation of the screw) without encroaching on the vertebral artery. (*Reproduced with permission from Currier BL, Todd LT, Maus TP, et al: Anatomic relationship of the internal carotid artery to the C1 vertebra: A case report of cervical reconstruction for chordoma and pilot study to assess the risk of screw fixation of the atlas. Spine 2003;28:E461-467.*)

Confusion exists in the distinction between the pars interarticularis (isthmus) and pedicle of C2 because the C2 superior facet is anterior to the inferior facet. The pedicle is considered the connecting tubular bone inferior to the superior facet and anteromedial to the transverse foramen. The isthmus is the narrower portion between the superior and inferior facets. There is no remarkable difference in bone density and trabecular bone orientation between the pedicle and the isthmus; however, there is greater stress concentration at the isthmus with hyperextension and axial loading. The mean optimal screw path for C1-C2 transarticular screws is 38.1 mm ± 2.2 mm (range, 34 to 43 mm). In most patients the use of 3.5-mm screws will be safe; however, in approximately 20% of patients 3.5 mm screws may be too large and there may be approximately 41% to 52% asymmetry between sides. At C2 there is an approximate 18% incidence of unilateral anomalous vertebral artery anatomy that results in a high-riding transverse foramen and narrowing of the C2 pedicle and lateral mass. The width of the superior surface of the isthmus averages 8.3 mm ± 1.5 mm (range, 3.3 to 12.6 mm), the width of the inferior surface averages 5.1 mm ± 1.2 mm (range, 1.3 to 8.5 mm), and the height of the isthmus averages 6.5 mm ± 1.5 mm (range, 2.7 to 10.1 mm). The width of the inferior surface of the isthmus is the most important measurement for avoiding injury to the vertebral artery.

Approximately 6% of cervical pedicle screws penetrate the pedicle cortex. The mean cervical pedicle heights and widths from C3-C7 vary from 6.0 to 6.5 mm and 4.7 to 5.3 mm, respectively. The superior border of the pedicle is in contact with the superior traversing nerve; however, the mean distance between the pedicle and inferior nerve roots ranges from 1.4 to 1.6 mm. The pedicle heights at all levels are significantly greater for males than for females, and are greater between the widths at C4 and C6. The inner diameters of the pedicles at C7, T1, and T2 in the medial to lateral plane average 5.2, 6.3, and 5.5 mm with medial angulation of 34°, 30°, and 26°, respectively.

## Osseous Anatomy for Occipital Fixation

The thickest bone in the external occipital protuberance measures 11.5 to 15.1 mm in males and 9.7 to 12.0 mm in females. The thickness decreases to less than 8 mm at a distance greater than 2 cm lateral to the external occipital protuberance. The placement of posterior occipital fixation presents the risk of injury to the confluence of sinuses and transverse sinuses located immediately beneath the thickest portions of the occiput; therefore, it is suggested that screw placement is safer at least 2 cm below the superior nuchal line. Anterior halo pins should be placed 1 cm above and lateral to the middle of the eyebrow in the occiput. The pins are placed laterally because the supraorbital and supratrochlear nerves are located over the medial half of the eyebrow. The temporal fossa contains the muscles of mastication and is thin, making pin penetration possible. Halos and Gardner Wells tongs should be placed above the pinna of the ear but below the equator of the skull.

## Osseous Anatomy for Thoracic Fixation

The thoracic vertebral body increases in size from rostral to caudal. The pedicles are oval with the cephalocaudad height larger than the mediolateral width at the isthmus. The pedicle wall is two to three times thicker medially than laterally. The thoracic pedicle diameter in the transverse plane, on average, can be less than 5 mm and may be even smaller in deformed spines, such as in patients with scoliosis or kyphosis. The narrowest pedicle widths are usually between T3-9 and may be less than 5 mm in 80% of patients. On average, T5 has the narrowest pedicle diameter; however, T7 on the concave side of a scoliotic spine also may be abnormally narrow. Additionally, pedicle morphology varies among people of different races and thus preoperative CT scans are recommended for accurate determination of implant size. The pedicle-rib unit has a significantly wider width and chord length than the pedicles, therefore, extrapedicular screw fixation may be an alternative option for patients in whom the pedicles are too small. Costotransverse screw fixation is also an option. To avoid the intercostal vessels, costotransverse screw trajectories should be oriented parallel to the sagittal plane, and angled 80° to 90° toward the upper portion of the rib relative to the frontal plane for T1-4, and 50° to 70° for T5-T10 starting at the posterior center of the transverse process. Screw lengths gradually decrease from 19.7 mm at T1 to 13.9 mm at T4-5 before increasing to 16.3 mm at T10. The anteromedial angulation ranges from 0.3° at T12 to 13.9° at T4. The mean distance from the pedicle to the superior nerve root ranges from 1.97 to 3.9 mm from T1-T12, whereas the mean distance to the inferior root ranges from 1.7 mm to 3.7 mm. The mean distance between the pedicle and dural sac is 1.5 mm.

## Osseous Anatomy for Lumbosacral Fixation

In the lumbar spine, the transverse pedicle width averages 18 mm at L5 but decreases more cephalad to an average of 9 mm at L1. The medial or transverse angulation is approximately 30° at L5 but only 12° at L1. The S1 pedicle can be broad, measuring on average approximately 19 mm (range, 16.7 to 22.0 mm) with an angle of approximately 39° (range, 30° to 48°) from midline. These numbers may vary among patients and should not be used as a substitute for actual measurements on preoperative axial and intraoperative radiographs before pedicle screw insertion. The mean distance between the pedicle and adjacent nerve root superiorly is 5.3 mm and 1.5 mm inferiorly in the lumbar spine. Thus the nerve root is at greatest risk for injury medially and inferiorly to the pedicle in the lumbar spine. The pedicle and transverse processes are the only bony posterior elements that are located at the same vertebral level. The midpoint of the transverse process usually approximates the cephalad-caudad location of the center of the pedicle. The lateral border of the pars approximates the medial border of the pedicle at L2-L4 but is in line with the center of the pedicle at L5. Anomalous fusions of the fifth lumbar vertebra to the sacrum (sacralization) should be noted; the presence of a cervical rib may be an indication of such fusions. Sacralization was found in 73.2% of patients with cervical ribs; 64.4% of patients with sacralization also had a cervical rib. For anterior fixation, the average lumbar vertebral body depth, width, and height increased from L1-L4; 26 mm, 36 mm, and 22 mm at L1, respectively; and 30 mm, 44 mm, and 23 mm at L4, respectively.

In the upper sacrum three distinct trabeculations are noted. One extends from the center of the sacral body anterolaterally, and the other two extend from the pedicle toward the auricular surface. The trabeculations coincide with weight transmission extending from the weight-bearing surfaces (body, facets, and alae) toward the auricular surface pointing in the general direction of the hips. The strongest part of the sacrum is the area where these trabeculations intersect (condensation

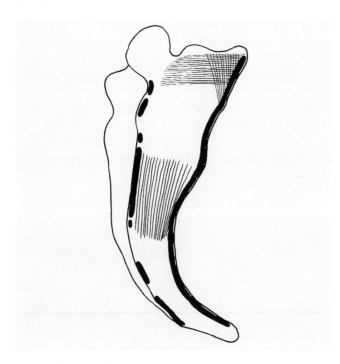

Figure 3 Illustration of a sagittal section in the midsacrum showing the main trabecular orientation. (*Reproduced with permission from Ebraheim N, Sabry FF, Nadim Y, Xu R, Yeasting RA: Internal architecture of the sacrum in the elderly: An anatomic and radiographic study. Spine 2000;25(3):292-297.*)

zone) in the cortical region above the S1 and S2 foramina in zone II (to counterbalance the weakness caused by the presence of the foramina). The junction between S2 and S3 where the condensation abruptly disappears is a weak area and is a common point of transverse sacral fractures. Zone 1 lateral to the foramina also is a weak area and a common location of longitudinal sacral fractures. The cortical thickness gradually decreased caudad from S1. The midanterior cortex of the sacral ala has the highest bone density and provides the best location for mechanical screw fixation (Figure 3).

## Cervical Spinal Ligaments

The ligaments of the spine are crucial for stability. The ligamentum nuchae is a continuation of the supraspinous ligament from C7 to the occipital protuberance. It is a two-part structure consisting of a dorsal raphe and a midline fascial septum and is formed from aponeurotic fibers of the underlying muscles. Interweaving of the right and left upper trapezius, splenius capitis, and rhomboid minor forms the dorsal raphe. The fascial septum consists of dense connective tissue and runs ventrally from the midline raphe to become confluent with the interspinous ligaments and atlantoaxial and atlantooccipital membranes. There are attachments in the midline between the nuchal ligament and the posterior spinal dura at the atlanto-occipital and atlantoaxial interval but none caudally. There also is a connective tissue bridge between the deep aspect of the rectus capitis

posterior minor muscle to the transverse fibers of the posterior atlanto-occipital membrane that extends laterally to blend with the perivascular tissue of the vertebral arteries. These attachments can be identified on MRI scans. In 1929, the series of fibrous strands (ligamentum craniale durae matris spinalis) between the dura mater and the posterior border of the atlanto-occipital joints, the edge of the foramen magnum, the posterior arch of the atlas, and the arch of the axis was described. Anterior attachments of the posterior longitudinal ligaments and the dura also exist. The meningovertebral ligaments anchor the dura to the vertebral canal throughout the spine. This anatomy may explain some forms of cervicogenic headaches.

The posterior longitudinal ligament runs intimately with the posterior aspect of the vertebral body throughout the spine and has two loosely connected layers. The anterior layer covers the anulus fibrosus and the posterior layer covers the dura. In the cervical spine the posterior longitudinal ligament attaches laterally to the posterior end of the uncinate process where it separates into two fibroligamentous bundles. One layer covers the lateral aspect of the uncinate process and the other covers the vascular contents of the foramen transversarium. The uncinate process and its covering ligamentous structures may offer some protection to the neurovascular structures during anterior cervical decompression.

## Thoracolumbar Spinal Ligaments

The supraspinous and interspinous ligaments are formed from muscle tendons and aponeuroses along the length of the thoracic and lumbar spine, resulting in regional differences in their connective tissue architecture. In the thoracic spine, the supraspinous ligament may have been formed from spinal attachments from the trapezius, rhomboideus major, and splenius cervicis combined with the deep fascia. The posterior layer of the thoracolumbar fascia makes a major contribution to the formation of the supraspinous and interspinous ligaments in the lower thoracic spine. In the lumbar spine, the posterior layer of the thoracolumbar fascia, longissimus thoracis, and multifidus combine to form the supraspinous and interspinous ligaments. Bursae exist within the interspinous ligaments that may become inflamed with aging and repetitive hyperextension (Baastrup's disease).

## Cervical Spine Blood Vessels

Safe surgical approaches to the cervical spine require a thorough knowledge of the neurovascular anatomy. The paired vertebral arteries originate off the first segment of the subclavian arteries and travel between the scalene and longus colli muscles. They enter the transverse foramen of C6 in 95% of patients and in 5% at C7 before ascending the spine slightly medial of the midline of the lateral masses. Anteriorly, the distance between the vertebral arteries decreases cephalad from 27.4 mm (± 2.3 mm) at C6 to 22.6 mm (± 1.8 mm) at C3. The distance between the lateral border of the uncinate process and the medial border of the transverse foramen also decreases from a mean of 3.3 mm (± 1 mm) at C6 to 1.7 mm (± 0.8 mm) at C4. The distance from the medial border of the longus colli muscle and the ipsilateral vertebral artery decreases from C2-C5 before increasing at C5-6. Vertebral veins travel anteromedial to the artery and are more likely to be injured first. The artery may anomalously erode into the vertebral body making a loop before exiting, which predisposes it to injury during corpectomy. Approaches to the lower anterior cervicothoracic junction will need to mobilize the brachiocephalic vein in most patients. The left brachiocephalic vein is located at T1 and T2 in 80% of patients, and the aortic arch is at T2 and T3 in 90%. The thoracic duct empties into the systemic venous system from C7 to T2.

Posteriorly, each artery takes a variable loop inside the ipsilateral C2 foramen on the inferior aspect of the C2 superior facet and extends toward the midline at an average 14.6 mm from the middle of the C2 vertebral body. The artery exits the C2 transverse foramen abruptly at 35° to 40° laterally to enter the ipsilateral transverse foramen of C1 approximately 7.2 mm from the lateral end of the C2 ganglion and 15.3 mm from the dura. The artery curves posteromedially along the lateral mass and posterior C1 arch to travel within the vertebral artery groove. There is a dynamic relationship between the artery and the groove on C1 such that the artery may not always travel within the groove. It then travels beneath the posterior atlanto-occipital membrane before penetrating the dura and arachnoid to enter the foramen magnum where the pair of arteries unite to form the basilar artery. One of the vertebral arteries is usually dominant. Prior to formation of the basilar artery, each vertebral artery gives off branches that form the anterior and posterior spinal arteries that supply the upper aspects of the cervical spinal cord. The spinal arteries are small in the subaxial spine; therefore, the cervical cord derives additional blood supply from branches of the vertebral, deep cervical, ascending cervical, and at times the highest intercostals arteries. The anterior spinal artery runs uninterrupted along the cord between the vertebral arteries, the arteria radicularis magna (artery of Adamkiewicz), and the posterior intercostals and lumbar arteries.

## Thoracolumbar Spinal Blood Vessels

The inferior thoracic and superior lumbar regions of the spinal cord are primarily supplied by the great anterior radicular artery or arteria radicularis magna. In 80% of patients this artery arises from the left side off an inferior intercostal artery and enters the intervertebral fo-

ramina near the costotransverse joints, accompanying one of the ventral roots of T9 to T12. Other times this artery may originate from a superior lumbar artery and therefore may enter the canal anywhere from T5 to L5. The great anterior radicular artery most likely serves as the main blood supply for the inferior two thirds of the anterior cord. To limit the risk of injury to this artery or collaterals, ligature of a vessel close to the foramen should be avoided during anterior approaches to the spine and care should be taken when disarticulating a costotransverse or costovertebral joint.

Radicular branches off the aortic segmental vessels travel lateral to the intervertebral foramen and run dorsocaudal, inferior to the spinal nerve and lateral to the superior facet of the vertebra below. These arteries branch into lateral and intermediate branches that penetrate the back muscles, and a medial branch that travels close to the pars interarticularis to anastomose with the contralateral artery posterior to the spinous processes. Segmental veins run parallel to the arterial paths.

The use of an anterior exposure to the lumbosacral region is anticipated to increase with the use of disk replacement devices; however, the use of this approach risks injury to multiple neurovascular structures that need to be manipulated for adequate exposure to the disk spaces (Figure 4). Usually on the left side of the middle of L4, the abdominal aorta divides into visceral, parietal, and terminal branches and becomes the right and left common iliac arteries and the middle sacral artery. The bifurcation is variable and can occur anywhere from L3 to the lower border of L5. The left common iliac vein averages 12 mm from midline and 33.5 mm from the right common iliac artery. The middle sacral artery averages 2.5 mm in width and, because of its variable location, is a poor anatomic landmark for locating the midline of L5-S1. Single or multiple iliolumbar veins usually drain the lower lumbar region before passing behind the psoas major muscle into the common iliac vein and act as a tether during anterior exposure of L4-5. Ligature of this vein is often required for exposure; however, ligature presents the risk of injury to the obturator nerve that courses superficially approximately 1.5 to 2.76 cm laterally and to the lumbosacral trunk, which is approximately 2.5 cm lateral and deep, but may be less than 1 cm in some patients.

## Nerves and Plexuses

There are 31 pairs of spinal nerves: 8 cervical, 12 thoracic, 5 lumbar, 5 sacral, and 1 coccygeal. The spinal nerves are mixed and consist of the dorsal sensory fibers and ventral fibers. The anterior primary division (ventral ramus) and posterior primary division (dorsal ramus) of the mixed spinal nerve, the recurrent meningeal (sinuvertebral) nerve, and the sensory fibers that course through the sympathetic nervous system provide sensa-

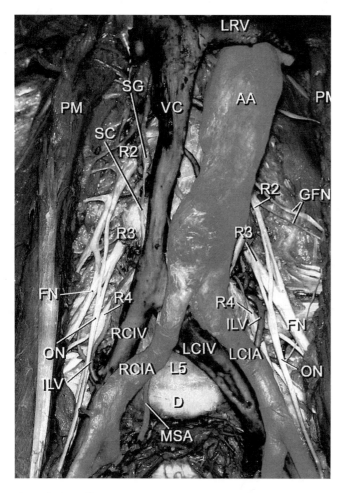

Figure 4 View of the neurovascular anatomy ventral to the lumbar spine. AA, abdominal aorta; D, Disk; FN, femoral nerve; GFN, genitofemoral nerve; ILV, iliolumbar vein; L, Lumbar; LCIA, left common iliac artery; LCIV, left common iliac vein; LRV, left renal vein; MSA, middle sacral artery; ON, obturator nerve; PM, psoas muscle; R2, second nerve root; R3, third nerve root; R4, fourth nerve root; RCIA, right common iliac artery; RCIV, right common iliac vein; SC, sympathetic chain; SG, sympathetic ganglion; VC, vena cava. (*Reproduced with permission from Pait GT, Elias AJ, Tribelll R: Thoracic, lumbar, and sacral spine anatomy for endoscopic surgery. Neurosurgery 2002;51(5): S2-67-S2-78.*)

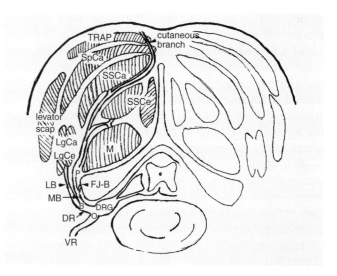

Figure 5 Axial view of the posterior cervical spine highlighting the course of the dorsal rami and the muscles. SSCa, semispinalis capitis; SSCe, semispinalis cervicis; M, multifidus; LgCa, longissimus capitis; LgCe, longissimus cervicis; DRG, dorsal root ganglion; VR, ventral ramus; DR, dorsal ramus; LB, lateral branch; FJ-B, facet joint branch; O, origin of the DR; B, branching point of DR into LB and medial branch; P, point at which the medial branch reaches the lateral edge of the multifidus. (*Reproduced with permission from Zhang J, Tsuzuki N, Hirabayashi S, Saiki K, Fujita K: Surgical anatomy of the nerves and muscles in the posterior cervical spine: A guide for avoiding inadvertent nerve injuries during the posterior approach. Spine 2003; 28(13):1379-1384.*)

tion to the spinal elements. Many of the nerves and plexuses are at risk for injury when approaching the spine during surgery.

## Cervical Spine

During anterior cervical spine surgery the recurrent and superior laryngeal nerves are particularly at risk for injury. The recurrent laryngeal nerve is a medial branch of the vagus nerve (cranial nerve X) outside the carotid sheath that predictably runs in the tracheoesophageal groove on the left after turning beneath the aortic arch. On the right this nerve is more variable, often curving beneath the subclavian artery, and will likely cross the surgical field. In 50% of patients the right recurrent laryngeal nerve reaches the tracheoesophageal groove at C5-6. Injury to this nerve or the vagus nerve can lead to vocal cord paralysis but often manifests as temporary

hoarseness. The superior laryngeal nerve originates from the vagus nerve in the carotid sheath an average 20 mm (range, 5 to 32 mm) proximal to the bifurcation of the carotid artery, and after traveling approximately 15 mm (range, 3 to 20 mm) bifurcates into internal (sensory) and external (motor) branches. Distally, the internal branch is located around C3-4, courses close to the superior laryngeal artery, and inserts into the thyrohyoid membrane within 1 cm superior to the artery. It innervates the mucosa of the larynx and has an important sensory reflex that serves to protect the lungs from aspiration.

During posterior cervical spine procedures, a precise knowledge of the cervical dorsal rami anatomy and the innervating patterns of the paravertebral muscles may help avoid inadvertent neural injuries. Such injuries may explain symptoms after posterior neck surgeries. Each medial branch from the dorsal rami of the C3-C8 spinal nerves passes through an anatomic tunnel dorsolateral to the facet joint (Figure 5). The base of the tunnel is a bony gutter between neighboring facets, and the roof is the tendon of the semispinalis capitis. The nerve branch is lax in the tunnel and is most susceptible to iatrogenic injury. Cutaneous branches from the dorsal rami are found adjacent to each spinous process bilaterally below the C2 spinous process with few discernible larger cutaneous nerves below the C5 or C6 spinous process. Except for the greater occipital nerve at C2 (medial branch of C2) and the third occipital nerve (superficial median branch of C3), the cutaneous nerves at each spinous process below C3 are small with diameters smaller than 2 mm. Cutaneous nerves may be cut during a middorsal skin incision. Intermuscular branches of medial branches run among paravertebral muscles and can be injured in an intermuscular release. Approaches to the lateral aspect of the facet joints will encounter trunks of the median branches directly in the surgical field after releasing the paravertebral muscles from the spine. The median branches accompany blood vessels; the use of electrical cautery may inadvertently destroy the nerve sheaths of median branches. Excessive lateral retraction can overstretch the median branches within the anatomic tunnel.

Injury to the spinal accessory nerve can occur with lateral dissection or excessive traction on the shoulders with contralateral neck rotation and results in ipsilateral shoulder droop, loss of shoulder elevation, and pain. This nerve crosses obliquely across the posterior triangle on the surface of the levator scapula muscle, through the posterior border of the sternocleidomastoid muscle 50.7 mm (± 12.9 mm) below the tip of the mastoid process, and reaches the anterior border of the trapezius 49.8 mm (± 5.9 mm) above the clavicle.

## Thoracolumbar Spine

In the thoracolumbar spine, each nerve is connected to a lumbar sympathetic ganglion by one or two rami. During dorsomedian surgical approaches, exposure lateral to the facets may injure medial branches of the posterior rami, which may cause segmental muscle atrophy, pain, and instability (Figure 6). The medial branch of the posterior ramus courses from the cranial adjacent segment over the transverse process and lateral to the pars interarticularis where it is attached by fibers of the intertransverse ligament to the periosteum lateral to the facet. In the lumbar spine, added attachments to the mamilloaccessory ligament are present. These attachments tether the nerve; therefore, wide exposure creates the risk of rupture.

The first three lumbar nerves and part of the fourth unite to form the lumbar plexus. In 50% of patients, a small branch of the 12th thoracic nerve (subcostal nerve) contributes to the lumbar plexus. Part of the fourth and fifth nerve form the lumbosacral trunk, which takes part in the formation of the sacral plexus. A nerve that is involved in the formation of two plexuses is called a furcal nerve. The lumbar plexus lies in the posterior aspect of the psoas muscle just anterior to the transverse processes and medial border of the quadratus lumborum. The first lumbar nerve splits into superior and inferior branches after receiving contribution from the 12th thoracic nerve. The superior branch redivides into the iliohypogastric and ilioinguinal nerves. The smaller inferior branch unites with a small superior

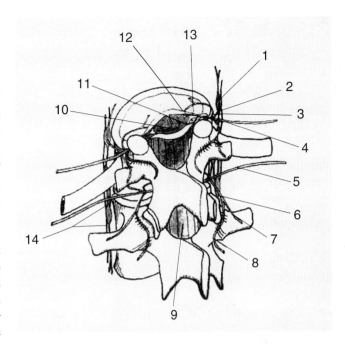

Figure 6    The nervous system of the thoracolumbar spine. 1) Ganglion of sympathetic trunk; 2) Ramus communicans; 3) Meningeal branch; 4) Spinal nerve; 5) Anterior ramus of spinal nerve; 6) Posterior ramus of spinal nerve; 7) Lateral branch of posterior ramus of spinal nerve; 9) Dura mater; 10) Spinal cord; 11) Dorsal root of spinal nerve; 12) Spinal ganglion; 13) Ventral root of spinal nerve; 14) Interganglionic branches. (*Reproduced with permission from Boelderl A, Daniaux H, Kathrein A, Maurer H: Danger of damaging the medial branches of the posterior rami of the spinal nerves during a dorsomedian approach to the spine. Clin Anat 2002;5:77-81.*)

branch of the second lumbar nerve to form the genitofemoral nerve. Anterior surgical approaches to the lumbar spine may injure these nerves. The iliohypogastric nerve provides sensation to the skin of the gluteal and hypogastric regions. The ilioinguinal nerve innervates the skin of the upper and medial part of the thigh, root of the penis and scrotum in males, and mons pubis and labium majus in females. Injury to these nerves may be confirmed by injection of local anesthetic approximately 3 cm medial to the anterior superior iliac spine (ASIS). The genitofemoral nerve may divide into a genital and femoral branch. The genital branch is small and enters the inguinal canal at the deep inguinal ring to supply the cremaster muscle and skin and fascia of the scrotum and adjacent thigh.

## Sympathetic Division of the Autonomic Nervous System

The preganglionic neurons of the sympathetic nervous system have cell bodies in the thoracic spinal cord and the first two to three lumbar cord levels. The postganglionic neurons have cell bodies that are generally arranged in a chain of ganglia (sympathetic trunk or chain) on the anterolateral surfaces of the vertebral body. There are 22 ganglia in each of the two trunks extending from the coccyx to the base of the skull: 3 cervical, 11 thoracic, 4 lumbar, and 4 sacral. In the cervical spine the sympathetic

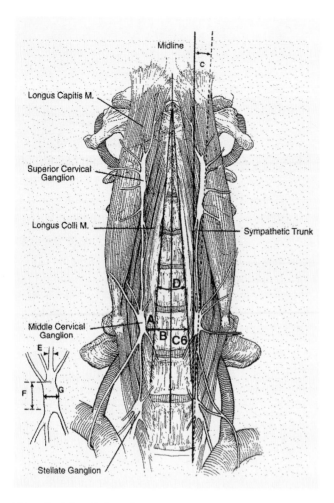

**Figure 7** Schematic illustrating measurements of the sympathetic trunk (ST); A, Distance between the ST and the medial border of the longus collis (LC) muscle at C6. B, Distance between the medial borders of the LC muscle. C, Angle of the ST relative to the midline. D, Angle between the medial borders of the LC muscle. E, Diameter of the St at C6. F, Length of the middle cervical ganglion. G, Width of the middle cervical ganglion. (*Reproduced with permission from Ebraheim NA, Lu J, Yang H, Heck BE, Yeasting RA: Vulnerabiity of the sympathetic trunk during the anterior approach to the lower cervical spine. Spine 2000;25(13):1603-1606.*)

trunk lies anterior to the longus capitis muscles and the transverse process, and posterior to the carotid sheath. Injury to postganglionic neurons or the sympathetic trunk may result in Horner's syndrome characterized by ptosis, ipsilateral meiosis, and anhydrosis. In the cervical spine, the sympathetic trunk runs in a superior and lateral direction and converges caudally, with an average angle of 10.4° (± 3.8°) relative to the midline and on average 10.6 mm (± 2.6 mm) from the medial border of the longus colli. The sympathetic trunk is most vulnerable at C6 where it is closer to the medial border of the longus colli during anterior cervical approaches (Figure 7). The superior cervical ganglion is located at C2-3 and is the largest. The middle ganglion, which measures 9.7 mm long (± 2.1 mm) and 5.2 mm wide (± 1.3 mm) is usually located at C6 but can be variable and absent in 61% of patients. The inferior (stellate) ganglion is located lateral to the longus colli

muscle between the base of the C7 transverse process and the neck of the first rib. The trunks rest over the rib heads in the thoracic spine and along the ventrolateral surfaces of the lumbar vertebra. On the right of the lumbar spine, the sympathetic trunk lies under the inferior vena cava and on the left it is overlapped by the lymph nodes along the aorta. There may be as many as six and as few as two ganglia on the sympathetic chain. The ganglia rest against the bodies or intervertebral disks of the corresponding vertebra. The ganglia of the second lumbar vertebra may be the largest. Relative to the transverse processes, there is a safe zone anterior to the lumbar nerves and posterior to the sympathetic trunk that measured 22 mm in the transverse dimension at the T12-L1 disk region and 25 mm at the L4-5 disk region. The genitofemoral nerve runs close to the lateral margin of the L2-3 disk region. Tissue dissection during anterior approaches to the lumbar spine should proceed from left to right to decrease the risk of injury to the superior hypogastric plexus (causing retrograde ejaculation) as it crosses anterior to the L5-S1 disk space.

## Piriformis Anatomy

The piriformis muscles and fibrovascular structures may cause compression of the sciatic nerve as it exits the sciatic notch, resulting in sciatica. The piriformis muscle is flat, pyramid-shaped, and broadly originates from the ventrolateral surface of the sacrum from the S2-S4 vertebrae and is innervated by branches from L5, S1, and S2 nerve roots. From the point of origin of the piriformis muscle, it passes through the greater notch and dorsal to the sciatic nerve before inserting on the superomedial aspect of the greater trochanter of the femur. The superior gluteal nerve and artery travel above the piriformis to supply the gluteus medius and minimus whereas the inferior gluteal nerve and artery lie below and supply the gluteus maximus muscle. The sciatic nerve consists of branches from the L3 to S3 nerve roots and usually courses beneath the piriformis muscle and dorsal to the gemelli muscles. In approximately 20% of the population, the piriformis muscle belly is split with one or more parts of the sciatic nerve dividing the muscle belly itself. In 10% of the population, the tibial and peroneal divisions of the sciatic nerve are not enclosed in a sheath. Usually, the peroneal portion splits the piriformis muscle belly, although it is rare for the tibial division to split the piriformis muscle belly. The intersection of the piriformis muscle and the sciatic nerve is approximately midpoint between the top of the greater trochanter and the ischium.

## Bone Graft Anatomy

The iliac crest and fibula are common sites of bone graft harvest for spinal fusion. A more vertical incision placed laterally within 68 mm of the posterior iliac spine or 8 cm from midline, along with directing bone graft harvesting more parallel to the iliac crest will limit complications to the superior cluneal nerves and superior gluteal vessels. Preserving the inner cortex and limiting harvesting to 4 cm from the posterior superior iliac spine will avoid violation of the sacroiliac spine. The lateral femoral cutaneous nerve supplies skin sensation to the anterolateral thigh and has variable positions relative to the ASIS. This nerve can be avoided in most patients by dissecting on the outer cortex and staying more than 3 cm posterior from the ASIS. This technique also leaves enough bone to decrease the risk of avulsion fractures of the ASIS by the sartorius muscle and injury to the inguinal ligament attachment. The lateral cutaneous branch of the T12 subcostal nerve may lie as close as 6 cm from the ASIS. The ilioinguinal and iliohypogastric nerves can be injured with retraction of the iliacus muscle during dissection on the inner wall of the ilium. Fibular bone-graft harvesting can cause injury to the peroneal nerves in the proximal third of the fibula and the peroneal vessels in the middle third of the fibula. Staying greater than 10 cm above the ankle will avoid ankle instability.

## Summary

Knowledge of the main anatomic elements surrounding the nonpathologic spine is essential for the physician to make correct diagnoses and render safe and efficacious surgical and nonsurgical treatment. Identification of anatomic landmarks and adjacent neurovascular structures helps facilitate safe placement of instrumentation in the spine.

## Annotated Bibliography

Dong Y: Hong Xia, Jianyi L: Quantitative anatomy of the lateral mass of the atlas. *Spine* 2003;28:860-863.

Specimens from the atlas of 30 fresh cadavers were used to measure the dimensions of the lateral mass for posterior screw fixation. The mean width of the lateral mass of the atlas is 15.47 mm (± 1.19 mm), the mean thickness is 17.21 mm (± 0.93 mm), the mean height is 14.09 mm (± 1.92 mm), the mean transverse diameter of the atlantoaxial joint surface 17.90 mm (± 1.18 mm), the mean longitudinal diameter of the atlantoaxial joint articular surface 15.63 mm (± 1.04 mm), and the obliquity of the facet atlantoaxial joint in coronary plane is 34.57° (± 3.77°).

Kwon BK, Song F, Morrison WB, et al: Morphologic evaluation of cervical spine anatomy with computed tomography: Anterior cervical plate fixation considerations. *J Spinal Disord Tech* 2004;17:102-107.

The authors used CT studies of the cervical spine of 50 males and 50 females to determine anatomic parameters relevant to anterior cervical plating. Widths of the vertebral bodies measured 24.6 mm (± 2.4 mm) in males and 23.0 mm

(± 2.4 mm) in females. The narrowest measurements were 17 mm in males and 14 mm in females. The average midsagittal diameter of each vertebral body in males was approximately 17 to 18 mm with the smallest being 13 mm. In females the average midsagittal AP diameter was 15 to 16 mm, with the smallest being 10 mm.

Lu J, Ebraheim NA, Georgiadis GM, Yang H, Yeasting RA: Anatomic considerations of the vertebral artery: Implications for anterior decompression of the cervical spine. *J Spinal Disord* 1998;11:233-236.

Measurements of the vertebral artery relative to the medial margin of the longus colli and the anterior margin of the vertebral body from C6 to C3 were performed. The average angle of the vertebral artery relative to midline was 4.3° (± 2.6°). The average distance between the medial margin of the longus colli and medial border of the vertebral artery decreased from C6 (11.5 mm ± 1.0 mm) to C3 (9.0mm ± 1.3 mm). The average distance between the anterior margin of the vertebral body and the vertebral artery increased from C6 (7.2 mm ± 1.9 mm) to C3 (9.6 mm ± 2.1 mm). The distance between the medial borders of the longus colli decreased from C6 (13.8 mm ± 2.2 mm) to C3 (7.9 mm ± 2.2 mm).

McLain R, Ferrara L, Kabins M: Pedicle morphology in the upper thoracic spine: Limits to safe screw placement in older patients. *Spine* 2002;27:2467-2471.

T1-6 vertebrae from 18 human cadavers age 62 to 85 years were measured showing that 25% of T1 pedicles, 17% of T2, and 42% of T3 pedicles were narrower than 5.5 mm. It was also found that 61% of T4 pedicles were too small to accept a 5.5 mm screw, as were 67% of T5, and 75% of T6 pedicles. The pedicle diameter of 33% of T4 and 25% of T5 were smaller than 4.5 mm. Pedicles become increasingly narrow and oblong in the T4-6 cross sections. Craniocaudal heights were fairly consistent from T1-T6 but the distance from the facet cortex to the anterior vertebral body cortex increased from T1-6. Safe screw lengths ranged from 30 mm at T1 and T2, 35 mm at T4-5, to 40 mm at T5-6.

Okan B: An anatomic and morphometric study of C2 nerve root ganglion and its corresponding foramen. *Spine* 2004;29:495-499.

The dimensions and location of the C2 ganglion in relation to adjacent structures with head motions were assessed in 20 cadaveric cervical spines. The shape of the ganglion was oval in 70%, spindle-like in 20%, and spherical in 10%. The height was 4.97 mm (± 0.92 mm) on the right and 4.6 mm (± 0.84 mm) on the left. The C2 ganglion lies in the C1-2 intervertebral space, bordered superiorly by the posterior arch of the atlas, inferiorly by the lamina of the axis, anteriorly by the lateral atlantoaxial joint and its fibrous capsule, and posteriorly by the anterior edge of the ligamentum flavum. The ganglion occupied 50% to 65% of the intervertebral space respectively with neutral and hyperextension with opposite head rotation positions. There was no bone contact or impact to the ganglion with normal limited or forced hyperextension and rotation head motions. This result may contradict prior reports of impaction of the C2 ganglion with head motion as a cause of cervicogenic headaches.

Weiner BK, Walker M, Wiley W, McCulloch JA: The lateral buttress: An anatomic feature of the lumbar pars interarticularis. *Spine* 2002;27:E385-E387.

A morphometric study was performed on the lateral buttress region of the L1-L5 pars interarticularis on 10 dried lumbar spines. The surface area of the buttresses at L1-3 was similar, measuring approximately 80 mm$^2$ (± 10 mm$^2$). At L4, it measured 50 mm$^2$ (± 10 mm$^2$), and at L5 it measured 15 mm$^2$ (± 5 mm$^2$). These differences were statistically significant and approximated to a 40% and 80% smaller surface area at L4 and L5 respectively, compared to upper levels. This finding may explain the higher incidence of spondylolysis and iatrogenic instability at the L4 and L5 levels. C

## Classic Bibliography

Ebraheim NA, Lu J, Brown JA, Biyani A, Yeasting RA: Vulnerability of vertebral artery in anterolateral decompression for cervical spondylosis. *Clin Orthop Relat Res* 1996;322:146-151.

Fardon DF, Garfin SR, Abitol JJ, Bodem SD, Herkowitz HN, Mayer TG (eds): *Orthopaedic Knowledge Update: Spine.* Rosemont, IL, American Academy of Orthopaedic Surgeons, 2002.

Goel A, Laheri V: Plate and screw fixation for atlanto-axial subluxation. *Acta Neurochir (Wien)* 1994;129:47-53.

Gupta S, Goel A: Quantitative anatomy of the lateral masses of the atlas and axis vertebrae. *Neurol India* 2000;48:120-125.

Phillips FM, Phillips CS, Wetzel TF, Gelinas C: Occipito-cervical neutral position: Possible surgical implications. *Spine* 1999;24:775-778.

Robinson DR: Piriformis syndrome in relation to sciatic pain. *Am J Surg* 1947;73:435-439.

Xu R, Kang A, Ebraheim NA, Yeasting RA: Anatomic relations between the cervical pedicle and the adjacent neural structures. *Spine* 1999;24:451-454.

# Chapter 3

# Biomechanics of the Spine

Avinash G. Patwardhan, PhD

Ioannis N. Gaitanis, MD

Leonard I. Voronov, MD, PhD

## Physiologic Loads

Mechanical loading of the spine is an important factor in the etiology of spinal disorders and it also affects the outcome of treatments of these disorders. The loads on the human spine are produced by gravitational forces resulting from the mass of body segments, external forces and moments induced by a physical activity, and by muscle tension. These loads are shared by the osseoligamentous tissues and muscles of the spine. Tensile forces in the paraspinal muscles, which exert a compressive load on the spine, balance the moments created by gravitational and external loads (Figure 1). Because these muscles have a small moment arm from the spinal segment, they amplify the compressive load on the osseoligamentous spine.

The human spine is subjected to large compressive preloads during activities of daily living. The internal compressive forces on the ligamentous spine have been estimated for different physical tasks using kinematic and electromyographic data in conjunction with three-dimensional biomechanical models. The compressive force on the human lumbar spine is estimated to range from 200 to 300 N during supine and recumbent postures to 1,400 N during relaxed standing with the trunk flexed 30°. The compressive force may be substantially larger when an individual is holding a weight in their hands in the static standing posture, and even more so when the individual is doing dynamic lifting. The human cervical spine also withstands substantial compressive preloads in vivo. The cervical preload approaches three times the weight of the head because of muscle coactivation forces in balancing the head in the neutral posture. The compressive preload on the cervical spine increases during flexion, extension, and other activities of daily living, and is estimated to reach 1,200 N in activities involving maximal isometric muscle efforts. In normal individuals, the spine sustains these loads without injury or instability.

The preload, produced by muscles, can be considered an "external" compressive load that acts on the spinal segments in vivo during the performance of differ-

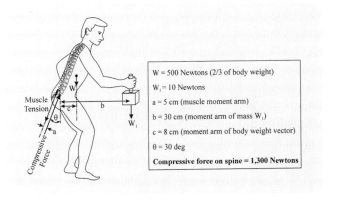

Figure 1  Loads on the spine. The compressive force acting on the spine is magnified by the small moment arm of the muscles. *(Adapted from Mow VC, Flatow EL, Ateshian GA: Biomechanics, in Buckwalter JA, Einhorn TA, Simon SR (eds): Orthopaedic Basic Science, ed 2, Rosemont, IL, American Academy of Orthopaedic Surgeons, 2000, p 141).*

ent activities of daily living. The mechanical response of healthy, degenerated, or injured spinal segments will be influenced by this preload. The implants used to restore stability to the unstable spinal column must be sufficiently strong and rigid to withstand these physiologic loads.

## Stability of the Spinal Column

### Load-Bearing Ability of the Osteoligamentous Spine

In the absence of muscle forces, the osteoligamentous spine cannot support vertical compressive loads of in vivo magnitude. Studies in which a vertical load was applied at the cephalic end of the cervical, thoracolumbar, or lumbar spine specimens showed buckling of the spines at load levels well below those seen in vivo. The stability of the spine, characterized by a critical load (maximum load carrying capacity, or Euler buckling load of the spinal column), was determined by these experiments. When the load exceeded the critical value, the spine, constrained to move only in the frontal plane in these experiments, became unstable and buckled. The cervical spine buckled at a vertical load of approximately 10 N, the thoracolumbar spine at 20 N, and the

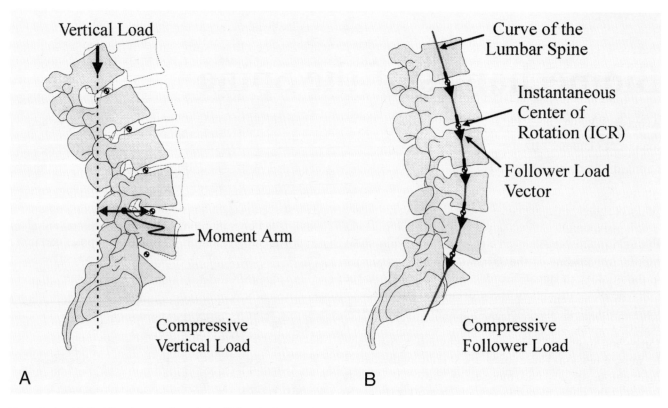

**Figure 2**  **A** and **B,** Depiction of compressive vertical and follower load vectors. The compressive follower load vector in the sagittal plane passes through the flexion-extension instantaneous center of rotation of each segment, thereby minimizing the coupled flexion/extension angular changes.

lumbar spine at 88 N, all well below the compressive loads expected in vivo during activities of daily living. When a compressive load is applied in a vertical direction to a multisegment spine specimen, segmental bending moments and shear forces are induced because of the inherent curvature of the spine. This load application causes large changes in the specimen's posture at relatively small loads. Further loading can cause damage to the soft tissue or bony structures. Thus, in the absence of muscles, the osteoligamentous spine alone cannot support vertical compressive loads of the magnitude that occur in vivo.

### Role of Muscles
The observation that the ligamentous spine is unstable at low vertical compressive loads has led many investigators to postulate various mechanisms by which the spine could withstand physiologic compressive loads. Some researchers have modeled the muscles as springs to explain the role of muscles in preventing a buckling instability of the spinal column. Simulation of active muscle forces in experiments on the ligamentous spine is difficult because of the large number of muscles and the uncertainty in load sharing among the various muscles during different activities. The simulated muscle actions must provide stability to the ligamentous spine to carry compressive loads while simultaneously permitting

mobility needed to perform the activities of daily living.

Recent analysis using muscle models of the trunk supports the argument that the individual spinal segments or functional spinal units (FSUs) are subjected to nearly pure compressive loads in vivo. Attempts to determine joint loads based on the assumption of a vertical load on the spine have resulted in serious overprediction of shear forces on the FSU. The calculations of these spine models, taking into consideration the activity of paraspinal and abdominal muscles, showed that in weight-holding tasks the compressive force on the lumbosacral disk increased with increasing trunk inclination and the amount of weight lifted, whereas the maximum AP shear force remained small (about 20% to 25% of the compressive force). The obliquity of the pars lumborum extensors allows them to share anterior shear forces resulting from lifting a load. When these muscles are activated to contribute a balancing extensor moment, they help to offset the anterior shear force on the lumbar FSU.

### Stability of the Spinal Column Under a Follower Load
It could be reasoned that coactivation of trunk muscles could alter the direction of the internal compressive force vector such that its path followed the lordotic and kyphotic curves of the spine, passing through the instantaneous center of rotation of each segment (Figure 2).

This scenario would minimize the segmental bending moments and shear forces induced by the compressive load, thereby allowing the ligamentous spine to support loads that would otherwise cause buckling, and would provide a greater margin of safety against both instability and tissue injury. The load vector described above is called a "follower load."

Experiments on human cadaveric specimens of lumbar (L1-L5), thoracolumbar (T2-sacrum), and cervical (C2-C7) spines as well as mathematical models have demonstrated that: (1) the ligamentous spine with multiple motion segments can withstand physiologic compressive loads without tissue injury or instability if the compressive load vector is applied along a follower load path approximating the curve of the ligamentous spine; (2) the ligamentous spine subjected to compressive preloads of in vivo magnitude along the follower load path permits physiologic mobility under flexion-extension moments; and (3) the follower preload simulates the resultant vector of muscles that allow the spine to support physiologic compressive loads. Intradiskal pressures in human cadaveric lumbar spines under a follower preload are comparable to those measured in vivo, and the spinal stability is increased without compromising its mobility in flexion-extension and lateral bending. A superimposed follower preload renders the in vitro loading of the ligamentous spine with pure moments more physiologic.

The follower load concept suggests a new hypothesis for the role of muscle coactivation in providing in vivo spinal stability. Coactivation of trunk muscles (for example, the lumbar multifidus, longissimus pars lumborum, iliocostalis pars lumborum) could alter the direction of the resultant internal force such that its path follows the curve of the spine (follower load path), thereby allowing the ligamentous spine to support compressive loads that would otherwise cause buckling of the column. Muscle dysfunction can induce abnormal shear forces at the lumbar FSU, leading to segmental instability in the presence of disk degeneration. On the other hand, a compressive follower preload produced by coordinated muscle action could stabilize shear instability in a degenerative FSU. This finding suggests a role for muscle conditioning and therapy in treating degenerative conditions of the spine.

## Stability of the Functional Spinal Unit
### Three-Joint Complex
A spinal motion segment is the smallest functional unit of the osteoligamentous spine and exhibits the generic characteristics of the spine. The FSU consists of two vertebral bodies connected by an intervertebral disk, facet joints, and ligaments (except at the C1-C2 segment where there is no intervertebral disk). The FSU could be viewed as a three-joint complex consisting of the disk

(a cartilaginous joint) and two facets joints (synovial joints). A dynamic relationship exists between the intervertebral disk and facet joints in sharing physiologic loads.

The intervertebral disk carries substantial loads because of gravitational and muscle forces. It is the major anterior load-bearing element in axial compression and flexion. In the young healthy spine, load transmission from vertebra to vertebra occurs primarily through the nucleus pulposus of the disks. As load is applied to the healthy disk, forces are distributed equally in all directions from within the nucleus, placing the anulus fibrosus fibers in tension. The collagen fibers of the anulus fibrosus are well suited to resisting tension along the fiber direction. The pressure in the nucleus pulposus stretches the fibers in the anulus fibrosus, and the resistance of the fibers to tensile loading allows the anulus fibrosus to contribute to load sharing. The anulus fibrosus is well suited to resisting torsion because of the characteristic orientation of fibers in each layer. Fiber strains rarely exceed 6% under physiologic flexion and extension moments and 8.5% under physiologic axial rotation. The intervertebral disk provides most of the motion segment's stiffness in compression, whereas ligaments and facets contribute significantly in resisting bending moment and axial torsion.

Facet joints provide a posterior load path and have an important role in determining the limits of motion in the FSU. Biomechanical studies demonstrated that facets in the lumbar spine carry 10% to 20% of the compressive load when a person is standing upright. The proportion of the total load shared by the disk increases with flexion. Load transmission through the articular facet surfaces as well as through the tips of the inferior facets in extension relieves some of the load on the intervertebral disk. The maintenance of cervical and lumbar lordosis helps to reduce the load on the disk, whereas flexion increases disk loading. The contribution of the facet joints to the stability of an FSU is also dependent on the capsular ligament and the level within the spine. For example, thoracic facets have a limited capsular reinforcement, which facilitates axial rotation, in contrast to the lumbar spine in which the facet capsule is well developed to stabilize the spine against rotation and lateral bending.

### Segmental Instability
Injuries, degeneration, and surgical procedures can significantly alter the normal load sharing between the components of an FSU, and can cause abnormal motion response under physiologic loads. Instability is quantified in terms of a loss of stiffness or an increase in flexibility of an FSU. Stiffness of an FSU is a measure of how much load is required to produce a given motion. Flexibility is the inverse of stiffness; it is a measure of

the motion produced by a given load. An FSU is unstable if the stiffness is too small or flexibility is too large. It is helpful to think about FSU instability in terms of macroinstabilities and microinstabilities.

### Macroinstability

Macroinstability implies gross disruption of the spinal column (such as instability caused by a fracture) leading to disruption in load transmission from one vertebra to another. Macroinstability can lead to a progression of the deformity at the injury site and neurologic deficit. Examples of macroinstability include instability caused by injuries of the thoracolumbar spine such as compression fracture, fracture-dislocation, traumatic spondylolisthesis, and burst fracture as well as tumors, infections, and iatrogenic causes. To appreciate the severity of clinical and biomechanical macroinstability it is helpful to think about the spine as a structure made of three load-bearing columns. The anterior column is formed by the anterior longitudinal ligament, anterior anulus fibrosus, and anterior part of the vertebral body. The middle column is formed by the posterior longitudinal ligament, posterior anulus fibrosus, and posterior wall of the vertebral body. The posterior column is formed by the posterior arch, supraspinous and interspinous ligaments, facet joints, and ligamentum flavum. Compression fracture involves failure of the anterior column with the middle column being totally intact. The burst fracture involves failure of both the anterior and middle columns. The seat belt injuries represent failure of the middle and posterior columns. The fracture-dislocation injury represents failure of all three load-bearing columns.

The severity of macroinstability, which has a detrimental effect on the load-carrying capacity of the spine, is influenced by the number of columns disrupted. The disruption of a single column (such as the anterior column caused by a compression fracture) results in a minimal loss of load-carrying capacity. The instability associated with a two-column disruption (such as that caused by a burst fracture or a flexion-distraction seat belt injury) is more severe. Burst fractures cause significant instability (loss of stiffness relative to intact segment) in flexion, lateral bending, and axial rotation. The injured segments undergo excessively large motion as compared with the intact or uninjured segment for the same amount of load. If in addition to the two-column burst fracture the facets are disrupted, a significantly larger loss of stiffness may be seen in axial rotation. A fracture-dislocation is an example of a three-column disruption, and is at the high end of the macroinstability spectrum.

### Microinstability

In contrast to fractures, the instability associated with degenerative disorders of the lumbar spine can be viewed as microinstability. Failure or degeneration of any one element of the three-joint complex can alter the normal load sharing between these elements, leading to symptoms of back and leg pain. It also may set into motion a chain reaction (degenerative cascade) leading to degeneration and pain at other elements of the FSU.

Disk degeneration is believed to precede all other changes within the aging FSU. Degenerative changes in a disk are associated with a loss of proteoglycans in the nucleus that, in turn, leads to a decrease in the ability of the nucleus to generate fluid pressure. With disk dehydration and narrowing of the disk space, the annular fibers of the disk are no longer subjected to the same tensile stresses as would be found in a healthy disk with the hydrated nucleus. Instead, the anulus fibrosus in a degenerated disk is more likely to bear the axial load under direct compression from the vertebra above. Early degenerative changes in the disk render the FSU more flexible. Facet degeneration is most commonly a result of the segmental instability. As narrowing of the disk space occurs as a result of degeneration, the facets begin to undergo subluxation until the tips of the inferior facets impinge on the lamina below, causing the facets to increase their share of load transmission. Typically, the patient having facet syndrome will have symptoms aggravated by an extension maneuver because facet loading increases in extension. Increased peak pressures within the facet joint may give rise to degeneration of the joint cartilage; a thinning of the cartilage may cause capsular ligament laxity and allow abnormal motion or hypermobility of the facet joints. Cartilage degeneration seems to further increase the segmental movements that already were increased with disk degeneration. The final stage of the degenerative cascade is associated with attempted stabilization. The abnormal pressure and focal degeneration give rise to formation of bony hypertrophy and osteophytes and a decrease in segmental mobility. Occasionally, an uneven collapse of the disk space may cause acute angular deformities within the three-joint complex; the patient may report both neurogenic and low back pain.

During the process of three-joint complex degeneration, surgical intervention may be necessary to alleviate disabling symptoms. The combination of the surgical procedure (such as diskectomy, facetectomy, foraminotomy, and laminectomy) and the phase of degeneration will affect the biomechanical stability of the FSU and the clinical outcome. Biomechanical studies on human cadaveric spines showed that disruption of the ligamentum flavum and posterolateral annular integrity and removal of the nucleus content, simulating partial diskectomy for disk herniations, significantly increase primary motions in flexion, axial rotation, and lateral bending. Significant changes to motion of the FSU occur with removal of the nucleus pulposus as opposed to the removal of the anulus fibrosus. Hemilaminotomy with partial diskectomy increases angular motion over that seen in the intact FSU. Unilateral hemifacetectomy has little effect on the angular motion in flexion-extension and lateral bending, but may cause a small increase in axial rotation. Subsequent partial diskectomy significantly increases the angular motion in flexion-extension without a preload (Figure 3); however, a physiologic compressive preload of 400 N tends to reduce the instability produced after diskectomy. Diskectomy also significantly increases angular motion in axial rotation in the absence of a compressive preload. Hemilaminotomy with partial diskectomy is the gold standard for the surgical treatment of symptomatic radiculopathy caused by a herniated disk. Although diskectomy is quite effective in relieving radicular symptoms, persistent mechanical low back pain is not uncommon. The back pain may relate to disk degeneration and the ensuing altered kinematics at the involved segment, which may be exacerbated by surgical treatment. However, the true source of back pain remains unknown despite many attempts at defining it. The nonphysiologic motions may lead to altered stresses across the motion segment stabilizers including the facet joints as well as the supporting musculoligamentous structures, which could potentially contribute to postdiskectomy mechanical back pain.

Procedures performed for pathologies in the late degenerative phase, such as decompressive laminectomy or facetectomy for degenerative spondylolisthesis, also may lead to instability. Significant instability may result from bilateral hemifacetectomy. Unilateral or bilateral total facetectomy was shown to produce an increase in the segmental motion of 65% in flexion, 78% in extension, 15% in lateral bending, and 126% in rotation. These procedures may require postdecompression stabilization.

## Biomechanics of Stabilization
### Spinal Fusion

If surgical stabilization is indicated, the most appropriate fusion construct must be determined. Options range from uninstrumented fusion to fusion aided by the combination of anterior and posterior instrumentation.

### The Role of Spinal Instrumentation in Fusion Enhancement

There is consensus in the literature concerning the ideal mechanical environment to promote spinal fusion; a greater degree of immobilization of adjacent vertebrae enhances the chances of obtaining a solid bony fusion. Spinal instrumentation increases the rigidity of segments at the fusion site, thereby reducing the relative motion between the vertebrae during the biologic healing process. Animal studies have shown that a successful posterolateral fusion is more likely to be achieved in the presence of spinal instrumentation, and that stiffer constructs result in stiffer fusion masses. Posterior spinal

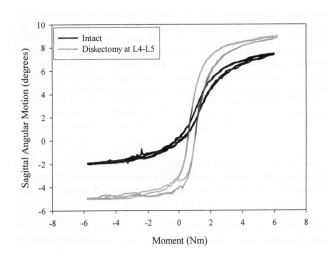

**Figure 3** Moment versus angular displacement curve for an L4-L5 segment: intact, and after unilateral hemifacetectomy with partial diskectomy

implants typically act as tension band devices. When the load-bearing function of the anterior column is not compromised to the degree that would not allow adequate load transfer, posterior stabilization systems can enhance spinal stability. Posterior instrumentation typically consists of two longitudinal components (such as plates or rods) with segmental attachments to the vertebrae to form a solid construct. The rigidity of the construct depends on the size and shape of the longitudinal components, the number of vertebrae spanned by the implant, the method of their attachment to the vertebrae, and the cross links between the longitudinal components.

Implants that use wires or hooks to attach the longitudinal components to the vertebrae can resist tensile forces but cannot effectively resist angular deformity caused by loads experienced during activities of daily living in the presence of compromised load-bearing ability of the anterior column. On the other hand, spinal instrumentation that uses transpedicular screws has the ability to resist both compressive and tensile forces, as well as bending moments. Because transpedicular screws span all three columns, they can transfer compressive loads and bending moment from the anterior column, through the pedicle, to the longitudinal components of the instrumentation. Thus, fixation using transpedicular screws results in more rigid constructs than sublaminar wire or hooks. However, in the presence of failure of anterior elements as a load-sharing component, the possibility of failure (loosening or breakage) of the screws is high. This situation is common in highly comminuted fractures of the vertebral body, treated by hyperdistraction with posterior instrumentation.

### The Role of Anterior Support

Although posterior instrumented fusions provide rigid fixation, they do not provide complete anterior column support. Transpedicular fixation allows three-column bony purchase; however, reports indicate the potential for continued micromotion in the intervertebral space, which provides a possible explanation for persisting back pain despite solid fusion. Furthermore, in the presence of chronic instability, the risk of screw loosening or breakage is a possibility if the anterior column support is lacking. This lack of support should also be considered in stabilizing the macroinstability associated with substantial disruption of two of the three load-bearing columns. To enhance stability it may be necessary to augment the load-bearing capacity of the anterior column (for example, using an interbody spacer such as a cage), thus providing the anterior support to allow posterior instrumentation to act as a tension band.

Can an interbody fusion device be used as a stand-alone device? In the early postoperative period, the stability of a stand-alone interbody device depends primarily on the compressive forces on the interbody implant that are produced by tension in the remaining lateral and posterolateral anulus fibrosus and ligaments resulting from disk-space distraction. A recent biomechanical study showed that the disk-space distraction force (and hence the compressive force on the interbody device) significantly increased in proportion to the degree of distraction. However, the distraction force reduced in magnitude by more than 20% in the first 15 minutes because of stress relaxation of the soft tissues, suggesting that the "tightness of fit" that the surgeon notes immediately after insertion of the interbody cage will degrade in the very early postoperative period. Furthermore, excessive disk-space distraction can result in changes in spinal alignment and stretching or tearing of the posterior ligaments and facet capsules. Distraction of the facet joints can cause pain and loss of segmental stiffness or hypermobility in extension. If disk-space distraction is inadequate, the compressive preload on the interbody implant may not be sufficient and may result in motion at the implant-bone interface in the early postoperative period, leading to delayed fusion and/or pseudarthrosis and, in some instances, dislodgement or migration of the fusion cage itself.

Supplemental fixation using translaminar facet screws or pedicle screws enhances the stability of the FSU treated with interbody cages. Fusion constructs that provide interbody support (anterior lumbar interbody fusion, posterior lumbar interbody fusion, and transforaminal lumbar interbody fusion cages) in conjunction with supplemental posterior fixation (pedicle screws or translaminar facet screws) have comparable stability in flexion-extension, lateral bending, and axial rotation.

## Nonfusion Devices

When a lumbar motion segment is fused, stresses on the adjacent segments may increase, thus increasing the risk of future injury. Biomechanical studies have reported increased motion and stresses in the adjacent segments (proximal or distal to the fusion) with application of compression, bending, and torsional loads. This altered mechanical environment may lead to accelerated degeneration of adjacent levels, which may become symptomatic. Many clinical studies report the increased incidence of facet and/or disk degeneration, segmental instability, and spinal stenosis at adjacent levels.

### Dynamic Posterior Stabilization Devices

In an attempt to eliminate the aforementioned problems inherent to fusion surgery, the concept of dynamically stabilizing an unstable FSU has been proposed to reduce abnormal painful movement while preserving some degree of motion. A suggested indication for dynamic posterior stabilization has been to restore near-normal motion after destabilization of the motion segment by surgical facetectomy and diskectomy. Some dynamic posterior stabilization devices are designed to be implanted between the spinous processes to induce an amount of flexion in the spinal unit, thus reducing the symptoms of neurogenic claudication. A metallic oval spacer (x-stop), when implanted between spinous processes, showed substantially reduced flexion-extension motion at the implanted segment, whereas motions in axial rotation and lateral bending were unaffected. A silicone interspinous process spacer that is secured using an interspinous process cable, called the device for intervertebral assisted motion (DIAM, Medtronic, Minneapolis, MN), was shown to be effective in reducing the increased segmental motions in flexion and extension after diskectomy. The angular motion was restored to below the level of the intact segment in flexion-extension without completely eliminating segmental mobility. The total residual flexion-extension angular motion after DIAM insertion was 75% of an intact FSU without a preload and 47% of an intact FSU under a 450 N preload. In lateral bending, DIAM reduced the increased motion induced by diskectomy, thereby bringing the range of motion close to that of the intact spine. However, in axial rotation the DIAM did not restore the rotational range of motion to the intact level. The relative ineffectiveness of the posterior dynamic stabilization devices implanted between the spinous processes in controlling rotation is not unexpected because the device is placed close to the torsional axis of rotation of the lumbar segment with diskectomy. In addition, intimate contact between the articular processes of the facet joint is essential for controlling rotational motion. Insertion of such devices between the interspinous processes may cause facet joint distraction, making the joint less effective at resisting axial rotation moments.

An alternative posteriorly applied nonfusion system, the DYNESYS system (Zimmer, Warsaw, IN), is composed of polycarbonate urethane spacers between pedi-

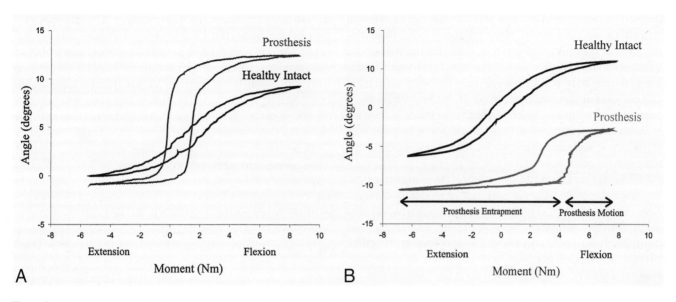

Figure 4  **A,** Moment versus angular displacement curve for an L4-L5 segment: healthy, intact FSU after TDR. **B,** Moment versus angular displacement curve for an L5-S1 segment: healthy, intact FSU after TDR.

cle screw heads to resist compression, and polyethylene-terephthalate cords that run through the hollow core of the spacers to resist tension. The DYNESYS system was shown to reduce the range of motion in a destabilized FSU below the magnitude of the intact FSU for flexion and lateral bending; however, the stabilizing effect of the DYNESYS system approached that of the internal fixator, suggesting that the DYNESYS system may be too stiff to allow for dynamic stabilization. In axial rotation the DYNESYS system increased motion compared with the intact spine.

### Motion Preservation Devices

Total disk replacement (TDR) has been recommended to reduce pain of presumed discogenic origin while preserving spinal motion, and to reduce the likelihood of accelerated adjacent level degeneration that has been reported following lumbar arthrodesis surgery. One of the objectives of TDR for degenerative disk disease is to allow replication of the natural biomechanics of a healthy intervertebral disk under physiologic loads. The design of a TDR, its implanted position within the disk space, and the presence and quality of the soft tissue and muscular structures are among the factors that determine how well the natural biomechanics are replicated. The biomechanical assessment of a TDR should address two questions: (1) Does a TDR restore normal load-displacement behavior of a spinal segment under physiologic loads? (2) How do the prosthesis components move relative to each other under physiologic loads when implanted in a spinal segment?

The motion response to physiologic loads of a spinal segment implanted with a TDR should be evaluated in terms of both the quantity of motion (range of motion) as well as the quality of motion (centers of rotation, neutral zone, and the pattern of intervertebral load-displacement curves).

The pattern of intervertebral load-displacement curves for implanted segments should be compared with that of healthy spinal segments. A healthy spinal segment displays a gradually changing angular motion pattern with gradual moment application (Figure 3). The motion response of an intact segment to applied moments is governed by bony and soft-tissue constraints. The disruption of some of these structures, most notably the anterior longitudinal ligament and the anterior anulus fibrosus, during the anterior insertion of a TDR decreases this constraint. As a result, a larger angular travel may be seen for the same applied moment for the TDR case when compared with the intact case (Figure 4, A). Any entrapment or locking of the prosthesis over a portion of the sagittal plane motion would be reflected in the relatively flat portion of the load-displacement curves in the presence of a preload (Figure 4, B). Once the entrapment is released, a large angular change would occur, reflected in the sharp rise of the load-displacement curves (Figure 4, B). The effect that these intervertebral motion patterns will have on the long-term outcome is not known, but nonuniform motion patterns could influence the wear behavior of the implant, and may also influence the load-sharing within the implanted segment and at adjacent levels.

The total joint experience in wear and survivorship of implants suggests that careful assessment of component motions under in vivo loading may provide important information to surgeons and manufacturers to decrease implant related long-term complications (such as wear, disintegration or fracture, dislodgment, loosening, or nonmovement). The prosthesis component motion patterns may have implications to component wear under in vivo physiologic loads and load sharing within the implanted and adjacent levels. Failure to provide normal load-sharing may result in hypertrophic bone formation or accelerated facet degeneration. If the prosthesis components are subject to wear either from shear, compression, or a combination of these forces, or if motion patterns are abnormal, the goal of saving adjacent levels may not be achieved.

Clinical measurement of vertebral motion using flexion and extension films is commonly performed to assess the function of TDR. However, this measurement may not be adequate because it demonstrates end points only. It does not allow the clinician to visualize prosthesis component motion throughout a given motion cycle. Sequential imaging showing the pattern of motion could be helpful in assessing the quality of motion that may affect the survivorship of the implant components and long-term results.

Articulated disk prostheses rely on physiologic compressive preload to function as a bearing. In the absence of adequate compressive preload, a separation of the upper prosthesis end plate from the bearing surface in extension can be observed. This separation demonstrates the importance of muscle loading in maintaining TDR function for an articulated device.

In a disk prosthesis that has two articulating surfaces for angular motion (for example, the Charité prosthesis [DePuy Spine, Raynham, MA] with two metal end plates and a mobile core), angulation between the upper and lower end plates can be the result of angulation between the upper end plate and the core, angulation between the lower end plate and the core, or angulation between both end plates and the core. If the predominant angular motion within the prosthesis occurs at only one of the two articulations when full contact of all three components is reached, it will have obvious implications to the quality of motion.

Factors likely to affect the function of the prosthesis include implant placement, segmental lordosis, an intraoperative change in lordosis, and magnitude of physiologic compressive preload on the implant. Although the patient's overall sagittal alignment and balance may be preserved in the short term, the increase in segmental lordosis after TDR and alteration in the alignment of adjacent segments may influence long-term outcome.

### Spinal Orthoses
Orthoses have been used as nonsurgical alternatives to spinal fusion in some patients with microinstability and macroinstability and as postoperative adjuncts to protect the surgical constructs used for stabilizing macroinstability in the thoracolumbar spine. The postoperative orthosis should limit the gross motion of the trunk during activities of normal daily living, thereby protecting

the surgical construct from large loads created from motion of the torso until solid biologic fusion occurs. Another function of a postoperative orthosis is to protect the surgical construct from the planes of motion in which the construct may be vulnerable to failure. For most surgical constructs these motions are flexion and/or torsion. The molded thoracolumbosacral orthosis provides the most overall restriction of trunk motion in flexion-extension, lateral bending, and axial rotation. The corset provides an intermediate degree of gross motion restriction whereas the elastic corset is only minimally restrictive. A custom-molded thoracolumbosacral orthosis reduces intervertebral motion in the lumbar spine; however, it is more effective in reducing motion at the upper lumbar levels than at lower levels. A thigh extension may be needed to further limit motion at the lower lumbar and lumbosacral levels. Thus, by appropriate selection of a postoperative orthosis it is possible to augment the surgical construct used in stabilizing macroinstabilities.

Cervical orthoses are primarily used to limit flexion/extension, rotation, lateral bending, and translational motion in the cervical spine. For the upper cervical spine (occiput-C2), four-poster orthoses are best for reducing flexion/extension motion. The two-poster orthoses are also effective in reducing flexion; however, these orthoses have limited effectiveness in lateral bending and rotation. To immobilize odontoid injuries, the halo is clearly superior, as it will limit motions in all planes. The halo is not significantly better than the four-poster orthosis at immobilizing the midcervical spine (C3-C5). Rigid collars provide a moderate amount of immobilization at the midcervical levels, but tend to lose effectiveness at the upper (occiput-C2) and lower cervical segments (C6-C7). To achieve immobilization in flexion/extension at the lower cervical segments, the four-poster is the most effective orthosis, whereas the two-poster is effective for flexion alone. For all planes in the upper and lower cervical spine, the halo is the best orthosis, whereas rigid collars are acceptable for microinstabilities in the midcervical spine.

## Summary
The primary biomechanical functions of the spinal column are to support the substantial loads induced during activities of daily living while allowing physiologic mobility. In an individual with a normal spine, the spine performs these functions without injury to bones, soft tissues, or neurologic structures. To understand the biomechanical functions of the spine, it is important to understand the role played by muscles and healthy FSUs in maintaining the stability of the spinal column. It is also important to understand the effects of injuries, degeneration, and surgical procedures on load sharing between the components of an FSU. Spinal fusion im-

plants as well as nonfusion devices are available to stabilize an unstable spine.

## Annotated Bibliography

### Physiologic Loads

Wilke HJ, Rohlmann A, Neller S, Graichen F, Claes L, Bergmann G: A novel approach to determine trunk muscle forces during flexion and extension: A comparison of data from a in vitro experiment and in vivo measurements. *Spine* 2003;28:2585-2593.

This article presents the results of an in vitro study to determine the magnitude of trunk muscle forces during flexion and extension. The study accounted for body weight, local and global muscles, and forces resulting from the support of the abdominal soft tissues in different postures.

### Stability of the Spinal Column

Arjmand N, Shirazi-Adl A: Model and in vivo studies on human trunk load partitioning and stability in isometric forward flexions. *J Biomech* 2006;39:510-521.

This study used a combined in vivo and finite element modeling approach to determine muscle forces and spinal internal loads. The passive resistance of both the ligamentous spine and trunk musculature contributes to the equilibrium and stability of the spinal column.

Patwardhan AG, Havey R, Carandang G, et al: Effect of compressive follower preload on the flexion-extension response of the human lumbar spine. *J Orthop Res* 2003; 21:540-546.

This study showed that the load displacement response of the lumbar spine is affected by the magnitude of the follower preload and the preload path. An optimized preload path allows the spine to support compressive preloads while allowing physiologic mobility in flexion-extension.

### Stability of the Functional Spinal Unit

Frei H, Oxland TR, Nolte LP: Thoracolumbar spine mechanics contrasted under compression and shear loading. *J Orthop Res* 2002;20:1333-1338.

The mechanics of the thoracolumbar FSU under compression and shear-type loads were contrasted in this study. Load transfer in compression was via the production of high disk pressures; whereas in shear, the mechanism appears to be via the anulus fibrosus without the development of significant disk pressure.

Rohlmann A, Neller S, Claes L, Bergmann G, Wilke HJ: Influence of a follower load on intradiscal pressure and intersegmental rotation of the lumbar spine. *Spine* 2001; 26:E557-E561.

Intradiskal pressure and intervertebral motions measured in lumbar spines loaded with pure moments, with and without a compressive preload, suggest that superimposed follower preload renders spinal loading with pure moments more physiologic.

Rohlmann A, Zander T, Schmidt H, Wilke HJ, Bergmann G: Analysis of the influence of disc degeneration on the mechanical behavior of a lumbar motion segment using the finite element method. *J Biomech*, in press.

A mildly degenerated disk increases intervertebral rotation in the three main anatomic planes. With increasing disk degeneration, intervertebral rotation is decreased. Intradiskal pressure is lower whereas facet joint force and stress in the anulus fibrosus are higher in a degenerated disk compared with a healthy disk.

Shirazi-Adl A: Analysis of large compression loads on lumbar spine in flexion and in torsion using a novel wrapping element. *J Biomech* 2006;39:267-275.

This finite element modeling study showed that compressive preloads up to 2,700 N significantly stiffened the load-displacement response of the lumbar spine in flexion and in axial rotation, and also increased intradiskal pressure, facet contact forces, and maximum disk fiber strain.

### Biomechanics of Stabilization

Gavin TM, Carandang G, Havey RM, Flanagan P, Ghanayem AJ, Patwardhan AG: Biomechanical analysis of cervical orthoses in flexion and extension: A comparison of cervical collars and cervical thoracic orthoses. *J Rehabil Res Dev* 2003;40:527-538.

Cervical intervertebral motion in flexion-extension was measured in 20 healthy volunteers. Each orthosis significantly reduced intervertebral motion in flexion and extension. The cervical thoracic orthoses provided significantly more restriction of motion compared with the rigid collars.

Lindsey DP, Swanson KE, Fuchs P, Hsu KY, Zucherman JF, Yerby SA: The effects of an interspinous implant on the kinematics of the instrumented and adjacent levels in the lumbar spine. *Spine* 2003;28:2192-2197.

This study showed that an interspinous spacer significantly reduces flexion-extension range of motion in lumbar spine specimens, whereas axial rotation and lateral bending ranges of motion are not affected.

O'Leary P, Lorenz M, Nicolakis M, et al: Response of Charité total disc replacement under physiologic loads: Prosthesis component motion patterns. *Spine J* 2005;5: 590-599.

The Charité TDR restored near normal quantity of flexion-extension range of motion in lumbar spine specimens under a physiologic preload; however, the quality of motion differed from the intact FSU. The function of the Charité TDR is influenced by implant placement, intraoperative change in lordosis, and compressive preload magnitude.

Patwardhan A, Carandang G, Ghanayem A, et al: Compressive preload improves the stability of the anterior lumbar interbody fusion (ALIF) cage construct. *J Bone Joint Surg Am* 2003;85-A:1749-1756.

This study suggests that the lumbar FSU treated with anterior lumbar interbody fusion cages is relatively less stable under conditions of low external compressive preload. The magnitude of preload required to achieve stabilization with stand-alone cages may be only partially achieved by annular pretensioning.

Schmoelz W, Huber FJ, Nydegger T, Dipl-Ing, Claes L, Wilke HJ: Dynamic stabilization of the lumbar spine and its effects on adjacent segments: An in vitro experiment. *J Spinal Disord Tech* 2003;16:418-423.

This article presents the results of a study that compared the kinematics of lumbar FSUs stabilized using a posteriorly applied nonfusion system, DYNESYS, with an internal fixator. For the bridged segment, the DYNESYS stabilized the FSU and was more flexible than the internal fixator, particularly in extension.

Senegas J: Mechanical supplementation by non-rigid fixation in degenerative intervertebral segments: The Wallis system. *Eur Spine J* 2002;11:S164-S169.

The author describes the design rationale and clinical trials of an interspinous implant for nonrigid stabilization of lumbar FSUs.

Vander Kooi D, Abad G, Basford JR, Maus TP, Yaszemski MJ, Kaufman KR: Lumbar spine stabilization with a thoracolumbosacral orthosis: Evaluation with video fluoroscopy. *Spine* 2004;29:100-104.

This study assessed the effect of thoracolumbosacral orthoses on lumbar spine motion in healthy individuals. The authors concluded that a custom molded thoracolumbosacral orthoses reduces both total L3-L5 motion and intervertebral motion in the lower lumbar spine. These effects are enhanced if a thigh extension is used.

## Classic Bibliography

Abumi K, Panjabi MM, Kramer KM, Duranceau J, Oxland T, Crisco JJ: Biomechanical evaluation of lumbar spinal stability after graded facetectomies. *Spine* 1990; 15:1142-1147.

Fujiwara A, Lim TH, An HS, et al: The effect of disc degeneration and facet joint osteoarthritis on the segmental flexibility of the lumbar spine. *Spine* 2000;25:3036-3044.

Goel VK, Nishiyama K, Weinstein J, Liu YK: Mechanical properties of lumbar spinal motion segments as affected by partial disc removal. *Spine* 1986;11:1008-1012.

Han JS, Goel VK, Ahn JY, et al: Loads in the spinal structures during lifting: Development of a three-dimensional comprehensive biomechanical model. *Eur Spine J* 1995;4:153-168.

Krismer M, Haid C, Behensky H, Kapfinger P, Landauer F, Rachbauer F: Motion in lumbar functional spine units during side bending and axial rotation moments depending on the degree of disc degeneration. *Spine* 2000; 25:2020-2027.

Panjabi M, Cholewicki J, Nibu K, Grauer J, Babat LB, Dvorak J: Critical load of the human cervical spine: An in vitro experimental study. *Clin Biomech (Bristol, Avon)* 1998;13:11-17.

Patwardhan A, Havey R, Ghanayem A, et al: Load carrying capacity of the human cervical spine in compression is increased under a follower load. *Spine* 2000;25: 1548-1554.

Patwardhan A, Havey R, Meade K, Lee B, Dunlap B: A follower load increases the load-carrying capacity of the lumbar spine in compression. *Spine* 1999;24:1003-1009.

Shono Y, Kaneda K, Abumi K, McAfee PC, Cunningham BW: Stability of posterior spinal instrumentation and its effects on adjacent motion segments in the lumbosacral spine. *Spine* 1998;23:1550-1558.

Wilke HJ, Neef P, Caimi M, Hoogland T, Claes LE: New in vivo measurements of pressures in the intervertebral disc in daily life. *Spine* 1999;24:755-762.

# Chapter 4

# Pathophysiology of Degenerative Disk Disease and Related Symptoms

Raj D. Rao, MD

Vaibhav Bagaria, MD

## Disk Microanatomy and Physiology

The human intervertebral disk consists of three separate components: the inner gelatinous nucleus pulposus, the outer anulus fibrosus, and the cartilaginous end plates located superiorly and inferiorly. The nucleus pulposus is eccentrically situated closer to the posterior margin of the disk, and better developed in the cervical and lumbar regions than in the thoracic region. Histologically the nucleus contains cells suspended in a fibrous network, the extracellular matrix. These cells form approximately 1% of disk volume and are responsible for synthesizing the matrix constituents. In vitro studies show that these cells respond to changes in hydrostatic pressure, tensile strain, and fluid loss by altering the rate of synthesis of proteoglycan and collagen, and by altering the balance between proteases and their inhibitors.

The cells in the disk vary with age. In the newborn, the nucleus pulposus contains notochordal cells that are multinucleated, clustered, and appear vacuolated because of the presence of intracellular glycogen. These cells start disappearing soon after birth with the cell count dropping from $2,000/mm^2$ at 6 weeks of age to $100/mm^2$ at 1 year of age. By the end of the first decade, notochordal cells are replaced almost entirely by fibroblast-like cells, which are thought to have originated in the inner anulus fibrosus. These cells are ovoid with a large single nucleus, and often have a fibrous capsule around them; the entire entity is sometimes called a chondron.

Extracellular matrix is composed primarily of collagen, proteoglycans, and water. Collagen forms the strong fibrous framework anchoring the vertebral bodies and suspending cells and proteoglycan in the extracellular matrix. The predominant subtype of collagen in the anulus fibrosus is type I; type II is found in the nucleus. Type X collagen is found in aging and degenerating disks and may represent repair and remodeling of the matrix. Subtypes III, VI, IX, and XI are also found in the disk in small quantities.

Proteoglycans constitute 5% to 10% of wet disk weight. The primary proteoglycan is aggrecan, which be-

cause of its high anionic charge provides an osmotic gradient responsible for drawing water into the disk, maintaining disk turgor and height even under compressive loads. Other proteoglycans such as large aggregating versican and small low molecular weight decorin, biglycan, fibrimodulin, and luminican have also been found, with less clearly defined roles. The water content of the disk decreases from 90% in the first year of life to approximately 74% in the eighth decade, probably as a result of the change in content and nature of proteoglycans. Other disk components such as glycoproteins, fibronectin, and tenascin have a possible role in cell signaling and mechanotransduction.

The anulus fibrosus consists of approximately 25 concentric lamellae of collagen fibers increasing in thickness toward the center. The outer fibers attach to the vertebral bodies and periphery of the epiphyseal ring, and the inner fibers pass from one cartilage end plate to another. The strong anterior longitudinal ligament buttresses the anulus fibrosus anteriorly, whereas the posterior longitudinal ligament offers only weak reinforcement to the posterior anulus fibrosus. Peripheral fibers unite with the vertebral body as Sharpey's fibers. Individual layers of the anulus fibrosus contain parallel fibers, angled about 60° vertically and 120° to fibers in adjacent laminae (Figure 1). With age these fibers di-

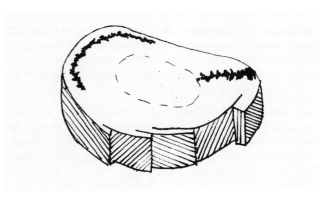

**Figure 1** Diagram showing lamellar architecture of the anulus fibrosus and pathoanatomy of radial and circumferential tears.

vide, bifurcate, and interdigitate, making the arrangement more complex. There is also a dense elastin fiber network between the collagen layers that contributes to resilience and elasticity during mechanical loading of disk tissue. Elastin forms about 1% to 2% of the dry weight of the intervertebral disk, and is richer in polar amino acids such as lysine and histidine than elastin present elsewhere. Thin elongated cells are found between layers of the anulus fibrosus, arranged parallel to the collagen fibrils. These cells create and regulate the extracellular matrix.

## Vertebral End Plate

In early life the end plate region consists of two cartilaginous portions: hyaline cartilage adjacent to the disk space and physeal cartilage adjacent to the vertebra. The physeal cartilage further differentiates into a circumferential ring apophysis that increases vertebral body breadth, and end plate cartilage responsible for vertical growth of the vertebral body. The hyaline cartilage is the interface between the disk and vertebral body and serves to transmit loads from the disk to the trabeculae and cortical rim of the vertebral body. The cartilaginous end plate decreases in thickness with age until it reaches approximately 0.6 mm, the average thickness in adults.

## Disk Nutrition

Large vascular channels traverse the end plate during early fetal life but diminish with birth until they have disappeared completely by age 4 to 6 years, making the disk one of the largest avascular tissues in the body. Cells in the center of the adult disk are as far as 8 mm from the nearest blood source. Nevertheless, disk tissue is vital and has a demonstrable rate of metabolic turnover. Disk tissue in adults derives its nutrition either from the vascular plexus of the anulus fibrosus or through vessels in subchondral bone adjacent to the hyaline cartilage of the end plate. Smaller molecules such as glucose, lactate, and oxygen are carried through the end plate in a flow-independent passive diffusion process. End plate permeability may decrease with age and degeneration, leading to a decrease in nutrient supply to the disk cells. Larger molecules such as long chain proteoglycans (> 40 kd) and cytokines responsible for regulation of cellular processes (10 to 40 kd), depend on flow-dependent active convective transport, an adenosine triphosphate-mediated process that relies on fluid pumping in and out of the disk. Approximately 85% of carbohydrate use in disk tissue occurs through an anaerobic pathway that results in two molecules of adenosine triphosphate per molecule of glucose, and produces lactic acid that results in an acidic environment in the disk. Oxidative phosphorylation accounts for 15% of total carbohydrate use in the disk. Physical environmental conditions such as the avascular nature of disk and the mechanical loads applied can affect disk cell metabolism and function.

## Degenerative Changes at the Disk Space

Degenerative changes begin in the disk by the end of the first decade of life. Several microscopic studies have shown that these degenerative changes cannot be differentiated from age-related changes in the disk. The nucleus, which is a glistening and gelatinous structure at birth, becomes less shiny and dry over time. The number of cells declines, and the concentration and diameter of collagen fibers increases. There is a change in the collagen architecture of the anulus fibrosus. There is a decrease in the number of lamellae, individual lamellae increase in thickness, and the space between lamellae increases, a phenomenon known as delamination. Small radial or circumferential tears appear in the anulus fibrosus (Figure 1) that eventually become more obvious clefts. Subchondral sclerosis occurs within the adjacent bone, and the hyaline cartilage of the end plate develops calcification and fissure formation.

A specific stimulus initiating the degenerative cascade within the disk is unknown. The common mechanism that brings about this degeneration is apoptosis, a distinct form of programmed cell death encoded into cellular DNA that can be modulated by factors such as the genetic makeup of the individual, mechanical loading, nutrient or growth factor deprivation, tumor necrosis factor, nitric oxide, and other physiochemical stresses.

Kirkaldy-Willis described the intervertebral articulation as a three-joint complex, comprising the disk anteriorly and the two facet joints posteriorly. Degenerative changes occur in a parallel fashion at all three components, with an initial painful stage giving way to hypermobility of the motion segment and an eventual stable stage (Figure 2). The cascade of degenerative changes at the facet joints resembles those occurring at any synovial joint, beginning with synovitis and progressing to articular cartilage loss, capsular redundancy, and joint subluxation. Eventually hypertrophic osteophytes form at the margins of the joint and periarticular fibrosis results in a stiff joint. At the disk, circumferential and radial tears progress to complete internal disruption of the disk with subsequent loss of disk height and annular laxity. Over time, osteophytes form at the disk margins, the disk is resorbed, and bony ankylosis results.

## Molecular Basis of Degeneration

The decreased vascularity across the end plate and its reduced porosity have an adverse effect on the viability and number of disk cells, and the synthesis and maintenance of disk matrix (Figure 3). Proteoglycans within the disk are decreased by up to 80% as a result of com-

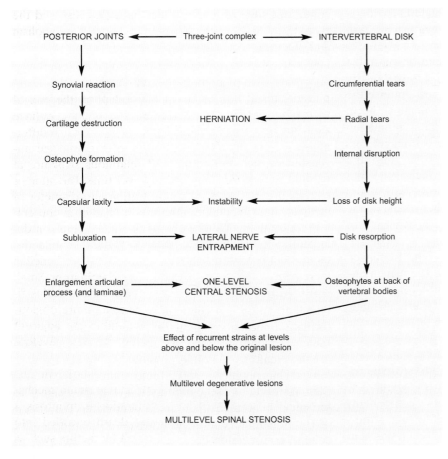

**Figure 2**  The spectrum of degenerative change that leads from minor strains to marked spondylosis and stenosis. *(Reproduced with permission from Kirkaldy-Willis WH, Wedge JH, Yong-Hing K, Reilly J: Pathology an pathogenesis of lumbar spondylosis and stenosis. Spine 1978;3:320.)*

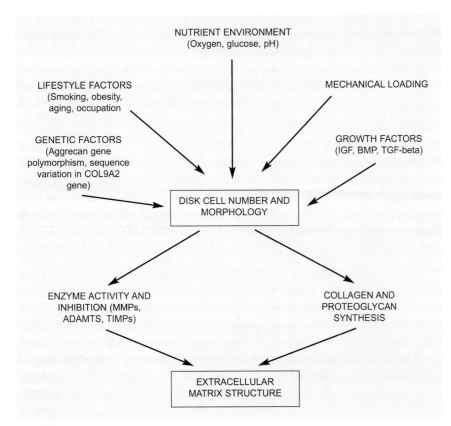

**Figure 3**  Factors influencing disk cell turnover and matrix structure. IGF = insulin-like growth factor; BMP = bone morphogenetic protein; TGF = Transforming growth factor; MMP = Matrix metalloproteinase, ADAMTS: a disintegrin and metalloproteinase with thrombospondin motifs; TIMPS = tissue inhibitor of matrix metalloproteinase.

promised cell function. The larger aggregated proteoglycans undergo fragmentation, and nonaggregated proteoglycans increase. A change in the relative proportions of matrix chondroitin sulfate and keratan sulfate occurs, with greater amounts of keratan sulfate present with increasing age. These changes diminish the hydroscopic property of the matrix and result in a net decrease in water content of the disk. The accumulation of degraded macromolecules physically further impairs diffusion through the disk.

Although absolute quantities of collagen do not change much, there is a change in the distribution and type of collagen. The fibrocyte-like cells present in the outer anulus fibrosus at the end of the first decade of life synthesize collagen type I, replacing the more pliable collagen type II of younger disks. Type I collagen begins to appear in the nucleus and type II collagen disappears from the end plates. Types I and VI increase in quantity whereas types III and VI, which are normally pericellular, are distributed more widely throughout the matrix.

Turnover of disk matrix is regulated by matrix metalloproteinases (MMPs) and their inhibitors: tissue inhibitors of matrix metalloproteinases (TIMPs). The MMPs responsible for degradation of the components of extracellular matrix can be divided into four groups of enzymes: collagenases, gelatinases, stromelysins, and membrane-type MMPs. Degenerative disks show increased production of MMPs in response to abnormal physical stresses. The inhibitory control of TIMPs on MMPs diminishes with degeneration. The complex signaling pathways that lead to these changes are mediated by proinflammatory and anti-inflammatory cytokines.

In addition to MMPs, other proteases such as aggrecanases (ADAMTS, a disintegrin and metalloproteinase with thrombospondin motifs) and cathepsins have been implicated in degradation of the extracellular matrix. Growth factors and cytokines such as fibroblast growth factor, tumor growth factor β, tumor necrosis factor α, and interleukins (IL)-1 and -6 have also been demonstrated in the disk and are believed to be important regulators of the extracellular matrix. Degenerative disks show increased levels of tumor necrosis factor α and IL-1 and IL-6. IL-1 increases production of nitric oxide, IL-6, MMPs, and prostaglandin $E_2$, all of which are pain mediators.

Other anabolic regulators, such as polypeptide growth factor, insulin-like growth factor, transforming growth factor β, and bone morphogenetic protein-7, counteract the degenerative process. New techniques involving direct injection of growth factors into the nucleus pulposus or anulus fibrosus, or transplantation of disk cells transfected with therapeutic genes by viral and nonviral genes are being investigated as potential therapeutic interventions.

## Mechanisms of Radicular and Axial Pain

Pain is the result of intense or potentially damaging stimulation of specialized primary sensory neurons. Usually, a specific spatiotemporal pattern of stimulation is interpreted as pain by higher cerebral centers. These patterns result not just from physical phenomena such as mechanical deformation, pressure, puncture, or tension but also from chemical phenomena such as alterations in pH, local concentration of inflammatogenic substances such as serotonin, bradykinin, histamine, potassium ions, prostaglandins, and substance P. Repeated stimulation or chemical release can sensitize peripheral sensory neurons and lower their threshold for activation. Alteration in threshold levels by these substances most likely results from phosphorylation of terminal membrane bound proteins.

### Radicular Pain

Disk herniation is a common source of mechanical deformation and an inflammatory response that results in radicular pain and nerve dysfunction. Mechanical compression leads to anatomic, physiologic, and electrophysiologic changes in the nerve root. Anatomically, the superficial parts of the compressed nerve are subject to greater displacement than the deeper parts. The effects of compression are most pronounced at the edge of the zone of compression because of greater shearing across different layers of the displaced nerve at this site. Physiologically, higher intraneural tension within the compressed nerve compromises arterial and venous blood flow and nutrition of the compressed nerve. The microvascular permeability increases, resulting in edema. Long-standing edema can cause intraneural fibrosis. In a study involving compression of the cauda equina in pigs, rapid onset of compression led to more pronounced effects on neural nutrition, microvascular permeability, and impulse propagation.

The fact that the nucleus pulposus is largely avascular has led to the theory that disk-related inflammation may in part be an autoimmune response to antigens present in the nucleus. Exposure of the nerve root to autologous nucleus pulposus results in epineural and endoneural accumulation of inflammatory mediators. Herniated lumbar disks in culture media spontaneously produce increased amounts of nitric oxide, prostaglandin $E_2$, and IL-6. These findings have been corroborated in studies of homogenates of disk tissue obtained from patients undergoing surgery for disk herniation where inflammatory cytokines IL-1 α, IL-1 β, IL-6, tumor necrosis factor α and granulocyte-macrophage colony stimulating factors were found. Cytokine-producing cells such as macrophages, fibroblasts, endothelial cells, and chondrocytes were also detected by immunohistologic staining. The cytokines secreted by these cells induce microvascular thrombus formation and increased permeability. Proinflammatory cytokines are indirectly responsible for pain production because of increased prostaglandin $E_2$ production, which has an important role in sensitization of nociceptors. Cytokines such as IL-1 α, interferon α, and tumor necrosis factor α are directly neurotoxic. Tumor necrosis factor α applied topically has been shown to cause demyelination, wallerian degeneration, and decreased conduction velocity of the neurons.

The dorsal root ganglion is associated with both axial and radicular pain (Figure 4). The dorsal root ganglion is exquisitely sensitive to direct pressure, resulting in prolonged discharges after brief compression, and is capable of spontaneously generating ectopic discharges similar to those from mechanical stimuli. Continued pain and paresthesia may result from cross excitation of other neurons in the dorsal root ganglion by afterdischarges. Various polypeptide amines associated with nociception are synthesized within the dorsal root ganglion. The capillaries of the dorsal root ganglion are fenestrated, making it susceptible to edema and inflammation. In the absence of direct compression, sensitization and pain generation at the dorsal root ganglion may still result from chemical mediators that spread from disk material into the tissues and fluids immediately adjacent to it. Biologic changes following compression of primary sensory neurons of dorsal root ganglia were studied in mongrel dogs; axonal flow was impaired and there was central chromatolysis of the neurons. At the cellular level there was a triad of increased nuclear clefting, increased density of nuclear pores, and the aggregation of metabolic organelles. Although these actions were associated with a decrease in substance P, calcitonin gene-related protein, and somatostatin, there was an increase in the metabolism of structural proteins that maintain axonal integrity, such as nerve growth factor and lipids required for membrane synthesis.

Nerve roots are more susceptible to compression than peripheral nerves, possibly because connective tissue sheaths around dorsal nerve roots contain more loosely organized collagen. Unlike the dorsal root ganglion, nerve roots do not generate long-lasting excitatory discharges following compression unless they are inflamed. Nerve endings contained in the nervi nervorum may be the pain generators, and the chemical mediators released during tissue inflammation and damage sensitize these nerve endings to cause radicular pain. Acute exposure of the nerve root to the nucleus pulposus causes inflammation and compression, resulting in vesicular and vacuolar degeneration of the myelin sheath, infolding of myelin sheath into axonal cytoplasm, an increase in the number of sodium channels, and a greater intensity of ectopic discharges. In contrast, chronic exposure of the nerve root to the nucleus pulposus results in mechanical desensitization, possibly as a result of axonal degeneration.

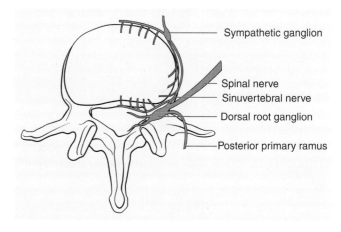

**Figure 4** Axial view of the lumbar vertebra showing the origin, course and structures innervated by the sinuvertebral nerve. (Reproduced from Rao R, David K: Lumbar degenerative disorders, in Vaccaro A (ed): Orthopaedic Knowledge Update 8. Rosemont, IL, American Academy of Orthopaedic Surgeons, 2005.)

## Axial Pain

Several structures are capable of producing axial symptoms along the posterior neck or back. In many patients, short-term, self-limited back and neck pain is caused by muscle strains. Myelinated A delta and unmyelinated C nerve fibers have been isolated from muscle tissue and are primarily associated with transport of nociceptive impulses. In patients with more persistent axial pain, the disk, facet joints, and dorsal root ganglia have all been implicated as pain sources.

Intradiskal injection of saline leads to reproducible pain patterns along the axial spine. The disk is innervated by the sinuvertebral nerve formed by branches from the ventral nerve root and sympathetic plexus (Figure 4). Nociceptive nerve fibers and free nerve endings have been seen in the superficial disk anulus fibrosus and adjacent posterior longitudinal ligament attachments. In degenerative or painful disks, these nerve fibers extend deeper into the anulus fibrosus and outer nucleus. Results from immunohistochemical studies have shown that substance P is present in neurons isolated from degenerative disks. Neurophysiologic experiments in the rabbit model suggest that the disk may also contain 'silent nociceptors' that are not readily excited in the normal state but respond to nociceptive chemicals or by-products of tissue damage in pathologic states. Discogenic back pain results from mechanical irritation of these nerve endings, or from chemical stimulation by substances including prostaglandin $E_2$, histamine-like-substances, lactic acid, potassium ions, and different polypeptide amines (substance P, calcitonin gene-related peptide, somatostatin).

Provocative injection of saline into the facet joints results in reproducible axial pain patterns that are relieved following injection of local anesthetic into the same joint. The facet joint is richly innervated by branches of the dorsal primary rami. Both free and encapsulated nerve endings have been found in the facet joint capsule. Nerve tissue immunoreactive for pain-related peptides has been isolated in facet joint synovial tissue, suggesting a role for the facet joint in pathogenesis of axial pain.

## Summary

The understanding of aging and degenerative processes at the human disk has dramatically increased over the past 10 years. Identification of nociceptive fibers in the peripheral disk and improved knowledge of nerve root pathophysiology provide better insight into axial and radicular pain mechanisms. Knowledge of these mechanisms allows more precise identification of pain generators in the clinical setting, and will eventually allow development of treatment modalities that prevent spondylotic changes.

## Annotated Bibliography

### Disk Microanatomy and Physiology

Ferguson SJ: Fluid flow and convective transport of solutes within the intervertebral disc. *J Biomech* 2004;37: 213-221.

 The physiology of fluid exchange and solute transport occurring in the intervertebral disk is described. The transport of low-weight solutes was independent of fluid flow.

### Degenerative Changes at the Disk Space

Ariga K: Mechanical stress induced apoptosis of end plate chondrocytes in organ cultured mouse intervertebral discs. *Spine* 2003;28:1528-1533.

 The author discusses the mechanism of cell signaling and initiation of cell death consequent to mechanical stress. Chondrocyte apoptosis was induced using static mechanical loads in a cultured cartilaginous end plate.

Boos N, Weissbach S, Rohrbach H, et al: Classification of age related changes in the lumbar intervertebral discs: 2002 Volvo award in basic science. *Spine* 2002;27: 2631-2644.

 The authors concluded that diminished blood supply to the intervertebral disk in the second decade of life appears to initiate tissue breakdown. Disk degeneration could not be histologically distinguished from aging.

### Molecular Basis of Degeneration

Le Maitre CL, Freemont AJ, Hoyland JA: Localization of degradative enzymes and their inhibitors in the degenerate human intervertebral disc. *J Pathol* 2004;204: 47-54.

 The authors describe various enzyme families and their location within the intervertebral disk. The authors believed that aggrecanases rather than matrix metalloproteinases may be a possible therapeutic target for inhibition of disk degeneration.

### Radicular Pain

Kobayashi S, Yoshizawa H, Yamada S: Pathology of lumbar nerve root compression: Part 1. Intraradicular inflammatory changes induced by mechanical compression. *J Orthop Res* 2004;22:170-179.

Kobayashi S, Yoshizawa H, Yamada S: Pathology of lumbar nerve root compression: Part 2. Morphological and immunohistochemical changes of dorsal root ganglion. *J Orthop Res* 2004;22:180-188.

 Inflammatory responses including wallerian degeneration, breakdown of the blood-nerve barrier, and the appearance of macrophages are important in the pathogenesis of radiculopathy.

Takahashi N, Yabuki, S, Aoki Y, Kikuchi S: Pathomechanisms of nerve root injury caused by disc herniation: An experimental study of mechanical compression and chemical irritation. *Spine* 2003;28:435-441.

 The authors studied the effects of compression and chemical irritation on cauda equina potentials and conduction velocities. They concluded that the combination of mechanical compression (mass effect of herniated disk) and chemical irritation (inflammation around nerve root) induces more nerve root injury than each factor by itself.

### Axial Pain

Kallakuri S, Singh A, Chen C, Cavanaugh JM: Demonstration of substance P, calcitonin gene-related peptide, and protein gene product 9.5 containing nerve fibers in human cervical facet joint capsules. *Spine* 2004;29:1182-1186.

 This study showed an abundance of protein gene product 9.5, substance P, and calcitonin gene-related peptide reactive nerve fibers within cervical facet joint capsules, lending credence to this structure as a source of pain.

Takegami K, Thonar EJ, An HS, Kamada H, Masuda K: Osteogenic protein-1 enhances matrix replenishment by intervertebral disc cells previously exposed to interleukin-1. *Spine* 2002;27:1318-1325.

 In a study of intervertebral disk cells cultured in alginate gel, the authors found that osteogenic protein-1 induced disk cells to replenish the matrix with glycoprotein.

## Classic Bibliography

Bogduk N, Tynan W, Wilson AS: The nerve supply to the human lumbar intervertebral discs. *J Anat* 1981;132:39-56.

Crock HV, Goldwasser M: Anatomic studies of the circulation in the region of the vertebral end plate in the adult grey hound dogs. *Spine* 1984;9:702-706.

Dwyer A, Aprill C, Bogduk N: Cervical zygapophyseal joint pain patterns: I. A study in normal volunteers. *Spine* 1990;15:453-457.

Freemont AJ, Peacock TE, Goupille P, et al: Nerve in growth into diseased intervertebral disc in chronic back pain. *Lancet* 1997;350:178-181.

Howe JF, Loeser JD, Calvin WH: Mechanosensitivity of dorsal root ganglia and chronically injured axons: A physiological basis for the radicular pain of nerve root compression. *Pain* 1977;3:25-41.

Kang JD, Stefanovic-Racic M, McIntyre LA, Georgescu HI, Evans CH: Toward a biochemical understanding of human intervertebral disc degeneration and herniation: Contributions of nitric oxide, interleukins, prostaglandin E2, and matrix metalloproteinases. *Spine* 1997;22:1065-1073.

Kirkaldy-Willis WH, Wedge JH, Yong-Hing R, Reilly J: Pathology and pathogenesis of lumbar spondylosis and stenosis. *Spine* 1978;3:319-328.

Naylor A: Intervertebral disc prolapse and degeneration: Biochemical and biophysical approach. *Spine* 1976;1:108-114.

Omarker K, Myers RR: Pathogenesis of sciatic pain: Role of herniated nucleus pulposus and deformation of spinal nerve root and dorsal root ganglion. *Pain* 1998;78:99-105.

# Chapter 5

# History and Physical Examination

Michael H. Haak, MD

## Focusing the Evaluation of Spine Problems

The history and physical examination of patients with spinal disorders is one of the most critical aspects of the evaluation. The history of the onset and description of the symptoms by the patient will be invaluable in guiding the physical examination and selection of other imaging and laboratory studies. The art and science of the history is to assist the patient in focusing on the significant symptom complaints so that a comprehensive assessment can proceed. The patient's description of the magnitude of the problem and the degree of functional impairment will guide the selection of treatment options to ensure that the "treatment" is appropriate to the "disease."

Many advances in the area of imaging have occurred over the past several years; these technologies allow for a more sensitive evaluation of spine anatomy. The sensitivity for many of these tests has led to the identification of many silent and asymptomatic lesions in the spine, many of which are not the cause of patient symptoms. Too often, the early application of advanced imaging techniques in the absence of focal examination findings and a pertinent and related history consistent with the symptom description by the patient will lead to misdiagnosis and poorly focused treatments. At a time when the clinical outcomes of many spine procedures are being called into question, it is especially critical that structural pathologies identified on CT and MRI studies be carefully matched to actual patient symptoms before surgical solutions are proposed and performed.

The appropriate and logical flow of a spine evaluation should be a comprehensive history, guided by physician questioning that elicits the symptoms, symptom onset, and evolution of the problem. Patient input can be expanded by the description and location of the pain through the use of pain diagrams and scoring systems, as well as surveying the degree of impairment in activities of daily living. The history should then lead to focused or comprehensive physical examination as appropriate; the patient's posture and stance, gait pattern and rhythm, as well as how the patient transitions through sitting-standing-bending patterns, help to determine which imaging modalities will be best suited to better delineate what is causing the patient's symptoms. Imaging studies such as plain radiographs, MRI, and CT should confirm and focus the working diagnosis that came from the history and physical examination. Diagnosis-specific treatment options can then be presented to the patient.

## History

Helping to focus the spine patient's "chief complaint" to a region of the spine will facilitate building the appropriate history. Although the spine has well-recognized anatomic segments, the patient is much more likely to mix terms for regional areas and symptoms when describing a specific complaint. "Hip" pain is a perfect example; anatomically motion-related groin and thigh pain will be mixed with descriptions of symptomatology in the area of the lateral thigh and greater trochanter, as well as in the posterior buttocks and thigh.

It is likely that spine patients will have either axial type symptoms, radicular symptoms involving the limbs, or a combination of both. Having the patient describe the regional area of symptoms or the starting point of radiating pains is a good beginning; more refined history taking will lead to a more specific and segmental diagnosis of the condition. The intensity of pain and how it varies with activities of daily living, as well as the symptom trend (getting better, getting worse, essentially unchanged since onset) will help in the assessment of functional impairment. This part of the history should also be used to explore psychosocial aspects of the problem. The onset of the condition while at work or as a result of a car crash, the impact on the patient's home life and family, possible pending litigation, and the success or failure of prior treatment are important factors to consider (Tables 1 and 2).

### Axial Neck, Mid-back, and Low Back Pain

There are some common threads in the potential sources of pain in the axial skeleton. The history should

## Table 1 | The Differential Diagnosis of Back Pain: Spinal Causes of Back Pain

**Structural**
 Segmental instability
 Discogenic pain, annular tears
 Facet joint arthropathy
 Muscle strain, ligament sprain
 Spondylolisthesis
 Spinal stenosis
 Fracture
  Infection
  Diskitis
  Vertebral osteomyelitis
 Inflammatory
  Ankylosing spondylitis
  Rheumatoid arthritis
 Tumors
  Primary
  Secondary, myeloma
**Endocrine**
 Osteomalacia
 Osteoporosis
 Acromegaly
**Hematologic**
 Sickle cell disease

*(Reproduced from McLain RF, Dudeney S: Clinical history and physical examination, in Fardon DF, Garfin SR (eds): Orthopaedic Knowledge Update Spine 2. Rosemont, IL American Academy of Orthopaedic Surgeons, 2002, pp 39-51.)*

## Table 2 | Extraspinal Causes of Back Pain

**Visceral**
 Renal calculus, urinary tract infection, pyelonephritis
 Duodenal ulcer
 Abdominal or thoracic aortic aneurysm
 Left atrial enlargement in mitral valve disease
 Pancreatitis
 Retroperitoneal neoplasm
 Biliary colic
 Gynecologic
 Etopic pregnancy
 Endometriosis
 Sickle cell crisis
**Drugs**
 Corticosteroids give osteoporosis and methysergide produces retroperitoneal fibrosis
 Nonsteroidal anti-inflammatory drugs may cause peptic ulcer disease or renal papillary necrosis
**Musculoskeletal**
 Hip disease
 Sacroiliac joint disease
 Scapulothoracic pain
 Psychogenic

*(Reproduced from McLain RF, Dudeney S: Clinical history and physical examination, in Fardon DF, Garfin SR (eds): Orthopaedic Knowledge Update Spine 2. Rosemont, IL American Academy of Orthopaedic Surgeons, 2002, pp 39-51.)*

focus on the location of the pain symptoms, the onset and possible mechanisms of onset, the character and intensity of the pain, and the duration and interval changes in the pain. Factors that aggravate the pain, or relieve it, also may be useful in final diagnosis.

The onset of the pain may be in association with a specific acute event or a series of events. The mechanism of a lifting event, a fall, or sports injury may explain why a certain part of the spine is injured. The difference between a low-speed twisting injury and a high-energy motor vehicle crash and its impact on the spine can occasionally be judged by other associated musculoskeletal injuries. The impact of chronic degenerative conditions in the spine may proceed over years and may present as a slow increase in symptoms; an acute event may exacerbate slowly and result in the development of degenerative conditions. Pain of insidious onset with a rapid progression in intensity should be aggressively evaluated for pathologic processes such as infection, primary or secondary tumor involvement, or osteopenic pathologic fractures. Conditions such as abdominal or thoracic aortic aneurysm, pancreatitis, cancer of the pancreas and kidney, and rectal and pelvic conditions can be the cause of pain referred to the back.

The duration of the pain may be both diagnostic as well as prognostic. An acute soft-tissue injury from a strain or sprain will usually improve or resolve over a period of days to weeks; an acute flare-up of degenerative problems can resolve over weeks to months. Patients with similar symptoms that flare up every couple of years probably have muscular weakness as a result of recurrent symptoms. Symptoms that occur more frequently, and to the level where the ability to work or perform activities of daily living is impaired, or that persist without improvement over a couple of months should be more carefully assessed.

The quality and intensity of the pain should be carefully evaluated as part of the patient's history. The use of a visual analog pain scale allows patients to classify pain intensity. This assessment can be correlated with posture or positioning and activities of daily living. Most mechanical pain in the neck, mid-back, and low back is of a focal, aching nature that is increased with activity and decreased with rest. Patients with degenerative conditions may experience some increased pain in the morning because of muscle and joint stiffness resulting from decreased movement during the sleep cycle; most patients with mechanical symptoms will notice an increase in pain with activity and as the day progresses. Infection and neoplasm characteristically cause deep, boring type pains that are not relieved by rest. Pain that is increased by axial load, flexion-extension, or exposure to vibration may be related to discogenic pain. Sitting in a car or operating vibrating machinery such as a forklift would be associated with increased low back pain in discogenic pain patients. Patients with ligamentous or osteoligamentous instability, such as spondylolisthesis, may have baseline aching pain with sharp stabbing pain and a sensation of "shifting" or "looseness" with motion. Catching or movement-related noise is more common in patients with degenerative cervical spine conditions, and may be a reflection of degenerative changes without true instability.

The mechanical stresses of flexion and extension are preferentially stressing structures in the front or back of the spine. Flexion increases the axial load on the disk, and increased pain in flexion or with activities in the flexion bias suggests mechanical dysfunction of the disk. Radiating pain along the muscle course (sclerotomal pain) with flexion passively stretches inflamed and irritated muscles in a strain type situation. Extension loads the posterior structures; increased neck or low back pain may be caused by a facet syndrome. Muscle pains that increase with extension may also reflect a muscle strain with increased tension as the posterior musculature tightens to carry out its mechanical function. These muscle pains may radiate to the attachment points on the skull or on the pelvis. Injury to the thoracic spine, where the primary motion function is rotation, may cause mechanical pain when the patient does twisting and turning activities. Flexion and extension in the thoracic spine are limited because of the ribs and chest wall; increased pain here with flexion and extension may be a reflection of pathologic motion allowed by compression fracture and ligamentous laxity because of increasing kyphotic deformity.

Severe pain at night or pain unrelieved by rest may be associated with tumor or infection. Other classic features such as fever, chills, weight loss, malaise, and a history of recent of previous infection or previous malignancy may be present. Although most patients have some morning stiffness, prolonged or severe pain and stiffness lasting more than 1 hour may be suggestive of inflammatory conditions such as rheumatoid arthritis or ankylosing spondylitis. A careful family history may be helpful in patients who may have collagen vascular disorders.

## Neurogenic Pain

Pathologic conditions affecting the spinal cord or nerve roots are generally associated with radicular symptoms into the arms or legs. Thoracic involvement is more difficult to assess, because only sensory function is readily testable. Focal compression of a single root will generally lead to nerve dysfunction in that single root distribution; focal changes in sensation and/or motor strength can be elicited from the patient's history. More diffuse

compression, such as that found in spinal stenosis, may lead to more diffuse symptoms manifesting themselves over many dermatomes, and leading functionally to more global and bilateral symptoms. These more diffuse conditions will generally cause difficulties with hand and arm function, or gait and balance disturbances.

Neurogenic disturbances in the cervical spine can lead to either focal or diffuse symptoms. Compression of a single root will lead to radiating pain in that dermatome, along with potential sensory, motor, and reflex changes. Motor dysfunction is likely to be described by patients as "arm weakness"; it is important to try to localize which functions are diminished and then confirm them with the physical examination. Sensory dysfunction is generally described as "numbness," although it is more likely to reflect some degree of hypesthesia or dysesthesia. Some patients may have associated neck pain, and radiating pain with rotation or neck tilt. Cervical spinal stenosis can also lead to upper extremity (and in some instances lower extremity) complaints. Patients are more likely to describe diffuse dysesthesia and clumsiness in both arms. Pain is less likely to be of a sharp radicular type with a dermatomal distribution; it is generally more aching and involving the entire arm and hand. Patients with more extensive myelopathic symptoms will report tiredness and walking and balance issues in the lower extremities.

Radicular symptoms in the thoracic spine are not seen as frequently as in the neck and low back. Radiating, band-like symptoms following the rib distribution and then extending down into the abdomen have been described. These patients may have a history of other intrathoracic or intra-abdominal sources of pain. Herpes zoster (shingles) is another condition that may cause neurogenic type pain in the thoracic nerve root distribution; it is characterized by a burning pain that predates the onset of vesicular lesions in the same distribution. Thoracic myelopathy caused by degenerative change, fracture and progressive kyphotic deformity, and other structural pathology would manifest itself in the lower extremity in a pattern similar to cervical myelopathy.

Radicular symptoms emanating from the lumbar region are fairly common; a herniated disk with nerve root compression may be the most common reason for back and leg symptoms in patients age 20 to 50 years. Single nerve root compression will lead to neurogenic symptoms (sensory change, reflex alteration, muscle weakness, or fatigue) in either the sciatic or femoral distribution. Most of the single root compressions are unilateral. A very large midline herniation may lead to bilateral symptoms; cauda equina syndrome may be associated with perineal sensory loss, bilateral leg weakness, urinary retention and overflow incontinence, and loss of voluntary bowel control. Although generally acute, these symptoms can develop over time in a chronic variant. Several other extraspinal causes of

**Table 3 | Extraspinal Causes of Radicular Pain**

**Intrapelvic extraneural compression**
Tumors
Psoas hematoma
Endometriosis
Abscess
Aneurysms

**Extrapelvic extraneural compression**
Gluteal artery aneurysm
Pseudoaneurysms
Tumor
Abscess
Piriformis muscle syndrome
Avulsion fractures of the greater tuberosity

**Intraneural**
Diabetes mellitus
Tumors of neural origin
Fibrosis of the sciatic nerve

*(Reproduced from McLain RF, Dudeney S: Clinical history and physical examination, in Fardon DF, Garfin SR (eds): Orthopaedic Knowledge Update Spine 2. Rosemont, IL American Academy of Orthopaedic Surgeons, 2002, pp 39-51.)*

radicular pain in the lower extremities need to be considered in the differential diagnosis; some of these can be confirmed by the physical examination (Table 3).

Neurogenic claudication is a classic symptom of lumbar spinal stenosis. Patients report progressive loss of walking ability, with a progressive decrease in the length of time they can stand or the distance they can negotiate. The pain and dysesthesia occur with walking or standing, and are relieved by bending or sitting. Leaning forward over a cart or a walker allows patients to ambulate further or stand longer; activities requiring extension or maintaining an upright spine (such as walking downhill) generally exacerbate the symptoms. These patients must be evaluated for possible vascular claudication as a source of the walking problems; however, patients with vascular symptoms usually will not have leg pain with standing at rest, and their leg pain resolves when walking is halted for 1 or 2 minutes. Descriptions of color changes in the lower extremity because of changes in blood flow usually occur in patients with vascular symptoms.

*Completing the Picture*

Once the patient has provided a good description of their chief complaint, and an adequate regional history has been provided, the patient's history should be completed with an assessment of the degree of impairment they are experiencing, as well as a family history, review of systems (respiratory, cardiac, gastrointestinal, etc.), a surgical history, and then a social history that includes work and job history. These factors will serve to complete the picture of how the patient's condition may be related to associated medical problems, previous treatment including surgery, and family, social, and occupational issues.

Use of a pain diagram and visual analog pain scores will provide a good picture of the level and magnitude of the pain the patient is experiencing from their own perspective. A listing of usual everyday activities and the patient's assessment of their ability to perform these tasks will give the evaluating physician a measure of the patient's limitations as a result of the pain. Limitations in performing work-related duties or if the patient is off work or confined to bed is a measure of how disabled the patient is; the degree to which other factors such as on-the-job injury or other work-related factors play a role may provide some insight into how the patient views their limitations or disabled status.

A review of systems (respiratory, cardiac, gastrointestinal, etc.), including a family history, may elicit other medical conditions and factors that play a role in the spinal condition. There are many medical contributors to both nerve dysfunction and the mechanical structural integrity of the spinal column. Other musculoskeletal conditions that limit normal lower or upper extremity functions may place additional stresses on the neck or low back; limitations and deformity of adjacent joints can cause peripheral nerve dysfunction. Because of the many medical contributors to axial and peripheral pain, careful assessment of the cardiovascular, pulmonary, gastrointestinal, genitourinary, and endocrine systems is necessary. Psychologic and psychiatric issues have been shown to play a significant role in a patient's response to spinal pain; a history of psychiatric illness and treatment, along with questions about the symptoms of secondary depression resulting from the spine condition, should be carefully assessed and factored into the treatment plan.

The family and social history may provide additional insight into the contributors to the patient's condition, as well as assessing the patient's resources and support for the treatment plan. An occupational history and current job status, along with information about job demands and requirements, will be important. Patients who enjoy their job and like their coworkers and supervisors will be more motivated to return to work after treatment. Because some jobs are physically demanding, even spine patients whose treatment was successful may not be capable of returning to heavy physical work. An assessment of health risks such as smoking, alcohol consumption, and the use of chronic pain medicine can help to judge the patient's ability to change health habits to optimize treatments or surgery.

**Physical Examination**

The physical examination of the spine will be used to corroborate the patient's history of the condition and symptoms; circumstances will often dictate whether the physician may need to perform a screening examination or one that is comprehensive.

The screening examination of the spine is necessary in the acute care setting, when prompt evaluation of the multiple trauma patient who requires intensive resuscitation is needed, and the patient requires additional urgent diagnostic testing or emergency surgical treatment. In this situation, a brief and concise examination should focus on identifying spinal conditions that could worsen during the course of other urgent treatment and testing (Table 4). This examination should be completed rapidly with a goal of identifying existing and possible injuries; the findings should lead to precautions or temporary measures of stabilization to prevent further damage to the spine and spinal cord. Injuries that cannot be confirmed or ruled out will require further evaluation when the patient is clinically stable.

Comprehensive testing is indicated in the spine patient who is clinically stable and is able to cooperate with the examination. In these patients, the goal of the examination is to determine objective findings that might match the patient's symptomatic complaints. The history and symptoms will lead to a differential diagnosis—the examination will narrow the differential diagnosis and lead to treatment options. The spine examination should elucidate the findings associated with common spinal conditions; a more subtle and intensive examination may be needed for patients with extensive medical and surgical histories. The examination includes evaluation of musculoskeletal abnormalities adjacent to the spine in areas such as the shoulders, pelvis, hips, and knees. It also should include evaluation of the neurologic and vascular systems.

The manner of examination, with repetitive testing of the same area or function, may be indicated where the accuracy of the findings is made questionable by the patient's potential for secondary gain. The examination should focus on the regional area of interest and is shaped by the patient's symptoms; examination findings will dictate what further physical examination testing should be done to obtain a working diagnosis. The extent and location of physical findings will be the focus of the examination; not all possible physical testing will be needed for all patients.

### The Screening Examination

The goal of the screening examination is to quickly identify existing or potential injuries in the cervical, thoracic, and lumbar spine that could lead to additional injury to the spine or spinal cord while the patient undergoes further evaluation and treatment. In the trauma and emergency department setting, the medical team should assume that a spinal injury has occurred and use provisional cervical immobilization and spinal precau-

**Table 4 | Screening Examination**

Rapidly survey airway, breathing, and circulation and initiate resuscitation as necessary.

Immobilize the neck in a collar and the spine on a backboard if not already done.

Obtain history from patient or transport personnel.

Mechanism of injury (fall, motor vehicle accident, speed of collision, ejection from the vehicle).

Neck or back pain, weakness, numbness, or paralysis at time of accident.

Previous illnesses including medications and allergies.

When the patient last ate or drank.

Assess for loss of consciousness, altered mental status, and cooperation.

Examine for facial, head, or neck contusions or lacerations that would indicate a likelihood of cervical spine injury.

Examine for seatbelt marks on the flanks.

Determine neurologic function before directly examining the spine.

Can the patient demonstrate voluntary motion of hands and feet?

Does patient have sensation on each side, at all dermatomes?

Are reflexes normal?

Does rectal examination reveal normal anal tone and perianal sensation?

*(Reproduced from McLain RF, Dudeney S: Clinical history and physical examination, in Fardon DF, Garfin SR (eds): Orthopaedic Knowledge Update Spine 2. Rosemont, IL American Academy of Orthopaedic Surgeons, 2002, pp 39-51.)*

tions during the evaluation. A careful stepwise examination by the spine surgeon is performed with a goal to identify potentially dangerous injuries and determine if any neurologic deficits are present. Initial radiographs taken in the emergency room should provisionally confirm injuries, although definitive evaluation and diagnostic testing should be performed after urgent and initial resuscitation have been completed and the patient's condition has been stabilized. A rectal examination by the spine specialist is mandatory to confirm evidence of spinal shock and/or sacral sparing; one should not rely on a rectal examination performed by other members of the trauma team.

The visual inspection should begin at the cervical spine; head trauma, facial trauma, laceration, or bruising in this area should alert the physician to the potential for cervical spine injury. Careful palpation of the cervical spine, while maintaining gentle in-line traction, may reveal a palpable bony step-off or gapping in the spinous processes. This finding would suggest a malalignment or instability, although the absence of this finding does not confirm stability. Spinal precautions should be observed during the log roll maneuver needed to complete the examination of the thoracic and lumbar spine. Critical to the screening examination is a prompt determination of the patient's neurologic function (Table 5). Dermatomal motor and sensory testing in the awake and cooperative patient should be performed and the results recorded using a standardized scoring sheet; the neurologic classification

## Table 5 | Neurologic Function Determination

**Function appears intact**

Palpate each interspinous ligament and check for increased interspinous distance or loss of resistance suggesting interspinous ligament rupture.

Inspect the skin for abrasions, and inspect/palpate for focal kyphosis. Evaluate focal pain, spasm.

Note any apprehension the patient may have to motion. A patient in the emergency department with a complete cervical disruption may have the sensation that his or her head is going to fall off if it is not supported with the patient's hands. Never discount the patient's sense of apprehension.

**Deficit is found**

Determine whether the injury is complete or incomplete, and whether spinal shock is present.

If quadriplegia or paraplegia is present, evaluate for signs of sacral sparing, signifying an incomplete lesion.

If injury appears complete, confirm presence of spinal shock by testing the bulbocavernosus reflex. The return of the bulbocavernosus reflex (anal contraction on squeezing the glans penis or pulling on the Foley urinary catheter) signifies the end of spinal shock. Only when spinal shock has resolved can a valid assessment be made as to whether a lesion is truly complete or incomplete.

*(Reproduced from McLain RF, Dudeney S: Clinical history and physical examination, in Fardon DF, Garfin SR (eds): Orthopaedic Knowledge Update Spine 2. Rosemont, IL American Academy of Orthopaedic Surgeons, 2002, pp 39-51.*

scoring used by the American Spinal Injury Association has been clinically validated and is currently used in many settings. The neurologic examination will need to be repeated at intervals, and the standardized approach allows direct comparison (Figure 1).

The results of the screening examination should suggest the appropriate diagnostic studies to evaluate areas of potential injury and should be prioritized based on the patient's clinical condition. The injured spine should be considered unstable and provisionally immobilized and protected until definitive assessment is possible. The cervical spine, particularly in the obtunded, unconscious patient, should not be cleared (declared free from injury and stable) until later, when the patient can cooperate with the examination and definitive diagnostic testing can be done.

### The Comprehensive Examination

The goal of the comprehensive spinal examination is to carefully evaluate and define structural spinal and spinally based neurologic pathologies. In conjunction with the patient's symptomatology, results of the examination should then allow the physician to suggest which diagnostic modalities would serve to better define the condition, and lead to treatment options.

### *Cervical Spine*

The comprehensive examination of the cervical spine focuses on the mechanical and structural characteristics of the cervical segment and the neurologic function of the spinal cord and nerve roots in this region. Lower oropharyngeal pathologies and anterior soft-tissue conditions, as well as peripheral sources of pain in the shoulder girdle and arm, must be evaluated. The neurologic examination of the upper and lower extremities should attempt to differentiate between central compression, cervical radicular compression, and peripheral nerve compression in the arm itself. The physician must be aware of the potential for compression in several locations (double crush syndrome) that might manifest as upper extremity neurologic impairment.

The cervical examination should begin with a visual inspection of the neck and shoulder girdle; the patient's posture should be assessed in the sitting and standing position to determine the resting alignment of the cervical spine. The patient's gait should be assessed; balance and proprioceptive conditions can stem from central cerebellar sources, compression of the posterior columns of the spinal cord, or from medical peripheral neuropathy. Cervical myelopathic compression often leads to lower extremity dysfunction such as a stiff or spastic gait pattern.

Palpation of the cervical spine structures and range of motion testing of the cervical spine should be done with the patient in a comfortable sitting position. The posterior structures, including the spinous processes, midline paraspinal musculature along its entire course, and the bilateral trapezial muscles, should be assessed. Pain located at the muscle insertions or trigger point areas of muscular irritation in the muscle body often will be noted in the setting of sprain injuries. Assessment of the anterior cervical spine should include palpation of the midline tracheal cartilage, anterior lymph nodes, thyroid gland, and carotid pulses. Laterally, the temporomandibular joints and preauricular regions should be palpated. Notable asymmetry or palpation tenderness in these extraspinal structures should not be overlooked as a source of "neck" pain.

Active cervical range of motion should assess all six planes of motion: flexion, extension, right and left lateral bending, and right and left rotation. The total flexion-extension arc in young patients should be about 100°. Normal motion consists of flexion of the chin down to the chest, and neck extension straight up, with the patient looking toward the ceiling. Rotation should be approximately 70° bilaterally; lateral bend tilting the ear to the shoulder while looking straight ahead should normally be about 40° bilaterally. Asymmetry may be noted in the face of structural pathology or soft-tissue injury. The location of pain with motion and its intensity during motion or at the end range should be noted. Radiating arm and leg symptoms may be noted in some patients with compressive radiculopathy or myelopathy; several provocative range-of-motion maneuvers should be included in the examination to help elucidate these

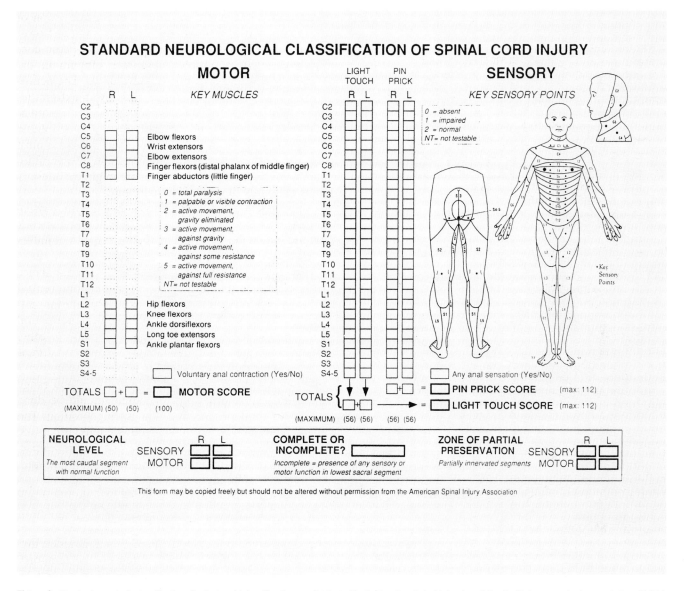

**Figure 1** Standard neurologic classification of spinal cord injury. The diagram distributed by the American Spinal Injury Association facilitates accurate documentation of initial neurologic status and provides a means of monitoring changes as they occur with time following the injury, which assists in determining the prognosis of spinal injuries. (*Reproduced with permission from the American Spinal Injury Association.*)

conditions. Age-related degenerative changes may cause some decreased motion and this occurrence may be a consideration when assessing the expected normal range. Resistive muscle strength testing should be performed in conjunction with the range-of-motion evaluation.

The cervical examination continues with a careful musculoskeletal and neurologic examination of the upper extremities (Figure 2 and 3). Visual inspection may reveal muscle mass asymmetry or loss of tone, arm and hand postures suggestive of weakness or dysfunction, or other signs of peripheral sources of pathology. The upper extremity should be assessed for muscle tone, motor strength, sensation, and deep tendon reflexes. Use of the bilateral limbs for comparison may facilitate the identi-

fication of the level of neurologic involvement; the sensory and reflex examination should be symmetric. Subtle strength differences may exist even in normal patients when the dominant and nondominant extremities are compared. Although the classic dermatomal levels are generally accurate, the physician should be aware of some cross- and multilevel innervations to motor, sensory, and reflex levels.

In the patient with a neurologic deficit, the physical examination is the critical tool in identification of the location and level of the injury or lesion. The source of upper extremity neurologic dysfunction can be the peripheral nerve, brachial plexus, cervical nerve root, and spinal cord. Neurologic dysfunction in the brachial plexus will frequently be associated with a penetrating

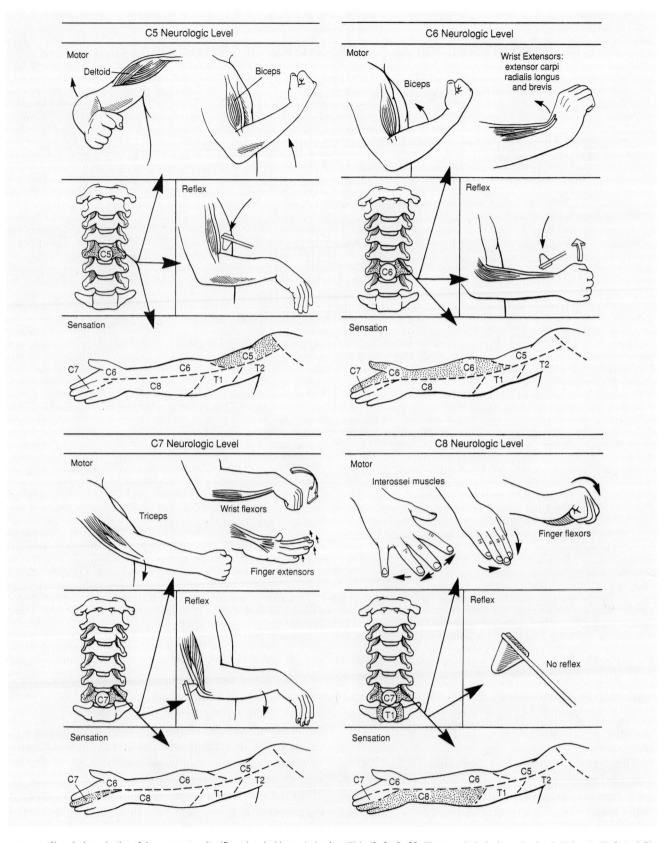

**Figure 2** Neurologic evaluation of the upper extremity. (*Reproduced with permission from Klein JD, Garfin SR: History and physical examination, in Weinstein JN, Rydevik BL, Sonntag VKG (eds): Essentials of the Spine. New York, NY, Raven Press, 1995, pp 71-95.*)

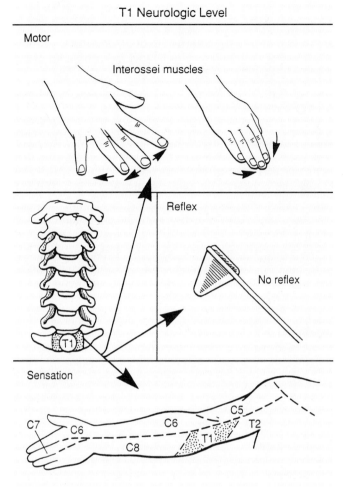

T1 Neurologic Level

Motor

Interossei muscles

Reflex

No reflex

Sensation

**Figure 3** Neurologic examination of the upper extremity, the T1 neurologic level. (*Reproduced with permission from Klein JD, Garfin SR: History and physical examination, in Weinstein JN, Rydevik BL, Sonntag VKG (eds):* Essentials of the Spine. *New York, NY, Raven Press, 1995, pp 71-95.*)

function. It is therefore critical to check the common locations of peripheral nerve entrapment for the radial, median, and ulnar nerves in the arm and hand; the most common locations are for the ulnar and median nerve at the wrist, and the ulnar and radial nerves at the elbow. Percussion tenderness over the nerve entrapment (Tinel's sign) with reproduction or increase of the sensory dysfunction is strongly suggestive of peripheral nerve root compression. Hyperflexion positioning (Phalen's test) will reproduce or enhance symptoms because of increased intracompartmental pressures around the nerve and diminished blood supply. It is important that the physician keep in mind the potential for a double crush syndrome with compression of both the cervical root and the peripheral nerve. The pattern of sensory and motor loss may also identify the level of the nerve lesion. In patients with carpal tunnel syndrome, there should be sensory sparing of the thenar eminence because of the more superficial course of the cutaneous nerve; in those with C6 radiculopathy, the entire dermatome should be equally affected. Ulnar nerve compression will affect the ulnar side sensory function; compression at the wrist affects the ulnar digits to the hand, and compression at the elbow leads to a larger sensory deficit that extends proximally. Compression at the cubital tunnel will affect the ulnar flexors to the finger and wrist, as well as the interossei that would be affected by entrapment at the wrist.

Radiculopathy resulting from compression of a single cervical root is commonly seen with cervical disk herniation and cervical degenerative disk disease. It generally produces a single level deficit with normal motor and sensory functions at the levels above and below the lesion. This condition is usually unilateral, although a larger compressive lesion in the cervical spine may create enough tension for bilateral symptoms and findings. Physical findings correlating with the root affected include flaccid weakness or paralysis, atrophy of the muscles supplied, diminished or lost deep tendon reflex of the muscle supplied, and sensory dysfunction of the cutaneous dermatome supplied. Painful sensation can occasionally be accentuated by extension or lateral bend to the symptomatic side; symptoms may be relieved by manual cervical traction. Adduction at the shoulder or placing the arm on top of the head may also relieve symptoms by decreasing the tension on the cervical root.

Cervical myelopathy resulting from pathologic compression of the spinal cord will produce a myriad of both easily observable and very subtle signs of neurologic dysfunction. Significant compression of the cord will generally lead to examination findings in the upper and lower extremities (Table 6). The extent of the compression may broaden the examination findings to include both the upper and lower extremity, whereas the duration of the compression over time will lead to additional subtle findings. Decreased vibratory sense and proprioception distal to

injury of the region or trauma involving the shoulder girdle. Thoracic outlet syndrome, a condition caused by vascular and neural structure compression in the area between the interscalene triangle and the inferior border of the axilla, may be caused by congenital soft-tissue bands, anomalous upper rib structures, or trauma. The condition can be confirmed on examination noting a pulse pressure loss or decreased blood pressure reading during Adson's maneuver. The tested arm is abducted, extended, and externally rotated; the patient is asked to take a deep breath and rotate the head toward the examined arm. Compression of the subclavian artery and adjacent brachial plexus causes a drop in palpated radial pulse pressure and reproduction of the neurologic symptoms.

In patients with upper extremity neurologic deficit, it is important to distinguish between peripheral nerve lesions and cervical root lesions. Patients with both lesions may report similar upper extremity symptoms and dys-

## Table 6 | Signs of Myelopathy

| Sign | Comment |
| --- | --- |
| Hyperreflexia | Upper motor neuron mediated response |
| Myelopathy of the hand | Difficulty with finger extension and abduction of ulnar digits |
| Hoffman's sign | Rapid extension of the middle finger leads to involuntary flexion of thumb and other fingers |
| Scapulohumeral reflex | Tap on scapular spine, scapula elevates or humerus abducts |
| Ankle, patellar clonus | Rapid end-range extension causes multiple repetitive flexion-extension wavering |
| Crossed adductor response | Tap on medial femoral condyle, contralateral limb adducts |
| Babinski sign | Scrape pointed object along lateral plantar border. Abnormal response is great toe extension and less toe flexion and splaying. |
| Oppenheim's test | Scrape nail or pointed object over tibial crest. Abnormal response same as with Babinski sign. |

the compressive lesion may be early signs of myelopathy. Some of the findings are intermittent and positional; repeated flexion and extension of the cervical spine may bring on positive findings not noted at rest. Lhermitte's sign (passive flexion and compression of the neck) may cause radiating, shock-like pain into the upper and lower extremities. Spinal cord compression above C4 may manifest with a hyperreflexic scapulohumeral reflex; striking the acromion or scapular spine with the patient seated may elicit scapular elevation or humeral abduction. Cervical stenosis and myelopathy between C4 and T1 generally will demonstrate abnormal motor, sensory, and reflex findings in both the upper and lower extremity. Myelopathic findings in the lower extremity only are suggestive of a lesion between T1 and L2. Findings common to all levels of myelopathy include weakness or paralysis with little loss of muscle volume (atrophy resulting from disuse), hyperreflexia, and an abnormal plantar response (Babinski reflex or Oppenheim reflex). Neurologic symptoms that are progressive, either rapidly in the setting of trauma, tumor, or infection, or with slower development in the face of degenerative changes, should alert the physician to the need for aggressive further evaluation with imaging modalities to assess the extent of compression.

### The Thoracolumbar Spine

The thoracic and lumbar spine should be examined together, both for anatomic and structural abnormalities, as well as functional deficits in the comprehensive evaluation.

The examination should begin with an assessment of the patient's posture and gait. If possible, observation of how the patient achieves the sitting position, the position of comfort assumed once seated, and the transition from sitting to standing to move to the examination table all provide information about the patient's condition. A significant antalgic gait favoring one leg or the other is strongly suggestive of nerve root irritation or lower extremity weakness; other causes may be concomitant hip or knee issues that can be confused with radicular type pain. Patients with L3-L4 weakness (quadriceps muscle) may attempt to stabilize the knee in the stance phase of gait by hyperextension. L5 involvement (hip abductors/gluteus medius) may manifest itself as lateralizing over the hip joint in the stance phase in an attempt to substitute adductors for weak hip stabilizers. Patients with weak S1 innervated muscles (hip extensors/gluteus maximus) will sometimes hyperextend the lumbar spine and push the pelvis forward in stance to compensate.

The contours of the thoracolumbar spine should be examined while the patient is standing and while in the forward bending position. Asymmetry of the shoulder height, uneven scapular contours, contralateral side prominence of the structures of the thoracic and lumbar spine, and either structural or apparent pelvic obliquity may be associated with scoliosis. A history of scoliosis as a child or gradual development of asymmetry as part of the degenerative disk process may be factors in the history. A significant prominence visually in the thoracic or thoracolumbar junction may be associated with kyphosis, with or without scoliosis. The plumb line examination should be used in deformity evaluation to determine the sagittal and coronal plane balance in the standing patient. The structural components of the deformity are best assessed with radiographs; these radiographs should be compared with previous films to document whether the curve is stable or progressive. The flexibility of the curve can be assessed on right and left side bending films in patients with scoliosis, whereas flexion and extension films may demonstrate whether a kyphotic curve is rigid and structural or flexible and postural. A painful, rapidly progressive curve should trigger further evaluation to rule out a more acute, pathologic process such as tumor, infection, or pathologic fracture.

Range-of-motion testing of the thoracic and lumbar spine can be performed with visual inspection of the spinal contours. Observation of the rhythm of movement, whether it is smooth or halting and jerky should be recorded. Because of the constraints of the rib cage, movement in the thoracic spine is primarily left and right rotation. The pelvis should be stabilized in stance, and the rotation recorded qualitatively compared with the contralateral side or measured in degrees; there may be a symmetric relative contribution from the lumbar spine

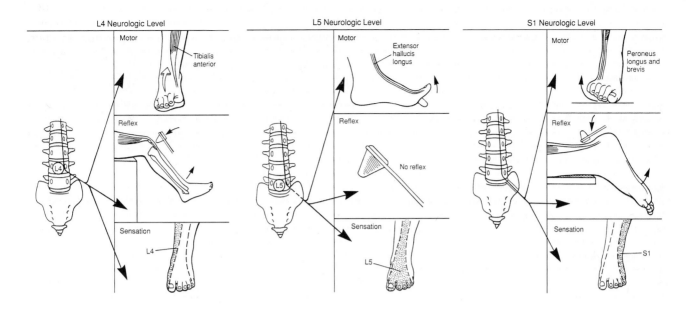

Figure 4   Neurologic evaluation of the lower extremity. (*Reproduced with permission from Klein JD, Garfin SR: History and physical examination, in Weinstein JN, Rydevik BL, Sonntag VKG (eds): Essentials of the Spine. New York, NY, Raven Press, 1995, pp 71-95.*)

that would be difficult to measure and subtract from the thoracic assessment. The range of motion for the lumbar spine should be evaluated for flexion, extension, and lateral bending bilaterally. This assessment can be described as an angular measurement or in qualitative terms (lateral bend compared with the opposite side). Flexion should be evaluated with the knees and hips in neutral position; most adults will not be able to touch their toes or the floor, and the distance from the fingertips to the floor can be used as a repeatable measurement. Schober's test can provide quantitative data; it is performed by measuring the excursion in flexion of the lumbar segment from the sacroiliac dimples to a midline point 10 cm proximal to them. The expected normal increase in this dimension is 5 cm with the patient fully flexed forward.

A symmetric palpation examination of the bony prominences and muscular structures should be performed in conjunction with range-of-motion testing. The presence of pain over bony prominences should be noted; evaluation of the soft tissues for scars from previous surgery, masses, muscle spasm, and soft-tissue trigger points can be compared with the contralateral side, aiding in the identification of pathology. In the thoracic spine, asymmetry or winging of the scapula may suggest neurologic dysfunction of the shoulder girdle musculature. Although thoracic radicular compression is rare, nerve root compression may manifest as a band or stripe of dysesthesia or hypesthesia, and sensory alteration can be checked from T4 to T12 with a disposable cotton swab in comparison with the contralateral side. An exaggerated pain response to light touch in the af-

fected or adjacent area may be the first confirmatory physical examination finding of nonorganic factors; these factors will be discussed further in the section on psychosocial aspects of the comprehensive examination.

Upon completion of the evaluation of the thoracolumbar spine, the examination continues with evaluation of the bilateral lower extremities, including complete neurologic testing (Figure 4). The lower extremity examination includes both a sitting and supine component; some of the neurologic testing should be repeated in both positions to confirm the validity of the patient's symptoms and findings. The seated component of the examination should take place with the patient sitting comfortably on the examination table. Range-of-motion testing for the hips, knees, and ankles should be recorded, with the contralateral limb serving as a comparison. Osteoarthritis of the hip, suggested by limited motion, may reproduce groin, pelvic, or back pain on examination. A seated straight-leg raise can be accomplished while checking lower extremity joint range of motion and may reproduce radicular symptoms suggestive of nerve root compression; these symptomatic complaints will be rechecked and confirmed in the supine position. Motor strength testing in the lower extremity should include hip flexors and extensors, hip adduction and abduction, knee flexion and extension, foot and ankle flexion, extension, adduction, and abduction. The results of static strength testing should be matched with functional strength testing to include toe walking (ankle flexors), heel walking (ankle and foot extensors), and deep knee bend (knee extensors). Single-leg stance may demonstrate pelvic girdle muscle weakness (Trendelen-

## Table 7 | Provocative Tests

| Test | Comments |
|------|----------|
| Straight-leg raise (SLR): sitting and supine | Must produce radicular symptoms in the distribution of the provoked root; for sciatic nerve, that means pain distal to the knee |
| Lasègue's sign | SLR radiculopathy aggravated by ankle dorsiflexion |
| Contralateral SLR | Well-leg SLR puts tension on involved root from opposite direction |
| Kernig's test | The neck is flexed chin to chest. The hip is flexed to 90°, and the leg is then extended similar to SLR; radiculopathy is reproduced. |
| Bowstring sign | SLR radiculopathy aggravated by applying pressure over popliteal fossa |
| Femoral stretch test | Prone patient; examiner stretches femoral nerve roots to test L2- L4 irritation |
| Naffziger's test | Compression of neck veins for 10 seconds with patient lying supine; coughing then reproduces radiculopathy |
| Milgram's test | Patient raises both legs 3 inches off the examining table and holds this position for 30 seconds; radiculopathy may be reproduced |

*(Reproduced from McLain RF, Dudeney S: Clinical history and physical examination, in Fardon DF, Garfin SR (eds): Orthopaedic Knowledge Update Spine 2. Rosemont, IL American Academy of Orthopaedic Surgeons, 2002, pp 39-51.)*

burg's sign). Sensory testing to light touch with a disposable cotton swab should be performed in a dermatomal pattern from L1 to S1. In patients with unilateral symptoms, the contralateral limb may serve as the control; patients with spinal stenosis or bilateral involvement may demonstrate asymmetric deficits. Knee and ankle deep tendon reflexes should be elicited, realizing that joint surgery such as total knee replacement may eliminate or alter the reflex. Hyperreflexia should be noted; the presence of a positive Babinski reflex or Oppenheim reflex in conjunction with ankle clonus is suggestive of a spinal cord level compression.

The supine examination allows for clinical corroboration of lower extremity findings noted in the initial seated examination, as well as examination of the thoracic innervated anterior abdominal musculature. The patient is asked to tighten the abdominal musculature by performing a partial sit-up. Visual asymmetry of the rectus abdominis muscles in the upper portion of the abdomen (innervated by T5-T10) or lower portion of the abdomen (innervated by T10-L1), along with a positive Beevor's sign (shift of the umbilicus away from the weak side) suggests radicular compression in the thoracic spine. The presence of the superficial abdominal reflex (a shift of the umbilicus toward the abdominal quadrant that is lightly stroked) is normal; its absence, because it is an upper motor neuron reflex, may reflect

spinal cord compression in the thoracic spine. Compression of the spinal cord in the thoracic spine may cause myelopathic reflexes in the lower extremities similar to cervical myelopathy. The supine position offers the most patient comfort when evaluating for tension signs or symptoms of nerve root compression. Range of motion of the hip and knee can be reassessed; the sacroiliac joints can be stressed by compressing the iliac wings and performing the Fabere test (flexion, abduction, external rotation in extension) on the hip and pelvis. Active and passive straight-leg raising testing is performed to elicit the signs and symptoms of nerve root compression; many tests have been described and may corroborate findings as well as suggest the level of compression.

The patient's degree of active participation and possible nonorganic issues can be assessed with Hoover's test. The patient is asked to perform a straight-leg raise while the examiner's hand is cupped under the heel of the contralateral leg; the examiner should feel pressure as the patient stabilizes the lower extremity to raise the leg. Straight-leg raising symptoms occur when the maneuver places additional stretch on the compressed nerve, pulling it forward anatomically onto the compressing structure. For nerves in the sciatic distribution, a positive straight-leg raise sign should cause radiating symptoms distal to the knee. The increased tension generally occurs between 20° and 70° of passive elevation. The "reverse" straight-leg raise sign with radicular complaints into the thigh when the hip on the symptomatic side is extended in the lateral decubitus or prone position is suggestive of compression of nerve roots in the femoral nerve distribution. Several variants of stretch or nerve root tension signs have been developed and are useful clinically in determining the level of compression and confirming the consistency and veracity of the patient's symptoms (Table 7).

The psychosocial factors associated with spinal disorders must be assessed as part of both the history and physical examination process. Preliminary information can be gained from the patient's description of how the injury occurred, particularly if it is work related or caused by an accident. A minor injury causing a severe disability, symptoms out of proportion to the structural problem, and inconsistent findings on the examination should alert the examiner to spend additional time evaluating the patient's psychologic and social situation. If the injury is work related, the patient's job, work status, and job satisfaction should be evaluated. The presence of or potential for litigation should be considered as part of the history. Multiple inconsistencies in the physical examination findings should lead the examiner to include the tests and signs developed by Waddell to help in evaluating patients who are exaggerating or magnifying their symptoms.

Waddell's pain behavior findings include nonanatomic pain distributions, pain out of proportion to the stimulus, and exaggerated behaviors such as grimacing, moaning, and vocalization such as crying or calling out. These behaviors may be present with normal actions or during the tests. The skin roll test can be performed in any position; it consists of gently rolling the loose skin of the low back between the examiner's index finger and thumb while asking the patient to describe any radiating leg pain complaints. The twist test is performed while the patient is standing with the feet together. The examiner holds the patient's pelvis and hips and gently rotates the patient to the left and right. The actual rotation occurs through the knees, with no motion occurring through the spine; the patient is asked to describe any back pain symptoms. The head compression test places about 5 lb of force on the patient's head and the patient is asked if there is an increase in their back pain: this degree of axial loading is not sufficient to place a significant or destabilizing load on the lumbar spine. The flip test is useful to assess the consistency of straight-leg raise symptoms in those patients with radicular complaints. In the seated patient, the symptomatic leg is raised directly in front of the patient as part of the assessment of the lower extremity range of motion; this maneuver creates a 90° straight-leg raise and increased nerve root tension. The patient will note radiating leg pain, and perhaps lean back to lessen the straight leg raise effect. The absence of radicular complaints during the sitting straight-leg raise, and the presence of radiating pain complaints during supine testing are incongruent and the test considered positive.

Although most patients may exhibit one or two pain behaviors or test findings, patients with three or more findings demonstrate a poor response to treatment unless the cause of the abnormal pain behaviors can be discovered and addressed. It may be necessary to schedule a follow-up examination because of subtle examination findings and the complexity of the spinal problem; additional information may come to light with a more in-depth doctor-patient relationship. The aspects of the psychosocial examination in spine patients are usually not entirely concrete, so it is important to make a full and careful assessment before drawing conclusions about a patient's motives and veracity.

## Summary

Most patients with spinal complaints are likely to have a history and physical examination findings that are compatible. A good doctor-patient relationship evolves from open and honest exchange of medical information. It is critical not to disrupt this working relationship by suspecting that many or most patients are intentionally providing false or misleading symptoms and examination findings. It is part of the art of medicine to develop a sense for when the history and physical examination

are not congruent and to judiciously use these testing techniques.

## Annotated Bibliography

Clark CR, Benzel EC, Currier BL, Dormans JP, Dvorak J, Eismont FJ: *The Cervical Spine*, ed 4. Philadelphia, PA, Lippincott, Williams & Wilkins, 2004.
    This book is the definitive text on the cervical spine compiled by the editorial board of the Cervical Spine Research Society.

Herkowitz HH, Dvorak J, Bell GR, Nordin M, Grob D: *The Lumbar Spine*, ed 3. Philadelphia, PA, Lipincott, Williams & Wilkins, 2004.
    This book addresses all aspects of lumbar spine disorders. History and physical examination testing and findings are located in the chapters on specific disorders of the lumbar spine.

## Classic Bibliography

Hoppenfeld S, Jutton R (eds): *Orthopaedic Neurology: A Diagnostic Guide to Neurologic Levels*. Philadelphia, PA, Lippincott, 1977.

Macnab I, McCullogh JA (eds): *Neck Ache and Shoulder Pain*. Baltimore, MD, Williams & Wilkins, 1994.

McCullough JA, Transfeldt E, Macnab I (eds): *Macnab's Backache*, ed 3. Baltimore, MD, Williams & Wilkins, 1997.

Nitschke JE, Nattrass CL, Disler PB, Chou MJ, Ooi KT: Reliability of the American Medical Association Guides' model for measuring spinal range of motion: Its implication for whole-person impairment rating. *Spine* 1999;24:262-268.

Ono K, Ebara S, Fuji T, Yonenobu K, Fujiwara K, Yamashita K: Myelopathy hand: New clinical signs of cervical cord damage. *J Bone Joint Surg Br* 1987;69:215-219.

Sanders RJ, Haug CE: *Thoracic Outlet Syndrome: A Common Sequelae of Neck Injuries*. Philadelphia, PA, JB Lippincott, 1991.

Shimizu T, Shimada H, Shirakura K: Scapulohumeral reflex (Shimizu): Its clinical significance and testing maneuver. *Spine* 1993;18:2182-2190.

Waddell G, McCulloch JA, Kummell E, Venner RM: Nonorganic physical signs in low back pain. *Spine* 1980; 5:117-125.

Wolfe R, Borenstein D, Wiesel S (eds): *Low Back Pain: A Comprehensive Approach*, ed 3. Charlottesville, VA, Matthew Bender & Company, 2000.

# Chapter 6

# Spinal Imaging: Radiographs, Computed Tomography, and Magnetic Resonance Imaging

Warren D. Yu, MD

Susan Lai Williams, MD

## Introduction

Radiographic imaging studies have an important role in the diagnosis and treatment of spinal diseases. A thorough and accurate patient history and physical examination remain the standard in the assessment of spinal disorders. Imaging studies help to verify or refute the presumed diagnosis and guide further treatment. It has been well established that an accurate diagnosis based on the patient's history and physical examination, confirmed by imaging studies, and free of confounding psychosocial issues provides the greatest opportunity for a favorable outcome when surgical management is elected. Caution should be used before performing any examination because numerous studies have shown a high rate of abnormal findings in asymptomatic individuals. One study reported abnormal MRI findings of the lumbar spine in 30% of asymptomatic volunteers. Furthermore, there is a correlation between age and the increasing incidence of asymptomatic abnormal radiographic findings with 75% of asymptomatic patients in their seventh decade exhibiting degenerative changes on plain radiography. A careful history and physical examination is imperative to prevent unnecessary workup and treatment of an incidental finding.

## Plain Radiography

As in most areas of orthopaedic practice, plain radiography remains the best initial study to evaluate the patient. It provides a view of the overall alignment of a spinal segment and gross features of the bony elements. Standard initial views include standing AP and lateral views with the addition of two oblique views if a pars interarticularis defect or facet pathology is suspected. Lateral radiographs with the patient positioned in flexion and extension can help assess stability in traumatic injuries or in patients with spondylolisthesis. Unless the history or physical examination arouses suspicion of infection, tumor, trauma, or neurologic compression, it is reasonable for the patient to undergo a 4- to 6-week course of nonsurgical treatment before obtaining radiographic films because common causes of neck and back pain (such as muscle sprains and strains) are not apparent on radiographs and typically resolve with time.

In degenerative disk disease, disk space narrowing with sclerosis of the end plates and osteophytes can be seen. Frequently, these degenerative findings are present in asymptomatic patients. One study reported that 25% of asymptomatic patients in their fifth decade had degenerative findings and this number increased to 75% by the seventh decade. The significance of such degenerative findings should be determined by clinical correlation.

In spondylolisthesis, the relationship between adjacent vertebral bodies will display a disruption in normal alignment. The rostral vertebral body can be slipped anterior (anterolisthesis) or posterior (retrolisthesis) to the caudal vertebral body. Dynamic radiographs with the patient in flexion or extension can show exacerbation or correction of the slippage. The severity of spondylolisthesis is described on the lateral radiograph as the percentage of overhang in comparison with the width of the vertebral body.

The radiographic evaluation of scoliosis begins with full-length standing posteroanterior and lateral radiographs. The Cobb angle is measured between the line at the superior end plate of the most proximal body and the inferior end plate of the most distal body involved in the curve. In pediatric scoliosis, a Cobb angle of 20° to 30° can progress and should be followed with serial radiographs. Adult scoliosis is defined as a skeletally mature patient with a Cobb angle of 10° or greater. According to a recent study, in an attempt to define clinically significant radiographic measurements, lateral listhesis (maximal lateral overhang), L3 and L4 obliquity (the angle between superior end plate and horizontal of S1), lumbar lordosis, and thoracolumbar kyphosis significantly correlated with the pain scores of patients.

Traumatic or osteoporotic compression fractures are readily diagnosed on plain radiographs by loss of vertebral body height as is typically seen on a lateral radiograph. The loss of height is reported as a percentage loss compared with an adjacent unaffected vertebral body or as the relative anterior vertebral body height compared with the posterior body height. In patients with traumatic compression fractures, a loss of 50% is considered potentially unstable. Traumatic compression fractures should be further studied to distinguish them from burst fractures and to identify potential injury to the posterior elements that would imply instability. Findings on plain radiographs that suggest posterior injury include an increase in interpedicular or interspinous process distance, or traumatic spondylolisthesis. Osteoporotic compression fractures can be treated symptomatically. Additional studies to distinguish between acute and old fractures may be important if treatment with vertebroplasty or kyphoplasty is considered. The importance of obtaining weight-bearing radiographs in patients found to have compression or burst fractures in the thoracolumbar junction has been shown in a recent study. Twenty-eight patients with fractures between T11-L2 were assessed with both supine and standing radiographs. A mean supine Cobb angle of 11° increased to 18° on standing radiographs and a mean anterior vertebral compression increased from 34% to 46%. The treatment plan changed from nonsurgical to surgical in 7 of the 28 patients.

There is growing interest in determining which patients in the emergency department or trauma setting require radiographic cervical spine evaluations. Two main studies introduced criteria for radiographic evaluation. The National Emergency X-Radiography Utilization Study (NEXUS) defined five criteria that determined if a patient had no risk of cervical spine trauma and thus did not require radiographic evaluation. The five NEXUS criteria are: absence of posterior midline tenderness, absence of focal neurologic deficit, normal level of alertness, no evidence of intoxication, and absence of painful distracting injury. These criteria had a sensitivity of 99.6% for significant injury and a specificity of 12.9%. The Canadian C-Spine Rule was developed after the NEXUS criteria and identified three instances in which radiography was not indicated. (1) No high-risk factors present including age older than 64 years, dangerous mechanism (such as a fall from a height of 3 m or 5 stairs, axial load to the head [diving accident], high-speed vehicle crash [at 60 mph, rollover, or ejection from the vehicle], bicycle collision, motorized recreational vehicle crash), or paresthesias in the extremities. (2) The presence of low-risk factors such as low speed rear-end vehicle crash, patient in sitting position in the emergency department, patient ambulatory at any time, delayed onset of neck pain, and absence of midline cervical tenderness. (3) A patient who has the ability to rotate the neck actively 45° to the left and right. The Canadian study had a sensitivity of 100% and specificity of 42.5%.

The most important difference between the two studies was in the specificity of the prediction rules. The difference in specificity (12.9% versus 42.5%) implies that the Canadian C-Spine Rule could potentially decrease unnecessary cervical radiographs by a greater proportion. The NEXUS criteria have shown acceptability because the validation study involved several centers. However, the NEXUS study examined only five criteria and did not evaluate other potentially useful criteria. The Canadian study was more methodologically rigorous in its development and exhibits a higher specificity; however, it has not been validated.

Primary tumors or metastatic lesions of the spine may be seen on plain radiographs. It should be remembered that lytic lesions of the spine are not detected by plain radiographs until a significant amount of cancellous bone has been lost. CT or MRI may be indicated in a patient with a history of cancer who is reporting neck or back pain, even if plain radiographs do not show any abnormalities.

## Computed Tomography

CT uses ionizing radiation to provide images to evaluate both bony elements and soft tissues. CT provides the equivalent of cross-sectional radiographs of the spine. Traditional CT is performed by passing a pencil-thin collimated x-ray beam through the body as the x-ray tube is rotated around the body. As the x-ray tube is rotated, the detector on the opposite side of the body detects the remaining x-ray beam that has not been absorbed by the intervening tissues and records its position. The computer divides each cross section of the body using a grid. The information collected is used to compute the amount of x-ray absorption for each square within the grid, allowing construction of a cross-sectional image based on the radiopacity of the various tissues. Data from the scanning can be further manipulated to provide sagittal and coronal reconstructions.

Innovations in CT technology have included helical (spiral) CT and multidetector helical CT. In traditional CT, the patient is moved through the gantry incrementally, stopping to allow acquisition of data for each cross section. In helical CT, the patient moves through the gantry in a continuous motion and data are acquired by the continuously rotating x-ray beam and the detector in a helical pattern. This continuous data acquisition allows more flexibility in image reconstruction, shorter scanning time, and decreased motion artifact. Multidetector helical CT uses multiple detectors to simultaneously collect data, allowing multiple CT cross-sections to be obtained with each x-ray tube rotation; this method results in faster scanning.

Axial cross-sectional images can be reformatted to provide coronal, sagittal, and three-dimensional images (Figure 1, *A*). Sagittal images provide an overview of multiple levels and are helpful in determining which levels are affected by disease or trauma. Gross encroachment on the neural elements can be seen. Disk and ver-

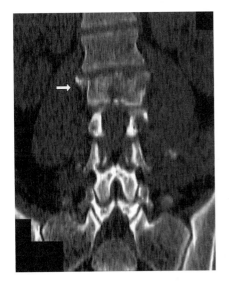 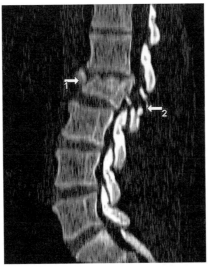 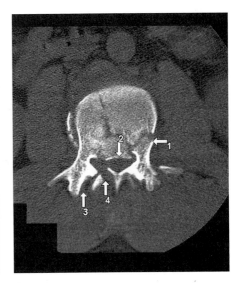

Figure 1  **A,** CT coronal reconstruction of a patient with comminuted L2 burst fracture (*arrow*). The patient was injured after falling two stories. **B,** CT sagittal reconstruction. Kyphosis, comminution, and loss of height of the L2 vertebral body is shown with evidence of retropulsion of bone into the spinal canal (*arrow 1*). Posterior injury is evidenced by the presence of widened facet and lamina fracture (*arrow 2*). **C,** Axial CT of the L2 vertebral body. Pedicle fracture (*arrow 1*), retropulsed bony fragments (*arrow 2*), dislocated facet (*arrow 3*), and lamina fracture (*arrow 4*) are well delineated.

tebral body height also can be evaluated. Once the abnormal segments are identified, axial images at those levels can be further examined to assess the relationship of the disease to posterior elements and the foramen. Three-dimensional reconstructions can take into account all of this information and present it as one image. Bony anatomy is very well seen on a CT scan; however, the detail of the soft tissue is not as well defined as on images obtained from MRI. If the imaging sections are too thick (> 3 mm), findings such as foraminal stenosis or a pars interarticularis fracture may be missed.

CT is ideal for delineation of bony anatomy and pathology in the spine. As the resolution and speed of CT scanners has improved in recent years, CT has become more commonly used, especially in the trauma setting.

### CT in Trauma
In patients with spinal trauma, a CT scan is helpful in further defining fractures seen on plain radiographs (Figure 1, *B*). Moreover, if adequate cervical spine radiographs are not possible because of body habitus, then CT is the next diagnostic step. Fractures of the vertebral body, pedicle, lamina, transverse process, spinous process, and/or the facets are well delineated on CT (Figure 1, *C*). CT is superior to MRI in detecting fractures, particularly those involving the cortical bone in the posterior spine such as the lamina, transverse process, and spinous process. Cortical bone is well detected on CT; on MRI, bone has a low water content and thus appears as a void adjacent to soft tissues, which have high water content. Fractures of the vertebral body can be further differentiated between stable and unstable fractures

based on stability of the posterior elements and the presence of bony injury to the middle column.

Multiple studies have shown the usefulness of CT in trauma patients suspected of having cervical spine injury. CT is capable of showing injuries not seen on plain radiographs. Various authors have advocated the use of CT in addition to plain radiography; some have even advocated the replacement of plain radiography with CT. Concerns regarding the liberal use of CT have centered mostly on the increased cost and radiation exposure. One study found a greater than 14-fold increase in the radiation dose to the thyroid in helical CT compared with plain radiography.

In a recent study, the cost-effectiveness of cervical spine CT compared with plain radiography in trauma patients undergoing CT of the head was investigated. Patients were divided into three risk groups for cervical spine fracture: high risk (> 10% chance of fracture), moderate risk (4% to 10% chance of fracture), and low risk (< 4% chance of fracture). CT detected a greater number of fractures than plain radiography in all groups. In high-risk patients, CT was cost-effective and lowered the probability of paralysis. In patients with moderate risk, the increased cost of CT was marginal and acceptable. In low-risk patients, CT was not cost-effective and radiography was the preferred option. Because the cost-effectiveness of imaging is dependent on the probability for cervical spine fracture, optimization of imaging in the cervical spine requires classification of patients by different levels of risk. The Harborview high-risk cervical spine criteria were formulated from a review of 304 randomly selected patients with spine fractures. The goal of this clinical decision rule is to

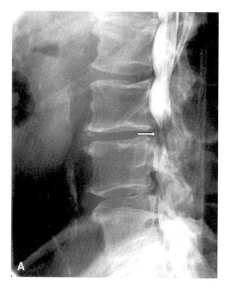 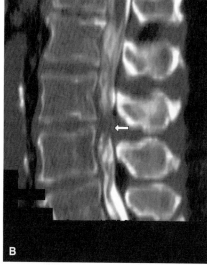 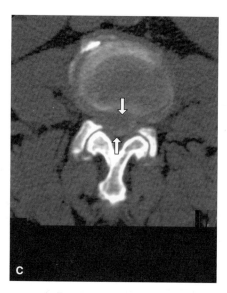

Figure 2  **A,** Myelogram of lumbar spine showing dye cutoff at L3-4 level (*arrow*) secondary to large central disk herniation. **B,** Sagittal reconstruction CT myelography showing dye cutoff at L3-4 level (*arrow*). **C,** Axial postcontrast CT at L3-4 shows large posterior disk herniation (*down arrow*) with minimal contrast within the remaining canal (*up arrow*).

identify patients with greater than a 5% risk of cervical spine injury and to use CT as the initial screening modality for these patients. The presence of any of the following criteria indicates a patient at sufficiently high risk to warrant the initial use of CT to evaluate the cervical spine: the involvement of a high-energy injury mechanism including high-speed (> 35 mph) motor vehicle or motorcycle crash, motor vehicle crash with death at the scene, fall from a height greater than 10 feet; or the involvement of a high-risk clinical parameter including significant head injury, neurologic signs or symptoms referable to the cervical spine, or pelvic or multiple extremity fractures. This decision rule has been validated.

### CT in Degenerative Disease

In degenerative spinal disease, CT can show the severity and location of stenosis. Central stenosis is defined by AP canal diameter of less than 10 mm or a cross-sectional area of less than 100 mm$^2$ as measured on CT. The cause of canal narrowing can be seen on CT and can be the result of hypertrophic or redundant ligamentum flavum, facet hypertrophy, or varying stages of disk degeneration. Evaluation with MRI often is needed to assess the integrity of the disk, to evaluate the foramina, and to visualize abnormalities in the neural elements. Because MRI has superior ability in visualizing soft tissues and given its lack of ionizing radiation, plain CT has been largely supplanted in the evaluation of degenerative disease of the spine. However, CT is superior to MRI in distinguishing between bony versus soft-tissue neural compression and can provide valuable additional information for surgical planning. In ossification of the posterior longitudinal ligament, high-resolution CT can

provide a better assessment than MRI, especially early in the disease process when MRI findings can be equivocal.

CT is commonly used with intrathecal contrast (CT myelography) for evaluation of the degenerative spine when the results of MRI are ambiguous or when MRI cannot be performed, such as in the postoperative evaluation of patients with persistent pain after the implantation of hardware or in patients with pacemakers. CT myelography is an invasive procedure performed by injection of water-soluble contrast within the cerebrospinal fluid. The contrast helps distinguish between disk margins, the thecal sac, and ligamentum flavum, and can show the degree of stenosis by delineating the amount of cerebrospinal fluid surrounding the spinal cord (Figure 2). In a 1999 study of patients with cervical spine disease, only moderate concordance between MRI and CT myelography was found; thus, it was suggested that CT myelography may yield additional valuable information in patients who had difficult or ambiguous findings when first evaluated with MRI. When CT of the cervical spine is performed, the use of oblique reformation can be especially helpful in evaluating the neural foramen. Oblique reformation in a plane perpendicular to the long axis of the neural foramen significantly reduces interobserver variability and increases observer confidence in the assessment of neural foraminal stenosis.

### Other Applications of CT

Plain radiography remains the cost-effective standard for assessing hardware placement postoperatively. CT can be helpful in assessing the position of pedicle screws when radiographic findings are equivocal and in patients with new neurologic deficits and/or pain. In both the cervical and lumbar spine, the accuracy of CT is between 80% and 90% for determining whether the screws are within bone when correlated to gross dissection results. This level of accuracy can be compared with an accuracy of approximately 60% using the findings from plain radiographs of the lumbar spine. In patients with persistent back pain after fusion, CT along with reformatted images remains the best noninvasive diagnostic measure to assess fusion.

Because of its superior ability to depict bony pathology, CT is commonly used as an adjunct to MRI to evaluate bone destruction in patients with tumors or infections. In one study, the combination of multidetector CT and MRI was found to be superior to MRI alone or MRI with plain radiography for the staging of multiple myeloma.

## Magnetic Resonance Imaging

Similar to CT, MRI allows visualization of the spine in cross-sections; however, it does so without the use of ionizing radiation. Whereas CT produces images based on the density of various tissues, MRI produces images based on free water content; its magnetic properties produce superior soft-tissue contrast.

The patient is placed in a powerful magnetic field during MRI. A small percentage of the body's hydrogen atoms, which constitute tiny magnets, become aligned with the external magnetic field. Radio waves in a particular sequence of short pulses are then passed through the body, causing a change in the direction of magnetization of the atoms. Each pulse causes hydrogen atoms in the patient's tissues to emit a responding pulse of radio waves characteristic of the intrinsic physical properties of the tissue. The radio waves are detected and used to deduce their location to create the cross-sectional images. Factors affecting the appearance of various tissues are the density of protons, the chemical environment of the protons, and the magnetic field strength of the scanner. The time it takes for the hydrogen atoms to return to equilibrium is called relaxation time. There are two relaxation times during MRI: T1 (longitudinal relaxation time) and T2 (transverse relaxation time). T1 and T2 relaxation times are intrinsic physical properties of tissue.

Several different MRI techniques are available to optimize visualization of different tissues and disease processes. Various sequences are produced by manipulating the strength of the radiofrequency (RF) pulses, the interval between pulses, repetition time, and echo time. Repetition time is the time between successive RF pulses and echo time is the time between the RF pulse and the recording of the signal. By manipulating these variables, images can be weighted to emphasize the T1, T2, gradient echo, or proton density characteristics of a tissue.

T1-weighted images use short echo time and repetition time and allow evaluation of anatomic detail including osseous structures, disk, and soft tissue. T1-weighted images are ideal for evaluating tissues containing fat, subacute hematoma, and proteinaceous fluids because these tissues appear white on T1-weighted images. T2-weighted images use long echo time and repetition time and are used primarily to evaluate the cerebrospinal fluid, the spinal cord, and to enhance conspicuous lesions. T2-weighted images are very sensitive to pathologic changes in tissue in which water content is increased and therefore tend to enhance and delineate pathologic processes such as cysts, inflammation, and tumors.

Gradient echo images appear like T2-weighted images because the cerebrospinal fluid appears bright; however, the technique of gradient echo images is sensitive to local inhomogeneities of the magnetic field, resulting in exaggerated signal loss. The products of blood breakdown cause local field distortions resulting in signal loss, making this technique very sensitive for the detection of blood.

Several considerations are necessary before a patient undergoes MRI. Because of the strong magnetic field of an MRI machine, absolute contraindications include ferromagnetic cerebral aneurysm clips, cardiac pacemakers, infusion pumps, certain heart valves, metallic foreign bodies in the eye or spine, and ferromagnetic cochlear or ocular implants.

Open MRI systems are becoming more popular because of improving quality. Many patients have problems with claustrophobia and children can find the closed MRI procedure intimidating. However, most open MRI machines are low-field strength MRI systems (0.3 to 0.5 tesla) and do not provide images at as high a resolution as those of closed MRI systems with high-field strength (usually 1.0 to 1.5 tesla).

Spine pathology represents a dynamic condition and symptoms often occur in the erect position; however, most advanced imaging studies are performed with the patient in the relaxed, supine position. With improvements in machinery and computing efficiency, the use of dynamic and weighted MRIs is currently being explored and should provide the clinician with a better understanding of the anatomy and pathology of disorders with the goal of tailoring treatments to pathology based on static, dynamic, and positional factors. The importance of spinal loading and posture in MRI has been reported by several authors. In a 2001 study, axial loading MRI and CT myelogram evaluations were performed on 172 patients. Criteria for additional valuable information was defined as (1) a significant reduction of the dural sac cross-section (15 mm$^2$) to areas smaller than 75 mm$^2$ (the borderline value for canal stenosis); or (2) a suspected disk herniation, lateral recess, or foraminal stenosis, or a intraspinal synovial cyst detected with the patient in a relaxed position that changes to an obvious manifestation during loading. Additional valuable information was found in 29% of patients. Additional information increased to 69% in patients with neurogenic claudication, 14% in patients with sciatica, and decreased to 0% in patients with back pain only.

### MRI in Trauma

Although plain radiography and CT are the dominant modalities in the evaluation of spinal trauma, MRI is being used more often, especially for patients with injury to the cervical spine. The primary reasons for obtaining an MRI scan of the cervical spine in a trauma patient include the need for evaluation of spinal cord injury or ligamentous instability, or the situation in which there is an indeterminate clinical examination (such as an obtunded patient or a patient with negative CT and plain radiography with persistent neurologic deficit). MRI provides the best visualization of the soft tissues, intervertebral disks, spinal cord, ligaments, and hematoma. In patients with spinal cord injury, assessment of the spinal cord is important because the presence of hemorrhage versus edema in the cord has prognostic significance. Patients with edema have a much greater chance of functional recovery than those with hemorrhage.

In the acute phase after cervical trauma, MRI is very sensitive to soft-tissue injury. Although there is little disagreement that MRI is sensitive to cervical ligamentous injury, its use in determining actual spinal instability from benign ligamentous injury is debatable. The actual existence of some of the observed injuries has been called into question. One study found that discontinuity of the "black stripe" representing cervical ligaments on T1-weighted images, considered a sign of ligamentous rupture, was a common finding on MRI scans performed on nontrauma patients being examined for degenerative disease. Another study examined patients who underwent CT scanning, plain radiography, and MRI. When CT scanning and radiography detected no fractures or signs of instability, MRI did not contribute information for determining cervical stability. However, MRI has shown a virtual absence of false-negative results; negative findings on a cervical spine MRI scan can be used as a reliable indication of the absence of injury and has been used successfully to determine that the cervical spine is clear of injury without adverse consequences.

MRI of the cervical spine has been shown to be valuable in the evaluation of suspected cervical spine injury in pediatric trauma patients. The pattern, frequency, and mechanism of spinal trauma differ between the pediatric and adult patient populations. Children have relatively large heads with less well developed neck musculature and lax ligaments compared with adults. Other unique anatomic features of children include incomplete ossification of the physes and apophyses, wedge-shaped

vertebrae, and shallow facet joints. Furthermore, the clinical evaluation of cervical spine injuries in pediatric patients is challenging because of unique mechanisms of injury, restricted patient evaluation, and limited patient cooperation. In a study of 237 children, MRI was required to define the diagnosis or clear the cervical spine in 31% of patients because of inconclusive clinical and radiographic evaluation. Another study found a protocol calling for a cervical spine MRI scan for clearance of the existence of injury in children who could not be cleared within 72 hours. The information provided by the MRI scans was cost-effective and allowed shorter hospital stays.

### MRI in Degenerative Disease

MRI is used routinely in the evaluation of degenerative diseases of the spine because of its ability to accurately delineate soft-tissue structures such as intervertebral disks, facet joints, uncovertebral joints, spinal ligaments, and neural elements. Furthermore, the ability of MRI to detect subtle abnormalities in both soft tissue and bone tissue provides great sensitivity in detecting pathology and results in both the widespread use and abuse of MRI. It has been well documented that MRI shows abnormalities in a large percentage of asymptomatic individuals. In one study of the lumbar spine, 22% of asymptomatic individuals younger than 60 years and 36% of those older than 60 years had a disk herniation on MRI scan. More than 50% of those 60 years or older had abnormal scans. Similarly, 19% of asymptomatic individuals have abnormal scans of the cervical spine. Therefore, correlation with clinical findings is imperative when using MRI for evaluating degenerative disease in the spine. Furthermore, abnormalities seen on the MRI scans of asymptomatic patients were not predictive of the development or duration of low back pain 7 years after initial imaging.

In the normal intervertebral disk, the nucleus pulposus appears bright on T2-weighted images because of its high water content. The annular fibers and the anterior and posterior longitudinal ligaments appear dark. As spinal degeneration progresses, decreased signal intensity from the nucleus as well as the intranuclear clefts appear. Annular fissures can lead to a generalized bulge of the disk contour. Disk herniations result from displacement of nuclear, annular, or end-plate material through tears in the annular fibers. A contained disk herniation is one in which the herniated material is still contained within the posterior longitudinal ligament. Extrusion occurs when the herniation has broken through the posterior longitudinal ligament but is still in continuity with its disk of origin. A sequestration occurs when the herniated fragment is separated from the parent disk. Care must be exercised in interpretation of disk abnormalities on MRI scans because of the frequency of abnormal findings in asymptomatic individuals. However, most herniations seen in

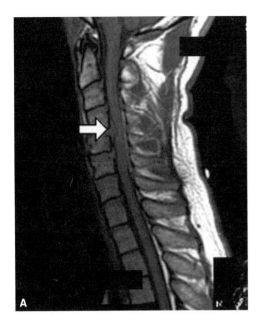 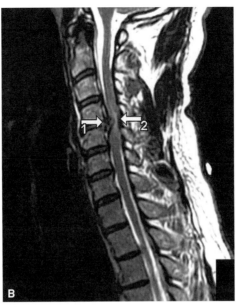

Figure 3 **A,** T1-weighted MRI scan showing large central disk herniation at C4-5 (*arrow*) with isointense appearance of spinal cord. **B,** T2-weighted MRI scan showing large central disk herniation at C4-5 (*arrow 2*) with increased signal within spinal cord posterior to disk (*arrow 1*).

asymptomatic individuals are contained and do not displace or compress nerve roots. Extruded herniation is rare in the asymptomatic population. In those patients whose MRI scans show disk degeneration without herniation, diskography can be used to further assess the disk as the possible source of pain.

Spinal stenosis is defined as narrowing of the central spinal canal, lateral recess, or neural foramina by either osseous or soft-tissue structures. Stenosis can be caused by a variety of abnormalities such as thickened ligamenta flava, hypertrophied facets and facet capsules, prominent epidural fat, a herniated disk, and osteophytes projecting off vertebral body end plates. In the cervical spine, degenerative changes in the uncovertebral joints can result in stenosis of the neural foramen and central canal stenosis can be amplified by the development of retrolisthesis. MRI has largely supplanted CT myelography as a primary screening method for cervical spondylotic radiculopathy and myelopathy because of its high soft-tissue contrast discrimination, multiplanar display, and its ability to image the spinal cord. Several studies have documented that MRI findings correlate well to surgical findings. Despite the advantages of MRI, differentiation of disks and osteophytes remain problematic in areas such as the foramen; MRI is often complemented by CT myelography. It is reasonable to begin an imaging evaluation with noninvasive MRI. However, CT myelography may provide valuable additional information in difficult or ambiguous cases and may aid in surgical planning.

In patients with cervical myelopathy, MRI provides the best assessment of spinal cord injury. Signal changes of the spinal cord on MRI in cervical compression myelopathy are believed to reflect pathologic changes in the spinal cord, and to be indicative of the prognosis.

Low-signal changes on T1-weighted sequences indicate a poor prognosis, whereas high-signal changes on T2-weighted images include a broad spectrum of pathology with varying recuperative potentials and are therefore nonspecific (Figure 3).

Stenosis in the lumbar spine involves many of the same structural abnormalities and MRI remains the dominant imaging method. Loss of disk height and anterolisthesis can further contribute to stenosis of the neural foramen in the lumbar spine. A recent study compared the relative contributions of MRI and CT myelography in surgical planning for lumbar stenosis. Surgeons expressed a general preference for MRI over CT myelography. However, the surgical plans derived from review of CT myelograms alone were much closer to plans derived from both studies together than were plans derived from the review of the MRI scans alone. It was concluded that the two modalities were complementary. Some investigators have found that axial loading during MRI can reveal stenosis not seen on MRI scans taken with the patient in a relaxed, supine position. Axial loading during MRI in patients with neurogenic claudication, in whom the greatest difference was found, has been proposed.

*MRI in the Postoperative Spine*

MRI is the modality of choice for imaging the postoperative spine. Scar tissue and disk material appear hypointense or isointense on T1-weighted imaging. The addition of gadolinium contrast on T1-weighted images can be used to help differentiate between scar tissue, which is vascular and thus enhances as a hyperintense image, and the disk, which is avascular and remains hypointense. The contrast between scar tissue and the disk can be improved by the use of an ionic rather than a nonionic contrast medium.

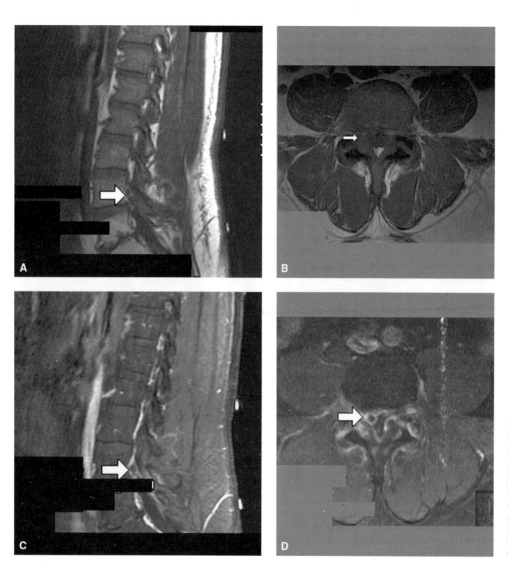

Figure 4 Pregadolinium and postgadolinium T1-weighted studies of the lumbar spine. Isointense homogenous mass (*arrow*) behind the body of L4 seen on sagittal **(A)** and axial **(B)** T1-weighted MRI scans are suggestive of an epidural abscess. **C,** Ring enhancement of a lesion (*arrow*) behind the body of L4 in the lateral recess is characteristic of epidural abscess seen on the sagittal T1-wieghted MRI scan with gadolinium contrast. **D,** Axial view of the ring enhancement lesion (*arrow*).

Several studies have shown that MRI scans taken in the immediate postoperative period show persistent abnormalities and do not correlate with patient symptoms. These abnormalities are believed to be a hematoma, normal healing immature scar tissue, or granulation tissue. Therefore, unless clinical findings strongly suggest evidence of a new or recurrent pathology such as a recurrent disk herniation or infection, postoperative MRI in the 3 months following surgery should be avoided.

Metal implants from surgery result in void artifacts obscuring the adjacent tissue. Generally, stainless steel implants generate greater artifact than titanium implants. The use of fast spin-echo sequences without fat saturation can minimize the amount of artifact caused by metallic implants.

## MRI in Tumors and Infection

Contrast-enhanced MRI is the study of choice for spinal cord, intradural-extramedullary, and extradural tumors. Osseous metastases, on the other hand, are routinely evaluated with nonenhanced MRI. A fat-suppression sequence should be used when attempting to detect marrow lesions. In tumors of the spine, MRI is an important imaging study to determine the location and extent of disease. The location of a spinal tumor gives important clues to possible diagnoses. For example, lymphoma and plasmacytoma often occur in the vertebral bodies. Osteochondroma often affects the posterior structures. Chordoma characteristically is located in the sacrum or upper cervical spine. MRI also can reveal the involvement of surrounding soft tissues and neural elements. It can distinguish between intradural and extradural involvement, which may be more difficult to distinguish on a CT scan.

MRI is the study of choice to diagnose diskitis, vertebral osteomyelitis, and epidural abscess. Although findings can be present on plain radiography, these occur late in the disease process. Bone scans can show increased activity, but do not differentiate between degeneration, infection, or tumor. In patients with diskitis,

MRI shows increased signal intensity on T2-weighted images within the disk space along with end-plate edema. In vertebral osteomyelitis, T2-weighted images show increased signal intensity within the disk and vertebral bodies with erosion of the end plate and paraspinal soft-tissue inflammation. Epidural abscess associated with vertebral osteomyelitis are best seen with T1-weighted gadolinium-enhanced MRI, which shows a ring-enhancing lesion within the spinal canal (Figure 4). The following findings have a high sensitivity for spinal infection: paraspinal or epidural inflammation, disk enhancement with contrast, increased disk signal intensity on T2-weighted images, and vertebral end-plate erosion. Commonly, MRI findings lag behind clinical improvement in a patient; therefore, other parameters should be used to assess progress. It should be noted that nonpyogenic osteomyelitis, such as tuberculosis and brucellosis, often spares the disk, appearing as skip lesions on MRI.

## Summary

Several imaging modalities are available for the evaluation of spinal disorders and each has a designated role in the workup of a patient and a specific place in the temporal sequence of clinical evaluation. Each of these studies should be used to confirm the clinical impression derived from the patient history and physical examination. It is imperative to distinguish findings that are clinically significant from those likely to be a part of the natural aging process. It is important to be mindful of the prevalence of abnormal findings in asymptomatic individuals. The results on imaging alone should not be relied on for treatment decisions.

Advances in technology, availability of imaging modalities, speed of scanning, and patient awareness have led to greater use of advanced imaging studies in many areas of spinal care including spine trauma and spine surgery. The role of imaging in the evaluation and treatment of spinal disorders will continue to evolve based on studies evaluating the clinical usefulness and cost-effectiveness of each method.

## Annotated Bibliography
### Plain Radiography

Blackmore CC: Evidence-based imaging evaluation of the cervical spine in trauma. *Neuroimaging Clin North Am* 2003;13:283-291.

This article discusses the evidence supporting cervical spine imaging in trauma patients. This discussion focuses on determining which patients should undergo imaging and what imaging modalities should be used. A summary of the evidence on diagnostic test performance, clinical prediction rules, and cost-effectiveness is included.

Mehta JS, Reed MR, McVie JL, Sanderson PL: Weight-bearing radiographs in thoracolumbar fractures: Do they influence management? *Spine* 2004;29:564-567.

In 28 patients with fractures between T11-L2 who were to receive nonsurgical treatment based on current criteria, radiographs were obtained while the patients were supine and erect. After analysis of erect radiographs, surgical treatment was chosen for 7 of the 28 patients.

Schwab FJ, Smith VA, Bisemi M, Gamez L, Farcy JC, Pagali M: Adult scoliosis: A quantitative radiographic and clinical analysis. *Spine* 2002;27:387-392.

This study of 95 patients with adolescent idiopathic scoliosis of the adult or de novo degenerative scoliosis correlated measurements from full-length radiographs with visual analog pain scores. Of the measurements taken, lateral vertebral olisthy, L3 and L4 end-plate obliquity angles, lumbar lordosis, and thoracolumbar kyphosis were significantly correlated with the pain scores.

### Computed Tomography

Griffen MM, Frykberg ER, Kerwin AJ, et al: Radiographic clearance of blunt cervical spine injury: Plain radiograph or computed tomography scan? *J Trauma* 2003;55:222-227.

In this study, 1,199 patients with blunt trauma who were at risk for cervical spine injuries had radiography and CT. Of the 9.5% of patients in whom injury was detected, 3.2% had negative findings on radiographs and positive findings on CT scans. All remaining patients had positive radiographs and CT scans. The authors concluded that CT should replace radiography for the evaluation of the cervical spine in patients with blunt trauma.

Learch TJ, Massie JB, Pathria MN, Ahlgren BA, Garfin SR: Assessment of pedicle screw placement utilizing conventional radiography and computed tomography: A proposed systematic approach to improve accuracy of interpretation. *Spine* 2004;29:767-773.

Three cadaver lumbar spines were instrumented bilaterally from L1-L5. Seven directions of deliberate misplacement as well as correct placement were randomly performed. Accuracy for identifying screw locations as in or out of the pedicle was 63% using radiographs and 87% using CT scans, compared with the findings from dissection. A systemic approach to image interpretation was developed.

Roberts CC, McDaniel NT, Krupinski EA, Erly WK: Oblique reformation in cervical spine computed tomography: A new look at an old friend. *Spine* 2003;28:167-170.

Cervical spine CT images in 19 patients with neural foraminal stenosis were reformatted in an oblique plane perpendicular to the long axis of the right and left neural foramina. Rates of agreement on the degree of stenosis and confidence ratings were significantly higher in seven independent observers using oblique reformations compared with axial images.

## Magnetic Resonance Imaging

Borenstein DG, O'Mara JW Jr, Boden SD, et al: The value of magnetic resonance imaging of the lumbar spine to predict low-back pain in asymptomatic subjects: A seven-year follow-up study. *J Bone Joint Surg Am* 2001;83-A:1306-1311.

Findings from MRI scans (performed 7 years earlier) of the lumbar spines of 76 asymptomatic individuals with no history of back pain were not predictive of the development or duration of low back pain.

Flynn J, Closkey R, Mahboubi S, Dormans J: Role of magnetic resonance imaging in the assessment of pediatric cervical spine injuries. *J Pediatr Orthop* 2002;22: 573-577.

The authors studied 237 consecutive children, 74 of whom were evaluated by MRI. Criteria for MRI were (1) an obtunded or nonverbal child suspected of having a cervical spine injury; (2) equivocal films; (3) neurologic symptoms without radiographic findings; or (4) an inability to clear the cervical spine within 3 days. MRI confirmed the plain radiography diagnosis in 66% of children and altered the diagnosis in 34%. MRI is valuable in the evaluation of potential cervical spine injuries, especially in obtunded children with equivocal plain radiographs.

Frank JB, Lim CK, Flynn JM, Dormans JP: The efficacy of magnetic resonance imaging in pediatric cervical spine clearance. *Spine* 2002;27:1176-1179.

Patients were evaluated before and after the institution of a protocol to perform MRI of the cervical spine when patients with injuries to the cervical spine could not be cleared within 72 hours of injury. The protocol led to a reduction in the amount of time required for cervical spine clearance, stay in the intensive care unit, length of hospitalization, and total cost. The authors concluded that in obtunded and intubated pediatric trauma patients with suspected cervical spine injury, the clearance protocol was effective and cost-efficient.

Horn EM, Lekovic GP, Feiz-Erfan I, Sonntag VK, Theodore N: Cervical magnetic resonance imaging abnormalities not predictive of cervical spine instability in traumatically injured patients. *J Neurosurg Spine* 2004;1: 39-42.

This study reviewed 6,328 patient admitted through the trauma service. Of 166 patients in whom CT scanning and radiography showed normal findings, 70 had undergone MRI that revealed abnormal findings. MRI results in these patients revealed poor correlation with true instability of the cervical spine. The authors concluded that if CT and radiographs show no fractures or signs of instability, MRI is not helpful in determining cervical instability and may lead to unnecessary testing.

Ledermann HP, Schweitzer ME, Morrison WB, Carrino JA: MR Imaging findings in spinal infections: Rules or myths. *Radiology* 2003;228:506-514.

Contrast-enhanced spinal MRI scans were obtained in 46 patients with spinal infection. Criteria with good to excellent sensitivity (84.1% to 97.7%) included the presence of paraspinal or epidural inflammation, disk enhancement, hyperintensity or fluid-equivalent disk signal intensity on T2-weighted images, and erosion or destruction of at least one vertebral end plate. Criteria with low sensitivity (29.5% to 52.3%) included decreased height of the intervertebral space and disk hypointensity on T1-weighted images.

Morio Y, Teshima R, Nagashima H, Nawata K, Yamasaki D, Nanjo Y: Correlation between operative outcomes of cervical compression myelopathy and MRI of the spinal cord. *Spine* 2001;26:1238-1245.

MRI scans of patients with cervical compression myelopathy were retrospectively analyzed in comparison with surgical outcomes. The low-signal intensity changes on T1-weighted sequences indicated a poor prognosis. The authors speculate that high-signal intensity changes on T2-weighted images include a broad spectrum of compressive myelomalacic pathologies and reflect a broad spectrum of spinal cord recuperative potentials.

Saifuddin A, Green R, White J: Magnetic resonance imaging of the cervical ligaments in the absence of trauma. *Spine* 2003;28:1686-1692.

Twenty patients undergoing MRI for cervical degenerative disk disease were examined using sagittal images. On T1-weighted images, 74% to 79% of anterior longitudinal ligaments, 36% to 74% of posterior longitudinal ligaments, 63% to 65% of ligamenta flava, and 35% to 60% of apical ligaments were visualized. The authors conclude that discontinuity of the "black stripe" on a T1-weighted sequence cannot be used as a reliable isolated sign of ligament rupture because the spinal ligaments are commonly not visualized.

Willen J, Danielson B: The diagnostic effect from axial loading of the lumbar spine during computed tomography and magnetic resonance imaging in patients with degenerative disorders. *Spine* 2001;26:2607-2614.

In this study, 50 patients undergoing CT myelography and 122 patients undergoing MRI were imaged both in relaxed and axially loaded modes. Additional valuable information was found in 29% of patients during examination in the axial loaded mode and in 69% of the subgroup of patients with neurogenic claudication. The authors concluded that axially loaded imaging frequently adds additional valuable information compared with conventional imaging, especially in patients with neurogenic claudication.

## Classic Bibliography

Blackmore CC, Ramsey SD, Mann FA, Deyo RA: Cervical spine screening with CT in trauma patients: A cost-effectiveness analysis. *Radiology* 1999;212:117-125.

Boden SD, Davis DO, Dina TS, Patronas NJ, Wiesel SW: Abnormal magnetic resonance scans of the lumbar spine in asymptomatic subjects: A prospective investigation. *J Bone Joint Surg* 1990;72:403-408.

Friedenberg ZB, Miller WT: Degenerative disc disease of the cervical spine: A comparative study of asymptomatic and symptomatic patients. *J Bone Joint Surg* 1963; 45:1171-1178.

Gehweiler JA Jr, Daffner RH: Low back pain: The controversy of radiologic evaluation. *AJR Am J Roentgenol* 1983;140:109-112.

Hayes MA, Howard TC, Gruel CR, et al: Roentgenographic evaluation of lumbar spine flexion-extension in asymptomatic individuals. *Spine* 1989;14:327-331.

Jackson RP, Cain JE Jr, Jacobs RR, et al: The neuroradiographic diagnosis of lumbar herniated nucleus pulposus: II. A comparison of computed tomography (CT), myelography, CT-myelography, and magnetic resonance imaging. *Spine* 1989;14:1362-1367.

Ross JS, Masaryk TJ, Schrader M, Gentili A, Bohlman H, Modic MT: MR imaging of the postoperative lumbar spine: Assessment with gadopentetate dimeglumine. *AJNR Am J Neuroradiol* 1990;11:771-776.

Schaefer DM, Flanders AE, Osterholm JL, Northrup BE: Prognostic significance of magnetic resonance imaging in the acute phase cervical spine injury. *J Neurosurg* 1992;76:218-223.

Shafaie FF, Wippold FJ II, Gado M, Pilgram TK, Riew KD: Comparison of computed tomography myelography and magnetic resonance imaging in the evaluation of cervical spondylotic myelopathy and radiculopathy. *Spine* 1999;24:1781-1785.

Wiesel SW, Tsourmas N, Feffer HL, et al: A study of computer assisted tomography: I. The incidence of positive CAT scans in an asymptomatic group of patients. *Spine* 1984;9:549-551.

# Chapter 7

# Interventional Diagnostic Imagery

George E. Charuk, DO

## Introduction

It has been said that nearly everyone will experience back pain sometime during their lifetime. Most patients will recover within 3 to 4 weeks from this self-limiting condition. However, approximately 10% of patients remain refractory to nonsurgical care. One of many difficulties in dealing with back pain is determining a proper diagnosis. A back disorder such as a disk herniation tends to superimpose on preexisting diseases such as mechanical low back pain, degenerative spinal conditions, and deconditioning. Nonspecific back pain of 6 weeks or shorter duration has a favorable natural outcome. The reason to intervene within the first 6 weeks is to shorten the period of disability.

## Pain Definitions

Axial back pain refers to pain located primarily in the region of the axial skeleton. Axial pain may or may not be associated somatic referred pain. Somatic pain is pain that arises from noxious stimulations of one or more musculoskeletal components of the body. Characteristically, somatic pain is deep, diffuse, aching in quality, and difficult to localize. Somatic referred pain is usually characterized by pain in a wide area, in a fixed location, and with indistinguishable boundaries. Referred pain is pain perceived in a region innervated by nerves other than those that innervate the actual source of pain. Referred pain can occur anywhere in the lower limbs, usually more proximal than distal. In contradistinction, radicular pain arises as a result of irritation of a spinal nerve or its roots. Radicular pain is characteristically shooting and band-like and travels in a narrow band, but in a nondermatomal pattern. Disk herniations are the most common cause of radicular pain. Most back pain is axial, with approximately 12% of patients having features of radicular pain.

Radicular pain is not produced by compression of healthy nerve roots. Compression produces only paresthesias and then numbness. Lumbar radicular pain can be produced by traction of nerve roots that have previously been affected by inflammation.

Inflammation is emerging as the cardinal pathologic process that underlies the mechanism of radicular pain. A variety of inflammatory agents have been shown to irritate lumbar nerve roots, including phospholipase $A_2$, which causes spontaneous activity in the neurons of the dorsal root ganglion. This irritation is the likely mechanism for radicular pain.

In a study of patient response to steroids and the duration of radicular pain as a predictor of surgical outcomes, it was found that if a steroid was injected into a patient's symptomatic nerve root and provided temporary pain relief, regardless of the duration of the patient's pain (1 year or less), these patients had a better surgical outcome in comparison with those patients who did not receive the steroids. Other evidence shows epidural steroid injections are more effective than placebo, local anesthetic alone, or bed rest for nerve root irritation or inflammation. Favorable outcomes are more common in patients with acute pain conditions rather than chronic pain states. Of those patients who responded favorably, more than 90% did so within 6 days of receiving the injection.

## Mechanism of Benefit

Although steroids have been found to be beneficial, the mechanism by which they provide benefit has not been identified. Controversy remains regarding the most beneficial route for administering epidural steroid injections, dosing with steroids, and the optimal number of injections. Proposed theories include the anti-inflammatory effect (blocking phospholipase $A_2$ activity), the neural membrane stabilization effect, modulation of peripheral nociceptor C-fiber input, and suppression of neuropeptides.

The use of fluoroscopy allows for visual feedback and ensures the placement of medication in the desired target location. Fluoroscopy also allows for the use of smaller diameter needles that limit tissue damage and accidental intravascular or intrathecal placement.

Epidural steroid injections are used for the treatment of radiculopathies with injection of either corticosteroids

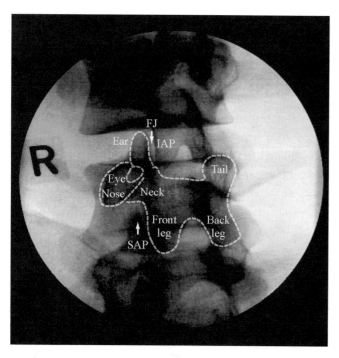

Figure 1  Right anterior oblique view of the lumbar spine. The outline resembles the form of a Scottish terrier (Scotty dog sign). SAP = left superior articular process, IAP = left inferior articular process, FJ = facet joint, Nose = left transverse process, Eye = left pedrile, Ear = left superior articular process, Front leg = left interior articular process, Neck = left parainterarticular process, Tail = right traverse process, Back leg = superimposed right inferior articular process and right superior articular process.

alone or a solution containing corticosteroids. The injection of long-acting corticosteroids into the epidural space allows the medicine to remain in the affected region for a longer period of time. The desired effects are decreased inflammation and improved pain control. Epidural steroids have been used in the treatment of lumbosacral radicular pain since 1952. The use of epidural steroid injections has not been without controversy. In a 1995 study, questions were raised about the rationale and efficacy of these injections. Because steroids are anti-inflammatory agents and work for sciatica, whether the benefits of steroids are derived from the reduction of nerve root inflammation was questioned (Figure 1).

## Spine Imaging

Advances in spine imaging have allowed better visualization of spinal anatomy and the associated disease process. These clearer images have led to improved treatments of acute disk herniations, foraminal stenosis, central spinal stenosis, and facet arthropathies. As technology has improved (for example, the use of soft-tissue contrasts), MRI can be used to identify more anatomic and pathologic findings; however, these findings do not always coincide with the patient's clinical signs and symptoms. There have been many published studies of asymptomatic patients with significant disk disease that has been identified on imaging studies.

MRI provides information on degenerative changes occurring in a disk. T1-weighted images are helpful in detecting fat and act as a natural contrast for epidural and spinal lesions. On T1-weighted MRI scans, fat appears bright whereas fluid is dark. On T2-weighted images, fluid is bright. On T2-weighted MRI scans, the nucleus pulposus and inner layers of the anulus fibrosus are bright and provide high signal intensity. In contrast, the outer layers of the normal anulus fibrosus are dark and show low signal intensity. In a degenerative disk, there is disorganization of the nucleus pulposus and anulus fibrosus. The resultant loss of integrity between the nucleus pulposus and anulus fibrosus appear as reduced signal intensity on T2-weighted MRI scans. The disk maintains a slightly diminished height and, with ongoing degeneration, the nucleus pulposus is replaced with fibrous tissue, leading to decreased signal intensity.

In addition to disk desiccation, T2-weighted images can show high-intensity zones and Modic changes. High-intensity zones are areas of hyperintense signal without the periphery of the disk in the region of the anulus fibrosus. These zones tend to occur more posteriorly than anteriorly. A 1992 study correlated the presence of an annular tear with an 85% chance of pain reproduction on diskography. Modic changes were described as vertebral marrow end-plate findings in association with degenerative disk disease.

An annular fissure is a focal disruption of the fibers of the anulus fibrosus. Three types of fissures have been described: concentric, transverse, and radial. An annular fissure closer to the nucleus pulposus may lead to dehydration and decreased signal intensity.

Historically, the radiologic nomenclature for disk pathology had been confusing. In 2001 a combined task force of the North American Spine Society, American Society of Spine Radiology, and American Society of Neuroradiology standardized the language regarding disk pathology. A localized, circumferential, diffuse, symmetric extension of a disk beyond the adjacent vertebral end plate is defined as a disk bulge. A focal herniation involves less than 25% of the circumference, a broad-based herniation involves from 25% to 50% of the disk circumference, and a symmetric bulging disk involves 50% to 100% of the disk circumference. A disk protrusion is a focal asymmetric extension of the intervertebral disk extending beyond the margin of the adjacent vertebrae. The posterior margin of the disk is greater than the AP dimension. A disk extrusion by definition has a greater distance between the edges of the disk material than the distance at the posterior margin. A sequestered disk occurs when the displaced disk material has lost any continuity with the parent disk.

In a 2001 study, 67 asymptomatic patients with no history of back pain underwent MRI of the lumbar spine. Of the 67 patients, 31% had identifiable abnormalities of a disk or the spinal cord. A questionnaire about the development and duration of low back pain over a 7-year period was sent to the 67 patients and MRI was repeated for 31 patients. The repeat MRI findings showed a greater frequency of disk herniation, bulging, degeneration, and spinal stenosis. Despite the presence of a disk herniation or degenerative disk, the development of low back pain was not predicted.

In another recent study, 148 patients without low back pain were assessed. Demographics, comorbidity, functional status, and quality of life were reviewed. Sixty-nine of the patients (46%) never experienced back pain. MRI scans of the lumbar spine were obtained, with 83% of patients showing moderate to severe dessication of one or more disks, and 32% had at least one disk protrusion with 6% having one or more disk extrusions. It can be concluded from this study that abnormal MRI findings do not always correlate with patient symptomatology.

## Treatments for and Causes of Low Back Pain

Several different theories regarding lumbosacral disk herniation with radicular symptoms have been proposed. These theories involve the resorption of lumbar herniated disk fragments; asymptomatic lumbar disk pathology, including herniation; and the inflammatory component of low back and/or radicular pain in the presence of disk herniation. An inflammatory reaction may be necessary to cause symptoms, even in the presence of mechanical compression.

High levels of phospholipase $A_2$ have been found adjacent to symptomatic lumbar disk herniations. Phospholipase $A_2$ propagates an inflammatory cascade by liberation of arachidonic acid that results in both chemotactic and noncellular mediated responses through leukotrienes, platelet activation factor, and prostaglandins. This inflammatory cascade may lead to back pain and radiculopathy even in the absence of any extension of disk material into the spine. Inflammatory substances in the epidural space also may directly or indirectly induce increased vascular permeability of endoneural blood vessels. Neuropeptides, such as substance P, are activated and released from dorsal root ganglion after noxious mechanical stimulation supporting the neurogenic inflammatory theory for pain generation.

Diagnostic and therapeutic spinal injections are discussed in detail in chapter 16.

### Epidural Steroid Injections

Epidural steroids have been administered via different routes with differing effects. Although the spread of the medicine cannot be controlled by the physician, certain techniques are believed to allow the corticosteroid solution to migrate more anteriorly than posteriorly.

One well-documented difficulty with epidural steroid injections is consistent placement of the injection. In a classic double-blinded study, placement of epidural nee-

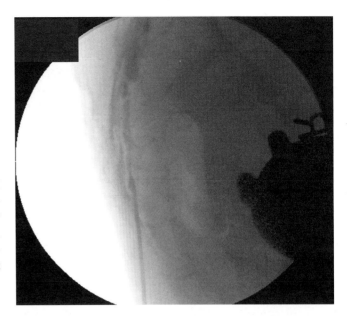

Figure 2   Image of caudal epidural steroid injection with a contrast agent.

dles was incorrect in 25% of patients, with placement being superficial to the vertebral canal. The use of fluoroscopy improved the success rate for injections. Early epidural steroid injections were administered using the caudal route, via the sacral hiatus. This approach requires 10 mL or more of injected fluid to ensure that the desired lumbar nerve roots will be reached (Figure 2). The advantages to a caudal approach are ease of administration and limited risk of dural puncture.

### Interlaminar Steroid Injections

Interlaminar epidural steroid injection places the medication in the posterior epidural space. The interlaminar approach involves insertion of a Tuohy epidural needle between the laminae of adjacent vertebrae. Once penetration through the ligamentum flavum occurs, there is loss of resistance noted with a glass syringe. Confirmatory placement with nonionic contrast agent under fluoroscopic imaging shows an even diffusion of contrast into the epidural space. As confirmation is obtained, either steroids or a steroid solution is injected. After injection, the medicine travels the path of least resistance and may be affected by epidural ligaments and epidural scarring. The improper penetration of epidurally administered steroids to the locus of the nerve root irritation may result in a poor outcome (Figure 3).

Interlaminar epidural steroid injections can achieve localized spread to targeted pathologic regions by injections made at the same or adjacent levels, or by using a catheter to reach the desired level. The use of a catheter has been found helpful in higher cervical lesions where the epidural space is smaller.

In a 2001 study, 160 patients with unilateral symptoms of sciatica lasting for 1 month and 6 months were ran-

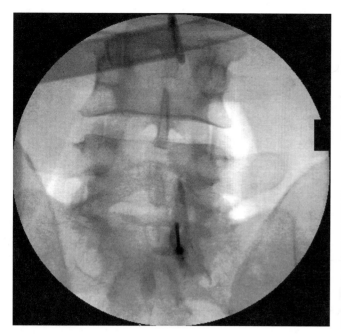

Figure 3   AP fluoroscopic image of an interlaminar approach.

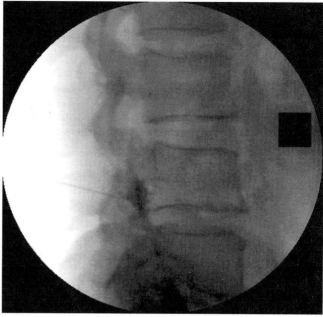

Figure 4   Lateral fluoroscopic image showing contrast agent with lumbar epidural space.

domized for double-blind injections with a methyl-prednisolone-bupivacaine combination or saline. Outcomes were periodically measured over 1 year and statistically significant improvement was noted in leg pain, straight-leg raising, lumbar flexion, and patient satisfaction after 2 weeks in the patients who received the steroids. However, the initial advantage disappeared at 1-year follow-up.

## Transforaminal Steroid Injections

The intended target for transforaminal steroid injections is the posteromedial aspect of the superior articular process at the waist of the foramen in the oblique view (Figure 4). The placement of a needle in a "safe triangle" with the base being the inferior border of the pedicle, the medial side being the exiting spinal nerve, and the lateral side being the lateral border of the vertebral body has been described.

Fluoroscopy allows for visualization and controlled needle placement. A 2000 study of the complications of fluoroscopically-guided transforaminal lumbar epidural steroid injections involved 207 patients who received 322 injections. Complications per injection included 10 transient nonpositional headaches that resolved within 24 hours (3.1%), 8 incidences of increased back pain (2.4%), 2 episodes of increased leg pain (2.4%), 4 episodes of facial flushing (1.2%), 1 vasovagal reaction (0.3%), 1 instance of increased blood glucose (258 mg/dL) in an insulin-dependent diabetic patient (0.3%), and 1 episode of intrasurgical hypertension (0.3%). No dural punctures occurred.

## Selective Nerve Root Blocks

Selective nerve root block (SNRB) has both diagnostic and therapeutic benefits. The procedure is designed to deliver an anesthetic agent and/or corticosteroid to the extra dural segment of the nerve. SNRB is helpful in patients who have radicular pain, an equivocal neurologic examination, and nonspecific findings with imagery. Compared with epidural steroid injections, SNRB delivers a low volume of concentrated medication over the involved nerve root sleeve. SNRB should elicit the radicular pain in the distribution of the nerve root injected. If the pain produced is inconsistent with the patient's typical pain, the needle can be moved to another level in an effort to elicit the radicular pain.

Studies have shown that a steroid injected into the patient's symptomatic nerve root should provide temporary pain relief and that those patients who receive this treatment have a more favorable surgical outcome. Also noted was that for patients with pain of less than 1 year duration, positive surgical results occurred in 89%. For patients with pain lasting more than 1 year and with positive response to steroids injected into the symptomatic nerve root, the positive surgical results slightly decreased to 85%. Of those patients who did not respond to steroid injections and had pain for more than 1 year, 95% had poor surgical outcomes. SNRB injections provide therapeutic benefits and also provide prognostic information regarding the surgical outcomes for some patients.

A 2000 study compared nonsurgical treatments of patients with degenerative lumbar radicular pain with disk herniation or central and foraminal spinal stenosis confirmed by MRI or CT myelography. Patients were randomized to receive a SNRB with either bupivacaine alone or bupivacaine with betamethasone. At 13- to 28-month follow-up, 20 of the 28 patients receiving bupivacaine with betamethasone opted not to have surgery, and 9 of 27 patients who received bupivacaine alone opted not to have surgery.

## Diskography

Historically, the mechanical model was used to view a herniated nucleus pulposus as a posterolateral prolapse with direct nerve root compression. Newer concepts of spinal pain expand the explanation beyond the simple mechanical mode. Focus is now being placed on inflammatory mediators within the nucleus and low-pressure (chemical) activation of annular nociceptors.

A position paper on diskography by the North American Spine Society states that, "discography is indicated in the evaluation of patients with unremitting spinal pain, with or without extremity pain, of greater than 4 months duration, when the pain has been unresponsive to all appropriate methods of conservative therapy." Before diskography is performed, patients should have undergone investigation with other modalities, which have failed to explain the source of pain. These other modalities should include but are not limited to CT and MRI and/or myelography. In these circumstances, diskography, especially when followed by CT, may be the only study capable of providing a diagnosis by permitting a precise description of the internal anatomy of a disk and a detailed determination of the integrity of the substructures of the disk. The observations of the anatomy may be complemented by the critical physiologic induction of pain, which is recognized by the patient as similar to or identical with the clinical findings. By including multiple levels in the study, the patient can control the evaluation of the reliability of the pain response.

Diskography also is indicated for patients who have failed to respond to surgery, those with possible painful pseudarthrosis, symptomatic disk, and recurrent disk herniation. Diskography may also be used to investigate dye patterns before percutaneous procedures, secondary internal disk disruptions, and pseudarthrosis.

Diskography is the injection of contrast material into the nucleus pulposus of an intervertebral disk. During the procedure, the examiner attempts to ascertain the patient's response to pain (provocation/analgesia) and the disk morphology with radiographic imaging and/or CT. The information obtained should include the resistance to the injection, the amount of contrast injected, the pattern of dye distribution (diffuse, location of fissures, extravasation, herniations, Schmorl's nodes), and the pain response.

The primary goal of diskography is to determine whether discogenic pain is the source of the patient's back pain. Diskography can relate a patient's pain symptoms to radiographic findings. The second goal of diskography is to identify the disk level causing the pain. The key question is whether the pain produced by performing a diskography coincides with the patient's pain.

Complications related to diskography include diskitis, spinal headaches, meningitis, intrathecal hemorrhage, and arachnoiditis. Older studies have shown that diskitis occurred in 3 of 61 patients studied with an incidence of 4.92%. In reviewing 15 studies the overall incidence was less than 0.25%.

### Facet Joint Injections

Facet joints or zygapophysial joints have been implicated as one of the causes of back pain. The facet joint is a synovial joint allowing motion of the spine for flexion, extension, and rotation. It has been shown that in the lordotic posture of patients with lumbar spondylolysis, the lumbar facets are weight bearing and resist compressive forces. Extension past normal limits can cause the interior facet to slide past the superior facet to contact laminae. An overloaded zygapophysial joint can stretch and even rupture the joint capsule.

Facet joint pathology is often diagnosed by the process of exclusion. Localized placement of anesthetic into the facet joint with elimination of pain implicates the facet joint as the source of dysfunction. Usually facet joint pathology is not limited to one level. The cascade of disk degeneration often leads to multilevel facet involvement.

The facet joint is identified under fluoroscopic guidance in an oblique position by identifying the inferior articular process of the upper vertebrae and superior articular process of the lower vertebrae. Facet joint injection is routinely performed with a 3.5-in spinal needle (either 22 or 25 gauge) that is placed in the plane of the x-ray beam. The target zone is the inferior portion of the inferior articulating process. The needle is repositioned and redirected. After joint penetration is perceived, 0.2 mL of contrast is injected which allows for visualization of the joint capsule. Once confirmed fluoroscopically, 1.0 to 1.5 mL of a steroid or steroid solution is injected.

### Sacroiliac Joint Injections

The sacroiliac (SI) joint is formed into a true synovial joint by the union of the sacrum and the iliac bone. The SI joint was once believed to be the most common cause of sciatica. SI joint discomfort is well known and recognized as a source of lumbosacral pain during pregnancy. The symptoms usually occur in the second trimester with the presence of pain over the SI joints. SI joint

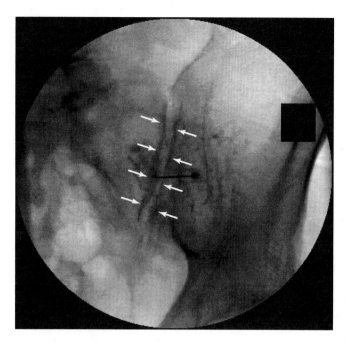

**Figure 5**  Image of the SI joint with contrast agent.

pain may have a radicular component. Radiation of pain can occur into the inguinal region, posterior thigh, or lower abdominal quadrant. Pain may be reproduced with overload activities such as prolonged standing or walking, transitional movements, and unsupported sitting.

Diagnostic values of the SI stress tests were assessed in a study of 85 patients with 12 widely used clinical tests and compared with those with intra-articular anesthesia injection. The clinical tests failed to substantiate diagnostic value. It has been found that a diagnosis of primary sacroiliitis was made with alleviation of symptoms following an injection of lidocaine and steroids.

SI joint injections have both a diagnostic and therapeutic benefit for patients. The SI joint is identified using fluoroscopic guidance. Using a posteroinferior to anterosuperior approach, a 32-gauge, 3.5-inch spinal needle is inserted. The needle is advanced into the posteroinferior aspect of the SI joint. After joint penetration is perceived (with a spongy feel), 0.2 mL of contrast material is injected to allow for visualization of the joint. This process is followed with injection of either anesthetic alone (for diagnostic purposes) or together with steroid for therapeutic purposes (Figure 5).

Current research is investigating the lumbopelvic muscle recruitment needed to stabilize the pelvis in patients with SI joint pain. Abnormal muscle recruitment may lead to pelvic obliquity, which in turn could affect the position of the innominate in relation to the sacrum. Therefore, rehabilitation of a patient with SI joint dysfunction should focus primarily on joint position; how-

ever, the support of muscular structures should also be considered.

## Summary

The nonsurgical treatment of low back pain has taken center stage in the era of managed care and fiscal restraint. The demographics of an aging, active baby boomer population has contributed to the increasing prevalence of back pain in patients. Studies show that with the proper placement of anti-inflammatory medication, pain can be managed and patient function can be improved. By regulating the inflammatory and neurogenic mediator response, improving patient function and aerobic tolerance, reconditioning the weakened secondary muscular support structures, and improving general physical fitness, patients may experience fewer symptomatic exacerbations and lead more fulfilling pain-free lives.

## Annotated Bibliography
### Spine Imaging

Borenstein D, O'Mara J, Boden S, et al: The value of magnetic resonance imaging of the lumbar spine to predict low back pain in asymptomatic subjects: A seven-year follow-up study. *J Bone Joint Surg* 2001;83:1306-1311.

In 67 asymptomatic patients with no history of back pain who underwent MRI of the lumbar spine the development of low back pain was not predicted, despite the presence of a disk herniation or degenerative disk.

Fardon DF, Milette PC: Combined Task Forces of the North American Spine Society, American Society of Spine Radiology, and American Society of Neuroradiology: Nomenclature and classification of lumbar disc pathology: Recommendations of the Combined task Forces of the North American Spine Society, American Society of Spine Radiology, and American Society of Neuroradiology. *Spine* 2001;26:E93-E113.

Nomenclature and classification of lumbar disk pathology were set forth with standardization of terms. This article includes a discussion of anatomic zones and levels of disk fragments to be used for consistency among clinicians.

Jarvik J, Hollingsworth W, Heagerty P, Maynor D, Deyo R: The Longitudinal Assessment of Imaging and Disability of the Back (LAID Back) Study. *Spine* 2001;26: 1158-1166.

Results from this study of 48 patients without low back pain showed that abnormal MRI findings do not always correlate with patient symptomatology.

### Treatments For and Causes of Low Back Pain

Botwin KP, Gruber R, Bouchlas CG, et al: Fluoroscopically guided lumbar transforaminal epidural steroid injections in degenerative lumbar stenosis: An outcome study. *Am J Phys Med Rehabil* 2002;81:898-905.

This study involved 34 patients with unilateral radicular pain from degenerative spinal stenosis who did not improve after nonsurgical treatment with physical therapy, anti-inflammatory drugs, and analgesics. These patients received fluoroscopically-guided lumbar transforaminal epidural steroid injections with 12 mg of betamethasone and 2 mL of 1% preservative free lidocaine. An average of 1.9 injections were administered per patient. At 1-year follow-up, 75% of patients had successful long-term outcomes with a 50% reduction between preinjection and postinjection pain scores. Sixty-four percent of the patients had improved walking tolerance and 57% had improved standing tolerance.

Vad V, Bhat A, Lutz G, Cammisa F: Transforaminal epidural steroid injections in lumbosacral radiculopathy: A prospective randomized study. *Spine* 2002;27:11-16.

The authors studied 50 patients with lumbosacral radiculopathy secondary to a herniated nucleus pulposus. Patients were divided into two groups: group one was treated with transforaminal epidural steroid injections and group two was treated with trigger point injections. Two patients were lost to follow-up. Of the 25 patients who received transforaminal epidural steroid injections, 21 (84%) showed improvement. Of the 23 patients who received trigger point injections, 11 (48%) showed improvement.

*Diskography*

Hungerford B, Gilleard W, Hodges D: Evidence of altered lumbopelvic muscle recruitment in the presence of sacroiliac joint pain. *Spine* 2003;28:1593-1600.

A difference of muscle activation in patients with SI joint pain compared with a control group was noted using electromyography. The onset of activity of the oblique internus abdominis, multifidus, and a gluteus maximus were delayed whereas the biceps femoris was activated early. Muscle imbalance can disrupt load transference through the pelvis.

Igarashi A, Kikuchi S, Konno S, Olmarker K: Inflammatory cytokines released from the facet joint tissue in degenerative lumbar spine disorders. *Spine* 2004;29:2091-2095.

Forty patients were studied to determine if the pain associated with degenerative lumbar spinal disorders was caused by chemical factors. Joint cartilage and synovial tissues were harvested during surgery from the facet joint. Results showed a higher level of inflammatory cytokines in the facet joint of patients with lumbar spinal stenosis than in those with lumbar disk herniations.

Karppinen J, Malmivaara A, Kurunlahti M, et al: Periradicular infiltration for sciatica. *Spine* 2001;26:1059-1067.

Transforaminal epidural steroid injection is done with a large concentration of steroid, placed in the vicinity of the irritated nerve root. This study examined 160 patients with sciat-ica who had unilateral symptoms lasting from 1 to 6 months with no prior surgery and who were treated with either a methylprednisolone bupivacaine combination or with saline. Recovery in the first 2 weeks was better in the group receiving the steroid injection with regard to leg pain; however, at 6 months the patients treated with saline had less back and leg pain.

## Classic Bibliography

April CN, Bogduk N: High intensity zone: A diagnostic sign of painful lumbar disc on magnetic resonance imaging. *Br J Radiol* 1992;65:361-369.

Boden SD, McCowin PR, Davis DO, Dina TS, Mark AS, Wiesel S: Abnormal magnetic resonance scans of the lumbar spine in assymptomatic subjects: A prospective investigation. *J Bone Joint Surg Am* 1990;72:1178-1184.

Bogduk N: Spine update: Epidural steroids. *Spine* 1995; 20:845-848.

Boos N, Rieder R, Schede V, Spratt KF, Summer N, Aebi M: The diagnostic accuracy of magnetic resonance imaging, work perceptions, and psychological factors in identifying somatic disc herniations. *Spine* 1995;20:2613-2625.

Botwin KP, Gruber R, Bouchlas C, Torres-Ramos F, Freeman T, Slaten W: Complications of fluoroscopically guided transforaminal lumbar epidural injections. *Arch Phys Med Rehabil* 2000;81:1045-10.

Bush K, Hiller S: A controlled study of caudal epidural injections of triamcinolone plus procaine for the management of sciatica. *Spine* 1991;16:572-575.

Derby R, Bogduk N: Precision percutaneous blocking procedures for localizing spinal pain: Part 2. The lumbar neuroxial compartment. *Pain Digest* 1993;3:175-188.

Derby R, Kine G, Saal J, et al: Response to steroid and duration of radicular pain as predictors of surgical outcome. *Spine* 1992;17(suppl 6):S176-S183.

Dreyfuss P, Michael Sen M, Pauza K: The value of medical history and physical examination in diagnosing sacroiliac joint pain. *Spine* 1996;21:2594-2602.

Fraser RD, Osti OL, Vernon-Roberts B: Discitis after discography: The role of prophylactic antibiotics. *J Bone Joint Surg Br* 1990;72:271-274.

Guyar RD, Ohnmeiss DD: Lumbar discography. *Spine J* 2003;3(suppl 3):11S-27S.

Holt EP Jr: The question of lumbar discography. *J Bone Joint Surg Am* 1968;50:720-726.

Jensen MC, Brant-Zawadzki MN, Obuchowski N, Modic MT, Malkasian D, Ross JS: Magnetic resonance imaging of the lumbar spine in people without back pain. *N Engl J Med* 1994;331:69-73.

McCarron R, Wimpee M, Hudkins P, et al: The inflammatory effect of nucleus pulposus: A possible element in the pathogenesis of low back pain. *Spine* 1987;12:760-764.

Nachemson AL, Jonsson E: *Neck and Back Pain.* Philadelphia, PA, Lippincott, 2000.

North Am Spine Society: Position paper on discography: The executive committee of the NASS. *Spine* 1988;13:1343.

Riew D, Yin Y, Gilula L, et al: The effect of nerve root injections on the need for operative treatment of lumbar radicular pain. *J Bone Joint Surg Am* 2000;82-A: 1589-1593.

Weinstein SM, Herring SA, Derby R: Contemporary concepts in spine care: Epidural steroid injections. *Spine* 1995;20:1842.

White AH: Injection techniques for the diagnosis and treatment of low back pain. *Orthop Clin North Am* 1983;14:553-567.

Yang KH, King AI: Mechanism of facet load transmission as a hypothesis for low back pain. *Spine* 1984;9:557-565.

# Chapter 8

# Clinical Neurophysiology

Aleksandar Beric, MD, DSc

## Introduction

Clinical neurophysiology is a branch of the neurosciences; however, its relationship with orthopaedics, and especially the spine, has been both dynamic and historic. Since the first clinical applications of electromyography (EMG) and nerve conduction (NC) studies in the 1950s, these procedures have been used in the diagnosis of disorders of the spine. Somatosensory-evoked potentials (SSEPs) were a stepping stone in the development of intraoperative monitoring, and were initially used to prevent the neurologic complications of scoliosis surgery. In the early 1990s, the development of this more affordable and portable diagnostic and monitoring instrumentation led to a rapid expansion of the field of clinical neurophysiology and of its usefulness in offices and operating rooms. More knowledge has been acquired about the indications and limitations of these stimulation and recording methods; however, an increase in the misuse and abuse of these techniques has also occurred. This chapter will review the current uses of various clinical neurophysiology techniques and will discuss the limitations of such techniques.

## Electromyography and Nerve Conduction Studies

Although EMG is discussed first in this chapter, NC studies are always obtained first in the clinical setting. It is necessary to establish that the peripheral nerves are functioning properly before a needle EMG examination is performed. Most of the relevant abnormalities in EMG and NC studies of spinal disorders are found in the EMG study. However, because of a large differential of EMG abnormalities, it is absolutely necessary to exclude certain disorders including plexopathy, spinal amyotrophy, and frequently, carpal tunnel syndrome. These disorders can masquerade as radiculopathy, or may be present in addition to radiculopathy such as double-crush syndrome (for example, C6 radiculopathy and carpal tunnel syndrome). Because they have a typical NC presentation, these disorders can be excluded or confirmed by proper NC studies.

Cervical spine disorders leading to chronic radiculopathies have a special relevance to EMG and NC studies. If there is a repetitive root compression or injury it will lead to a series of events that will have a repetitive nature, but will be cumulative. Usually a clinical examination is insensitive to mild cumulative changes because there will be no detection of weakness, sensory loss, or reflex abnormalities because the mild root injury will be compensated for by collateral reinnervation. Reinnervation occurs when the remaining noninjured nerve fibers sprout at the muscle level and reinnervate neighboring muscle fibers that were denervated by root injury or compression. Therefore, after 6 to 8 weeks there will be complete remission and no clinical signs of previous injury. When collateral reinnervation takes place, however, there is a reorganization of the motor units with a typical EMG signature of large neurogenic units. After the next mild injury, this process will be repeated and there will be more collateral reinnervation, with larger motor units and fewer separate units present. This process results in a paucity of motor units; the remaining units have large amplitudes as a sign that they are taking over fibers dropped by damaged (denervated) nerve fibers. A muscle biopsy of a patient with this condition would show typical changes in the fiber grouping. A less invasive EMG, however, can show the exact underlying nerve-muscle changes. The main importance of this concept is that after a certain number of relapses, or a large enough initial injury, there will be no reserve for collateral reinnervation. As a result, the next injury, which could be smaller than the initial injury, will lead to disproportionate clinical findings, such as weakness, that will be permanent. This situation is considered an exception to the neurologists' rule for nonsurgical treatment, and is an indication for surgery.

Several other disorders that may have similar primary symptomatology are treated nonsurgically. If there are incidental, coexisting cervical spine changes that are nonconsequential, surgery may be postponed or not performed. These situations include ulnar neuropathy at the elbow as opposed to chronic C8 and/or T1 radiculopathy, Parsonage-Turner brachial plexopathy as opposed to acute midcervical radiculopathy, monomelic amyotrophy as opposed to chronic low cervical radiculopathy, or carpal tunnel syndrome as opposed to C6 radiculopathy.

Lumbar spine pathology has been examined extensively using EMG and NC studies and results have shown a limited usefulness for these studies; however, despite such findings, extensive misuse of clinical neurophysiologic techniques has occurred. Spinal surgeons do not perform surgery based on EMG and/or NC findings; instead radiologic and morphologic techniques are used as a basis for a surgical plan. EMG and NC studies should not be used in an initial workup for patients with acute radiculopathy unless MRI and clinical findings do not correlate or the entire clinical picture is atypical. In these instances, an EMG and/or NC study can be useful in confirming particular disorders such as diabetic monoradiculopathy versus compressive disk pathology. Also, sensory-motor polyneuropathy can be present together with spinal pathology, especially in elderly patients. Polyneuropathy can be minimally symptomatic, or its clinical presentation can be confounded and dominated by spinal pathology. The appearance of bilateral foot numbness on the first postoperative day is not an unusual initial symptomatic presentation of an ongoing underlying polyneuropathy. This coincidental symptomatic presentation is inconsequential if it does not lead to emergency resurgery or to a series of urgent diagnostic tests. Therefore, EMG and/or NC studies may be used in a preoperative workup of a patient scheduled for potentially complex back surgery.

A well established "law" in clinical neurophysiology is that sensory nerve action potentials (SNAPs) are normal in radiculopathies. There have been rare descriptions of far lateral root compressions that may lead to a ganglion injury or dysfunction and can cause a drop in SNAP amplitude. This concept is convincing but clinically exceptional; therefore, it is not a mainstream concern. Another issue concerns the presence of scarce denervation in lumbar paraspinal muscles, mainly characterized by the finding of positive sharp waves in an otherwise normal appendicular EMG of a middle-aged or elderly patient. This condition should be considered a normal variant; however, such a finding is often labeled abnormal and specific root pathologies are inferred. This interpretation is widespread in the EMG and NC studies of patients with no-fault insurance plans and in patients treated nonsurgically, but not in other patient populations. In addition, there is no consensus that a proper single root abnormality can be diagnosed by using only a paraspinal EMG. Because appendicular abnormalities must be present for a definitive diagnosis, a mainstream neurophysiologist would label isolated paraspinal abnormality as a lumbosacral irritation. The anatomic concept of posterior rami injury is sensible; however, the translation of paraspinal abnormalities or

normal EMG paraspinal variants into the explanation concerning the cause of back pain is too simplistic and therefore misleading. Such a misconception could lead to unwarranted surgery.

Thoracoabdominal radiculopathies are rare and difficult to confirm. There has been progress in obtaining EMGs of abdominal and thoracic paraspinal muscles that provides an opportunity to confirm radiculopathy at any level of the spine. Further EMG studies are needed because the findings may be relevant for intraoperative monitoring for screw stimulation at the thoracic and upper lumbar levels.

## Somatosensory-Evoked Potentials

SSEPs have limited diagnostic use in spinal disorders. Despite their noninvasive character and potential for assessing every spinal segment, SSEPs are known to be nonsensitive and nonspecific. Nonspecificity can be improved by recording peripheral, spinal, and cortical responses simultaneously, which effectively localizes the site of the abnormality.

Unfortunately, there is no cure for the lack of sensitivity of SSEPs in spinal disorders. Abnormal SSEP results are seen only in patients with moderately severe radiculopathies in which clinical findings are clear. For patients with spinal cord injuries, SSEPs do not provide any more insight into a diagnosis than a thorough clinical examination. There is, however, one exception. In slowly progressing, chronic conditions such as lumbar spinal stenosis there is a cumulative characteristic of sensory abnormalities that is not clinically transparent; SSEPs can be useful in confirming or excluding other pathologies beyond spinal stenosis.

Although the application of SSEPs is somewhat limited, they are the single most important technique in neurosurgery and orthopaedic intraoperative monitoring. Knowledge and experience in using SSEPs exceeds that of all other intraoperative monitoring techniques.

## Intraoperative Monitoring

There are two main techniques in spine monitoring, SSEPs and motor-evoked potentials (MEPs). Significant advancements have been made in screw stimulation, although the traditional neurogenic MEPs (NMEPs) are now almost obsolete. Spinal cord direct recordings and stimulations are special forms of SSEPs and MEPs that are mainly used for monitoring during the removal of spine tumors.

### SSEPs in Intraoperative Monitoring

SSEPs have a long history of use in intraoperative monitoring, especially in scoliosis surgery. Since the late 1970s when lower extremity SSEPs were more thoroughly studied, intraoperative monitoring exploited the use of the fundamental principle of clinical neurophysiology—that the emerging lesion can be instantly detected if the presumed lesion is between the stimulating and recording setup along the assessed pathway. Therefore, any lesion between the wrist and the cortex, or between the ankle and the cortex (for tibial nerve stimulation), can be detected with routine median nerve stimulation. This concept is too simplistic because the extent of the lesion and the underlying pathology and pathophysiology of the lesion play a role in sensitivity as well as in timing the length of the period after occurrence that the injury or lesion can be detected.

Incremental advancements have taken place in the understanding and application of peroneal nerve stimulation. At first, the knee was stimulated, but it was soon discovered that the tibial nerve at the ankle is technically easier to approach. Because of less movement of the leg during stimulation and larger SSEP amplitude, this new placement produced more reliable cortical responses. Later, because of improvements in instrumentation and a continued expansion of knowledge of SSEPs, large peripheral nerves were stimulated, including the ulnar, radial, saphenous, peroneal nerve at the knee, and the superficial peroneal nerve at the ankle.

During the 1990s, so-called dermatomal SSEPs became popular and were primarily used to detect single root dysfunction along the spinal segments. As discussed previously, the use of these SSEPs failed because of sensitivity and specificity issues. However, the use of SSEPs provided an opportunity to expand intraoperative monitoring to different spinal segments and to other spine and orthopaedic surgeries. Although sensory nerves represent some dermatome, better responses are always obtained when stimulating the nerve instead of only the skin area within the presumed dermatome. Essentially, a sensory or mixed nerve is chosen that has a particular dermatomal distribution, such as the superficial peroneal nerve for L5 dermatome or the saphenous nerve for L4 dermatome. The size of the input plays a role, as these cortical responses are generally small and are adversely affected by anesthesia. The general rule that bigger is better holds true for intraoperative monitoring with SSEPs. Distal stimulation is usually more reliable because cortical representation for the hand and foot is larger and denser than, for example, the shoulder or upper thigh. The bigger the neuronal cortical generator, the larger are the SSEPs. It is not surprising that median and ulnar nerve stimulation at the wrist, and tibial nerve stimulation at the ankle produce the most reliable intraoperative monitoring responses and have the least amount of false positive results. This is again a much too simplistic explanation because other factors also are important—namely the pathway that is being tested in respect to the outcome that is being monitored.

Cortical SSEPs can be difficult to record in children, and especially in infants, because their brain is more sensitive to anesthetic agents. The electroencephalo-

graphic waves of children and infants can be of large amplitude and fluctuating, thus obliterating a small SSEP response in large electroencephalographic amplitude (electroencephalographic waves are considered biologic "noise" for SSEP recording). A reasonable substitute for use in thoracolumbar surgeries is simultaneous recordings of cervical spinal cord afferent sensory responses (cervical SSEPs). These responses are generated by passing axons that are less influenced by anesthesia, in contrast to the multisynaptic organization of the sensory cortex generators. However, these cervical SSEPs are much smaller because they are not generated by synapses and are usually recorded only with tibial nerve stimulation and not with stimulation of smaller segmental nerves or with dermatomal stimulation. Therefore, cervical SSEPs are useful in scoliosis surgery, but rarely useful in lumbar instrumentation. In adults, the distance from the dorsal column generator to the needle or surface recording electrode is larger than in children, resulting in inherently small cervical SSEPs that are unrepeatable and that consequently cannot be monitored. It is important to note that after upper extremity stimulation, cervical SSEPs (median nerve SSEPs) are both axonal and synaptic-dorsal horn, and therefore larger and easier to record. The complication arises from the fact that for cervical and cranial surgeries, cervical SSEPs represent input, as they are generated below the surgical site and therefore do not qualify for monitoring based on the fundamental principle that the potential injury site has to be between the stimulating and recording setup.

The primary concern in scoliosis surgery is postoperative leg weakness; however, sensory afferent pathways are tested with SSEPs. It is not surprising that isolated anterior spinal artery events that would lead to catastrophic paraplegia may not be detected by SSEPs. Fortunately, most spinal ischemic events caused by overcorrection in scoliosis surgery lead to some indirect changes of the sensory system. In this instance, changes in SSEPs, although temporary, can be seen and reported to the surgeon. If partial, sudden changes in SSEPs occur within 20 to 30 minutes of correction, these changes should prompt a reconsideration of the correction and an immediate wake-up test. Monitoring of the motor system is recommended to avoid false negative monitoring.

### Motor-Evoked Potentials
Recording of MEPs is not as simple as recording SSEPs. The first transcranial MEPs in humans were obtained in the mid 1980s, some 20 years later than SSEPs were first obtained. MEPs required different stimulation parameters, recording techniques, anesthesia, and essentially completely different intraoperative monitoring. For many years MEPs were considered high-risk proce-

dures, and the U.S. Food and Drug Administration and Institutional Review Board protocols interfered with progress in this field. Within the past 2 to 3 years, the U.S. Food and Drug Administration approved the Digitimer stimulator (Digitimer Ltd, Hertfordshire, UK) for clinical use, followed by approval for instruments from Axon Systems (Hauppauge, NY) and Cadwell Laboratories (Kennewick, WA). Today, the same intraoperative monitoring instrument can be used to record both SSEPs and MEPs without an additional stimulator, connections, or approvals.

Experience is important for monitoring MEPs and SSEPs. An incremental learning process is inherent to MEP monitoring. The larger the cortical motor representation of the muscle group, the easier it is to achieve a reliable response. Furthermore, intrinsic muscle responses of the hand are easiest to obtain. Leg responses are much more difficult to obtain; however, the densest corticospinal fibers are in the tibialis anterior and foot muscles, which provide the best opportunity to obtain leg responses. The tibialis anterior muscles can be used because foot drop is the most relevant deficit that can be detected. Reliable monitoring of upper extremity MEPs approaches the reliability of SSEPs (over 90%) in approximately 97% to 98% of surgeries that can be monitored. However, the yield of lower extremity MEPs, even in patients without preoperative neurologic deficit, is not much higher than 80%.

There are many reasons for these differences in reliability. The anatomy of the leg motor cortex, density of corticospinal fibers, and the age of the patient all play a role. The maturity of the motor system in regards to myelination and synaptic organization is even more critical in MEPs than for SSEPs. Lower extremity SSEPs are very difficult to record during the first 1 to 2 years of life, whereas MEPs often cannot be reliably recorded for intraoperative monitoring until the patient is 5 to 7 years of age. The type of anesthesia used in the surgery is a major factor that can be controlled. It is a requirement to use total intravenous anesthesia to reliably monitor MEPs. There are, of course, exceptions where consistent MEPs can be obtained with inhalation and combined anesthesia. This fact, however, does not justify the 25% to 30% yield of MEPs with inhalation or combined anesthesia compared with the at least 80% yield achieved with total intravenous anesthesia.

Transcranial MEPs are difficult to obtain in the lower extremities and it is impossible to use them for segmental motor-monitoring (for example, to differentiate reliably L3 from L5 dysfunction). However, in some patients, reliable multiple muscle-segmental MEP monitoring is possible. These patients represent an exception; therefore, the use of MEPs for segmental motor-monitoring are not considered a routine procedure. However, recordings from the deltoid or biceps brachii

muscle are feasible and are possible in cervical spine surgeries.

NMEPs are, conceptionally, completely different than transcranial MEPs. For some time, NMEPs have been used as a substitute for transcranial MEPs in scoliosis surgeries. It is important to note that NMEPs are not purely or mainly motor responses that are related to corticospinal tract function. Therefore, NMEPs are simply another modality similar to SSEP. Traditionally, NMEPs were used as an add-on technique to the routine SSEPs.

### Segmental Root-Pedicle Screw Stimulation

With the advent of the use of pedicle screws for lumbar instrumentation and the use of screws instead of hooks for scoliosis surgery there is a need for reliable monitoring of the proximity of the screw to the neighboring root. Imaging is always used; however, independent neurophysiologic confirmation of the proximity, or lack of root proximity, is desirable and considered routine monitoring. As with all other monitoring techniques, segmental root-pedicle screw stimulation is not a simple procedure. Reliable results of basic threshold behavior from different abdominal and paraspinal muscles for abdominal and upper lumbar segments do not exist. The approach and criteria for L4, L5, and S1 roots are extended to all other segmental levels without rigorous assessment of the potential for false negatives such as obtaining a high-passable threshold, even when a screw is close to the root. This situation can occur if the muscle that is being recorded has insufficient representation of the presumed root that is in the proximity to the stimulated screw. This situation occurs with multisegmental muscles, such as abdominal muscles.

A further explanation of false negativity and false positivity is needed. In general, personnel performing intraoperative monitoring are not concerned about false positive readings, unless they are very frequent. Sporadic false positive readings are a good test of emergency protocol, preparing anesthesiologists and surgeons to act promptly under emergency circumstances. False positive readings do not directly harm the patient, but may indirectly prolong the surgery, cause a modification of the surgical approach, or require a wake-up test for the patient. If false positive readings are recognized quickly, however, they keep the surgical team alert and ready to act when truly needed. When screw stimulation is used, there are no false positive readings if the technique is sound. A compound muscle action can be obtained if the corresponding root is stimulated. Therefore, an artificially low threshold cannot be obtained to qualify for false positive screw stimulation (for example, appearing closer to the root than in actuality). There are many instances where false negative readings can easily be obtained in a practice using daily intraoperative monitoring. For instance, if the electrode is not in the right muscle, or not close enough to muscle fibers (for example, in superficial fat tissue) a false negative reading can occur. The same result will occur if the recording electrode is electrically suboptimal (high impedance), or if the stimulating electrode has a partial contact. If more than the target screw is stimulated (for example, interconnecting rods and electrically nonconducting metal-like structures), an elevated threshold will occur. Consequently, the stimulation current would appear as a passable threshold, while the screw could be very close to the root.

Another important factor in segmental root-pedicle screw stimulation is neuromuscular blockade. If the components of anesthetic agents are analyzed separately, it appears that if blockade, halogenated inhalation agents, or nitrous oxide in high doses (over 50%) are administered, these anesthetic agents will promptly disappear from the bloodstream and will not influence monitoring. This result is an oversimplification of findings usually tested in small experimental animal models. In reality, MEPs and compound muscle actions in children and some adults can be depressed for a much longer time and in an unpredictable fashion. Therefore, it is a safe practice to exclude neuromuscular blockade from surgeries using MEPs and to allow at least 45 to 60 minutes of washout of the blocking agent before screw stimulation. Although reports exist that MEPs, screw stimulation, or similar modalities can be reliably monitored with almost any agent and combination, to eliminate or decrease false negative readings as much as possible, the use of total intravenous anesthesia and the absence of neuromuscular blockade should be the common practice.

A new trend in the manufacture of intraoperative monitoring instruments is to provide instrumentation that does not require the presence of a technician to perform intraoperative monitoring during screw stimulation. An assistant still needs to place electrodes and connect the stimulator, and the surgeon must stimulate the screw. The only advantage to these new systems is that the threshold can be measured by a computer algorithm and not manually by intraoperative monitoring personnel. The disadvantages are that the people preparing the recording may not be fully qualified, and the surgeon must trust the computer to provide the readings. This technique may be faster because there is less quality control. However, the important question concerns the reliability of this new technology. In the event of difficulties with the system, no one will be available to troubleshoot the problems. Properly trained personnel, versatile instruments that can monitor all needed intraoperative modalities, and adequate professional supervision are necessary.

## Annotated Bibliography

Jones SJ, Buonamassa S, Crockard HA: Two cases of quadriparesis following anterior cervical disectomy, with normal perioperative somatosensory evoked potentials. *J Neurol Neurosurg Psychiatry* 2003;74:273-276.

An uncommon failure of perioperative SSEP monitoring to detect iatrogenic lesions causing temporary quadriparesis during straightforward cervical surgery is discussed in this article. Despite the normally low incidence of false negative results, SSEP monitoring failed to detect an iatrogenic lesion causing moderate to severe, although temporary, motor impairment. Monitoring of MEPs may be considered an alternative to monitoring of SSEPs during anterior cervical procedures, whereas combined monitoring of SSEPs and MEPs may be the ideal.

Legatt A: D: Current practice of motor evoked potential monitoring: Results of a survey. *J Clin Neurophysiol* 2002;19:454-460.

Centers responding to a survey of MEP monitoring practices predominantly used transcranial electrical brain stimulation (TCES) with brief pulse trains and/or spinal cord stimulation to elicit MEPs; transcranial magnetic stimulation and single-pulse TCES were not techniques of choice. Most centers using TCES had patient exclusion criteria (for example, cochlear implants, cardiac pacemakers, prior craniotomy or skull fracture, history of seizures). Adverse effects included rare tongue injuries or seizures from TCES, and minor bleeding from needle electrodes in muscle. MEPs suitable for monitoring were obtained in about 91.6% of patients overall. Most of the failures were attributed to technical factors; preexisting neurologic dysfunction precluded MEP monitoring in approximately 1.7% of patients. Almost all centers monitored SSEPs concurrently with MEPs. SSEPs and MEPs should be used together for optimal monitoring of the spinal cord.

Legatt AD, Emerson RG: Current practice of motor evoked potential monitoring: It's about time. *J Clin Neurophysiol* 2002;19:383-386.

This article discusses motor evoked potential monitoring and current practices.

## Classic Bibliography

Ben-David B, Haller G, Taylor P: Anterior spinal fusion complicated by paraplegia: A case report of a false-negative somatosensory-evoked potential. *Spine* 1987; 12:536-539.

Beric A: Transcranial electrical and magnetic stimulation, in E Niedermeyer, Lopes da Silva F (eds): *Electroencephalography.* Baltimore, MD, Williams & Wilkins, 1999, pp 836-850.

Chiappa KH: *Evoked Potentials in Clinical Medicine,* ed 2. New York, NY, Raven Press, 1990.

Dawson EG, Sherman JE, Kanim L, et al: Spinal cord monitoring: Results of the Scoliosis Research Society and the European Spinal Deformity Society Survey. *Spine* 1991;16:S361-S364.

Dumitru D, Dreyfus P: Dermatomal/segmental somatosensory evoked potential evaluation of L5/S1 unilateral/unilevel radiculopathies. *Muscle Nerve* 1996; 19:442-449.

Dumitru D: *Electrodiagnostic Medicine.* Philadelphia, PA, Hanley & Belfus Medical Publishers, 1995.

Jones S: Somatosensory evoked potentials II: Clinical observations and applications, in Halliday AM (ed): *Evoked Potentials in Clinical Testing,* ed 2. London, England, Churchill Livingstone, 1992, p 421.

Jones SJ, Harrison R, Koh KF, Mendoza N, Crockard HA: Motor evoked potential monitoring during spinal surgery: Responses of distal limb muscles to transcranial cortical stimulation with pulse trains. *Electroencephalogr Clin Neurophysiol* 1996;100:375-383.

Kimura J: *Electrodiagnosis in Disease of Nerve and Muscle: Principles and Practice,* ed 2. Philadelphia, PA, FA Davis, 1989.

Kothbauer, KF, Deletis V, Epstein FJ: Motor-evoked potential monitoring for intramedullary spinal cord tumor surgery: Correlation or clinical and neurophysiological data in a series of 100 consecutive procedures. *Neurosurg Focus* 1998;4:1-17.

Nuwer MR, Dawson EG, Carlson LG, Kanim LE, Sherman JE: Somatosensory evoked potential spinal cord monitoring reduces neurologic deficits after scoliosis surgery: Results of a large multicenter survey. *Electroencephalogr Clin Neurophysiol* 1995;96:6-11.

Zornow MH, Grafe MR, Tybor C, Swenson MR: Preservation of evoked potentials in a case of anterior spinal artery syndrome. *Electroencephalogr Clin Neurophysiol* 1990;77:137-139.

# Chapter 9

# Differential Diagnosis of Spinal Disorders

Christopher G. Furey, MD

## Introduction

The treatment of patients with spinal disorders begins with formulation of the appropriate diagnosis. It is essential to correlate the subjective and objective presentation with the pertinent findings from imaging studies and diagnostic modalities to reach the correct diagnosis. With the dramatic advancements of neuroimaging technology and their increased accessibility, physicians may tend to rely too heavily on imaging modalities in the course of patient evaluation. However, the appropriate diagnosis can usually be made based on conclusions derived from obtaining an in-depth medical history and a careful physical examination.

## History

The location of pain and its duration, severity, nature of onset, and aggravating factors help identify its etiology. Complaints of neck or back pain should always be clarified to identify associated arm or leg pain, paresthesias, or weakness. The duration and progression of symptoms over time should also be considered. Response to prior intervention, whether surgical or conservative, may frequently be overlooked in patients during their initial evaluation. Patient age, occupation, and activity level are frequent correlating factors in establishing diagnoses. Pertinent features of the medical history are especially important in establishing the correct diagnoses, especially when nonspinal entities play a role in pain or weakness.

## Physical Examination

A comprehensive physical examination is of utmost importance in all patients presenting for evaluation of spinal disorders. Initially, a general assessment of a patient should be made, with attention to identifying body habitus, general degree of vitality, and emotional appearance. Gait is easily evaluated and should be the first specific task requested of every patient. Inspection of each spinal region should be made to assess for alignment, deformity, and surgical scars. Active and passive motion should be assessed for the cervical, thoracic, and lumbosacral regions of the spine. Evaluation of each limb should include identification of deformity, joint range of motion, and muscle symmetry. A detailed neurologic examination should be conducted in both the upper and lower extremities and include assessment of muscle strength and sensation as well as reflex testing, including assessment of pathologic reflexes. Rectal tone and perineal sensation should be evaluated, especially in patients with acute neurologic deterioration. A vascular examination should include identification of pulses as well as skin temperature, color, and the quality and presence of ulcers. An abdominal examination is of particular importance to assess for the presence of masses, pulsations, adenopathy, tenderness, and occult causes of acute low back pain.

## Lumbar Spine

### Acute Low Back Pain

Low back pain is ubiquitous and ranks second only to upper respiratory infection in the frequency of requests for medical attention. Approximately 80% of the adult population will experience an episode of acute low back pain. The source of pain can be any musculoskeletal component of the spinal column. Pain may originate from the paraspinal musculature and tendons, longitudinal ligaments, facet joints, bone, intervertebral disks, and neural elements. The duration, severity, and presence of an inciting event are the most helpful features in identifying a cause.

Acute low back pain most commonly originates from a soft-tissue structure. Muscular strain or ligamentous sprain resulting from overuse or acute injury typically manifests as severe, self-limited pain with restricted mobility. These episodes often follow a particular inciting event. The branches of the sinuvertebral nerve innervate both the posterior longitudinal ligament and the anulus fibrosus; acute stretching of the posterior longitudinal ligament or tears in the anulus fibrosus are frequent causes of acute low back pain. Patients may frequently describe either a previous occurrence of acute low back pain or a history of chronic, episodic low back pain. Radiculopathy is generally associated with acute mechanical low back pain. Patients may experience referred gluteal muscular pain, which can be ipsilateral or bilateral; however, true radicular pain or paresthesias traveling below the buttock in a dermatomal pattern does not typically occur. A patient with an acute disk herniation may present with a prodrome of acute low back pain; however, the onset of radicular symptoms begins several days following the acute low back pain. Most mechanical pain occurs diffusely across the lumbar region with bilateral spasms. However, inflammation or injury of an isolated facet joint may cause more localized, ipsilateral pain, which is frequently referred to as a facet syndrome. Ipsilateral local tenderness over a fact joint that reproduces a patient's specific report of pain can confirm this particular diagnosis.

Aggravation of lumbar spondylosis is a common occurrence, typically in patients with a history of chronic, intermittent back pain. Exacerbation of axial low back pain is frequent and may be associated with overuse or minor injury. Again, true radiculopathy is uncommon in patients with isolated mechanical low back pain. In the absence of high-energy trauma, fractures of the lumbar spine are an uncommon cause of acute low back pain. In contrast, osteoporotic vertebral body compression fractures are increasingly more common with the aging of the population. These fractures can occur spontaneously or as a result of trivial or low-energy injuries. Abrupt onset of severe low back pain in an older patient or in a patient with risk factors for osteoporosis may indicate the presence of an acute compression fracture. Acute radiculopathy is not common in patients with osteoporotic fractures because retropulsion of bone into the spinal canal or neural foramen rarely occurs. However, preexisting spinal stenosis or deformity may be aggravated by an acute compression fracture and may produce more accelerated radicular symptoms.

Expansile lesions, whether infectious or neoplastic, weaken or disrupt bone to the point of fracture, elevate the longitudinal ligaments, and can compress neural elements. Special concern should be given to patients with acute low back pain when clinical symptoms raise the possibility of an underlying malignant neoplasm or infection. When vertebrae are affected by tumor or infection, pain is most often indolent, progressive, and severe. Night pain in particular is a red flag for the presence of a malignant neoplasm. Associated systemic reports of fever, chills, weight loss, loss of appetite, or malaise should heighten suspicion when these symptoms occur in conjunction with acute low back pain.

Although uncommon, visceral sources are serious causes of acute low back pain that require a high degree of suspicion and timely evaluation and intervention. Aortic aneurysm dissection, intra-abdominal or pelvic malignancy, pancreatitis, appendicitis, and peptic ulcer disease may have initial symptoms of acute, severe low back pain. Such diagnoses should be considered when specific history and physical examination findings suggest their presence.

Sacral insufficiency fractures typically affect elderly, osteoporotic individuals and manifest as severe low back and pelvic pain without true radiculopathy and generally with no inciting event. Diagnosis is best done with a high degree of suspicion and confirmed with MRI.

The sacroiliac joint is an uncommon source of low back pain. Pain caused by inflammation, injury, or arthrosis of the sacroiliac joint may cause ipsilateral, localized low back and buttock pain. Radiation may occur with change in position from sitting to standing or with rapid ambulation. Diagnosis is suggested by localized tenderness or with provocation by Patrick's test (fabere sign), in which pain is produced by flexion, abduction, and external rotation of the ipsilateral hip. Fluoroscopic-guided cortisone injections with cortisone and local anesthetic serve both diagnostic and therapeutic purposes.

### Lumbar Radiculopathy

Radicular leg pain and paresthesia is caused by irritation of lumbosacral nerve roots, with distribution occurring in a dermatomal fashion. Acute onset radiculopathy is most commonly the result of a disk herniation and typically affects young adults in the third and fourth decades of life. Direct mechanical pressure and chemical irritation of nerve roots have been implicated as causes for the resultant nerve response. Patients frequently report the spontaneous onset of severe leg pain, often with a prodrome of low back pain. Less commonly, a history of trivial trauma is reported as an inciting event. Radicular pain, usually with associated paresthesias, travels from the low back and buttock into the thigh, calf, and foot in a dermatomal fashion. Varying degrees of weakness may be noted both subjectively and objectively. Patients will often describe a sense of lower extremity weakness, but none is noted on objective evaluation. Additionally, acute sciatica may also preclude accurate assessment of motor strength during physical examination when patient cooperation is limited by pain. Symptoms from an acutely herniated disk are exacerbated by maneuvers that increase intrathecal pressure such as coughing, sneezing, and straining with bowel movements. Frequently, sitting is more bothersome than standing or walking in patients with acute sciatica.

Radiculopathy should be distinguished from localized buttock pain that is referred from an inflamed facet joint or anulus fibrosus pathology. These entities cause acute low back and buttock pain, but typically not radicular pain that travels into the thigh or below the knee.

Acute radiculopathy generally is unilateral, although central disk herniation may cause bilateral symptoms. A large lumbar disk herniation with severe compression of the thecal sac can produce the signs and symptoms of cauda equina syndrome. This entity is composed of severe back and leg pain, with varying degrees of leg weakness (unilateral or bilateral), decreased perineal sensation, and disturbance of bowel and bladder function. Emergent neuroimaging and surgical decompression is indicated in patients with cauda equina syndrome.

Less commonly, pathology within the retroperitoneum (such as tumor, abscess, or hematoma) will compress the lumbosacral plexus, causing acute radicular pain similar to that associated with an acutely herniated disk. Spontaneous retroperitoneal hematoma resulting from excessive anticoagulation is a rare cause of acute leg pain that should be addressed with prompt diagnosis and managed nonsurgically with correction of any persistent coagulopathy.

Chronic radicular pain is the result of nerve irritation commonly caused by spondylitic changes associated with spinal stenosis. Although patients may experience classic neurogenic claudication, radicular pain may also be seen with isolated or multilevel foraminal and lateral recess stenosis. If more than one level is involved, symptoms may occur at multiple dermatomal levels. Degenerative synovial cysts arising from facet joints can produce severe lateral recess and foraminal stenosis with resultant ipsilateral radicular symptoms. MRI is effective in identifying this less common type of stenosis. Patients with nerve-based tumors, both intradural and extradural, may present with varying degrees of radicular pain and neurologic deficit and require imaging with contrast (MRI or myelogram) to assist in distinguishing nerve-based tumors from extradural nerve compression caused by disk pathology and spondylytic changes.

### Piriformis Syndrome

Piriformis syndrome is an uncommon cause of radicular symptoms in which the sciatic nerve is directly compressed by the piriformis muscle, fibrous bands, or a leash of blood vessels distal to the sciatic notch. Patients with piriformis syndrome will report buttock and leg pain and paresthesias that are frequently exacerbated by prolonged sitting. Patients will report localized buttock tenderness with palpation of the sciatic notch or piriformis fossa. Tension signs, such as the straight-leg raise or femoral nerve stretch test, are negative. Appropriate diagnosis requires exclusion of lumbar pathology, MRI of the piriformis region, and diagnostic injection.

### Coccydynia

Coccydynia is localized pain in the coccyx that is frequently chronic and severe. Pain is aggravated with pro-

longed sitting on firm surfaces. Radiation generally does not occur proximally into the back or distally into the leg, but it may travel to the buttock or ischial tuberosity in either an ipsilateral or bilateral fashion. Localized, superficial tenderness or reproduction of pain with manipulation of a mobile coccygeal segment during rectal examination are common in patients with coccydynia. Plain radiography is rarely of diagnostic benefit, but increased signal on bone scanning typically correlates with the area of inflammation responsible for the pain. Localized injection with fluoroscopic guidance may be of both diagnostic and therapeutic benefit.

### Hip Pathology

Hip pathology can occasionally be confused with radiculopathy. Hip pain caused by arthritis, osteonecrosis, or labral pathology is generally localized to the groin, with extension to the anterior thigh. Pain is worse with weight bearing, climbing steps, or squatting to sit at a low level. Hip pathology is associated with an antalgic gait and limited, painful range of motion noted during physical examination. Hip pathology is not associated with the tension sign that occurs in patients with acute radiculopathy. Diagnostic injection, typically with fluoroscopic guidance, is an excellent tool to distinguish pain from upper lumbar nerve root compression and hip arthrosis causing groin and radiating thigh pain.

### Neurogenic Claudication

Lumbar spinal stenosis causes characteristic symptoms of leg pain and fatiguing with ambulation known as neurogenic claudication. Stenosis occurs most commonly in older patients who may also experience a varying degree of chronic, mechanical low back pain. Patients with neurogenic claudication are able to ambulate varying distances before leg pain becomes intolerable. Leg pain is generally eased by sitting or assuming a flexed posture (as occurs with pushing a grocery cart, walking up an incline, or pedaling a stationary bike). The flexed posture slightly increases the spinal canal diameter, thus transiently decreasing compression of the neural elements. The leg symptoms of spinal stenosis are generally not acute and may fluctuate over time. Acute deterioration of symptoms or function is uncommon. However, lumbar radiculopathy may coexist with neurogenic claudication if acute nerve root compression occurs with foraminal stenosis.

### Vascular Claudication

Vascular claudication caused by arterial insufficiency of the lower extremities is also a cause of leg pain that should be distinguished from spinal stenosis. The leg pain in vascular claudication occurs with ambulation, but it is often relieved simply by stopping and standing; riding a stationary bike in a flexed posture will not affect the leg pain. In addition, patients with vascular claudication may have leg pain at night that requires sitting and dangling the legs at the bedside. Consideration of a vascular etiology should also be given to patients with risk factors of vascular disease elsewhere, as well as patients who smoke and those with diabetes and hypertension.

### Chronic Low Back Pain

Chronic low back pain without radiculopathy is most commonly caused by degenerative conditions. The evolution of spondylosis typically begins in the third decade of life and progresses at varying rates in each patient. It is generally agreed that the degenerative process begins with the disk space, with dehydration and subsequent loss of disk height. With collapse of the disk space, osteophyte formation occurs. Facet arthrosis and ligamentum flavum hypertrophy develop to further restrict mobility and also may cause encroachment of the spinal canal and neural foramen. The symptoms include episodic low back pain and stiffness, which is often exacerbated by simple activity, slow to resolve, and frequently recurrent. In the absence of associated spinal stenosis, leg pain is not a feature of chronic mechanical back pain. In some patients, a specific pain generator may be identified. Facet syndrome is isolated low back pain caused by inflammation of an individual facet with resulting discrete, ipsilateral pain and occasional radiation into the buttock. Discrete facet block may help to address this entity diagnostically and therapeutically. When spondylosis is more diffuse, specific identification of the pain generator may not be possible.

Patients with chronic low back pain are often obese, have limited muscle mass, have poor aerobic conditioning, use tobacco, and have medical comorbidities. Although degenerative changes are not reversible, patients should be advised that addressing these aggravating factors can have a significant beneficial effect on chronic low back pain.

Special caution should be used when evaluating patients with chronic low back pain and potential secondary gain issues, which may benefit them if their pain is ongoing. Workers' compensation claims, personal injury litigation, and narcotic and muscle relaxant abuse are frequently encountered in such patients. The Waddell signs include five physical signs exhibited by patients with a nonorganic source for their pain. Nonorganic tenderness occurs in a nonanatomic distribution or with exaggerated response to light touch. Simulation tests are used to imply to a patient that a specific test is being performed, when in fact it is not; a positive response occurs when pain is recreated with axial rotation of the spine or compression on the top of the head. Distraction tests attempt to reproduce pain with maneuvers when a patient is distracted; for example, exaggerated pain is elicited during a supine straight-leg lift that is not repro-

duced when a patient extends the hip and knee while in a sitting position. Regional, nondermatomal disturbances of strength or sensation may be encountered and cannot be explained on a neuroanatomic basis. Finally, gross exaggeration of symptoms with emotional overreaction to benign maneuvers is the most common and statistically relevant Waddell sign.

When chronic low back pain is associated with any red-flag features, including weight loss, malaise, appetite loss, chronic cough and hemoptysis, change of bowel or bladder habits, and fevers or chills, consideration should be given to an accompanying neoplastic (vertebral metastatic disease) or infectious (diskitis/vertebral osteomyelitis) process.

## Cervical Spine
### Acute Neck Pain

Neck pain, like low back pain, is a source of discomfort experienced at some point by nearly every adult. The most common acute cause is soft-tissue injury or inflammation, which is generally the result of muscular or ligamentous strain. Aggravation of underlying degenerative conditions frequently occurs and can have sudden onset without preceding trauma. Such pain is generally self-limited, associated with limited motion, but not with radicular symptoms. Occasionally, pain will radiate in a sclerotomal (as opposed to dermatomal) pattern, traveling to one or both trapezial regions. Such pain can be anxiety provoking for some patients, but it generally resolves within days to weeks. This mechanical type of pain is relieved with anti-inflammatory medications, moist heat, and short periods of immobilization in a soft collar. When such localized acute neck pain persists or worsens over a period of several weeks or true radiculopathy is present, then the patient should be assessed for the presence of a more serious condition.

Acute cervical strain (whiplash) with neck pain and stiffness is often caused by motor vehicle accidents, typically rear-end collisions. Symptoms may be noted initially, but frequently it is not until a day later when the onset of the pain occurs. A constellation of symptoms can accompany whiplash injuries, including cervicothoracic or trapezial pain, headache, dysesthesias, paresthesias, and persistent stiffness. In most low-energy injury collisions, skeletal injuries or acute disk herniation are uncommon. However, plain radiography is justified to evaluate patients with persistent neck pain. Severe, persistent axial neck pain, true radiculopathy, or neurologic abnormalities may require the use of more advanced diagnostic imaging.

When axial neck pain is indolent or progressively severe, more ominous etiologies must be considered. Primary neoplasms and metastatic disease are less common in the cervical spine than elsewhere in the axial skeleton, but when they do occur, they can produce varying degrees of bone destruction, deformity, instability, and neurologic compromise. Neck pain in an individual with a history of malignancy or associated with malaise, cachexia, and weight loss should be evaluated with plain radiography and advanced diagnostic imaging to exclude the involvement of a malignant neoplasm.

Vertebral osteomyelitis and diskitis can be encountered in the cervical spine, but they are a less common cause of persistent, severe, progressive neck pain with associated evidence of bone destruction. An epidural abscess is a life-threatening entity that should be considered in an ill individual with severe neck pain with or without myelopathy or paralysis. Diagnosis is confirmed with MRI. An epidural abscess should be treated surgically with decompression from an anterior or posterior approach depending on the location of the abscess in relation to the spinal cord.

Visceral causes of neck pain, although rare, can occur. Tumors in the head and neck regions can cause axial neck pain, whereas involvement in or adjacent to the brachial plexus may cause radicular symptoms. Observation of neck masses, asymmetry, or adenopathy on examination may indicate the presence of an extraspinal problem. Coronary disease that can cause ischemia and result in neck pain similar in nature to angina is referred to as cervical angina.

## Cervical Radiculopathy

Radicular arm pain is most commonly caused by nerve root compression within the cervical spine. The source of compression is related to the acuity of the symptoms. Acute radiculopathy (dermatomal) is generally the result of a soft disk herniation. Most acute disk pathology occurs in a posterolateral fashion, causing varying degrees of nerve compression, but frequently referred pain will cause guarding that is exhibited as weakness. An acute foraminal disk herniation with severe nerve root compression may cause severe, radiating chest pain that can be confused with a cardiac or pulmonary condition.

Chronic cervical radiculopathy is generally caused by spondylosis, with disk and osteophyte complexes that result in varying degrees of central and neuroforaminal stenosis. Symptoms are frequently bilateral, depending on the location and severity of the underlying spondylosis. Chronic radiculopathy is usually accompanied by some degree of neck pain and limited motion. Facet arthrosis and degenerative disk disease may also contribute to headaches, which will frequently be an additional symptom of patients with chronic radiculopathy.

## Compressive Neuropathies of the Upper Extremities

Nerve compression elsewhere in the upper extremity may be confused with symptoms of cervical radiculopathy. Thoracic outlet syndrome, cubital tunnel syndrome, and carpal tunnel syndrome cause pain, paresthesias, and occasionally muscle weakness in the arm and hand. Double crush syndrome exists when more than one area of nerve compression exists simultaneously. Obtaining a thorough medical history and provocative findings on physical examination should be the first means in establishing a diagnosis.

Cervical radiculopathy is supported with a positive Spurling's test, in which radicular symptoms are reproduced with head compression when the neck is extended and rotated toward the side with radicular symptoms. A positive distraction test may help confirm cervical radiculopathy when axial distraction of the head and neck transiently relieves arm symptoms.

Thoracic outlet syndrome is implicated with a positive Adson's test, in which the radial pulse is diminished when the head is rotated toward the affected side while the arm is abducted, extended, and externally rotated. Similarly, a Tinel's sign at the cubital tunnel or at the carpal tunnel with a positive Phalen's test suggest nerve compression at the elbow or wrist, respectively. Neurodiagnostics may assist in diagnosis, but should be used to support rather than be the sole basis for a diagnosis.

## Brachial Plexus Pathology

Tumors or vascular anomalies around the shoulder girdle may cause compression or disruption of the brachial plexus, with resulting neurologic symptoms of the upper extremities. When persistent pain, paresthesias, or weakness occur without obvious cervical lesions, a brachial plexus lesion may be present. Diagnosis is generally confirmed with advanced imaging of the shoulder girdle using either MRI or CT.

Brachial neuritis or Parsonage-Turner syndrome is diagnosed in patients with symptoms of acute, unremitting pain originating from the shoulder girdle. The pain is ipsilateral, may radiate proximally into the neck and distally into the arm and forearm, and is frequently associated with weakness. The onset of pain is spontaneous and the etiology is unclear. Although the symptoms are self-limited and begin to resolve within weeks to months, the motor deficits can persist for more than 1 year before recovery begins. Advanced diagnostic imaging should be used to exclude the presence of compressive lesions within the cervical spine or brachial plexus. Neurodiagnostic testing can be used to assist with the diagnosis and assess the degree of recovery.

## Shoulder Pathology

Shoulder pathology may produce symptoms similar to those of cervical radiculopathy. Some patients may have components of both cervical radiculopathy and shoulder pathology. Rotator cuff problems can cause localized shoulder pain with radiation into the upper arm in addition to painful, limited motion. In general, rotator cuff pathology does not cause pain to radiate below the elbow, nor will it produce paresthesias. Large rotator cuff tears are frequently associated with significantly decreased range of motion and loss of strength. Glenohumeral arthrosis, with or without rotator cuff pathology, will cause pain, disturbance of function, and loss of motion. Plain radiography can be used to confirm the presence of shoulder pathology in patients with glenohumeral arthrosis. Diagnostic shoulder and subacromial injections with local anesthetic and corticosteroids can be of use both diagnostically and therapeutically in patients with shoulder pain.

### Cervical Myelopathy

The presence of cervical myelopathy should be considered in patients with unexplained extremity weakness, gait abnormality, or loss of coordination and dexterity. Spondylitic myelopathy is the most common cause of these symptoms; it typically occurs in older patients with degenerative changes within the cervical spine. Congenital canal stenosis can predispose certain patients to spinal cord compression and subsequent myelopathy. Acute, centrally herniated disks, if large enough, can produce spinal cord compression and myelopathy, although most disk herniations are smaller and posterolateral and responsible for radiculopathy instead.

Myelopathy is often indolent and not appreciated by the patient. Because neck and arm symptoms are not prominent features of cervical myelopathy, a patient may not seek medical care until neurologic symptoms are severe. A family member commonly becomes aware of the presence of weakness or gait abnormalities more so than the patient. Myelopathy can occur acutely because of large, soft cervical disk herniations, especially in young adults with rapidly progressive neurologic deficits.

Myeloradiculopathy is diagnosed in patients with pain and paresthesias in dermatomal fashion who also experience or display the signs and symptoms of myelopathy.

### Central Nervous System Disorders

Global weakness and gait abnormality should raise concern for the presence of inherent neurologic disorders in patients in whom spinal cord compression is not identified with neuroimaging. Demyelinating disorders (primarily multiple sclerosis) may present with previously unknown weakness, coordination problems, or bowel and bladder dysfunction. Pain may not be prominent in patients with demyelinating disorders. Transverse myelitis, which is thought to be a precursor of multiple sclerosis, may mimic radiculopathy with acute pain or paresthesias involving upper or lower extremities.

The symptoms of amyotrophic lateral sclerosis (Lou Gehrig's disease) include upper and lower extremity weakness in adults, without associated pain, which is similar to the presentation of patients with cervical spondylitic myelopathy. In contrast, patients with amyotrophic lateral sclerosis do not have the signs or symptoms of sensory abnormalities present with myelopathy.

### Summary

The correct diagnosis for most patients with spinal disorders can be obtained with a careful patient history and physical examination. Imaging modalities should be used judiciously to confirm the clinical diagnosis.

### Annotated Bibliography
#### History
Carragee EJ, Alamin TF, Miller J, et al: Provocative discography in volunteer subjects with mild persistent low back pain. *Spine J* 2002;2:25-34.

In this study, 36% of volunteer subjects who were not seeking medical attention for mild low back pain were found to have significant, concordant pain using diskography. The prevalence of concordant responses in minimally symptomatic volunteers questions the role of diskography in identifying clinically relevant pathology.

Soehle M, Wallenfang T: Spinal epidural abscesses: Clinical manifestations, prognostic factors, and outcomes. *Neurosurgery* 2002;51:79-87.

The authors provide a comprehensive, contemporary review of the features, potential diagnostic pitfalls, and expectations of surgical treatment of spinal epidural abscesses.

Tay B, Deckey J, Hu S: Spinal infections. *J Am Acad Orthop Surg* 2002;10:188-197.

The authors provide a current review of the clinical features of spinal osteomyelitis, diskitis, and epidural abscesses, with a discussion of appropriate diagnostic and treatment strategies.

#### Physical Examination
Dreyfuss P, Dreyer SJ, Cole A, Mayo K: Sacroiliac joint pain. *J Am Acad Orthop Surg* 2004;12:255-265.

The authors of this comprehensive review of sacroiliac pathology emphasize the etiology of the disease and discuss conservative and surgical management.

#### Lumbar Spine
Maigne JY, Chatellier G: Comparison of three manual coccydynia treatments: A pilot study. *Spine* 2001;26:E479-E484.

This is an insightful study of different techniques for the management of coccydynia by two authors with extensive experience in this area.

Miller P, Kendrick D, Bentley E, Fielding K: Cost-effectiveness of lumbar spine radiographs in primary care patients with low back pain. *Spine* 2002;27:2291-2297.

The authors of this prospective, randomized study found no difference in clinical outcomes in patients with low back pain who were referred for plain radiography on presentation to a primary care clinic and those who did not undergo radiography. Patient satisfaction, however, was greater in patients who had radiographs.

Modic M: Degenerative disc disease: Role of imaging. *Semin Spine Surg* 2001;13:258-267.

The author, a preeminent spinal radiologist, provides a detailed review of the imaging features of disk disease with emphasis on clinical correlation.

Schimandle JH, Boden SD: Cervical radiculopathy, in *Surgery of the Cervical Spine*, ed 1. Philadelphia, PA, WB Saunders, 2003, pp 89-111.

This is an exhaustive, contemporary review of cervical radiculopathy, its diagnosis, and treatment.

*Cervical Spine*

Bronfort G, Evans R, Nelson B, et al: A randomized clinical trial of exercise and spinal manipulation for patients with chronic neck pain. *Spine* 2001;26:788-799.

The authors of this prospective, randomized study found that an exercise regimen, with or without a highly technical program, was superior to manipulation in the treatment of a patients with chronic neck pain.

Vad VB, Bhat AL, Lutz GE, et al: Transforaminal epidural steroid injections lumbosacral radiculopathy: A prospective randomized study. *Spine* 2002;27:11-16.

The authors conducted this prospective, randomized study to compare fluoroscopic-guided, steroid nerve blocks with saline trigger point injections in patients with radiculopathy caused by disk herniation. They reported that significant improvement was noted with steroid injections, which supports their use as diagnostic and therapeutic tools.

## Classic Bibliography

Boden SD, Davis DO, Tina TS, et al: Abnormal magnetic resonance scans of the lumbar spine in asymptomatic patients: A prospective investigation. *J Bone Joint Surg Am* 1990;72:403-408.

Frymoyer JW: Back pain and sciatica. *N Engl J Med* 1988;318:291-300.

Lees F, Turner JW: Natural history and prognosis of cervical spondylosis. *Br Med J* 1963;5373:1607-1610.

Macnab I (ed): *Backache*. Baltimore, MD, Williams and Williams, 1977.

Von Korff M: Studying the natural history of back pain. *Spine* 1994;19(suppl. 18):2041S-2046S.

Waddell G, McCullough JA, Kummel E, et al: Nonorganic physical signs in low back pain. *Spine* 1980;5:117-125.

Weber H: Lumbar disc herniation: A controlled, prospective study with ten years of observation. *Spine* 1983; 8:131-140.

# Chapter 10

# Nomenclature and Coding

Bernard A. Pfeifer, MD

## Introduction

Proper treatment of the patient with spinal disorders requires correct communication on many levels. The physician must understand the nature, location, and character of the patient's symptoms in the context of cultural and social issues that may impact the patient's condition. Systematic and consistent recording and synthesis of the patient's symptoms and physical findings to a concise diagnosis is mandatory. This information must be communicated to the other members of the health care team in a commonly accepted language. If studies are to be used for guidance, consistent nomenclature must be used for comparison. With the expansion of the health care system, reimbursement as appropriate for the treatment rendered relies on correct conversion of the name (analog) to codes (digital) that can be used for mass processing of claims as well as large-scale demographic studies.

## Nomenclature

The North American Spine Society (NASS), along with the American Academy of Orthopaedic Surgeons, published a nomogram in an attempt to bring some consistency to the nomenclature. As with any first efforts, further improvements to clarify certain controversial topics, treatment recommendations, and standardization of classification and reporting were identified. A combined task force of NASS, the American Society of Neuroradiology and the American Society of Spine Radiology addressed these issues and their recommendations were published in 2001.

The following is a synopsis of some important concepts. A functional spinal unit consists of the vertebra and disk, and in strict terms is the bone-disk-bone at a single level. Parts of this unit that are anterior to the posterior longitudinal ligament are considered anterior structures (vertebral body, anterior longitudinal ligament, and disk). The posterior structures include the pedicles and lateral masses, transverse processes, zygoapophyseal joints (facet joints) consisting of the superior articulating process of the vertebra below and the

inferior articulating process of the vertebra above, pars interarticularis, lamina, spinous process, facet capsule, and interspinous ligaments. Nerve roots, cauda equina, and spinal cord are posterior but usually not considered posterior elements per se; muscle may be either posterior or anterior but usually is not discussed in this manner. The interlaminar space defines the space separating the lamina of adjacent segments and the term translaminar is considered less accurate in describing this area. The intervertebral foramen or neuroforamen defines the space through which the spinal nerve exits and for full description requires the level above and below as a prefix. Stenosis of the neuroforamen then would compress a single nerve root while a central stenosis compromises the vertebral canal and the spinal cord or cauda contained therein. By convention, less than one third occlusion of the cross-section of central canal is considered mild, one third to two thirds occlusion is considered moderate, and over two thirds occlusion of the section is considered severe.

Describing disk pathology has been the focus of much of the confusion of nomenclature. The guiding principle in describing the disk image is to avoid implying etiology. The disk has an anulus fibrosus consisting of laminates of collagen surrounding a proteoglycan nucleus. For description of the radiographic appearance, it is considered a two-dimensional structure having four quadrants. By convention, a focal herniation involves less than 25% of the circumference, a broad-based herniation between 25% and 50%, and a symmetric bulging disk 50% to 100%. The edges of the bony ring apophysis define the peripheral margin of the disk; the vertebral end plate (actually the terminal fibrocartilage portion of the disk) defines the cephalad and caudad extent of the disk. An intervertebral herniation is extension of disk material into the vertebral body beyond the limit of the end plate; for example, a Schmorl's node. Peripheral herniation can be divided into protrusion or extrusion. Protrusion is where the distance between the edges of the displaced disk material in any plane is less than the amount of displacement; that is, there is no waist to the displacement. Extrusion is where this distance is less in any one plane. Extrusion may be called sequestration if continuity between the fragment and the disk is lost and migration if it is displaced away from the area of extrusion with or without continuity with the remaining disk. A complete radiographic description of a disk herniation includes listing this morphology: whether it is contained within the anulus fibrosus, in continuity with the main disk, how it relates to the posterior longitudinal ligament, the volume herniated, and the composition and location of the herniation.

The NASS document recommended the term annular fissure be used rather than tear because the latter implied a traumatic etiology. However, the consensus document shows that the two terms are considered synonymous.

Invasive studies such as diskograms (diskography) may be required in addition to history and physical examination to evaluate the clinical relevance of these tears as well as high-intensity zones seen in the anulus fibrosus on MRI scans.

As the disk ages, fibrous tissue replaces nuclear material, the disk height is maintained, and the disk margins are maintained. These actions may be considered part of a normal process. The presence of anterior and lateral osteophytes also should be considered normal. The term applied to this normal aging process is spondylosis deformans. Significant radial tearing, gas within the center of the disk, narrowing of the disk space, end-plate erosions with osteosclerosis, bone marrow changes, and posterior osteophytes are signs of a pathologic disk degeneration. Degenerative disk disease is a clinical syndrome characterized by these morphologic changes and the symptoms thought to be related to them. Internal disk disruption is a symptom complex with the following criteria: no visible disk herniation may be seen on MRI or CT; during provocation diskography injection of the suspect disk with contrast must 'recreate' the patient's exact back and leg pain, and injection of at least one disk above or below the suspect disk must be nonpainful (a 'control disk'); grade 3 or 4 radial annular fissure must be demonstrated on CT diskography.

In order for a disk to be described as herniated, there must be a localized displacement of the nucleus or annular material beyond the disk space. A disk bulge is a generalized extension beyond the edges of the apophyses that usually extends greater than 50% of the circumference but is less than 3 mm beyond the edge of the apophysis. A disk protrusion describes a herniation and may be focal when it involves less than 25% of the circumference of the disk, or broad based when more than 25% is involved. Extrusion implies the material is forced through an opening. A sequestered disk has had its base severed from the parent structure, and may also be described as a free fragment. Containment of a disk fragment is defined by its relationship to the anulus fibrosus. Subligamentous, extraligamentous, and trans-

ligamentous or perforated refer to the relationship of the disk fragment to the posterior longitudinal ligament.

## Coding

As stated earlier, in order to understand a problem and apply statistical analysis, a correct method of classification is required. The International Classification of Diseases (ICD) is designed to classify morbidity and mortality for indexing of hospital records, statistical analysis, and data storage and retrieval.

This classification has undergone revisions approximately every 10 years; the ninth revision is in current use. The World Health Organization developed the system in collaboration with 10 international centers for the purpose of ensuring that the medical terms on death certificates are comparable and are appropriate for statistical analysis. As the practice of medicine becomes more complex, there will be the need for further refinement of these classification systems.

ICD-9 has three broad categories: diagnoses, procedures, and complications. It is designed to codify all of medicine from neoplasm to signs, symptoms, and ill-defined conditions. There are 17 chapters to the current volume of more than 8,000 codes. Each code has a main three-digit set followed by a decimal and a two-digit subset. Accuracy requires that all digits be completed. An example is herniated intervertebral disk:

722    Intervertebral disk disorders
722.1  Displacement of thoracic or lumbar intervertebral disk without myelopathy
722.10 Lumbar intervertebral disk without myelopathy. Lumbago or sciatica due to displacement of intervertebral disk
722.11 Thoracic intervertebral disk without myelopathy

The ICD-9 classification is available in three volumes. These are best used by looking up the alphabetical index first and then looking to the numeric code list for the optimal codes. This classification system is limited, especially for research. There is no laterality (left or right), acuity rating, or accommodation of temporal sequencing. In addition, this classification was not designed for outcomes, there is little logical or regional organization (no spine section), and there are very nonspecific codes. Nonetheless, it is the currently accepted system used for billing and reimbursement. To correct these shortcomings, ICD-10 has been introduced and was to have a gradual implementation from 1995 to 2003. It is also a three-volume set with 2,033 categories, 855 more than ICD-9. The categories are now alphanumeric six-character codes; the chapters have been rearranged and increased from 17 to 23. Notable changes include the addition of information relevant to managed care and ambulatory encounters, expanded injury codes, combination diagnosis and symptom codes, common fourth- and fifth-digit subclassifications, and laterality. An example of an ICD-10 code would be:

S12.1    Fracture of the second cervical vertebra
S12.10   Nondisplaced fracture of the second cervical vertebra
S12.11   Displaced fracture of the second cervical vertebra

The limited implementation of the ICD-10 system is probably related to reticence in changing the current computer billing systems already in place. Implementation will be based on the process for adoption of standards under the Health Insurance Portability and Accountability act of 1996 (HIPPA) and will have a 2-year window after publication in the Federal Register. As of this date, that has not happened.

Included in the ICD-9 system is a procedure code list. This is a four-digit system classifying surgical and other procedures. ICD-9 Procedure Coding System (PCS) is currently used for reporting under part A of Medicare; the part that applies to hospital reimbursement. It is not as specific as the American Medical Association's Current Procedural Terminology (CPT) codes. There are significant differences in the two systems that do not allow strict correlation and hence make database comparison complicated.

An example of the ICD-9 PCS code for hemilaminectomy for disk herniation is as follows:

80.51    Excision intervertebral disk
         Diskectomy
         Removal of Herniated Nucleus Pulposus
         Level:
             Cervical
             Thoracic
             Lumbar (lumbosacral)
         That by Laminotomy or hemilaminotomy
         That with decompression of spinal nerve root at same level
         Requires additional code for any concomitant decompression of
             Spinal nerve root at different level from excision site

For total laminectomy, one code covers many procedures, for example:

03.09    Other exploration and decompression of the spinal canal
         Decompression
             Laminectomy
             Laminotomy
             Expansile laminoplasty
             Exploration of spinal nerve root
             Foraminotomy

In comparing the two choices, one could ask should the codes 80.51 or 03.09 be used for the total laminectomy with facetectomy foraminotomy at the same level?

Most practitioners are familiar with the American Medical Association (AMA)-CPT as it is the current source of physician codes for procedures done for patient care, including evaluation and management. An agreement signed between the AMA and the Health Care Finance Administration (HCFA) in 1983 required the use of CPT for the reporting of physician's services. In 1986 this requirement was extended to state governments under the Medicaid program.

CPT is a five-digit system codifying the procedures done by physicians organized on a specialty basis. The procedures related to the structural spine (bone) are in the 20000 code series that are assigned to orthopaedic surgery. Hence, a one-level lumbar fusion without instrumentation would be coded 22612 with the addition of a bone graft code with either 20937 (iliac crest morcellized graft) or a 20936 (local bone graft). Codes for decompression of the neural elements would be in the 60000 series of codes assigned to neurologic surgery. A hemilaminectomy for disk would be coded 63030 whereas the total laminectomy for central stenosis with foraminotomy would be 63047.

This code system is dynamic and changes can be implemented. Any individual or organization can petition the AMA's CPT Editorial Panel for a code to describe a unique procedure. Procedures should be accepted (not experimental) and have peer-reviewed literature to support their use. Once the code has been applied for, the committee circulates requests for comments to all the member organizations. The editorial panel meets three times a year and seeks the input of both the applicant and the member representatives (CPT advisors). If a code is accepted, it will be placed in the CPT book for the following cycle (usually the calendar year). The committee has the option of designating a tracking code to a procedure are there are not enough data to consider the procedure mainstream.

Once a code has been designated, a relative value must be assigned. This is done by the Centers for Medicare and Medicaid Services (CMS) and published in a final rule generally released in the fall of the year. The AMA's Relative Value Update Committee (RUC) is the body responsible to advise the CMS on the appropriate value of a given procedure. The RUC consists of 23 members appointed by major national societies, 3 rotating seats whose members change every 2 years, chairs of the RUC, Practice Expense Advisory Committee, and the Health Professionals Advisory Committee, and AMA, American Osteopathic Association, and CPT Advisory Committee representatives for a total of 29 members. The committee meets three times a year. Once a code has been assigned, a level of interest form is circulated to the societies. Interest can include (1) to actively survey its members to create a code value, (2) commenting on the value suggested, or (3) no interest at all. The RUC has developed a survey instrument whereby the procedure is described in general terms and the surveyed person is asked to value both the time and intensity and select a comparison code from a list. For codes with a global period (all work in the care of the patient for either 0, 10, or 90 days); an additional request is asked for the number and levels of postoperative visits. These data are analyzed by a consensus panel of members of the societies that have expressed level one interest previously, and a summary form is submitted to the RUC for discussion. The RUC meeting is an open session attended by representatives of CMS, and the RUC will make a recommendation. Although CMS makes the ultimate decision and can seek whatever input it desires, this symbiosis between it and the RUC has resulted in over 95% of the RUC's recommendations being accepted by CMS.

This discussion applies only to the work component of the relative value unit (RVU) assigned to a code. The practice expense component RVU recommendation usually comes from a 'cross walking' of the practice expense from standards or from reference codes. Data upon which this is based comes from practice expense surveys performed in the past by the AMA with exceptions presented to the full RUC. The liability component of the RVU recommendation is made in a similar fashion.

CMS is mandated by Congress to review the values assigned to all codes every 5 years. This review is done with the RUC's cooperation and input.

HIPPA, when passed by Congress, changed significantly the complexity and stake of the practitioner in billing and coding issues. The legislation stated that the physician was responsible for correct coding (even if done by another individual or contractor) and allowed repercussions including triple damage fines and jail for incorrect coding. However, it is hoped that the need for good outcome assessment will motivate the physician to ensure that the codes used are correct. Each procedure that is performed must be associated with a correct, complete diagnosis. Any number of systems is available from both the professional societies as well as commercial entities.

The important financial consideration for optimal office practice is to have a closed loop system where the diagnosis code and the procedure code are submitted and the reimbursement tracked. Most insurance companies will send an Explanation of Benefits, a letter sent if there was believed to be an error of either type of code not supported by the chart documentation. The practitioner, to ascertain the accuracy of coding as well as the accountability of the insurer, should review Explanation of Benefit letters.

Correct coding facilitates registries of surgeries performed. Combined with results (especially maintained using standardized outcomes instruments), these registries can be especially helpful in internal performance reviews to maintain a level of excellence and assess new techniques. In addition, they can be powerful in negotiations with third-party providers.

## Annotated Bibliography

Fardon DF, Milette PC: Nomenclature and classification of lumbar disc pathology: Recommendations of the combined task forces of the North American Spine Society, American Society of Spine Radiology, and American Society of Neuroradiology. *Spine* 2001;26:E93-E113. Also on the web at http://www.asnr.org/spine_nomenclature/Discterms-dec_14.shtml. Accessed January 2006.
The information provided is the product of a three-society work group to be used as a reference for concise description of disk images.

American Medical Association: *Medicare RBRVS*. Chicago, IL, American Medical Association, 2005.
This text is an annual update of CPT codes and their values.

Fasciszewski T: Nomenclature and coding, in Fardon DF, Garfin SR (eds): *Orthopaedic Knowledge Update: Spine 2*. Rosemont, IL, American Academy of Orthopaedic Surgeons, 2002, pp 135-138.
A review of the coding system and its uses is presented.

## Classic Bibliography

Fardon DF (ed): *Disorders of the Spine: A Coding System for Diagnosis*. Philadelphia, PA, Hanley and Belfus, 1991.

Fardon DF, Herzog RJ, Mink JH, Simmons JD, Kahanovitz N, Haldeman S: Appendix: Nomenclature of lumbar disk disorders, in Garfin SR, Vaccaro AR (eds): *Orthopaedic Knowledge Update: Spine*. Rosemont, IL, American Academy of Orthopaedic Surgeons, 1997.

United States Department of Health and Human Services: *International Classification of Diseases Ninth Revision, Clinical Modification*, ed 5. Washington, DC, 1998; adapted and published by Practice Management Information Corporation, Los Angeles, and by St. Anthony's Publishing Company, Alexandria, Virginia, 1999.

# Chapter 11

# The Importance of Outcome Assessment in Orthopaedics: An Overview

Robert J. Gatchel, PhD, ABPP

Nancy D. Kishino, OTR, CVE

Alan Strezak, MD

## Introduction

In the United States, health care costs continue to increase at an alarming rate. Changes in health care policy and demands for better allocation of health resources resulted in greater pressure being placed on health care professionals to provide the most cost-effective treatment of pain-disability syndromes and to validate treatment efficacy. As a result, treatment-outcome monitoring has gained new importance in health care. Several publications are available to guide health care professionals in effectively conducting outcome assessments. Clinical research is important, with the concomitant increased emphasis on the use of well validated outcome measures. Monitoring of outcomes is important for three major reasons: (1) It is now customary for health care professionals to be monitored to determine the effectiveness of the treatments they provide, as well as patient satisfaction with these treatments. Often, a "scorecard" is maintained by third-party payers to monitor practitioners' efficacy. According to a recent study, many insurance companies require health care professionals to follow best-practice guidelines; however, not enough data are available to establish these guidelines. (2) Outcomes data are needed not only to provide third-party payers with demonstrations of treatment efficacy, but also can be used as an important marketing strategy to highlight the effectiveness of a particular treatment program. (3) Health care professionals also need to monitor such outcomes for quality assurance purposes within their own practice to maintain high-quality service.

Unfortunately, many health care professionals do not have the requisite background in conducting program or treatment evaluations because of a lack of knowledge about outcome methodology and statistical tools needed for such assessments. The purpose of this chapter is to provide an overview of the basic tools needed for such an evaluation, as well as to examine some of the important concepts involved in outcomes assessment.

## The Biopsychosocial Approach to Assessment

Before discussing outcome assessment methodology, it is important to first review the most commonly used and heuristic perspective to the understanding, assessment, and treatment of pain/disability disorders: the biopsychosocial model. This model views physical disorders, such as pain and disability, as the result of a complex and dynamic interaction among physiologic, psychologic, and social factors that perpetuate and may even worsen the clinical presentation. Each patient experiences pain or disability uniquely, as a result of the range of psychologic, social, and economic factors that can interact with physical pathology to modulate that patient's report of symptoms and subsequent disability. The development of this biopsychosocial approach has grown rapidly during the past decade. One recent study highlighted how people differ significantly in the frequency that they report physical symptoms, in their tendency to visit physicians when experiencing identical symptoms, and in their responses to the same treatments. Often, the nature of a patient's response to treatment has little to do with his or her objective physical condition. Disease is a term used to define an objective biologic event that involves the disruption of specific body structures or organ systems caused by anatomic, pathologic, or physiologic changes. Illness, in contrast, is generally defined as a subjective experience with self-attribution that a disease is present. An illness will produce physical discomfort, behavioral limitations, and psychosocial distress. Thus, illness refers to how a sick patient and their family members live with, and respond to, symptoms and disability. The distinction between disease and illness is analogous to the distinction made between pain and nociception. Nociception involves the stimulation of nerves that convey information about tissue damage to the brain. Pain, on the other hand, is a more objective perception that is the result of the transduction, transmission, and modulation of sensory input. This input may be filtered through a person's genetic composition, prior learning history, current physiologic status, and sociocultural influences. Pain or disability, therefore, cannot be comprehensively assessed without a full understanding of the individual who was exposed to the nociception. The biopsychosocial model focuses on illness, which is the result of a complex interaction of biologic, psychologic, and social factors. Thus, with this perspective, diversity in pain and illness expression (including its severity, duration, and psychosocial consequences) can be expected. The interrelationships among biologic changes, psychologic status, and the sociocultural context all need to be considered to fully understand the patient's reception and response to illness. The model for an assessment-treatment approach that focuses on only one of these core sets of factors will be incomplete.

With this biopsychosocial perspective in mind, several important issues need to be considered when determining the various measures to be used in outcomes assessment. Three broad categories of measures—physical, psychologic, and socioeconomic—have all been used to assess pain and disability. However, these three major measurement categories, or biopsychosocial referents, may not always be in agreement with one another when measuring pain or disability. Therefore, if a self-report measure is used as a primary index of pain and compared with the overt behavioral (some functional activity) or physiologic index of the same pain, direct overlap among all three measures cannot be expected. In addition, two different self-report measures of the same pain may not be as highly correlated as desired.

## Important Psychometric Properties of Assessment

Before discussing specific assessment methods, it should be noted that the common denominator of all such assessment methods is the quality of validity, reliability (reproducibility), and predictive value. Misunderstandings often arise over the appropriate use of assessment based on the ability to generalize the scientific reports of validity to the circumstances in which the provider is using the assessment method. These ambiguities can be minimized by examining the match between the clinical context in which a test is evaluated and the patient to whom it is applied in the clinical setting: the validity of a test is addressed by answering the question "valid for what?" For example, assessment methods may be valid for measuring specific biologic/physiologic states, but have no validity in predicting work readiness or risk of morbidity, impairment, disability, or mortality. In addition, the results of a test may or may not be valid for informing or clarifying treatment planning or work readiness. Moreover, within the confines of validity, the properties of accurate identification of test-positive (sensitivity) or test-negative (specificity) patients may be clinically important. At that point, predictive values (the sensitivity and specificity adjusted for disease prev-

alence in the population where the test is used) is the meaningful property that helps to direct assessment and treatment. A brief review of these basic concepts is presented in Table 1.

## General Illness Status Self-Report Measures

The Medical Outcomes Study 36-Item Short Form (SF-36) was developed for various uses in clinical practice and research. It is a good global index of patient functioning: it measures the functional status of the whole patient. It has good psychometric properties and is becoming a favorite tool of third-party payers for outcomes monitoring of patients with chronic medical conditions. The SF-36 has eight scales that measure health concepts: physical function; role limitation because of physical health problems; bodily pain; social functioning; general mental health; role limitation because of emotional problems; vitality; and general health perception. There are also two global summary or component scales: a physical component summary scale and a mental component summary scale. Low scores on the mental component scale are usually a good index of potential emotional distress; low scores on the physical component scale are usually a good index of potential physical function limitations. The advantages of the SF-36 are that it is brief (taking approximately 10 to 20 minutes to complete), and it divides health into distinct physical, social, and mental health components. An even shorter form, SF-12, is available. One shortcoming, however, is that the actual clinical usefulness of the SF-36 with individual patients is not well established because of the test's psychometric properties. However, it can be used to monitor overall group changes.

Before the popularity and widespread use of the SF-36, the Sickness Impact Profile was commonly used because it was designed to document the disability behavioral impact across a wide range of groups and illnesses of varying types and severities. It consists of 136 items contained within 12 scales ranging from physical, psychosocial, and independent (such as home management) categories. The Sickness Impact Profile measures characteristics such as self-care, emotional functioning, ambulation, and household, work, and other activities. It has good psychometric properties, but has been replaced by the shorter SF-36 measure which provides comparable assessment information but takes less time to administer.

## Disease-Specific Self-Report Measures
### The Oswestry Low Back Pain Disability Questionnaire

The Oswestry Low Back Pain Disability Questionnaire has strong psychometric properties and is the oldest and most thoroughly researched instrument designed to assess functional status and disability. Several studies have shown the Oswestry questionnaire to be an effective

## Table 1 | Important Psychometric Properties of a Test

| | |
|---|---|
| Reliability | Refers to the reproducibility of a test from one administration to the next. It can be expected that if a test is administered at two points in time, with no major intervening circumstances possibly affecting the construct or dimension that is being measured (eg, pain report or functioning), then the test-retest reliability should be high. If not, there may be flaws in the test that make it less than acceptable for use. |
| Validity | Refers to the appropriateness and usefulness of a particular test or measurement in making an inference about an individual's behavior (eg, the level of pain being experienced). If a test was designed to measure pain, then it should tap that quality. There are, in turn, different types of validity. |
| Predictive validity | Refers to whether test scores can predict subsequent measures or behaviors. For example, will a high score on Pain Test A predict whether a patient will require a greater amount of pain management? |
| Concurrent validity | Refers to whether test scores are correlated with other current measures or behaviors. For example, is a high score on Pain Test A correlated with the amount of pain medication that the patient is now taking, or to his or her level of activities of daily living, and so on? |
| Content validity | Refers to whether test scores are representative of the quality being measured. This is usually evaluated by having experts in the field of pain agree that a measure or test of pain is actually evaluating that quality. |
| Construct validity | Somewhat abstract and difficult to define. A construct is a theoretical phenomenon, such as anxiety, pain, intelligence, temperament, and so on. Construct validity is concerned with the extent to which a test relates to some objective behavior, as well as to the particular theoretical model at hand. Because of this two-way relationship between theory and practice, construct validity is actually a process. It serves both as a check on theory and as a spur to the same theory. For example, for the construct of pain, the theorist seeks to develop a measure of pain. Lacking a specific criterion, however, the theorist may have to use certain behaviors as indicators of pain (eg, self-report, grimacing, inability to work, pain medication use, etc). It may then be possible to formulate and test hypotheses about how pain, as it is measured on a test, does or does not relate to other behaviors in particular situations. On the basis of the findings, the theorist then progressively revises and refines the construct. Construct validation, therefore, involves systematically testing and revising hypotheses about a construct by examining the empirically found relationships among responses in different situations. It is a form of hypothesis testing and theory building. |
| Sensitivity | Refers to an important property of accurate identification of a test—test positive. That is to say, how many individuals who have a particular characteristic being evaluated by a test actually come out positive for that characteristic on the test. Sensitivity will be low if there are many "false positives" on the test. |
| Specificity | Related to sensitivity, but refers to how many individuals who do not have a particular characteristic being evaluated by a test actually come out negative for that characteristic on the test. Specificity will be low if there are many "false negatives" on the test. |

self-report instrument in detecting clinically meaningful change. However, several studies suggest a possible floor effect, such that extremely low scores may not be as accurate as more moderate or high scores. Also, most currently available disability indices (including the Oswestry questionnaire) focus primarily on the physical activities of daily living, with only minimal attention given to psychosocial concerns. In fact, no items on the Oswestry questionnaire directly inquire about the patient's emotional or psychologic state, despite the fact that research has indicated that psychologic factors play an integral role in the development and maintenance of disability.

### The Roland-Morris Disability Questionnaire

The Roland-Morris Disability Questionnaire has 24 items that help evaluate a patient's physical abilities, such as dressing, walking, and lifting. An abbreviated form consisting of only 11 items has recently been developed. The Roland-Morris Disability Questionnaire was originally intended to be used for research purposes, but it subsequently was found useful in clinical practice. It was derived from the 136-item Sickness Impact Profile, which was developed as a generic health status indicator for use in a variety of chronic diseases, but not specifically for back or musculoskeletal injury. Although the validity and reliability of the Roland-Morris Disability Questionnaire have been proven over time, the responsiveness of the instrument has been the subject of some scrutiny. It has been shown to be the least responsive measure to clinically meaningful change when compared with other prominent indices of functional status. In addition, the Roland-Morris Disability Questionnaire is less sensitive at detecting change when disability is classified as severe, likely a shortcoming that can be attributed to the two-level response format of the questionnaire.

### The Million Visual Analog Scale

The Million Visual Analog Scale (MVAS) is a 15-item measure designed to assess disability and physical functioning, and is useful primarily for patients with chronic low back pain disorders. It provides a simple, easy to understand format for patients. The instrument has been

## Table 2 | Various Categories of Physical Measures of Function

**Range of Motion**
  Two-inclinometer technique
  Three-dimensional digitizer

**Spine Strength**
  Biodex back attachment (Biodex Medical Systems, Shirley, NY)
  Cybex trunk extension-flexion unit (Lumex Corp, Ronkonkoma, NY)
  Isostation B-200 (Isotechnologies, Inc, Hillsborough, NC)
  Kin-Com Device (Biodex)
  Loredan Products back system (Biodex)
  Med-X cervical extension machine (Med-X 96 Inc, Ocala, FL)
  Med-X lumbar extension machine lifting capacity (Med-X 96 Inc)
  Cybex lift task
  Employment Potential Improvement Corporation lift capacity test
    (EPIC, Ballwin, MO)
  Ergonometric strength testing unit (EPIC)
  Loredan Products lift (Biodex)
  Progressive isoinertial lifting evaluation (PILE, Medline@cos.com)
  Work evaluation systems technology II unit (WEST) other tests of
    human performance capacity (WEST, Ft. Bragg, CA)
  Aerobic capacity
  California Functional Capacity Protocol (CAL-FCP, EPIC)
  Employment and Rehabilitation Institute of California (ERIC) Work
    Tolerance Screening

**Battery**
  Functional Capacity Evaluation (FCE)
  Treadmill exercise tolerance

the focus of few studies since its development and, as a result, very little is known about the psychometric properties of the MVAS outside of the results from the original validation study. In a recent study, MVAS scores were used to categorize patients into one of six groups: no reported disability (score of 0); mild disability (score of 1 to 40); moderate disability (score of 41 to 70); severe disability (score of 71 to 100); very severe disability (score of 101 to 130); and extreme disability (score of 131 to 150). Using this categorical method, it was found that this measurement was related to several important outcomes such as treatment dropout rate and level of depression, as well as 1-year socioeconomic outcomes (such as work return rate, work retention, and postrehabilitation surgeries). These results indicate that the use of the MVAS scores as categorical indices is effective in predicting treatment outcomes in patients with chronically disabling spine disorders.

### Pain Disability Questionnaire

One measure recently developed as a new measure of functional status that shows great promise for monitoring change in chronic musculoskeletal disorders is the Pain Disability Questionnaire (PDQ). The measurement of clinical outcomes is an essential element of any mus-

culoskeletal treatment. The PDQ yields a total functional disability score ranging from 0 to 150. The focus of the PDQ, much like other health inventories, is primarily on disability and function. Unlike most other measures, the PDQ is also designed for the full array of chronic disabling musculoskeletal disorders, rather than purely low back pain alone. Psychosocial variables, which recent studies have shown to play an integral role in the development and maintenance of chronic pain disability, form an important core of the PDQ. The psychometric properties of the PDQ are excellent, demonstrating stronger reliability, responsiveness, and validity relative to many other existing measures of functional status, such as the Oswestry, MVAS, and SF-36 instruments. A factor analysis of the PDQ revealed two independent factors that can be evaluated: a functional status component and a psychosocial component. Analyses demonstrated each of these two components to be valid in assessing their theorized constructs.

### Other Measures

Other indices, such as the Waddell Disability Index, the Low Back Outcome Score, the Quebec Back Pain Disability Scale, or the Functional Rating Index show promising beginnings, but have a small body of related literature in comparison to the Oswestry and Roland-Morris instruments. These less studied measures primarily assess activities of daily living, while placing little emphasis on psychosocial factors. Because of the lack of studies investigating these measures or describing their psychometric properties, their usefulness has not been sufficiently confirmed.

## Physical Measures of Functional Performance

Drawing from earlier summaries of various measures used for the quantification of physical function, a comprehensive overview of the various measures that can be used for documenting functional performance in patients, as well as the advantages and disadvantages of these various measures, has been compiled. Most of these measures are related specifically to spinal disability conditions, but many can also be used for other orthopaedic conditions. Table 2 lists the general categories, as well as the more specific tests in each category, that can be used.

## Objective Socioeconomic Outcome Evaluation Methods

Even before the increased interest in outcome assessment, some authors believed that the systematic tracking of socioeconomic outcomes was the best approach to document the effectiveness of a treatment program. This approach has helped other clinical researchers in their attempts to objectively evaluate treatment outcomes. Table 3 presents the basic dimensions and elements of the objective monitoring of socioeconomic outcomes.

## Assessment of Treatment Helpfulness

With the increased federal government scrutiny of health care utilization in the treatment of medical conditions over the past decade, there has now been an increased emphasis on evaluating patient satisfaction with this treatment as an important outcome measure. Thus, it is incumbent upon health care professionals to monitor patient satisfaction/perceived helpfulness of treatment as an important outcome variable. It should also be noted that measures of patient satisfaction correlate highly with treatment compliance and outcome. In addition, patient satisfaction can be an important variable in determining the economic success of a clinic. Because of these important issues, professional organizations such as the American Pain Society have recommended that the evaluation of patient satisfaction should be one feature of a total quality assurance program in pain settings. However, the measurement of patient satisfaction has received very little attention in the literature to date, attesting to the fact that there has been no widely used standardized measure of this variable until recently. In response to this need, the Treatment Helpfulness Questionnaire was developed as a reliable and valid measure for evaluating patients' perceptions of the helpfulness of various treatment modalities administered in multidisciplinary pain centers. The Treatment Helpfulness Questionnaire consists of patients' ratings along a 10-point scale (ranging from -5 for "extremely harmful" to +5 for "extremely helpful"). A "neutral" rating yields a score of zero. All scores are then calculated to the nearest tenth of a point. The following components of the treatment program are individually rated on this 10-point scale: the whole program; medical assessment and treatment; psychology assessment and treatment; physical therapy assessment and treatment; office visits with physicians; individual psychological therapy; medical diagnostic tests (tomography, electromyography); medical work abilities testing (functional capacity, impairment); patient education groups; and group counseling. The modalities can vary depending on the nature of the specific program and the goals of the evaluation and, thus, can be incorporated into the questionnaire.

## Formal Statistical Analysis of Assessment Outcomes

Once psychometrically sound outcome data are collected, the next major task is appropriate statistical analysis of these data. Unfortunately, many health care professionals do not have a background in conducting

**Table 3 | Major Socioeconomic Outcome Measures Used to Evaluate Effectiveness of Functional Restoration Effectiveness**

**Return-to-Work**
Work return
Work retention (at 1 year)

**Health Care Utilization**
Surgery to injured musculoskeletal area
Percent of patients visiting a new health care provider (continued care-and-documentation-seeking behaviors)
Number of visits to new health care providers

**Recurrent (Same Musculoskeletal Area) or New (Different Area) Injury Claims**
Percent with recurrent or new injury claims
Percent with injury claims involving work absence (lost time)

**Case Closure**
Resolution of legal/administrative disputes over permanent partial/total impairment or disability resulting from occupational injury
Resolution of related disputes (third-party personal injury or product liability claims)
Resolution of financial claims arising from perceived permanent disability (long-term disability, social security disability income, etc)

program or treatment evaluations because of the requisite experimental methodology and statistical tools needed for such evaluations. A database with appropriate psychometrically sound measures to use at baseline and follow-up evaluations should be established. Such data then need to be statistically analyzed. Templates or easy-to-follow reviews are now available for conducting treatment-outcome evaluations, and use of these materials is highly recommended. It also is highly recommended to gain familiarity with two basic statistical packages: SAS (Statistical Analysis System) and SPSS (Statistical Package for the Social Sciences). Both are PC-compatible and include manuals that provide a helpful guide for applying the various statistical techniques. Finally, most academic institutions have a biostatistician available for consultation. Such an individual can provide invaluable assistance in the initial design of an outcome study/program, as well as the final statistical analysis of the results.

## Summary

Treatment-outcome monitoring is essential in health care. Several helpful publications have been developed to guide health care professionals in effectively conducting outcome assessments. There are three important purposes for such outcome monitoring: to determine the effectiveness of the treatments provided; as a potentially important marketing strategy to highlight the effectiveness of one's treatment program; and for internal monitoring of outcomes for quality assurance purposes in one's own practices that will allow changes needed to maintain high-quality service. The biopsychosocial model is now the most widely used and heuristic perspective to the understanding, assessment, and treatment of pain/disability disorders. With this biopsychosocial perspective in mind, several important issues were considered when determining the various measures to be used in outcome assessment, such as the psychometric properties of reliability and validity. Once psychometrically sound outcomes data are collected, an important next task is to apply appropriate statistical analyses to the outcomes data.

## Annotated Bibliography

### General

Bourne RB, Maloney WJ, Wright JG: An AOA critical issue: The outcome of the outcomes movement. *J Bone Joint Surg Am* 2004;86-A:633-640.

This article reports the conclusions of an outcomes symposium sponsored by the American Orthopaedic Association and highlights the fact that the current outcomes movement revolutionized clinical research. There is now a demand for well validated outcomes measures.

Deyo RA: The role of outcomes and how to integrate them into your practice, in Herkowitz HN, Dvorak J, Bell G, Nordin M, Grob D (eds): *The Lumbar Spine*. Philadelphia, PA, Lippincott Williams & Wilkins, 2004.

This chapter emphasizes the importance of obtaining patient outcomes in a consistent manner. Guidance is provided concerning the use of a standard battery of instruments for measuring several dimensions of patient outcome.

Gatchel RJ: *A Compendium of Outcome Instruments for Assessment and Research of Spinal Disorders*. La Grange, IL, North American Spine Society, 2001.

This text discusses the most psychometrically sound measures and devices that can be used for measuring outcomes in patients receiving spinal care. Descriptions of the test, references, and examples of use are provided.

Gatchel RJ, Oordt MS: *Clinical Health Psychology and Primary Care: Practical Advice and Clinical Guidance for Successful Collaboration*. Washington, DC, American Psychological Association, 2003.

The important role of evidence-based outcomes in medicine is reviewed. Some of the most reliable measures that can be used in different medical specialties are presented.

Jackson DW: Quality orthopaedics: New incentives to practice "evidence-based medicine." *Orthopaedics Today* 2004;24:3.

This article discusses the fact that many third-party insurance payers are now demanding objective data that appropriate 'best practice' treatment guidelines followed by health care professionals.

Morley S, Williams AC: Conducting and evaluating treatment outcome studies, in Turk DC, Gatchel RJ (eds): *Psychological Approaches to Pain Management: A Practitioner's Handbook*. New York, NY, Guilford, 2002.

This chapter provides a comprehensive review of the best methodology to use in evaluating treatment outcomes, specifically in the area of pain and disability.

Pfeifer BA, Wong DA: Outcomes assessment and guidelines of care, in Fardon DF, Garfin SR, Abitbol JJ, Boden SD, Herkowitz HN, Mayer TG (eds): *Orthopaedic Knowledge Update: Spine 2*. Rosemont, IL, American Academy of Orthopaedic Surgeons, 2002.

With the increased demand for outcome assessment and reliable treatment guidelines, this chapter provides an overview of how to meet this demand.

Spratt KF: Outcomes assessment: Overview and specific tools, in Herkowitz HN, Dvorak J, Bell G, Nordin M, Grob D (eds): *The Lumbar Spine*. Philadelphia, PA, Lippincott Williams & Wilkins, 2004.

This chapter provides important information about how health care professionals can effectively conduct treatment outcomes assessments.

### The Biopsychosocial Approach to Assessment

Turk DC, Monarch ES: Biopsychosocial perspective on chronic pain, in Turk DC, Gatchel RJ (eds): *Psychological Approaches to Pain Management: A Practitioner's Handbook*. New York, NY, Guilford, 2002.

This chapter provides an overview of the biopsychosocial perspective of chronic pain. Physical disorders (pain and disability) are viewed as the result of a complex interaction among physiologic psychologic, and social factors that may perpetuate and even worsen the clinical presentation.

### Important Psychometric Properties of Assessment

Gatchel RJ: *Clinical Essentials of Pain Management*. Washington, DC, American Psychological Association, 2004.

This text provides a comprehensive review of the best assessment and treatment approaches in pain management.

### Disease-Specific Self-Report Measures

Anagnostis C, Mayer TG, Gatchel RJ, Proctor T: The Million Visual Analog Scale: Its utility for predicting tertiary rehabilitation outcomes. *Spine* 2003;28:1051-1060.

This study documented the clinical sensitivity of categorizing patients into one of six groups: no disability, mild disability, moderate disability, severe disability, very severe disability, and extreme disability. This method is more clinically meaningful than assigning a numerical score.

Anagnostis C, Gatchel RJ, Mayer TG: The development of a comprehensive biopsychosocial measure of disability for chronic musculoskeletal disorders: The Pain Dysfunction Questionnaire. *Spine* 2004;29:2290-2302.

This article discusses a new psychometrically-strong measure of pain and disability designed to measure the full array of musculoskeletal disorders rather than just low back pain; functional and psychosocial variables are also measured.

Feise RJ, Menke JM: A new valid and reliable instrument to measure the magnitude of clinical change in spinal conditions. *Spine* 2001;26:78-87.

The Oswestry Low Back Pain Disability Questionnaire is reviewed.

Stroud MW, McKnight PE, Jensen MP: Assessment of self-report of physical activity in patients with chronic pain: Development of an abbreviated Roland-Morris disability scale. *J Pain* 2004;5:257-263.

This study demonstrated that an abbreviated version of the Roland-Morris disability scale has good psychometri properties and can be used in place of the larger version to save time.

### Formal Statistical Analysis of Assessment Outcomes

Dorey F, Hildibrand AS, Wang JC: A practical guide to understanding statistical concepts in the spine literature. *SpineLine* May/June 2002:6-11.

This article reviews some of the basic ways that statistical methods can be used to answer important clinical questions encountered in the spine literature. Fundamentals of statistical analyses are provided.

## Classic Bibliography

Altman DG: *Practical Statistics for Medical Research.* London, England, Chapman and Hall, 1991.

Bergner M, Bobbit RA, Carter WB, Gibson BS: The sickness impact profile: Development and final version of a health status measure. *Med Care* 1981;19:787-805.

Beurskens AJ, de Vet HC, Koke AJ, van der Heijden, Knipschild PG: Measuring the functional status of patients with low back pain: Assessment of the quality of four disease-specific questionnaires. *Spine* 1995;20:1017-1028.

Chapman SL, Jamison RN, Sanders SH: Treatment Helpfulness Questionnaire: A measure of patient satisfaction with treatment modalities provided in chronic pain management programs. *Pain* 1996;68:349-361.

Fairbank JC, Couper J, Davies JB, O'Brien JP: The Oswestry low back pain disability questionnaire. *Physiotherapy* 1980;66:271-273.

Flores L, Gatchel RJ, Polatin PB: Objectification of functional improvement after nonoperative care. *Spine* 1997;22:1622-1633.

Fordyce WE, Roberts AH, Sternbach RA: The behavioral management of chronic pain: A response to critics. *Pain* 1985;22:113-125.

Gatchel RJ, Mayer TG: *Functional Restoration for Spinal Disorders: The Sports Medicine Approach.* Malvern, PA, Lea & Febiger, 1988.

Gatchel RJ, Polatin PB, Mayer TG, Robinson R, Dersh J: Use of the SF-36 health status survey with a chronically disabled back pain population: Strengths and limitations. *J Occup Rehabil* 1998;8:237-246.

Greenough CG, Fraser RD: Assessment of outcome in patients with low back pain. *Spine* 1992;17:36-41.

Gronblad M, Jarvinen E, Hurri H: Relationship of the Pain Disability Index (PDI) and the Oswestry Disability Questionnaire (ODQ) with three dynamic physical tests in a group of patients with chronic low-back pain and leg pain. *Clin J Pain* 1994;10:197-203.

Kaplan GM, Wurtele SK, Gillis D: Maximal effort during functional capacity evaluations: An examination of psychological factors. *Arch Phys Med Rehabil* 1996;77:161-164.

Kopec JA: Measuring functional outcomes in persons with back pain. *Spine* 2000;25:3110-3114.

Leclaire R, Blier F, Fortin L, Proulx R: A cross-sectional study comparing the Oswestry and Roland-Morris Functional Disability Scales in two populations of patients with low back pain of different levels of severity. *Spine* 1997;22:68-71.

Mayer TG, Gatchel RJ: *Functional Restoration for Spinal Disorders: The Sports Medicine Approach.* Malvern, PA, Lea & Febiger, 1988.

Mayer TG, Gatchel RJ, Polatin PB (eds): *Occupational Musculoskeletal Disorders: Function, Outcomes and Evidence.* Philadelphia, PA, Lippincott Williams & Wilkins, 2000.

Mayer TG, Prescott M, Gatchel RJ: Objective outcomes evaluation: Methods and evidence, in Mayer TG, Polatin PB, and Gatchel RJ (eds): *Occupational Musculoskeletal Disorders: Function, Outcomes and Evidence.* Philadelphia, PA, Lippincott Williams & Wilkins, 2000.

Pocock SJ: *Clinical Trials.* New York, NY, John Wiley, 1983.

Roland M, Fairbank J: The Roland-Morris Disability Questionnaire and the Oswestry Disability Questionnaire. *Spine* 2000;25:3115-3124.

Sackett DL, Haynes RB, Guyatt GH, Tugwell P: *Clinical Epidemiology: A Basic Science for Clinical Medicine.* Boston, MA, Little, Brown and Company, 1991.

Taylor SJ, Taylor AE, Foy MA, Fogg AJ: Responsiveness of common outcome measures for patients with low back pain. *Spine* 1999;24:1805-1812.

Turk DC: Assessment of patients reporting pain: An integrated perspective. *Lancet* 1999;353:1784-1788.

Von Korff M, Jensen MP, Karoly P: Assessing global pain severity by self-report in clinical and health services research. *Spine* 2000;25:3140-3151.

Waddell G, Main CJ: Assessment of severity in low back disorders. *Spine* 1984;9:204-208.

Ware JE, Sherbourne CD: The MOS 36-Item Short-Form Health Survey (SF-36). I: Conceptual framework and item selection. *Med Care* 1992;30:473-483.

# Chapter 12

# Disability Evaluation

Gunnar B. J. Andersson, MD, PhD

## Introduction

Although most patients with back disorders respond to treatment, some continue to experience pain and loss of function. It is sometimes necessary to quantify this loss of function, which may allow the patient to receive compensation from a variety of governmental and private insurance systems (Table 1). The treating or consulting physician may be asked to evaluate a patient for disability; this evaluation differs depending on the unique requirements and demands of each system. These requirements may include performing an examination, making a diagnosis, establishing causality, determining disease severity, providing an impairment rating, and commenting on the disability. In addition to the individual requirements of different systems, different states also have individual requirements even within the same system. The purpose of this chapter is to present relevant definitions and discuss the role of the orthopaedic surgeon in the disability evaluation process. The main principles used to evaluate back pain in the *American Medical Association Guides to the Evaluation of Permanent Impairment*, 5th Edition (the *Guides*) will be discussed. A detailed description of the *Guides* and other systems is beyond the scope of this chapter.

## Definitions

Most systems differentiate impairment from disability, but in layman's terms the definitions are sometimes blurred. An impairment rating is occasionally used as a disability rating, which can be misleading. The *Guides* defines impairment as "the loss of, loss of use of, or derangement of any body part, organ system or organ function." The impairment can lead to functional limitations or inability to perform activities of daily living. The loss may be anatomic (such as loss of a finger), functional (loss of movement of a finger joint), or both. Disability is defined in the *Guides* as "an allocation of an individual's capacity to meet personal, social, or occupational demands, or to meet statutory or regulatory requirements because of an impairment." Activity limitation is sometimes used to replace the word disability to

| Table 1 | Compensation Systems in the United States |
|---|
| Workers' Compensation System |
| Social Security Administration |
| Veterans Administration Benefit Program |
| Federal Employees' Compensation Act |
| Longshore and Harbor Workers' Compensation Act |
| Federal Black Lung Program |
| Federal Employers Disability Act |
| Jones Act |
| Private Insurances |
| Americans With Disabilities Act |
| Family Medical Leave Act |

avoid the stigma associated with the term. An example that illustrates the difference between impairment and disability is a loss of a finger, an impairment that may result in severe disability to a surgeon, but may result in little or no disability to a psychiatrist.

## Workers' Compensation

Workers' compensation is a state-based social insurance system that compensates workers who are injured on the job. Although variations in the systems exist between states, there are basic common principles. One important principle is the no-fault principle (no need to prove that the employer is at fault, and that the employee is not at fault). Employees are entitled to benefits for injuries that arise out of or in the course of employment. These benefits include wage replacement and medical and rehabilitation benefits. When maximum medical improvement (MMI) is reached and the patient is experiencing residual deficits from the injury, permanent partial and total benefits are paid. According to the *Guides*, MMI is defined as the stage in recovery when the medical condition has stabilized, and further recovery or deterioration is not anticipated, although over time there may be some expected change. This stage usually means that the patient's condition is not expected to change over the next 12 months or so. The type, level, and duration of benefits vary across states. Another common principle is that the workers' compensation system is the only remedy under the law for the employee against the employer for personal injury, disease, or death arising out of and in the course of employment. There are exceptions, such as when the employee can show that the employer intended for the employee to be injured, but in principle the employer's liability is limited. An employee can still sue a third party. For example, a faulty machine causing an injury because it malfunctions can result in a lawsuit against the manufacturer of the machine.

The physician plays several important roles in the workers' compensation system. One of these roles is related to causality. The physician will often be asked to provide an opinion as to whether the job activity caused the injury. It is important to recognize that the legal proof is only "50% more likely than not," which is of course different from the usual clinical proof. Some states require an assessment of the degree to which an impairment is related to a specific event when there are preexisting conditions or residual effects of earlier injuries. This analysis, called apportionment, requires that the physician document preexisting conditions, determine that the current impairment is greater because of the preexisting condition, and that the preexisting condition caused or contributed to the impairment. The physician also provides or directs treatment and rehabilitation. Once rehabilitation is completed the physician should help the patient return to gainful employment by determining when return to work is possible, if there are restrictions, and when MMI is reached.

## Rating Back and Neck Impairments

Impairments listed in the *Guides* are rated by percent of a whole person; 0% means no functional loss of an organ or body system and no limitations in performing activities of daily living; 100% implies a very severe loss of organ or body system function, making an individual completely dependent on others for self-care. Because the rating refers to the whole person, but the deficit may be regional (for example, the spine or hand), the *Guides* provides conversion tables. In patients who have multiple impairments, percentages for each impairment are determined. These percentages are then combined, rather than added, using a combined value chart. The *Guides* typically does not rate pain separately, but rather as part of the anatomic or functional abnormality. In other words, the impairment rating for the spine makes allowances for any accompanying pain. A discretionary 1% to 3% may be added to an impairment rating based on a physician's determination that the patient has a pain-related impairment that has increased the burden of his or her condition. For example, an individual may have had a diskectomy with complete relief of pain and excellent functional recovery, or may have residual pain and loss of

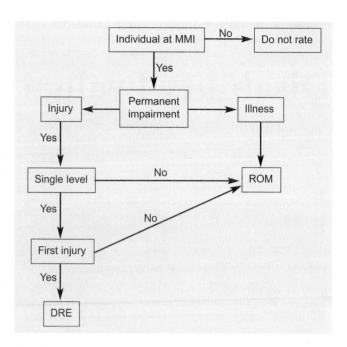

**Figure 1** *Impairment evaluation using the* AMA Guides. *(Adapted from* AMA Guides, *ed 5. Chicago, IL, AMA Press 2001).*

select neuromuscular function (for example, foot drop). Both conditions would be rated the same using the diagnosis-related estimates, discussed later in this chapter. The 3% increase in the impairment rating allows additional consideration of a less successful result. Although the *Guides* also has a chapter on pain, it is rarely applicable in a patient with a back or neck impairment.

## Rating Permanent Impairments of the Spine

Evaluation for the purposes of rating the impairment should include a comprehensive medical history; a review of (appropriate) records; a detailed description of the patient's current symptoms, and how these symptoms affect daily activities; a physical examination; and a review of imaging, electrophysiologic, laboratory and other tests (as available). Two methods are used to determine impairment: diagnosis-related estimates (DRE) or range of motion (ROM).

The DRE method is the primary method and should be used except when (1) the impairment is not caused by an injury, or its cause is completely unclear; (2) there is multilevel involvement in the same region of the spine (cervical, thoracic, or lumbar); (3) there is a change in the motion segment integrity at multiple levels in the same region of the spine; (4) there is radiculopathy caused by a new (recurrent) disk herniation; and (5) there is a statutory requirement to use the ROM method by jurisdiction. There are a few other very rare reasons to use the ROM method as described in the *Guides*. Figure 1 details the thought process used to determine which method to use.

Use of the DRE method requires knowledge of the definitions used to differentiate between categories. There are five categories for each region: Category 1: 0% impairment, no significant clinical findings; Category 2: 5% to 8% impairment, significant clinical findings or minor fracture; Category 3: 10% to 13% impairment, radiculopathy, or moderately severe fracture; Category 4: 20% to 23% impairment, instability or fusion, or severe fracture without neurologic compromise; and Category 5: 25% to 28% impairment, instability or fusion and radiculopathy or severe fracture with unilateral neurologic compromise. For example, for the lumbar region, a patient in Category 1 would have no significant clinical findings and no fracture at the time of MMI, whereas a Category 5 patient could have radiculopathy and loss of motion segment integrity (instability or fusion) with neurologic deficit, or a compression fracture of at least 50% of one vertebral body with unilateral neurologic compromise.

Use of the ROM model requires determining a diagnosis from a table in the *Guides*, measuring the ROM using one or two inclinometer(s), determining if there is a spinal nerve deficit, and combining the rating for all three components using specific tables.

## Rating Lumbosacral Corticospinal and Cauda Equina Injuries

Cauda equina syndrome refers to polyradicular symptoms arising from compression of the lumbosacral nerve roots located in the thecal sac. Corticospinal tract injury is defined as damage to the spinal cord. The most common location is at the conus (T12-L1), but higher levels are sometimes injured. Injuries to the cord and/or cauda equina are infrequent. After determining the neurologic level of involvement by identifying the lowest normally functioning nerve root, tables in the spine chapter and nervous system chapter of the *Guides* outline classifications of the neurologic impairment. The neurologic impairment rating is then combined with the appropriate diagnosis-related estimates category.

## Social Security Disability Insurance and Supplemental Security Income

Both Social Security Disability Insurance (SSDI) and Supplemental Security Income (SSI) are administered by the Social Security Administration (SSA). SSDI is a program for people who have worked (and paid into the system through the Federal Insurance Contributions Act) and who subsequently become disabled, whereas SSI is a supplementary income program for indigent individuals who are disabled. In both systems, qualification is based on medical evidence; however, in contrast to the workers' compensation program there is no consideration of how disability occurs. Disability in the SSDI and SSI systems is defined by the *Guides* as "an impairment that results from anatomical, physiological and psychological abnormalities which can be shown by medically acceptable clinical and laboratory diagnostic techniques."

Orthopaedic surgeons become involved in the SSA systems either as a treating physician asked to prepare a report, or as a consultant asked to perform an independent examination. Once an applicant has contacted the SSA office and filled out an application, nonmedical eligibilities are determined and the application is assigned to an adjudicator. The adjudicator collects available medical information, including the records from treating and consulting physicians, and may also ask the treating physician to write a report that summarizes the applicant's medical condition. The adjudicator documents objective abnormalities, and identifies activity limitations. A medical report for the SSA office should include the patient's medical history, clinical findings (physical examination), laboratory findings (radiographs, other imaging studies), diagnosis, treatment prescribed with response and prognosis, and a statement providing an opinion about what activities the patient can perform despite his or her impairment(s). For patients with back pain, this statement should describe the patient's ability to perform work-related activities such as sitting, standing, walking, lifting, carrying, handling objects, and traveling. Consultative examinations are required for about 40% of applicants. This examination involves obtaining a patient history, physical examination, and assessment of function based on objective findings. Consulting physicians are hired by the SSA. There is currently a shortage of orthopaedic surgeons performing this work.

An administrative peculiarity of the SSA system is the "listing of impairments" section of the disability program. The listing describes, for each body system, impairments that are severe enough to prevent a person from performing any gainful (occupational) activity. These impairments must have lasted, or be expected to last, for at least 12 months. If the criteria in the listing are met, no further evaluation is needed–the individual is disabled. If the criteria are not met, additional evaluation is required before a decision is made. The SSA impairment listing for the musculoskeletal system defines a functional loss as "either the inability to ambulate effectively on a sustained basis for any reason, including pain associated with the underlying musculoskeletal impairment, or the inability to perform fine or gross movements effectively on a sustained basis for any reason, including pain associated with the underlying musculoskeletal impairment." Disorders of the spine qualify under this listing when certain criteria are fulfilled.

## The Veterans Administration Disability Benefits

These benefits are provided both as monetary and nonmonetary assistance. Benefits are based on the inability to work. The physician is not required to supply an impairment or disability rating; a medical evaluation that includes a diagnosis and a description of the severity of the medical condition is provided. This information is then evaluated by a three-member board composed of two Veterans Administration officials and one independent physician.

## Federal Workers' Compensation Programs

Federal programs include the Federal Employees' Compensation Act, the Long Shore and Harbor Workers' Compensation Act, and the Federal Black Lung Program. The Federal Black Lung Program has no musculoskeletal implications and applies to coal miners who are totally disabled from pneumoconiosis.

The Federal Employees' Compensation Act covers civilian employees of the United States Government, such as postal workers. It excludes disability benefit claims involving the brain, heart, and spine. These exclusions are also true for the Long Shore and Harbor Workers' Act.

## The Federal Employers' Liability Act and the Jones Act

The Federal Employers' Liability Act provides benefits for interstate railroad workers who suffer work-related injuries. It is a highly adversarial system in which the employee must sue the employer in the state's civil court or in federal court, if they cannot reach a settlement for disability claims. The physician is required to examine the patient, establish a diagnosis, assign an impairment rating, and in some instances comment on potential disability. Physicians may be required to testify in a federal court. The Jones Act is very similar to the Federal Employers' Liability Act, but instead covers civilian sailors while in the service of a ship or vessel in navigable waters.

## Americans With Disabilities Act

This Act prohibits employment discrimination based on disability. Under this law, an employer must employ qualified individuals with disabilities who can perform the essential functions of the job and make reasonable accommodations if the person is disabled. Disability under the Americans With Disabilities Act is defined as any physical or mental impairment that substantially limits one or more of the major life activities. Reasonable accommodation is subject to a determination of whether the worker's disability imposes an undue hardship on the business. This hardship may be economical. Back impairments are very common reasons for accommodations and the physician must state the patient's restrictions so that it can be determined if accommodations can be made without causing undue hardship.

## Private Disability Programs

For patients with private disability insurance, the physician may be required to perform an evaluation to determine disability. The scope of this evaluation may vary depending on the insurer and the disability policy.

## Summary

The complexity of issues surrounding disability evaluation may require physicians to access the appropriate literature and participate in a training course. It is important to realize that physician involvement has significant medical and economic consequences for the patient and society. The relationship between the accident (if applicable) and the impairment needs to be established. The physician must also determine if impairment exists and, if applicable, assign a rating for the impairment. Physicians also may need to estimate an individual's capacity to perform activities of daily living and work.

## Annotated Bibliography

Cocchiarella L, Andersson GB (eds): *AMA Guides to the Evaluation of Permanent Impairment*, ed 5. Chicago, IL, AMA Press, 2001.

This book details the approach to the evaluation of permanent impairment used by many states.

*Disability Evaluation Under Social Security.* (Blue Book). Washington, DC, US Government Printing Office, 2003, pp 1-255. Social Security Administration, Office of Disability, SSA Pub. No 64-039, ICN 468600.

This book provides details on the SSA disability evaluation system.

## Classic Bibliography

*Consultative Examinations: A Guide for Health Professionals.* (Green Book). Washington, DC, US Government Printing Office, 1999, pp 1-74. Social Security Administration, SSA Pub. No. 64-025, ICN 954095.

This book provides information about how to perform consultative examinations for the SSA.

# Section 2

# Pain Treatments and Rehabilitation

Section Editor:
Joel M. Press, MD

# Chapter 13

# Pharmacologic Management of the Patient With Chronic Pain: An Update

Steven Stanos, DO

## Introduction

The International Association for the Study of Pain defines pain as "an unpleasant sensory and emotional experience associated with actual or potential tissue damage, or described in terms of such damage." Rational pharmacologic management of spine-related conditions must incorporate a more pragmatic understanding of pain. Pain is a subjective and individually personal experience, influenced by learning, the situation or context at hand, and other psychosocial variables. Pain is not merely the end product of peripheral receptor stimulation but a complicated dynamic process of neural signaling modification along ascending and descending peripheral, spinal cord, and brain networks.

Pain serves an adaptive function, warning to protect the body from harm, as well as a more maladaptive function, reflecting pathologic changes in the nervous system. Acute pain is time limited and usually occurs in response to a noxious event with stimulation of nociceptors and possible related tissue damage. Treatment is aimed at removing the underlying pathologic process. In contrast, pain is considered chronic if present 3 to 6 months after the initiating event and may or may not be associated with any obvious ongoing single noxious event or pathologic process. Chronic pain may differ from acute pain in that underlying tissue pathology or injury may not directly correlate with levels of pain. Whereas acute pain can be considered a physiologic response to tissue trauma or damage, chronic pain involves a more dynamic interplay of additional psychologic and behavioral mechanisms. Chronic pain is associated with disruption of sleep and normal daily function, ceases to serve any protective role, and becomes a source of ongoing suffering and disability. Rational polypharmacy implies a mechanistic approach to selecting and adjusting medications as a means of targeting specific sites along the complex pathways involved in the experience of pain.

The treatment of spine-related pain conditions may include active core stabilization exercises, body mechanics training, passive modalities, spinal injections, and sur-

gery. Comprehensive management of acute and chronic spinal pain also should include a rational pharmacologic approach and may include the use of nonsteroidal anti-inflammatory drugs (NSAIDs), oral steroids, and opioids. Over time, after unimodal treatments and/or interventional procedures have failed or levels of analgesia and function have reached a plateau, more comprehensive medication management may be necessary. A mechanistic approach to rational pharmacology is an important component in the management of acute and chronic pain. This approach incorporates the use of newer generation and traditional antidepressants, neuropathic and sleep agents, and chronic opioid medications.

Goals for pharmacotherapy should focus on maximizing independent physical function, decreasing pain, and improving the psychosocial state. It is important to review current updates in pharmacotherapy as applied to a broad range of spine-related conditions including neuropathic pain (a model for treatment of radiculopathy) and manifestations of chronic pain conditions (pain, affective distress, and sleep disturbance). Controversies related to the use of cyclooxygenase (COX)-2 inhibitors, pharmacologic use of opioids, and updates related to traditional and novel antidepressants, anticonvulsant medications, and topical analgesics also merit discussion.

## NSAIDs and COX-2 Inhibitors

Conventional or nonspecific NSAIDs have been used as first-line treatment for analgesia and inflammatory conditions including osteoarthritis and rheumatoid arthritis. Acute spinal pain may benefit from the anti-inflammatory effects of these agents as related to lumbar radiculopathy, facet joint irritation, and related soft-tissue injury. COX-1 and COX-2 isoforms catalyze the conversion of arachidonic acid to prostaglandins. More recent classification of NSAIDs includes (1) conventional or nonselective (NS-NSAID), those that inhibit both the COX-1 isoenzyme and the COX-2 isoenzyme; and (2) those that are more selective for the COX-2 isoenzyme (COX-2 inhibitors). Conventional

NS-NSAIDs were found to offer effective analgesic responses but are limited by potential upper gastrointestinal bleeding and ulceration, renal toxicities, and platelet dysfunction.

The isolation of COX-2 protein in the early 1990s led to the development and release of a new class of NSAIDs, the COX-2 inhibitors. The new oral COX-2 inhibitors include celecoxib, rofecoxib, and valdecoxib. Injectable COX-2 inhibitors, such as parecoxib, the prodrug of valdecoxib, is currently under study and awaiting approval for use in treatment of acute and perioperative pain states. COX-1 is constitutively expressed in most tissues and is responsible for homeostatic functions such as platelet aggregation and the maintenance of upper gastrointestinal mucosal integrity by producing protective prostaglandins. COX-2, a largely cytokine "inducible" constitutive isoenzyme, is primarily responsible for producing inflammation and pain. At the cellular level, animal and human models of COX-2 inhibition have demonstrated reduced central sensitization, a critical neuroplastic state underlying several chronic pain states.

Major randomized trials, including Vioxx Gastrointestinal Outcomes Research (VIGOR) and Celecoxib Long-Term Arthritis Safety Study (CLASS), demonstrated significant safety benefits in comparison with NS-NSAIDs with regard to reduced incidence of symptomatic gastric ulcers and renal toxicity. The use of COX-2 inhibitors during the perioperative period (preemptive analgesia and postoperative pain management) has led to significant opioid sparing effects, postoperative analgesia, and improved function. Despite billions of dollars in sales and widespread use of COX-2 inhibitor agents, questions and concerns emerged regarding potential increased risk of cardiac events including myocardial infarction and sudden cardiac death. Some have proposed that selective COX-2 inhibitors may decrease vascular prostacyclin ($PGI_2$) production, interfering with the balance between prothrombotic and antithrombotic eicosanoids (thromboxane $A_2$), increasing the likelihood of a prothrombotic state manifested by possible cardiac events. In October 2004, Merck voluntarily withdrew the coxib rofecoxib from the market after a trial involving the use of high-dose rofecoxib in the treatment of adenomatous polyp disease. An increased risk for serious cardiovascular events was found in patients taking the drug compared with those patients using a traditional NSAID. Other studies have found conflicting results with other agents and possible "class effects" with an increased incidence of myocardial and renal events. Subsequently, other studies demonstrated similar cardiac effects with naproxen, leading to the reassessment of the use of NS-NSAIDs and COX-2 inhibitors for management of chronic spinal and osteoarthritic conditions. More careful selection of these agents for long-term use has been recommended by the Food and Drug Administration (FDA). Relative risks versus potential benefits (analgesia, decreased stiffness, and improved function) should be examined on a patient-by-patient basis.

## Opioid Pharmacology

Opioid and opioid-like medications are potent analgesics. Opioids work by binding to opioid receptors (mu, delta, kappa), decreasing neural excitability and the subsequent release of excitatory neurotransmitters (serotonin, norepinephrine, substance P, and glutamate). Central effects of opioids primarily include actions at the brainstem (periaqueductal gray) and limbic areas, causing increased descending inhibition leading to possible analgesia and anxiolytic effects. Recent guidelines for acute treatment of pain with opioids in the postoperative and outpatient setting include consensus statements of the American Pain Society and the American Society of Anesthesiologists Task Force on Acute Pain Management.

### Chronic Opioid Analgesic Therapy

In the treatment of chronic spinal pain, chronic opioid analgesic therapy should incorporate the use of longer acting medications and the judicious use of short-acting medications for breakthrough pain episodes (Table 1). Maintaining steady serum levels with long-acting agents may help to maintain consistent opioid serum levels. Advantages related to consistent serum levels include convenient dosing schedules, more sustained analgesia, uninterrupted sleep, a decrease in the number of episodes of breakthrough pain, and less reliance on the daily use of short-acting opioids.

Controversy continues regarding the use of chronic opioid therapy for chronic spinal pain. Studies have demonstrated modest to moderate levels of analgesia in patients with chronic pain but levels are varied when examining improvement in functional status. Other studies have shown that chronic opioid therapy may lead to a so-called pain-opioid downhill spiral characterized by loss of functional capacity and a corresponding increase in depression. Studies to corroborate these findings found support for the downhill spiral but noted that opioid use alone did not account for the changes in patient function and mood. Instead, associated benzodiazepine use was found to be associated with functional decline, medical visitations, and disability days. Assessing a patient's individual psychosocial factors and analgesic response to chronic opioid analgesic therapy should incorporate goals of improved function and general quality of life.

### Opioid Analgesic Agents

Recent advancements in opioid management include novel oral delivery systems, and transmucosal oral and transdermal delivery systems (transdermal therapeutic system).

**Table 1 | Selected Clinical Pharmacokinetics of Commonly Used Oral Opioids**

| Drug | Approximate Time of Onset of Action (min) | Approximate Time to Peak Effect (h) | Approximate Duration of Effect (h) | Approximate Bioavailability (%) |
|---|---|---|---|---|
| Hydromorphone | 30 to 45 | 1.5 to 2 | 3 to 4 | 60 |
| Methadone | 30 | 2 to 3 | 6 to 12 | 80 |
| Morphine (immediate release, sublingual) | 30 to 45 | 1.5 to 2 | 3 to 4 | 30 |
| Morphine (long-acting) | | | | |
| MS Contin Oramorph SR, other generic products | 120 | 6 to 8 | 10 to 12 | 30 |
| Kadian | 120 | 8 to 12 | 18 to 24 | 30 |
| Avinza | 45 | 4 to 6 | 18 to 24 | 30 |
| Oxycodone (immediate release) | 20 to 45 | 1.5 to 2 | 3 to 4 | 80 |
| Oxycodone (controlled release) | 30 to 60 | 4 to 6 | 10 to 12 | 80 |
| Fentanyl (transmucosal) Actiq | 10 (after start of dose application) | 20 to 25 (after start of dose application) | 120 | 50 |

*(Adapted with permission from Strassels SA, McNicol E, Suleman R: Postoperative pain management: A practical review, part 1. Am J Health Syst Pharm 2005;62:1904-1916.)*

Extended-release morphine formulations include Avinza (Ligand Pharmaceuticals, San Diego, CA) and Kadian (Alpharma, Piscataway, NJ) designed for once-daily and twice-daily administration, respectively. These formulations contain immediate-release and extended-release beads that release morphine in a time-dependent manner, sustaining therapeutic concentrations over approximate 24- and 12-hour dosing intervals, respectively.

Sustained release oxycodone, OxyContin (Purdue Pharma LP, Stamford, CT), provides a bimodal release system, with bimodal peak serum release at 0.6 and 6.8 hours twice a day. A recent survey at a large university-based chronic pain clinic found that a significant number of patients on chronic sustained-release oxycodone management required dosing more often than twice daily (every 8 hours) (67%). Those patients required less frequently scheduled rescue or break-through opioid medication (21% versus 47% in the comparison group that received dosing every 12 hours), which may be the result of more sustained serum oxycodone levels provided by three times daily dosing. Sustained-release oxycodone has been found to provide significant analgesia in neuropathic pain states, countering the traditional view of limited effects of opioids in general neuropathic pain states. The average sustained doses in several studies were less than 100 mg/day. Sustained-release oxymorphone, the active metabolite of oxycodone, is presently undergoing phase III studies for use in opioid-tolerant patients.

Palladone (Purdue Pharma LP), a once-daily, extended-release hydromorphone capsule, was approved by the FDA in September 2004 for use in opioid-tolerant patients with persistent, moderate to severe pain. The product was voluntarily removed from the market in July 2005 because of concerns regarding potentially dangerous interactions with alcohol. This interaction could potentially cause dose dumping and rapid release of the hydromorphone into the bloodstream. A reformulation of Palladone is planned, with re-release in 2006 or 2007.

*Methadone*

Methadone has experienced a rebirth as a "novel" opioid analgesic. Long used in addiction treatment maintenance programs and still carrying a social stigma, this synthetic opioid has several potential advantages compared with other opioids. Its clinical use in pain management increased significantly after more widespread use in cancer pain management. Methadone hydrochloride is a relatively potent *N*-methyl-D-aspartate (NMDA) receptor antagonist. This excitatory amino acid has been implicated as a key factor in central sensitization and opioid tolerance mechanisms. Clinicians prescribing methadone should exercise caution. Methadone is highly protein bound and accumulates in tissues, with repeated dosing creating an extensive reservoir. Its half-life varies from 7 hours to 5 days. Dosing changes must be done at least every 5 to 6 days. A 1998 study described one of a small number of standardized conversion regimens for converting oral morphine equivalents to methadone. For example, with 24-hour doses less than 300 mg, a fixed dose one-tenth the actual morphine dose is administered every 3 hours as required for 5 days. On day 6, the amount taken over the previous 2 days is averaged to a daily dose, which is then taken twice daily on a regular, fixed schedule. Also, recent case reports of cardiac arrhythmias (torsade de pointes) have been reported in patients on methadone therapy for pain and in those in methadone maintenance programs.

Actiq (Cephalon, Fraser, PA) is used as an oral transmucosal delivery system of fentanyl in a solid drug matrix delivered on a stick. The lollipop is twirled in the oral mucosa, dissolving the fentanyl in the mouth over a 15-minute administration period. Peak serum levels occur within approximately 25 minutes of use. The highly lipholic character of fentanyl contributes to rapid absorption across the blood-brain barrier. Rapid onset of effect is also caused by bypassing the first-pass metabolism transmucosal route compared with traditional oral medications. Additional pipeline transmucosal opioids in development include effervescent-like medications delivered sublingually, similar to sublingual nitroglycerin.

### Transdermal Delivery

The use of transdermal delivery with agents such as fentanyl (Duragesic, Janssen Pharmaceutica LP, Titusville, NJ), has become more common in long-term opioid management of chronic spine-related and neuropathic pain conditions. Several studies have shown improved function, analgesia, and stable dosing (less than 100 µg/day) in patients with chronic pain. In a small number of patients, dosing may be required every 48 hours versus the recommended 72 hours because of patient variability in fentanyl metabolism. Other studies have reported mixed results in quality of life and psychosocial function. According to some studies, a decrease in constipation has been suggested with fentanyl in direct comparisons with sustained-release morphine. Aggressive treatment of opioid-induced constipation should be initiated at the start of treatment.

Future developments of sustained-release medications include the use of a matchstick-sized pump system (Chronogesic, Durect, Cupertino, CA), implanted subcutaneously to deliver sufentanil at a constant rate over several months. Another device allows on-demand drug administrations via iontophoresis of fentanyl. The patient-controlled transdermal system, using the E-TRANS delivery system (ALZA Corp, Mountain View, CA), is a programmed, self-adhesive system that may deliver fentanyl over a fixed period of time. In a postoperative pain study, patients were able to self-administer 40 µg of fentanyl on demand, up to six doses per hour.

### Legislative and Federal Scrutiny

The more liberal prescribing practices of the late 1990s have been slowed after the realization of an increased incidence of abuse and diversion of opioid medications. An increased focus on more comprehensive patient pain and psychologic assessment, as well as standardized office screening and monitoring practices (formal patient-physician contracts or treatment agreements) are becoming basic standards of practice for physicians choosing to prescribe opioids and other controlled substances. Patient-physician treatment agreements have been published by several national pain organizations, including the American Pain Society and the American Academy of Pain Medicine. The use of a trilateral opioid agreement has been proposed, which includes the collaboration of the patient's primary care physician, pain physician, and patient. Besides improving communication between providers, the agreement may act as a means of effectively transferring care and responsibility of long-term opioid management back to the primary care physician once the individual regimen is stabilized.

### Controversies Related to Chronic Opioid Analgesic Therapy

Several ongoing controversies have led to the reluctance of physicians to prescribe chronic opioids for painful spinal disorders. In addition to commonly recognized concerns about addiction, tolerance, and legislative scrutiny, the level of symptom relief and physical and psychologic functioning after chronic opioid analgesic therapy is another source of debate. Questions remain regarding impaired cognitive function, endocrine effects, and possible iatrogenic contribution of opioid-induced hypersensitivity with long-term high-dose opioid management.

#### Cognitive Function With Opioid Therapy

Conflicting results exist regarding the effects of chronic opioid analgesic therapy and psychomotor function. Studies of patients with chronic nonmalignant pain found evidence of impaired attention and deficits in psychomotor speed and working memory. Interestingly, these same findings may have resulted from related affective distress (depression, anxiety) and distraction caused by uncontrolled pain. Similar studies have examined the effects of opioids on driving ability and reaction time. A recent comprehensive review of studies found moderate, generally consistent evidence of no impairment of psychomotor abilities and inconclusive findings for no impairment in cognitive functioning in patients receiving long-term opioid treatment. Others have argued that transient cognitive and psychomotor impairment may be evident during dose titration or escalation only. Careful individual assessment and monitoring by the physician is recommended.

#### Endocrine Effects of Long-Term High-Dose Opioid Management

Animal models and some case study reviews in humans have suggested chronic high-dose opioid therapy may cause abnormalities in hypothalamic-pituitary-adrenal axis and hypothalamic-pituitary-gonadal secretion. Endocrine effects may include decreased testosterone,

**Table 2 | Anticonvulsant Primary Mechanisms**

| Anticonvulsant | Na$^+$ Channel Blockade | Ca$^{2+}$ Channel Blockade | Glutamate Antagonism | GABA Potentiation | Carbonic Anhydrase Inhibition |
|---|---|---|---|---|---|
| Gabapentin | | X | | X | |
| Lamotrogine | X | X | | | |
| Levetiracetam | | | | | |
| Oxcarmazapine | X | X | | | |
| Pregabalin | | X | | X | |
| Tiagabine | | | | X | |
| Topiramate | X | X | X | X | X |
| Zonisamide | X | X | X | X | X |

progesterone, and estradiol levels (decreased libido in men and women), amenorrhea, and reduced cortisol response to stress. The syndrome of opioid-induced androgen deficiency has been described in case studies and may require additional screening and treatment (testosterone supplementation) by the prescribing physician.

***Opioid Hyperalgesia: Possible Pronociceptive Effects***
Animal and human studies have shown that under certain circumstances, opioids may elicit unexpected changes in pain sensitivity manifested as hyperalgesia (abnormal or elevated pain in response to painful stimuli) and allodynia (abnormal intense pain in response to nonpainful stimuli). These possible pronociceptive effects of opioids are in contrast to more widely accepted and understood neural mechanisms of tolerance. Tolerance is characterized by receptor morphologic changes manifested by the need to increase dosage to maintain the opioids's analgesic effects. Repeated administration of opioids may contribute to tolerance, and also paradoxically lead to a pronociceptive cascade of events (opioid-induced abnormal pain sensitivity) representing a 'sensitization' process supported by evidence of increased spinal dynorphin (pronociceptive) pathways. Some pain specialists have suggested maintaining opioid doses at the lowest levels to achieve analgesia in contrast to more traditional views of aggressive dose escalation until appropriate analgesia is achieved as a means of limiting these possible cellular processes.

Activation of pronociceptive spinal glutamate occurs via the NMDA receptor. Blocking or inhibiting the NMDA receptor has been proposed as a possible target for medications to limit tolerance and sensitization. Opioids with possible NMDA antagonist effects include methadone and propoxyphene. Nonopioid NMDA antagonist medications include dextromethorphan, ketamine, and memantine. Formal efficacy studies of these medications used in this regard are pending.

## Antidepressants
### Tricyclic Antidepressants
Tricyclic antidepressants are effective agents in selected neuropathic pain states. Their use as both potent antidepressants and sedating medications may fit into several therapeutic targets related to symptom management of chronic pain syndrome (pain, depression, disturbed sleep). The initial use of these medications at night may be of benefit for the relatively potent serotonin and norepinephrine effects. Slow titration to higher antidepressant doses may lead to additional antidepressant effects and analgesia. Although selective serotonin reuptake inhibitors have proven effects as potent antidepressants and anxiolytics in patients with general anxiety and are associated with fewer side effects than traditional tricyclic antidepressants, limited analgesic effects have been reported.

### Anticonvulsants/Neuropathic Agents
The important pathophysiologic mechanism underlying chronic neuropathic pain is central sensitization. A mechanistic approach to pharmacotherapy has emerged. Understanding basic physiologic neurotransmitter changes may help target the use of a single or several anticonvulsants in the management of chronic neuropathic pain states including spinal radiculopathy (Table 2). The incorporation of newer generation anticonvulsants into outpatient management is practical because of their more favorable metabolic and interaction profiles compared with traditional anticonvulsants. New generation agents have limited enzyme induction, relatively longer half-lives, and strong protein binding, which limit the necessity of ongoing serum monitoring.

Gabapentin (Neurontin, Pfizer, New York, NY), approved for postherpetic neuralgia and diabetic peripheral neuropathy, has been used off-label for the treatment of spine-related pain conditions including radiculopathy, as well as migraine headache, spasticity, and several psychiatric conditions. Gabapentin, although structurally related to γ-aminobutyric acid (GABA), is an α2–delta ligand. The α2-delta receptor is a protein associated with neuronal voltage-gated calcium channels. Binding to this channel reduces presynaptic calcium influx into the cell at the dorsal horn, reducing the release of several neurotransmitters (glutamate, substance P, norepinephrine, and calcitonin gene-related peptide). Several indirect GABA-ergic mechanisms have also been proposed. Multiple studies have shown a significant reduction in pain and improved sleep, mood, and quality of life at dosages between 1800 mg/day to 3,600 mg/day. Side effects include somnolence and dizziness. Gabapentin's unique pharmacokinetics necessitate using higher doses compared with other second- and third-generation anticonvulsants. With escalating dose titration, the intestinal active transport absorption system becomes saturated, decreasing bioavailability, resulting in a nonlinear relationship between serum concentration and dosage. Thus, a significant increase in dosage is needed to produce a relative increase in therapeutic response.

Pregabalin (Lyrica, Pfizer), also an α2-delta ligand, is chemically related to gabapentin. However, pregabalin demonstrates linear pharmacokinetics, has a rapid onset of action (within 1 hour), a bioavailability of approximately 90%, and an affinity for the α2-γ subunit six times more potent compared with gabapentin. Pregabalin, the newest anticonvulsant, has been approved by the FDA for treating postherpetic neuralgia and diabetic peripheral neuropathy. In studies of patients with diabetic peripheral neuropathy and postherpetic neuralgia, the average dose of pregabalin was between 150 mg/day and 600 mg/day. Pregabalin's relative increased potency and linear pharmacokinetics may diminish the need for rapidly escalating dose titration and large sustained doses necessary to achieve therapeutic effects with gabapentin.

Tiagabine (Gabitril, Cephalon), a novel selective GABA reuptake inhibitor indicated for partial seizures, has also been used off-label for the treatment of chronic neuropathic pain and insomnia. Theoretically, increasing GABA levels at the synaptic cleft (dorsal horn and brain) may help to increase GABA's inhibitory effects on neuronal excitability. Increased GABA levels have been associated with improved sleep, characterized by increasing time in nonrapid eye movement stage III and stage IV sleep.

Topiramate and zonisomide are broad-spectrum anticonvulsants. Besides calcium and sodium channel effects, and additional proposed mechanisms including inhibition of carbonic anhydrase, antiglutamate also is responsible for significant weight loss. The mechanism of levetiracetam (Keppra), an agent with a chemical structure unrelated to other anticonvulsants, remains unclear but may include calcium channel effects. It is similar to gabapentin, having minimal drug-drug interactions, and is easily renally excreted.

### Serotonin/Norepinephrine Reuptake Inhibitors

The newest class of antidepressants, dual monoamine reuptake inhibitors, was developed for the treatment of depression with a goal of providing shorter onset of antidepressant effects and fewer adverse effects because of their relative selectivity. Mirtazapine is a potent antagonist of central α2 adrenergic receptors, an antagonist of 5-hydroxytryptamine (5-HT)2 and 5-HT3 receptors and enhances norepinephrine and serotonin (5-HT) neurotransmission. Mirtazapine is indicated for the treatment of depression and may be used to enhance the efficacy of selective serotonin reuptake inhibitors. Its relatively sedating effects may have additional benefits for improving sleep in patients with chronic pain. Venlafaxine is a potent reuptake inhibitor of 5-HT, with less potent effects on norepinephrine and dopamine. Higher doses (> 150 mg) have been found to have additional analgesic effects and may be efficacious in several neuropathic pain states. Duloxetine is a potent balanced reuptake inhibitor of both 5-HT and norepinephrine. It is indicated for depression, diabetic peripheral neuropathy, and postherpetic neuralgia.

### Topical Analgesics

The use of over-the-counter and prescription topical analgesics continues to increase. A better understanding of nociceptor physiology has led to a better understanding of thermosensation. Recently, a new class of thermosensitivity medications, the transreceptor protein channel family, has been identified. Capsaicin, the pungent agent found in chili peppers, acts via the vanilloid receptor, a transreceptor protein nonselective cation channel, causing the release of pronociceptive substance P and glutamate. Capsaicin is now marked in several analgesic creams. The cold and menthol sensitive receptor also has been identified and may contribute to a better understanding of cold thermosensation and possible development of targeted cold-producing analgesics.

Clinically, several prescription and over-the-counter topical therapies are available for the treatment of musculoskeletal and neuropathic pain. Prescription medications include lidocaine 5% patches for postherpetic neuralgia. Randomized placebo-controlled studies have demonstrated efficacy with the administration of 12-hour daily doses of medication to treat patients with postherpetic neuralgia. Recent studies examined potential risks for the use of multiple patches worn at the same time. No clinically relevant systemic effects were found with multiple patches worn 24 hours at a time. Although lidocaine's mechanism of action (peripheral sodium channel blockade) has long been understood, recent studies have demonstrated physiologic changes at the dorsal horn and changes in pain processing on functional MRI, implying possible central effects of patch use. Open-label studies in osteoarthritis with patch application locally over the affected joint demonstrated reduced stiffness and pain.

Over-the-counter topical analgesics include capsaicin (heat activated) and menthol-based products that cause cooling effects by inhibiting calcium currents and decreasing temperature thresholds). Pharmacologic studies of menthol have suggested a possible kappa opioid receptor effect, contributing additional analgesic properties to this substance. The use of topical tricyclic antidepressants, including doxpein (FDA approval for dermatologic eczema), has been more widespread in Europe in the management of neuropathic pain. Compounding pharmacies may serve a unique service to physicians in providing several medications individually compounded for topical use and include ketamine (NMDA receptor antagonist), gabapentin, and cyclobenzaprine.

The pharmacologic management of chronic low back pain includes a balanced approach focusing on maximizing analgesia and improving mood, sleep quality, and function. A rational polypharmacy approach should include the use of a wide range of pharmacologic agents individually selected, such as nonspecific NSAIDs, COX-2 inhibitors, anticonvulsants, short- and long-acting opioid analgesics, and topical agents.

## Annotated Bibliography
### NSAIDS and COX-2 Inhibitors
Cheng HF, Harris RC: Cyclooxygenases, the kidney, and hypertension. *Hypertension* 2004;43:525-530.

This article reviews the pharmacology of COX isoenzymes with an emphasis on discussing these agents and their effect on renal function, cardiac effects, and interactions with commonly used antihypertensive medications.

Kimmel SE, Berlin JA, Reily M, et al: Patients exposed to rofecoxib and celecoxib have different odds of nonfatal myocardial infraction. *Ann Intern Med* 2005;142:157-164.

The odds ratio for myocardial infarction among celecoxib users relative to NSAID users was 0.43 compared with an odds ratio of 1.16 in rofecoxib users.

Mukherjee D, Nissen SE, Topol EJ: Risk of cardiovascular events associated with selective COX-2 inhibitors. *JAMA* 2001;286:954-959.

This article reviewed major randomized trials of COX-2 inhibitors with respect to increased risk for cardiovascular events. VIGOR (rofecoxib) and CLASS (celecoxib) studies were associated with higher annualized rates of myocardial infarction compared with placebo.

Solomon DH, Schneeweiss S, Glynn RJ, et al: Relationship between selective cyclooxygenase-2 inhibitors and acute myocardial infarction in older adults. *Circulation* 2004;109:2068-2073.

Rofecoxib use was associated with a greater risk of myocardial infarction compared with NSAID and no NSAID use. A higher risk was seen with dosages of 25 mg or more.

### Opioids and Topical Analgesics
Ballantyne JC, Mao J: Opioid therapy for chronic pain. *N Engl J Med* 2003;349:1943-1953.

This article presents an update on the use of opioids for chronic pain. It includes a discussion of clinical efficacy studies, prolonged high-dose treatment, tolerance, opioid-induced sensitivity, and immune modulation. Protocols for therapy are suggested.

Bartleson JD: Evidence for and against the use of opioid analgesics for chronic nonmalignant low back pain: A review. *Pain Med* 2002;3:260-271.

This article presents a literature review of 13 studies that found scant evidence supporting the use of chronic opioid therapy in patients with low back pain. Treatment was associated with moderate side effects but low risk for abuse or addiction.

Dworkin RH, Backonja M, Rowbotham MC, et al: Advances in neuropathic pain: Diagnosis, mechanisms, and treatment recommendations. *Arch Neurol* 2003;60:1524-1534.

Evidence-based treatment recommendations for neuropathic pain are discussed.

Dworkin RH, Borbin AE, Young JP Jr, et al: Pregabalin for the treatment of postherpetic neuralgia: A randomized, placebo-controlled trial. *Neurology* 2003;60:1274-1283.

Significant pain relief was noted at week 1 in this randomized trial. Fifty percent of patients experienced a reduction in pain of almost 50% with a 600 mg per day dosage of pregabalin.

Fishbain DA, Cutler B, Rosomoff HL, Rosomoff RS: Are opioid-dependent/tolerant patients impaired in driving-related skills?: A structured evidence-based review. *J Pain Symptom Manage* 2003;25:559-577.

Opioid-related effects studied included psychomotor abilities, cognitive function, motor vehicle driving and accidents, and driving impairments.

Fishman SM, Mahajan G, Jung SW, Wilsdy BL: The trilateral opioid contract: Bridging the pain clinic and the primary care physician through the opioid contract. *J Pain Symptom Manage* 2002;24:335-344.

This article presents a study of the use of the trilateral opioid contract between the patient, physician, and pain specialist. Predictive factors for noncompliance included a history of psychiatric diagnosis. An example of a patient contract is included in the appendix section.

Marcus DA, Click RM: Sustained-release oxycodone dosing survey of chronic pain patients. *Clin J Pain* 2004; 20:363-366.

A mixed group of patients with chronic pain were studied. Sustained-release oxycodone was prescribed every 8 hours in 67% of patients. Patients on every 12-hours dosing used more short-acting opioids.

Milligan K, Lanteri-Minet M, Borchert K, et al: Evaluation of long-term efficacy and safety of transdermal fentanyl in the treatment of chronic noncancer pain. *J Pain* 2001;2:197-204.

A long-term prospective trial of more than 500 patients with chronic noncancer pain is discussed. Long-term pain control was associated with improved bodily pain scores on the Short Form-36 scale. Dosing of fentanyl averaged 90 μg/h over a 12-month period.

Sabatowski R, Galvez R, Cherry DA, et al: Pregabalin reduces pain and improves sleep and mood disturbances in patients with post-herpetic neuralgia: Results of a randomized placebo-controlled clinical trial. *Pain* 2004; 109:26-35.

Patients who received 150 or 300 mg/day pregabalin given three times per day showed improvements in relief of pain, sleeping habits, and quality of life.

Sawynok J: Topical and peripherally acting analgesics. *Pharmacol Rev* 2003;55:1-20.

A comprehensive review of peripheral and central pain signaling and a review of topical NSAIDs, capsaicin, local anesthetics, α-adrenoreceptor agonists, cannabinoids, and GABA agonists is presented.

## Classic Bibliography

Merskey H, Bogduk N (eds): *Classification of Chronic Pain: Descriptions of Chronic Pain Syndromes and Definitions of Pain Terms, ed 2.* Seattle, WA, IASP Press, 1994.

McQuay HJ, Tramer M, Nye BA, et al: A systematic review of antidepressants in neuropathic pain. *Pain* 1996; 68:217-227.

Morley JS, Makin MK: The use of methadone in cancer pain poorly responsive to other opioids. *Pain Rev* 1998; 5:51-58.

Schofferman J: Long-term opioid analgesics therapy for severe refractory lumbar spine pain. *Clin J Pain* 1999;15: 136-140.

Watson CP, Babul N: Efficacy of oxycodone in neuropathic pain: A randomized trial in postherpetic neuralgia. *Neurology* 1998;50:1837-1841.

Wheeler WL, Dickerson ED: Clinical application of methadone. *Am J Hosp Palliat Care* 2000;17:196-203.

# Chapter 14

# Manipulative Therapy

Natasha J. Kim, DC

John J. Triano, DC, PhD, FCCSC

## Introduction

The high prevalence of patients with back and neck pain places a significant financial burden on the health care system and is an important contributor to loss of productivity in the workplace. Following a differential diagnosis, nonsurgical management of back and neck pain commonly includes manual treatment methods such as massage, neuromuscular therapy (muscle energy and strain-counterstrain techniques), joint mobilization, and high velocity low amplitude (HVLA) manipulation to correct local and regional dysfunction of the spinal articulations and surrounding soft tissues. Manual therapy is used by chiropractors, osteopaths and, by referral in some instances, physical therapists with advanced training. Spinal manipulative therapy (SMT) is usually provided by chiropractors and is often used to treat either acute or chronic neck, thoracic, and low back pain, as well as related radicular pain and headaches. Evidence-based information derived from controlled clinical trials and systematic reviews over the past two decades have offered greater insight into the clinical role and benefits of SMT.

## Definitions of Manipulative Therapy and the Manipulable Lesion

SMT is a subgroup of manual methods involving several procedures generally classified as mobilization or HVLA manipulation. SMT is performed to correct local intersegmental or regional dysfunction of the spinal articulations and surrounding soft tissues. SMT uses the application of controlled loads (forces and moments) to the affected joint structures to reduce pain and to improve dysfunctional joint mechanics. Manipulative therapy achieves these goals by altering local mechanical joint stresses associated with the manipulable lesion. The components of a controlled load are determined by the physician and include the duration, speed, amplitude, and direction of the applied load, as well the patient's positioning at the time SMT is delivered to the manipulative lesion.

A current classification system of manipulative procedures is based on biomechanical characteristics including speed, mode of application, and type of load. Such a classification has clinical value through the relationship of mechanical stimulation of the tissues and the fundamental properties (stiffness and viscoelasticity) of the tissues that govern mechanical response to the loads reaching them. Slow-acting loads permit time-dependent effects involving the movement of tissues, fluid, or swelling from one compartment to another as well as influencing creep and dynamic creep within the structural components. More rapid methods induce motions that are more dependent on the relative stiffness of the individual tissues and the kinetic chain in a sequence of joint structures. Manipulative loads may be delivered externally through manual or mechanically assisted methods. Physician–induced procedures involve: (1) unloaded spinal motion, which includes continuous passive motion using motorized tables and manually applied flexion-distraction techniques; (2) mobilization, which includes manual application of rhythmic oscillation of incrementally varying grades of force without the use of an impulse thrust; and (3) HLVA methods, which involve direct contact over an underlying vertebra, focusing on bony prominences of the skull, vertebra, thorax, or pelvis followed by the delivery of a rapid but brief impulse thrust to the manipulative lesion without exceeding the vertebral joints' anatomic range of motion. In addition to physician-induced loads, SMT also may be administered as physician-guided patient muscle activation. This type of muscle activation is grouped into two categories designed to improve joint mobility by normalizing muscle tone and/or by addressing either the agonist or antagonist muscles. These categories are the neuromuscular release and counterstrain techniques.

The specific mechanism by which SMT improves joint and tissue mobility has not been completely determined. However, several explanations have been proposed: (1) release of entrapped meniscoid from the zygapophyseal joint; (2) release of interarticular or periarticular adhesions resulting from repetitive joint trauma, chronic inflammation, or immobilization; (3) reduction of muscle spasm via sudden stretch of periarticular soft tissue; and (4) inhibition of central sensitization by increasing neurochemical pain inhibitors, including β endorphins and substance P.

Although each of these mechanisms may be feasible and has circumstantial evidence to support its efficacy, none can explain the breadth of clinical presentations observed in practice. Recently, a more encompassing theory, intersegmental spinal buckling, has been proposed based on biomechanical evidence. This theory can better account for the observations of practice while enabling subgroups of response similar to the four mechanisms listed. Buckling appears to result in local changes that may involve remote effects. A cascade of biomechanical and/or inflammatory changes results in localized symptoms. Most intriguing is the fact that buckling occurs entirely within the normal range of motion. However, it is a disproportionate displacement for the load that is acting on the joint and is permitted by either the local tissues exceeding their local injury limits or by fatigued or inappropriate timing of the muscles controlling local equilibrium. The result is increased local tissue strain and restrictions in joint motion. Although operating within its normal range of motion, the joint is under increased stress disproportionate to what it would usually experience for the posture or task that the patient is undertaking.

Three types of events can cause buckling: (1) movement or increased load after a prolonged static posture; (2) a sudden overload incident; and (3) exposure to vibration while under load. The symptoms that arise from a buckling event depend on the tissue that is exposed to suprathreshold strains. For that reason, the clinical presentation can be quite varied with symptoms suggestive of injury to the facet, disk, ligaments, nerve, or muscle. This explains the variation in clinical presentation observed in patients responding to SMT. Structures that have undergone previous injury or those with degenerative or congenital abnormalities may be more susceptible to symptoms. When preexisting damage is present, the threshold for buckling is decreased and the total load necessary to reach the maximum displacement limit is reduced.

The mechanisms of spinal buckling are complex but will be covered briefly here. Recently, animal models simulating altered joint stress caused by experimentally induced restricted motion have been created. The early results have shown the development of intra-articular adhesions consistent with the theoretic effects of buckling. Continued restriction of motion leads to osteophytic formation similar to that of degenerative joint disease (Figure 1).

Stability of the spine occurs by coordinating the action of two sets of muscles to create appropriately timed regional and intersegmental stiffness in support of the upper body. The regional stabilizing group consists of the long torso muscles (abdominal and paraspinal) that tend to initiate movement and generate power and speed of motion. The local stabilizers are the smaller local muscles surrounding the spine (multifidus, rotators, intertransverse).

Biomechanical studies over the past two decades have shown that the intrinsic stiffness and viscoelastic properties of the passive tissues (bone, ligament, disk) offer significant influence on joint behavior (direction and limitation of motion) in an unexpected pattern; that is, the joint action at both the midrange (neutral zone) where little elastic resistance normally is found and at the extremes of motion where maximum resistance occurs. Thus, throughout most of the body's range of motion, the maintenance of stable and reliable function is dependent on multiarticular, multimuscle coordination and load sharing. Close cooperation between the regional and local stabilizers allows for controlled activity with a minimum of local tissue stress.

Before return to work and recreational activities, the body must strike a dynamic balance (equilibrium) by adopting postures and patterns of muscle recruitment that make the desired task feasible while keeping the local tissue deformation (strain) within tolerable ranges. Life experience shows that many tasks can be performed using one of several different postural configurations; however, many postures feel awkward and soon become uncomfortable as they promote stress concentration and extreme positions at one or more joints. Although these adaptations are feasible, they are not useful for prolonged periods because they tend to create local stiffness, pain, and possibly swelling.

The spine is a kinetic chain linkage that empowers motion while giving structural support to the upper body and protection to the spinal cord. Each task has a range of acceptable postural configurations where the local tissue stress remains below the injury threshold. As previously described, if a feasible but more stressful configuration is adopted, symptoms result. Awkward local joint configurations can be selected voluntarily. For example, workers attempting repairs beneath the dashboard of an automobile will assume strained but feasible positions that result in local aches and pains over time. Involuntarily sudden shifting within the joint as a result of momentary imbalances between the spinal stabilizers may occur but range of motion will remain normal. Arising from neural control error or from fatigue, these events correlate with mechanical buckling of the joint. Their existence has been studied in the laboratory and observed under fluoroscopy during lifting injury. In essence, the lesion is a local uncontrolled buckling event that shifts the joint configuration to one that is atypical for the task being performed. Stress is concentrated in one or more tissues and may exceed the injury threshold (Figure 2).

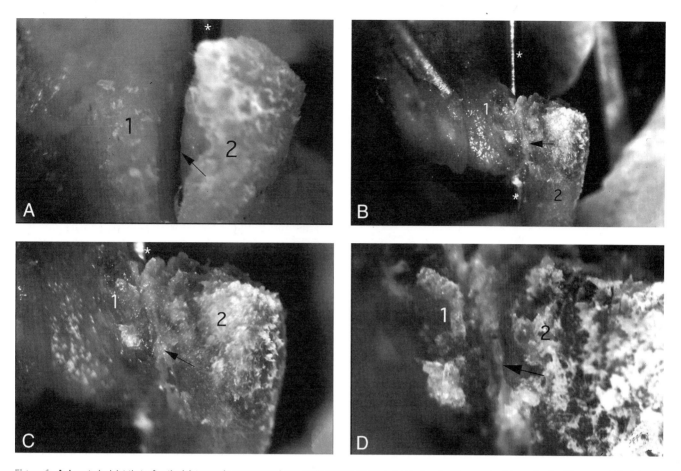

Figure 1 **A,** A control z-joint that, after the joint capsule was removed, was easily gapped by passing a small probe (*) approximately one fourth of the way into the joint. The arrow points to the opened joint space. The numbers 1 and 2 mark the caudad and cephalad articular processes respectively. **B, C,** and **D** present progressively larger magnifications of a z-joint that had been experimentally fixed for 12 weeks. The joint did not gap despite the inserted probe (*) being passed completely through the joint (joint capsule removed). The arrow points to intra-articular adhesions preventing gapping of the joint. The numbers 1 and 2 mark the caudad and cephalad articular processes respectively.

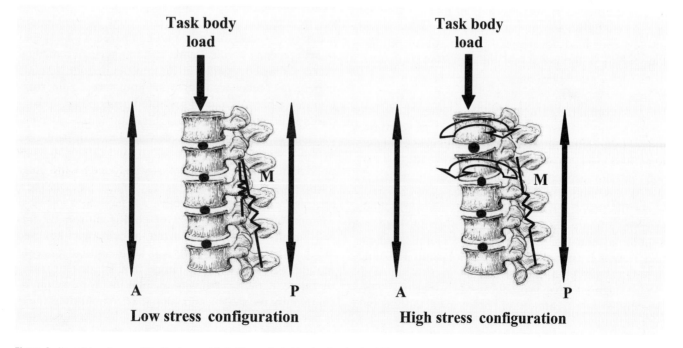

Figure 2 Normal, low stress configuration is associated with coordinated local and regional stabilizer muscle (M) balance. Fatigue or neural control error results in failure of coordinated muscle balance and a buckling event with high local tissue stress. A = anterior; P = posterior.

The result of stress concentration beyond injury threshold initially is a biomechanical phenomenon that may cause pain. Local symptoms predominate unless the involvement is extended by inflammatory or mechanical irritation of nerve endings or the root itself. Inflammatory irritation arises as a direct effect of the inflammatory response or release of neurotoxic byproducts such as phospholipase $A_2$ from an injured disk. Mechanical irritation generally arises secondary to coexisting pathology such as an osteophyte or disk bulge that is otherwise asymptomatic. Remote symptoms will develop by radiation or from direct neural involvement when it occurs. Nerve ending sensitization and proprioceptive signaling associated with altered biomechanical joint function may be a further trigger for remote changes through the development of central sensitization.

Selection of the appropriate type of procedure may be important to the treatment's effectiveness and safety. Factors to consider in patient-procedure matching include patient age, overall physical condition, coexisting pathology, and the effects of any prior surgical intervention affecting the area to be treated. Provocation testing, the test application of preliminary loads similar to those anticipated during the treatment, can help determine the sensitivity of the tissues, permitting modification of procedures as necessary. Acute edema, osteopenia, and weakened or unstable structures are conditions that may direct the use of one type of procedure over another. For example, severe osteopenia may warrant the use of mobilization or continuous passive motion over HVLA loading methods. The skilled physician is able to methodically vary the patient posture, direction of the loading vector, the impulse or cycle duration, and the speed of load development, all in consideration of the severity of the lesion and any comorbid pathology.

## Efficacy of SMT

Evidence supporting the clinical usefulness of SMT for symptomatic improvement of mechanical neck and back pain are derived from clinical trials and more recent systematic reviews. Although there is currently no clear consensus on aspects of effects of treatment with SMT, the preponderance of evidence has been favorable.

In the first rigorous systematic review of the literature on primary care management of acute low back pain in the adult, the US Agency for Health Care Policy and Research (now the Agency for Health Resources and Quality) developed guidelines in 1994 in which HVLA manipulative procedures were specifically recommended as a treatment of choice for acute low back pain in the absence of radiculopathy. Since that time, the preponderance of evidence from subsequent clinical trials, systematic reviews, and meta-analyses have continued to support the use of SMT for acute, subacute, and chronic back and neck pain against most established forms of therapeutic approaches.

### Efficacy of SMT for Neck Pain

SMT is commonly used in the management of neck pain, certain types of headaches, and radicular symptoms. Several studies have investigated the efficacy of cervical SMT used alone or in conjunction with modalities such as exercise, physical therapy, massage therapy, and medical management including medication and booklet advice. In a 1996 study, short-term benefits of SMT were found to be more effective than muscle relaxants and medical care for neck pain and headaches. There was minimal risk of SMT-associated complications. That same year, SMT was found to be appropriate for treating musculotendinous neck pain without radiculopathy.

In 2002, three separate clinical trials evaluating the benefit of SMT for neck pain were published. In one study, patients having nonspecific neck pain with or without radicular symptoms of at least 2 weeks in duration were randomized to receive manual therapy, physical therapy, or medical care. Most participants had neck pain for 12 weeks or less, and many had a prior history of neck pain with concomitant symptoms including cervicogenic headache and dizziness. All subjects were followed for 6 weeks and were assessed at 3 and 7 weeks. Outcome measures included perceived recovery ("completely recovered" and "much improved" were considered a success), functional disability, pain, improvement in range of motion, and general health status. At 7-week follow-up, the authors found that a significantly higher proportion of patients in the manual therapy group achieved a successful outcome compared with the patients receiving medical care. Patients receiving manual therapy showed significant improvement from baseline in perceived recovery, improvement of severe pain, rotation range of motion, and self-rated general health compared with patients receiving physical therapy. In comparison with the group receiving medical care, the manual therapy group demonstrated significant improvement in all parameters as was found in the comparison with the physical therapy group. Manual therapy also proved more effective for improving physical dysfunction, other measures of pain (for example, improvement in pain severity from the previous week and "bothersomeness" of pain), and all measured range of motion (flexion-extension, lateral flexion, rotation). Furthermore, patients receiving manual therapy and physical therapy required less analgesic treatment than those receiving medical care. Minor transient adverse effects such as headache, pain, or arm paresthesia and dizziness were reported in the manual therapy and physical therapy groups.

The role of SMT, specifically mobilization with manipulation, and the effect of using physical modalities in conjunction with manual techniques were addressed in another recent randomized study. Three hundred thirty-six patients with subacute and chronic neck pain with or without radicular symptoms and headaches lasting at least 3 weeks and no longer than 1 year, were randomized into the following treatment groups: (1) manipulation with or without heat; (2) manipulation with or without electrical stimulation; (3) mobilization with or without heat; and (4) mobilization with or without electrical stimulation. Subjects were interviewed at 4 weeks after the initiation of therapy to discuss any complications or side effects; questionnaires were completed for pain and disability measures at 2 weeks, 6 weeks, 3 months, and 6 months. The results showed cervical SMT in the form of mobilization and manipulation to be comparable in improving pain and disability at 6 months whether or not it was combined with heat or electrical stimulation. Although no serious complications occurred, patients undergoing manipulation often experienced minor discomfort during the first month of therapy compared with the patients who underwent cervical mobilization.

The third study from 2002 assessed SMT and exercise for the management of chronic cervicogenic headache and chronic neck pain. Two hundred participants were randomized into four treatment arms: (1) manipulative therapy group using HVLA technique and mobilization; (2) exercise therapy group incorporating low load endurance exercises including craniocervical flexion exercises, and stretching; (3) combination of manipulative therapy and exercise; or (4) control group receiving no treatment. Treatment lasted for 6 weeks and patients were followed up at baseline, week 7, and at 3, 6, and 12 months. The authors found a significant reduction in the intensity and frequency of headaches and neck pain at 12-month follow-up for patients in the combined SMT and exercise group compared with the control patients, but combined therapy was no better than SMT alone. No serious side effects were reported in either patient group. It appears either manual therapy alone or combined with exercise may provide benefits beyond the treatment period.

Based on recent clinical trials, SMT appears to offer clinical benefits for acute or chronic mechanical neck pain, even in patients with nonspecified forms of neck pain. However, two recently completed systematic reviews have reanalyzed data from earlier and more current clinical trials. In one 2004 review, criteria modified from the guidelines for acute low back pain from the US Agency for Health Care Policy and Research were used. The authors examined short-term (follow-up at ≤ 3 months) and long-term (> 3 months) trials. For acute neck pain, there was inconclusive evidence supporting the use of SMT. For chronic neck pain, the authors concluded there was moderate evidence suggesting that SMT was superior to general practitioner management and physical therapy over the short term, and most similar in pain relief compared with high technology rehabilitative exercise in studies having both short- and long-term follow-up. For studies including patients with acute and chronic neck pain, the results favoring use of SMT varied from moderate to superior when compared with physical therapy over both the short and long term. SMT was judged superior to medical care in the short term for improving neck pain.

The Cochrane Database published similar conclusions in 2004. Data were assessed from both randomized controlled trials and quasirandomized studies on the effectiveness of SMT for neck-related pain and concomitant radicular symptoms and headache. Strong evidence was available supporting multimodal care, including mobilization and/or HVLA manipulation when given with exercise. Improvements in pain, function, and global perceived effect for subacute and chronic mechanical neck pain were noted in patients with or without headaches. However, SMT was judged not to be better when administered alone or in combination with other modalities (for example, no treatment, placebo tablets, exercise, traction, massage, collar, galvanic current and ultrasound, ultraviolet light, mobilization, manipulation, and heat and/or electric stimulation, and analgesics). The relative efficacy of SMT for radicular symptoms was uncertain. Moderate evidence favored manipulative therapy in terms of cost effectiveness for the management of acute, subacute, and chronic neck pain with or without headache or radicular symptoms.

### Efficacy of SMT for Low Back Pain

Previous reports provide evidence that SMT may be more effective than medical care in improving pain and disability associated with symptomatic back pain. Medical care is defined as oral medication with other adjunctive therapy such as physical therapy, patient education, and exercise. In a 12-week randomized controlled trial, manipulative therapy was compared with standard medical care (medication, physical therapy, and physical modalities) in patients with subacute to chronic low back pain lasting from 3 weeks to 6 months, respectively. Both treatment groups showed comparable improvement in outcomes for pain and disability.

In a separate randomized study of SMT contrasted with standard medical care, 681 patients with subacute or chronic back pain received medication, and patient education with or without physical therapy or chiropractic care. Clinical outcomes for pain and disability were determined using follow-up questionnaires mailed to patients at 2 weeks, 6 weeks, and 6 months. At 6 months, the patients receiving chiropractic care demonstrated improvements comparable with those received by patients who underwent medical care without physical therapy for pain and disability. In the patients receiving physical therapy, there was a slight improvement in reduction of disability compared with medical care alone at the 6-month follow-up.

According to a 2003 study, SMT combined with medical therapy was shown to be more effective than medical therapy alone in treating low back pain. SMT combined with stabilizing exercises and medical consultation was compared with medical consultation alone (which included an educational booklet and self-management instructions) in patients with chronic low back pain. The combined therapy group experienced greater improvement in pain and disability than those in the physician consultation group at 5 months and at 1-year follow-up. This report was the first to suggest potential durability of combining SMT with medical therapy or patient education.

A separate randomized controlled trial done in 2003 found that patients with low back pain or radicular symptoms receiving SMT had significantly better outcomes for pain, disability, general health, and spinal range of motion than patients treated with exercise alone. Perhaps more importantly, patients who received manual therapy also showed better outcomes in returning to work full time upon follow-up. The latter finding is especially notable because patients in this study had experienced symptoms for more than 8 weeks and had been on sick leave from 8 weeks to less than 6 months.

SMT has also been compared with interventional procedures. In 40 patients with lumbar disk herniation and subsequent chronic radicular symptoms, SMT was compared with chemonucleolysis. The results showed significantly greater short-term improvement in low back pain and disability in the SMT group after 2 weeks. However, at 12 months, no differences in these outcome measures were found between the two treatment groups. Moreover, no serious adverse events occurred in the SMT group. Despite the relatively modest number of subjects included in the study, the findings suggest that SMT may be beneficial for some individuals with low back pain caused by disk herniation and radiculopathy, before more invasive procedures such as chemonucleolysis are used.

Several systematic reviews and meta-analyses on the role and benefit of SMT for low back pain have been published. In a 1997 systematic review, SMT was considered to be superior over placebo, general practitioner care, analgesic, bed rest, and massage for relief of chronic low back pain with or without leg pain. However, SMT was considered no more effective than exercise, physical modalities, massage, and medications for acute low back pain. An earlier systematic review concluded that SMT provided short-term benefit for acute and chronic low back pain and is associated with a low risk of therapy-related complications. The discordance

between these kinds of results from meta-analyses and the individual studies included in more modern reports is again observed.

In a 2004 systematic review, the authors rated several studies assessing low back pain and compared the efficacy of manipulation versus various therapeutic options using the modified guidelines for acute low back pain from the US Agency for Health Care Policy and Research. Among the included clinical trials, there were studies on acute and chronic low back pain (pain lasting less than 6 weeks or longer than 6 weeks, respectively) with length of follow-up categorized as either short-term (3 months or less) or long-term (more than 3 months) after starting therapy. Results from randomized clinical trials assessing acute low back pain only showed that SMT provided short-term pain relief when compared with mobilization or detuned diathermy, and there was limited evidence showing that patients receiving SMT experienced a faster recovery than those who received physical therapy. Studies examining patients with chronic low back pain only indicated that SMT was as effective as nonsteroidal anti-inflammatory drugs during short- and long-term follow-up. Additionally, studies indicated that SMT was as effective as physical modalities and general practitioner therapy in patients with short-term follow-up. Conversely, in patients with chronic low back pain followed up after less than 3 months, there was limited evidence favoring SMT over sham therapy or chemonucleolysis.

## Limitations of SMT Data From Clinical Trials and Systematic Reviews

Despite the rigorous study designs of several existing clinical trials and the relatively exhaustive systematic reviews on the clinical usefulness of SMT in the treatment of neck and back-related pain, the efforts are plagued with the same limitations that face the evaluation of most other forms of treatment. For instance, a high degree of clinical and pathologic heterogeneity exists in patients with neck and back pain in many clinical trials; clinical measures used in determining outcome often are not uniform. Additionally, differences in study design, diverse types of therapies evaluated across trials, difficulty in incorporating an adequate placebo arm in clinical trials, and variable length of follow-up all contribute to difficulty in making direct comparisons between trial data.

Finally, there is a lack of consensus on the appropriate objectives of treatment. Long-term outcomes are often expected with little consideration of the variable natural and treatment history of the underlying disorder. Late 20th century concepts that back pain is a self-limiting disorder that can be "cured" have proved to be too simplistic. Indeed, modern data suggest that many spine complaints are chronic, episodic disorders. If that

## Table 1 | Indications and Contraindications to SMT in the Management of Mechanical Neck and/or Back Pain

**Indications**

Local back or neck pain with and without radiating/radicular
  symptoms

Focal sensitivity to manual pressure, reproducing symptoms

Limited joint compliance
  Mid- or end-range joint play/altered end feel
  Overpressure testing

Reproduction of symptoms with provocation testing/range of motion

Myofascial restriction and hypertonicity

Nonspecific changes
  Local edema
  Altered tissue turgor
  Temperature change
  Color change

**Relative Contraindications: Modified Techniques May Be Used Based on Clinical Status**

Pregnancy

Spondylolisthesis

Midline disk herniation

Patients on anticoagulant therapy

**Contraindications From Local Pathology**

Cauda equina syndrome

Progressive neurologic compromise

Severe osteoporosis

Anatomic instability in the direction of instability

Acute inflammatory arthropathy

Osteomyelitis or metabolic bone weakening disease

Fracture

Primary or metastatic tumor

Vascular compromise (eg, vertebrobasilar insufficiency,
  thrombophlebitis, and thoracic or abdominal aneurysm require
  immediate consultation)

Visceral referred pain or significant psychosocial pathology

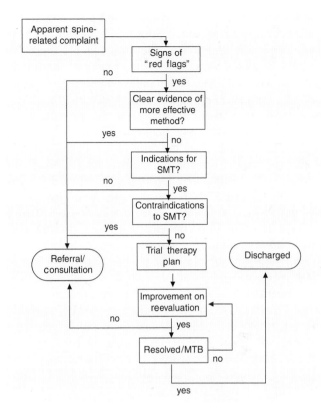

Figure 3 Clinical decision algorithm for administering SMT. Red flags represent findings suggesting emergent, urgent, or nonmusculoskeletal conditions requiring consultation for further diagnostic workup. MTB = maximum therapeutic benefit.

information holds true, widely spaced outcomes may well be irrelevant; the severity and rate of recovery from and recurrence of episodes may be more pertinent to the improvement of quality of life. Even under the concept of a self-limiting disorder, the late comparison of treatment effects is questionable. If it is expected that by a certain time, for example 12 months, the natural history of a condition would lead to resolution, why would an investigator rationally expect differences in results between any therapeutic efforts?

## Clinical Application of SMT for Mechanical Neck and Back-Related Pain

The preponderance of evidence shows that there are subgroups of patients with mechanical neck and back-related symptoms that benefit from the use of SMT, particularly in terms of symptomatic pain relief and im-

provement in levels of function with minimal iatrogenic adverse consequences.

The indications and contraindications for a trial of SMT are presented in Table 1. The algorithm in Figure 3 provides a simple sequence of clinical reasoning for treatment of the patient with SMT. Many clinical indications for SMT will become evident following an in-depth patient history and a thorough physical examination. A proper differential diagnosis for the cause of neck and back pain will allow selection of those mechanical causes most likely to respond to SMT while minimizing the risk of potential adverse events by excluding patients with contraindications.

Determining which type of procedure to administer is largely based on the clinical characteristics of the manipulative lesion and affected tissues, comorbid conditions, and patient tolerance. For instance, patients with chronic low back pain and underlying severe osteopenia may benefit from an unloaded spinal mobilization procedure such as continuous passive motion or flexion distraction. Alternatively, patients with chronic mechanical low back pain may require and tolerate higher loads given via HVLA techniques delivered manually or with the assistance of a mechanical device.

The duration and frequency of SMT sessions should vary according to the nature, duration, and severity of the specific condition being treated and according to the patient's willingness and compliance with the intensity and frequency of initiated therapy. Clinical improvement is expected within the first 2 weeks of treatment; patients with back and/or leg pain may require an average of 8 treatment sessions to reach maximal improvement, with a range of 1 to 40 sessions cited in the literature. Evidence from one randomized trial of patients with chronic nonspecific mechanical low back pain suggests that SMT given three to four times per week for 3 weeks may be the most appropriate treatment for this condition. Because SMT is customized to address both the patient and a specific underlying condition, it may be expected that some patients will respond more rapidly and require less frequent treatments.

A 4-week randomized controlled trial published in 2004 applied a previously described clinical prediction rule to successfully identify patients with low back pain who were most likely to benefit from SMT. Favorable predictors of better clinical outcome required patients to meet at least four of the following five criteria: (1) low back pain of less than 16 days' duration; (2) no radiating symptoms distal to the knee; (3) Fear-Avoidance Beliefs Questionnaire score less than 19 points; (4) at least one hypomobile lumbar segment; and (5) at least one hip with greater than 35° of internal rotation. Among patients having a favorable outcome, those receiving both exercise plus SMT had significant improvement in disability scores compared with patients receiving exercise only. In contrast, among patients with low back pain having three or less of the five favorable predictors, there was no significant improvement regardless of whether they received exercise only or exercise in addition to SMT. Thus, SMT may be beneficial when combined with exercise in patients having favorable outcome based on the clinical prediction rule.

In patients who are slow responders and who show temporary response but rapid regression (remaining particularly refractory to a typical course of traditional manipulative therapy [SMT for an approximate 4- to 6-week trial period with persistent pain and muscle guarding]), or in those patients who are too sensitive to local pressures from the treatment procedures, manipulation under joint anesthesia/analgesia may be a treatment option. With this technique, an anesthetic is injected fluoroscopically, with or without the use of a steroid, to suppress the underlying pain-generating structure. SMT is administered while the patient is still under the influence of the local anesthetic. A trial period of SMT may be warranted for six to eight sessions within the first 10 to 12 days after injection.

## Potential Complications Associated With SMT

As may be expected for any therapeutic procedure, there are potential complications associated with the use of SMT. The most commonly experienced adverse effects of SMT include minor muscle and joint discomfort, which may be either localized at or near the site of the manipulation. More intense reactions occur in up to one in seven patients. These reactions are self-limiting and resolve within 24 hours. In a single large prospective study, 465 patients receiving SMT administered by providers from any discipline were surveyed for adverse effects accompanying cervical, thoracic, or lumbar procedures. More than half of the patients reported experiencing a transient headache, stiffness, local or radiating discomfort, or fatigue. Women were more likely to report these adverse effects. Temporary headache, dizziness, and nausea were more likely to occur with cervical manipulation than with thoracic or lumbar manipulation. Findings from the Cochrane Database also showed that self-limiting adverse effects were reported in less than one third of all the included trials and consisted of local spine pain, transient headache, dizziness and ear symptoms, radicular pain, and distal paresthesia.

Serious complications, such as cauda equina syndrome and cerebral vascular accidents, are uncommon. Cauda equina syndrome typical occurs along with saddle anesthesia, bilateral leg weakness and sensory changes, and loss of bowel and bladder control. The risk of cauda equina syndrome is estimated to be no more than 1 in 100,000,000 lumbar procedures. According to the literature, most instances of cauda equina syndrome have been reported in patients receiving manipulation under general anesthesia who were unable to provide feedback during the procedure.

Estimates of the frequency of cerebral vascular incidents associated with SMT range from 1 in 1,000,000, to 1 in 3,850,000 manipulations. Conversely, the risk for a serious gastrointestinal event resulting from nonsteroidal anti-inflammatory drug use is 1 in 1,000 for all ages, 3.2 in 1,000 for patients older than 65 years, and 0.39 in 1,000 for those younger than 65 years. The largest retrospective review based on 69 medicolegal cases revealed the unpredictable nature of vertebrobasilar artery dissections. Although this topic is a great source of debate, the strength of the association of these complications with cervical manipulation is being questioned. The rate of occurrence of vertebrobasilar artery dissections appears to be the same in patients receiving manipulation treatment to the neck as in the general population. Symptoms of vertebrobasilar artery dissections arising after cervical spine manipulation generally have occurred within 2 to 4 hours of the procedure in 94% of patients and within 30 minutes to 1 hour in 75% of patients. The most common symptoms include loss of coordination, dizziness or vertigo, vomiting, dysphagia, dysarthria, visual disturbance, numbness, and nystagmus. Serious complications resulting from thoracic manipulation are even less common, possibly because of the inherent stability provided by the thoracic cage. Some of the complications reported include sprains at the costo-transverse and costovertebral articulations, rib fractures, and very rarely, fractures of the transverse process. For patients receiving manipulation under joint anesthesia/analgesia, there are the added risks inherent to local anesthetic, analgesic, and corticosteroid use in joint or muscle injections.

Both direct and indirect evidence indicates that extent of training and routine experience are factors related to successful outcome and relative risk of SMT procedures. For physicians attempting to integrate selected manipulation methods into medical management of low back pain following limited training through a series of weekend seminars, there was no added benefit. Training was intended to provide familiarity with the procedures, not to develop expert skills. Earlier research on skill development has demonstrated that skill among experienced operators is not transferable to unpracticed procedures, because HVLA procedures use unique bimanual, complex tasks often performed under different clinical circumstances to treat patients with local pathology or tissue injury. Like other clinical procedures requiring motor coordination and clinical integration, preparation and extent of training appear to play a significant role in provider proficiency.

Based on actuarial data, chiropractors perform approximately 94% of the manipulations done in the United States. Case series and case review literature reflect that approximately 46% to 80% (average, 62%) of complications associated with manipulation occur at the hands of chiropractors.

## Summary

The goal of SMT is to improve regional joint and soft-tissue dysfunction related to mechanical neck, mid-back, and low back pain. A recently devised classification system of SMT can be used to assist practitioners in identifying subgroups of patients who may derive the most benefit from SMT and to match types of procedures to patient needs. Findings from clinical trials and systematic reviews support a trial of SMT for patients who have no signs of 'red flags' (findings suggesting emergent, urgent, or nonmusculoskeletal conditions that require additional diagnostic workup) and no history of contraindications and appropriate differential diagnosis. Adverse effects from SMT are minimal and serious complications are rare. Adequate training and mentored experience are associated with increased effectiveness and decreased relative incidence of serious adverse events. Combining SMT with exercise and preventive lifestyle changes provide a long-term strategy for improved quality of life.

## Annotated Bibliography

*Definitions of Manipulative Therapy and the Manipulable Lesion*

Triano JJ: Biomechanics of spinal manipulative therapy. *Spine J* 2001;1:121-130.

This article discusses the biomechanics related to SMT, including unbuckling and its symptoms.

*Efficacy of SMT*

Andersson GB, Lucente T, Davis AM, et al: A comparison of osteopathic spinal manipulation with standard care for patients with low back pain. *N Engl J Med* 1999;341:1426-1431.

Patients with subacute and chronic low back pain (duration from 3 weeks to 6 months) were randomized to manual (osteopathic manipulation) or standard medical care groups and treated for 12 weeks. Pain decreased in both groups of patients; the manual treatment group used less medication and less physical therapy, with a satisfaction rate of greater than 90% for both groups.

Assendelft WJ, Morton SC, Yu EI, et al: Spinal manipulative therapy for low back pain: A meta-analysis of effectiveness relative to other therapies. *Ann Intern Med* 2003;138:871-881.

A meta-analysis of randomized controlled trials published from 1966 to 2000 found SMT was no better than general practitioner care, pain medication, physical therapy, exercise, or back school for treating acute and chronic low back pain. SMT was superior to sham or ineffective therapies for treating acute low back pain.

Aure OF, Nilsen JH, Vasseljen O: Manual therapy and exercise therapy in patients with chronic low back pain. *Spine* 2003;28:525-532.

Forty-nine sick-listed (symptoms lasting longer than 8 weeks, less than 6 months) patients with low back pain or radicular symptoms lasting longer than 8 weeks were randomized to either manual therapy or exercise and followed up to 1 year. In the manual therapy group, there was greater improvement for the year in all outcomes including pain relief/intensity, degree of disability, general health status, and ability to return to work.

Bronfort G, Haas M, Evans RL, et al: Efficacy of spinal manipulation and mobilization for low back pain and neck pain: A systematic review and best evidence synthesis. *Spine J* 2004;4:335-356.

The evidence supporting the use of SMT to treat acute neck pain was inconclusive. There was moderate evidence suggesting that SMT was superior to general practitioner management and physical therapy in the short-term treatment of chronic neck pain; study results indicated that the degree of pain relief was similar using SMT compared with high technology rehabilitative exercise in studies having both short- and long-term follow-up. For studies including patients with both acute and chronic neck pain, the results favoring use of SMT varied from moderate to superior when compared with physical therapy over both the short and long term. SMT was judged superior to medical care over the short term for improving neck pain. There was moderate evidence that SMT offered short-term relief of acute low back pain when compared with mobilization or detuned diathermy. There was moderate evidence that SMT was as effective as nonsteroidal anti-inflammatory drugs in treating patients with chronic low back pain having short- and long-term follow-up, and SMT was as effective as physical modalities and general practitioner therapy in patients with short-term follow-up.

Burton AK, Tillotson KM, Cleary J: Single-blind randomized controlled trial of chemonucleolysis and manipulation in the treatment of symptomatic lumbar disc herniation. *Eur Spine J* 2000;9:202-207.

Forty patients with chronic radicular symptoms received either osteopathic manipulation or chemonucleolysis. There was a statistically significant improvement in pain relief at 2 and 6 weeks and degree of disability at 2 weeks. At 12 months, both groups experienced fewer symptoms with no difference between groups. Manipulation was found to be more cost effective at 12 months. There were no serious complications.

Cagnie B, Vinck E, Beernaert A, et al: How common are side effects of spinal manipulation and can these side effects be predicted? *Man Ther* 2004;9:151-156.

Following the patient's first manipulation, common benign adverse effects reported included headache, stiffness, local and radiating discomfort and fatigue; these occurred within 4 hours following the treatment and dissipated within 24 hours. Reactions were considered transient and benign in nature. Women were more likely to report these reactions.

Gross AR, Hoving JL, Haines TA, et al: A Cochrane review of manipulation and mobilization for mechanical neck disorders. *Spine* 2004;29:1541-1548.

The use of multimodal management, most commonly combined manipulation/mobilization and exercise therapy, was advocated. There was no difference between manipulation/mobilization when performed alone or with other physical modalities. Efficacy for management of neck pain with radicular symptoms was uncertain. Thirty-one percent of patients experienced adverse effects such as transient headache, dizziness and ear symptoms, radicular pain and distal paresthesia, neck and thoracic pain.

Haas M, Groupp E, Kraemer DF: Dose-response for chiropractic care of chronic low back pain. *Spine J* 2004; 4:574-583.

Seventy-two patients with chronic mechanical low back pain, randomly assigned between 1 to 4 visits per week for 3 weeks, received either SMT or SMT with physical modalities. At week 4, patients experienced a greater reduction in

pain and disability, and three to four treatment sessions for 3 weeks provided relief.

Hoving JL, Koes BW, de Vet HCW, et al: Manual therapy, physical therapy, or continued care by a general practitioner for patients with neck pain: A randomized controlled trial. *Ann Intern Med* 2002;136:713-722.

Patients receiving manual therapy had greater success (68.3%) than with continued care (35.9%); decreased pain was also noted in patients receiving manual therapy over continued care. Patients receiving manual therapy and physical therapy required less medication use. Minor transient side effects such as headache, pain, or arm paresthesia and dizziness were reported in manual therapy and physical therapy patient groups.

Hurwitz EL, Morgenstern H, Harber P, et al: A randomized trial of medical care with and without physical therapy and chiropractic care with and without physical modalities for patients with low back pain: 6-month follow-up outcomes from the UCLA low back pain study. *Spine* 2002;27:2193-2204.

Patients were randomized to four groups: medical care with and without physical therapy, and chiropractic care with and without physical modalities. Patients experienced relief of pain and disability in both the chiropractic and medical treatment groups at 6 months, and slightly greater benefits from physical therapy, which was slightly more effective than medical care in reducing disability.

Hurwitz EL, Morgenstern H, Harber P, et al: A randomized trial of chiropractic manipulation and mobilization for patients with neck pain: Clinical outcomes from the UCLA neck-pain study. *Am J Public Health* 2002;92: 1634-1641.

Treatment arms included manipulation with or without heat, manipulation with or without electrical stimulation, mobilization with or without heat, and mobilization with or without electrical stimulation. Mobilization was comparable to manipulation (with/without modalities) for pain and disability at 6 months, with fewer adverse effects with mobilization.

Jull G, Trott P, Potter H, et al: A randomized controlled trial of exercise and manipulative therapy for cervicogenic headache. *Spine* 2002;27:1835-1843.

Patients with neck pain and headaches were randomized into manipulation, exercise, or combined manipulation/ exercise groups and followed up over 1 year. There was a reduction in frequency, intensity, and duration of headache as well as neck pain for patients in the combined manual therapy and exercise group at 12-month follow-up. In the patients receiving manual therapy, there was a significant decrease in frequency and intensity of headache at 12-month follow-up. Combined manipulation/exercise therapy provided a 10% greater chance of obtaining improvement.

Niemisto L, Lahtinen-Suopanki T, Rissanen P, et al: A randomized trial of combined manipulation, stabilizing exercises, and physician consultation compared to physician consultation alone for chronic low back pain. *Spine* 2003;28:2185-2191.

A randomized trial compared manipulation/exercise/ physician consultation treatment to physician consultation alone in patients with chronic low back pain. At 5-month and 1-year follow-up, there was a greater reduction in pain and disability for the patients who received manipulation/exercise/ physician treatment.

### Clinical Application of SMT for Mechanical Neck and Back-Related Pain

Childs JD, Fritz JM, Flynn TW, et al: A clinical prediction rule to identify patients with low back pain most likely to benefit from spinal manipulation: A validation study. *Ann Intern Med* 2004;141:920-928.

A previously described clinical prediction rule was applied during a 4-week randomized controlled trial to successfully identify patients with low back pain who were most likely to benefit from SMT. Favorable predictors of better clinical outcome required patients to meet at least four of five criteria. Among patients having favorable outcome, those receiving both exercise and SMT showed significant improvement in disability scores compared with patients receiving exercise only. In contrast, among patients with low back pain having no more than three of the five favorable predictors, there was no significant improvement regardless of whether they received exercise only or exercise and SMT. At 6-month follow-up, the exercise-only group had increased health care utilization, lost work time, and greater medication use because of back pain.

Kohlbeck FJ, Haldeman S: Medication-assisted spinal manipulation. *Spine J* 2002;2:288-302.

Manipulation can be used in conjunction with a fluoroscopically guided injection of an anesthetic and a steroid. Manipulation is performed immediately after the injection and then for a trial period while the medication has peak effect. Examples of medication-assisted procedures include manipulation under joint anesthesia/analgesia, manipulation under general anesthesia or sedation, manipulation under epidural anesthesia/analgesia, and manipulation with injectants and proliferant agents. More serious reported complications are related to manipulation under general anesthesia; no complications have been reported with manipulation under joint anesthesia/analgesia.

Triano JJ: Manipulation, in Cole A, Herring S (eds): *The Low Back Pain Handbook*, ed 2. Philadelphia, PA, Hanley & Belfus, 2003.

SMT may be beneficial in treating patients with low back pain and leg pain provided 'red flags' (findings suggesting urgent conditions requiring additional workup) are ruled out. Several SMT procedures varying in load type, application, and speed, can correct the manipulative lesion. At least eight treatment sessions may be necessary to bring about maximal im-

provement. Minor adverse effects usually resolve within 24 hours; severe complications are very rare.

### Potential Complications Associated With SMT

Curtis P, Carey T, Evans P, et al: Training primary care physicians to give limited manual therapy for low back pain: Patient outcomes. *Spine* 2000;25:2954-2960.

Thirty-one primary care physicians were trained to perform limited manual therapy techniques and optimal low back care (enhanced care) for patients with acute low back pain. Patients received either enhanced care alone or enhanced care with manual therapy. No difference was noted in Roland-Morris score, mean functional days to recovery, days absent from work, or patient satisfaction.

Haldeman S, Kohlbeck FJ, McGregor M: Unpredictability of cerebrovascular ischemia associated with cervical spine manipulation therapy: A review of sixty-four cases after cervical spine manipulation. *Spine* 2002;27:49-55.

The risk of cerebrovascular accident ranges from 1 in 400,000 to 500,000 to 1 in 3.85 million cervical spine manipulations and is considered unpredictable. In a review of 69 unpublished medicolegal records, the most common neurologic findings included nystagmus, visual disturbance, loss of consciousness, incoordination, dizziness/vertigo/nausea/vomiting, speech, numbness, and dysarthria/dysphagia. Onset of symptoms occurred within 2 days of manipulation in 94% of patients, and within 30 minutes in 75%.

McGregor M: Musculoskeletal complications of chiropractic practice, in Halderman S (ed): *Principles and Practice of Chiropractic*, ed 3. New York, NY, McGraw Hill, 2004, pp 1137-1147.

An overview of musculoskeletal complications in chiropractic practice is presented.

Triano JJ, Bougie J, Roger C, et al: Procedural skills in spinal manipulation: Do prerequisites matter? *Spine J* 2004;4:557-563.

Students were randomized into either a program with greater didactic training or greater emphasis on premanipulative laboratory skills. Students had no prior training in lumbar manipulation and were required to perform a specified lumbar technique. Results from the groups were also compared with results from patients who underwent manipulation performed by an expert doctor. A significant difference in measured parameters was noted between the greater skilled group and the expert doctor. Because of the complex nature of manipulation, students in the curriculum with greater emphasis on premanipulation techniques developed greater skills than students in the didactic program.

## Classic Bibliography

Bigos SJ (ed): *Acute Low Back Problem in Adults*. Rockville, MD, US Department of Health and Human

Services (Clinical Practice Guideline # 14: AHCPR Publication No. 95-0642), 1994.

Bronfort G: Spinal manipulation: Current state of research and its indications. *Neurol Clin* 1999;17:91-111.

Cassidy JD, Thiel HW, Kirkaldy-Willis WH: Side posture manipulation for lumbar intervertebral disk herniation. *J Manipulative Physiol Ther* 1993;2:96-103.

Cherkin DC, Deyo RA, Battie M, et al: A comparison of physical therapy, chiropractic manipulation, and provision of an educational booklet for the treatment of patients with low back pain. *N Engl J Med* 1998;339:1021-1029.

Cholewicki J, McGill SM: Lumbar posterior ligament involvement during extremely heavy lifts estimated from fluoroscopic measurements. *J Biomech* 1992;25:17-28.

Cohen E, Triano JJ, McGregor M, et al: Biomechanical performance of spinal manipulation therapy by newly trained vs practicing providers: Does experience transfer to unfamiliar procedures? *J Manipulative Physiol Ther* 1995;18:347-352.

Coulter ID, Hurwitz EL, Adams AH, et al: The appropriateness of manipulation and mobilization of the cervical spine. Santa Monica, CA, RAND Corporation Publication MR-781-CCR, 1996.

Crisco JJ, Panjabi MM, Yamamoto I, et al: Euler stability of the human ligamentous lumbar spine: Part II. Experiment. *Clin Biomech (Bristol, Avon)* 1992;7:27-32.

Eck JC, Circolone NJ: The use of spinal manipulation in the treatment of low back pain: A review of goals, patient selection, techniques, and risks. *J Orthop Sci* 2000; 5:411-417.

Gabriel SE, Jaakkimain L, Bombardier C: Risk for serious gastrointestinal complications related to use of nonsteroidal anti-inflammatory drugs: A meta-analysis. *Ann Intern Med* 1991;115:787-796.

Haldeman S, Rubinstein SM: Cauda equina syndrome in patients undergoing manipulation of the lumbar spine. *Spine* 1992;17:1469-1473.

Koes BW, Bouter LM, van Mameren H, et al: The effectiveness of manual therapy, physiotherapy, and treatment by the general practitioner for nonspecific back and neck complaints: A randomized clinical trial. *Spine* 1992;17:28-35.

Koes BW, Bouter LM, van Mameren H, et al: Randomised clinical trial of manipulative therapy and physiotherapy for persistent back and neck complaints: Results of one year follow-up. *BMJ* 1992;304:601-605.

Shekelle PG, Adams AH, Chassin MR, Hurwitz EL, Brook RH: Spinal manipulation for low-back pain. *Ann Intern Med* 1992;117:590-598.

van Tulder MW, Koes BW, Bouter LM: Conservative treatment of acute and chronic nonspecific low back pain: A systematic review of randomized controlled trials of the most common interventions. *Spine* 1997;22: 2128-2156.

Wilder DG, Pope MH, Frymoyer JW: The biomechanics of lumbar disc herniation and the effect of overload and instability. *J Spinal Disord* 1988;1:16-32.

# Chapter 15

# The Management of Low Back Pain: A Comprehensive Rehabilitation Program

Susan C. Sorosky, MD

Brad Sorosky, MD

Joel M. Press, MD

## Introduction

Low back pain (LBP) is a ubiquitous condition with a 60% to 90% lifetime incidence and a 5% annual incidence. It is the most common cause of disability in the United States in people younger than 45 years of age and is second to the common cold as the most frequent reason for visiting the doctor. The annual cost of managing LBP is estimated to be a staggering $56 billion. Although 90% of episodes resolve without medical attention in 6 to 12 weeks, 70% to 90% of patients with LBP have recurrent episodes. Despite a decrease in symptoms, these patients have anatomic and functional changes that increase their chance of reinjury. Therefore, it is essential that rehabilitation focuses not only on resolving the symptoms associated with injured and overloaded tissues but also on identifying and rehabilitating the unique associated biomechanical deficits and functional adaptations.

The benefits of exercise are profound and include improved cardiovascular fitness, muscle strength, flexibility, and endurance. Enhanced mood, increased pain tolerance, and better sleep also have been found to be related to exercise. There is also evidence that spine motion improves disk health through more efficient delivery of nutrients and removal of metabolic waste products. Exercise appears to be relatively safe in patients with LBP; there is no evidence that regular exercise increases the risk of additional back problems in patients with acute, subacute, or chronic LBP. Exercise appears to exert a neutral effect or may even slightly reduce the risk of future back injuries. On the other hand, bed rest has deleterious consequences in the setting of LBP, leading to decreased cardiovascular fitness, muscular strength, flexibility, bone density, and disk nutrition; increased spinal segment stiffness and depression are also associated with inactivity. There is no proven benefit of prolonged bed rest for patients with nonradicular pain. Therefore, no more than 2 days of absolute bed rest is recommended for patients with nonspecific LBP. Relative rest, which allows for short periods of rest between activities and helps minimize the negative effects of bed rest, is actually preferred.

There are several reasons why the clinician should choose rehabilitation techniques for patients with LBP. Rehabilitation techniques help resolve the clinical symptoms and signs created by a primary lumbar spine injury so that active treatment encouraging independence can be initiated as soon as possible, and the untoward effects of inactivity can be minimized. By addressing both the primary site of injury and secondary sites of dysfunction, rehabilitation restores function, returns patients to activity, and theoretically lessens the chance of recurrence, thus optimizing outcome. Specifically, rehabilitation after a lumbar spine injury may help decrease days lost from work or sports activities and may increase productivity. Rehabilitation of lumbar injuries must continue beyond resolution of symptoms so that all other aspects of the injury complex, including flexibility, strength, power, and endurance, are fully rehabilitated. A plan for prevention of recurrent episodes of LBP is developed based on the comprehensive rehabilitation program so that optimal physiologic and biomechanical fitness is maintained; therefore, the risk of injury is potentially minimized.

## Therapeutic Exercise and Cardiovascular Fitness, Flexibility, and Strength

In addition to reducing the intensity of back pain and the degree of disability related to back pain, the broad goals of a rehabilitation program are to improve cardiovascular fitness, flexibility, and strength, because deficits in all of these areas have been found in patients with LBP. Cardiovascular training can result in enhanced metabolism of free fatty acids, less body fat, increased insulin sensitivity, improved blood flow to muscles, higher maximal cardiac output, greater $Vo_{2max}$ (maximal oxygen consumption during exercise), lower heart rate for a given level of exertion, and reduced blood lactate accumulation and minute ventilation at a given submaximal level of exertion. In addition, studies suggest that individuals who are more physically fit may have LBP less often than individuals who do not exercise. On the other hand, aerobic conditioning is easily lost if a back injury results in more than 1 week of reduced activity. Specifically, $Vo_{2max}$, the best indicator of aerobic fitness, decreases by 25% after 3 weeks of bed rest. In addition, patients with chronic LBP have reduced aerobic capacity in comparison with healthy control patients; however, it is unclear whether LBP reduces fitness or if reduced fitness leads to LBP. Therefore, aerobic training is an important aspect of a comprehensive rehabilitation program. According to the American Heart Association (www.americanheart.org), in order to attain a high level of cardiovascular fitness, exercise should be performed for 30 to 60 minutes on most days of the week at 50% to 80% of one's maximum capacity. Improvements in cardiovascular fitness, as measured by a 10% to 20% increases in $Vo_{2max}$, usually can be noted within 8 to 12 weeks of training implementation. Many studies have found that patients with LBP are capable of improving their aerobic capabilities.

Rehabilitation for patients with LBP is also geared toward improving flexibility, which is defined as the ability to move a single joint or series of joints through an unrestricted pain-free range of motion. Flexibility is dependent on the extensibility of muscles and connective tissue that cross and surround a joint. General benefits of improved flexibility include increased available joint range of motion and reduced stress across one or more joints. Patients with LBP may report feeling "less stiff" and being able to perform activities of daily living (ADLs) and other work, sports, and/or leisure activities more comfortably. To produce normal lumbar motion, flexibility must be present in the hip flexors, hip extensors, hip rotators, adductors, abductors, hamstrings, quadriceps, and the gastrocnemius-soleus complex. A normal degree of flexibility of the hamstrings is required for appropriate lifting and bending postures; a flexibility deficit in the hamstrings appears to be a predisposing factor in the development of LBP. Particular muscles prone to tightness in patients with LBP include the erector spinae, tensor fascia latae, iliopsoas, quadratus lumborum, and hamstrings. Also, deficits in lead hip internal range of motion have been documented in golfers with LBP. Several methods of stretching exist, including static (steady force application over a period of 15 to 60 seconds); ballistic (use of rapid force in a repeated bouncing, throwing, or jerking maneuver); and proprioceptive neurofacilitation (techniques of hold-relax or contract-relax with or without agonist contraction). More recently, functional stretching, which includes activity and sport-specific stretches performed in a dynamic manner in multiple planes of movement, has come into favor. Despite the chosen stretching technique, rapid high-force stretches, which produce tissue recoil, should be avoided. Also, in patients with lumbar instability, end-range flexibility exercises should be avoided to prevent further dysfunction and pain. In general, stretching is effective in restoring normal trunk range of motion in patients with LBP. In patients with chronic LBP, flexibility training leads to a 20% average improvement in trunk flexibility.

The goal of a comprehensive rehabilitation program for LBP is to correct muscle weaknesses and imbalances with strengthening exercises. Strength training has been used as a successful strategy to reduce LBP and improve function. Other benefits include the potential for reduced risk of reinjury and an increased sense of well-being in patients with LBP. With complete bed rest, muscle has been shown to lose 1% to 3% of its strength per day and 10% to 15% per week during the first 2 weeks. Studies have shown that patients with chronic LBP have reduced strength and greater atrophy of the back muscles in comparison with healthy control patients. A 70% loss in trunk muscle strength was found in patients with lumbosacral pain persisting 6 months or longer. More globally, strength of the core muscles has been found to be preferentially affected in patients with LBP. Studies have reported that the multifidi muscles are atrophied in patients with LBP. A significant asymmetry in hip extensor strength was found in female athletes with LBP; there was an association between this strength imbalance and recurrence of LBP over the ensuing year. In addition to strength deficits, motor control abnormalities have been identified in the core musculature. Patients with LBP appear to have delayed activation of the transversus abdominis. One study reported, that compared with control patients, patients with LBP have delayed trunk muscle activation where the contraction of all trunk muscles precede that of the muscle responsible for lower limb movement; this delay was consistently and most significantly related to contraction of the transversus abdominis. Delayed firing and poor endurance of the gluteus maximus and medius have also been found in patients with LBP. In contrast to these findings that demonstrate the importance of individual core muscles, a more recent study reported that no muscle in isolation dominated in the enhancement of spine stability; each muscle's individual role was continuously changing across tasks. Therefore, it was proposed that global muscle activation by co-contraction of multiple agonist/antagonist muscles was preferable to training primarily "local" muscles. In addition to the core musculature, many other muscles are weak in patients with LBP, including the rectus femoris, vastus medialis and lateralis, tibialis anterior, and peroneus longus and brevis.

Strengthening exercises can be categorized into back extensor strengthening or core strengthening. Traditional strengthening of the back extensors is based on the progressive overload principle whereby increases in muscle strength are associated with muscular hypertrophy and enlargement of muscle cross-sectional area. Examples of this type of exercise include back extensor strengthening machines as well as roman chair exercises, which rely on one's own body weight to strengthen the back extensors. A typical strengthening routine is composed of three sets of 8 to 12 repetitions, performed once or twice a week; resistance should increase by no more than 10% per week. Studies have shown that such progressive resistance training results in improvements of 30% to 80% in volitional back muscle strength. It is unclear, however, whether these findings correlate with any functional benefits. In addition, although the human body functions in three cardinal planes (sagittal, frontal, and transverse), and back injury most commonly results from a combination of these motions, particularly flexion and torsion, these exercises are likely nonfunctional because they are performed solely in the sagittal plane.

Core strengthening is now favored among rehabilitation specialists and has come to supersede other therapeutic exercise regimens such as traditional back extensor strengthening. The core is the center of the functional kinetic chain and can be conceptualized as a "box" with the lumbar muscles (erector spinae and multifidi), abdominals, (transversus abdominis, internal oblique, external oblique, and rectus abdominis), hip girdle (iliopsoas, gluteus maximus and medius, hamstrings, and thoracodorsal fascia), and quadratus lumborum comprising the sides of the box. The diaphragm forms the top and the pelvic floor forms the bottom of the box. The core can be thought of as a muscular corset that works as a unit to stabilize the body and spine with and without limb movement. Core strengthening (also known as dynamic lumbar stabilization, motor control [neuromuscular] training, neutral spine control, and muscular fusion) describes the training of muscular control around the lumbar spine to maintain functional stability. This type of exercise is based on the belief that LBP is intimately linked with functional instability, defined as a significant decrease in the capacity of the stabilizing systems to maintain the neutral zone (the range in which internal resistance from active muscular control is minimal) within physiologic limits. Although intersegmental injury and intervertebral disk degeneration are associated with a larger neutral zone, muscular co-contraction of small intersegmental muscles and larger, more "global" muscles provide active stiffness or stability, thereby making the zone smaller. Rehabilitation of the core also allows the multisegmented spinal column to maintain its center of gravity through multiple ranges of motion, counteracting gravity and applied forces to decrease torsion and shear on spinal structures.

In contrast to progressive resistance training of the back extensors, which form part of the core, core strengthening involves more than simply making muscles strong. In fact, motor relearning of inhibited muscles may be more important than actual strengthening in patients with LBP. According to one study, muscular endurance, not absolute strength, is the most important factor in maintaining a "margin of safety" for stability. This study specifically reported that only a very small increase in the activation of the multifidi and abdominal muscles was required to stiffen spinal segments, including 5% of a maximum voluntary contraction for ADLs and 10% for rigorous activity. Contrary to the commonly held notion, core strengthening is not equivalent to sit-ups and pelvic tilts. Traditional sit-ups are unsafe because they cause increased compression loads on the lumbar spine; pelvic tilts may also increase spinal loading by decreasing lordosis. Moreover, these two traditional exercises are nonfunctional. Instead, with core strengthening, the focus is on a motor control model whereby specific deficits are identified and muscles then trained to provide dynamic stability and segmental control to the spine. Faulty movement patterns are targeted with the components of the movement isolated and retrained into functional tasks specific to the patient's needs. It is imperative that exercises progress from training isolated muscles to training as an integrated unit to facilitate functional activity. Studies demonstrating the efficacy of core strengthening in patients with LBP, along with a core strengthening protocol in the context of a comprehensive rehabilitation program for LBP, will be discussed in subsequent sections.

## Evidence-Based Approach to Specific Therapeutic Exercise Interventions for Specific LBP Diagnoses

Several advances have been made in the field of medicine to the understanding of identifying and managing pathology in the human body. For example, in the field of microbiology, hundreds of different disease-causing microorganisms have been discovered and specific antibiotics developed for treatment of each microorganism. As a result of this knowledge, no longer are all infections considered identical and managed simply with a course of penicillin. Similarly, musculoskeletal clinicians have also gained an appreciation of the various pain generators causing LBP, including muscles, ligaments, facet joints, intervertebral disks, and spinal nerves. Therefore, it makes no more sense to manage all causes of LBP with the same set of exercises as it does to treat all infections with penicillin.

Although specific therapeutic exercise interventions have been developed to address different diagnostic subsets of LBP, guidelines regarding the effectiveness of exercise for LBP, including the well-known Cochrane Database of Systematic Reviews, are sometimes confusing and controversial. According to the Cochrane Database, there is strong evidence that exercise therapy is no more effective than other active or even inactive treatments of acute LBP. In addition, there is conflicting evidence regarding the efficacy of exercise compared with inactive treatment for chronic LBP. Exercise therapy appears to be more effective than the usual care provided by the general practitioner and equally effective as conventional physiotherapy. The studies cited by such guidelines often contribute to misconceptions about the lack of efficacy of exercise for LBP because in many instances, a uniform exercise program was used irrespective of an ill-defined underlying condition. As a result, what is demonstrated is that nonspecific treatments of nonspecific diagnoses lead to nonspecific results. It is unreasonable to expect specific benefits from an exercise program if no specific diagnoses are made before initiation of the treatment arm of a study. Furthermore, a physical therapy program that is not individualized to each patient lessens the chance of successful rehabilitation of patients who have different causes of LBP. In summary, absence of proof because of methodologic flaws in the available literature is not equivalent to proof that exercise has no beneficial effect.

Better designed studies exist in which diagnostic subsets of patients with LBP are defined and treatments specific for these diagnoses are evaluated. For example, in the literature, back pain is not considered a nebulous entity but rather a presentation with many different etiologies including mechanical, flexion based (for example, disk herniation), extension based (for example, facet pathology, spinal stenosis), and instability mediated. In addition, as opposed to a blanket approach to physical therapy, specific therapeutic exercise protocols such as the McKenzie technique and core strengthening are evaluated in patients with LBP. In general, these studies show more promising results regarding the efficacy of therapeutic exercise for the management of LBP. For example, the effectiveness and medical costs of a classification approach to the rehabilitation of patients with acute, work-related LBP were compared with an approach based on the Agency for Health Care Policy Research guideline that advocates a more general approach for the first 4 weeks of rehabilitation. Joint mobilization or manipulation and spinal active range-of-motion exercises were assigned to those patients with unilateral symptoms who did not have signs of nerve root compression and positive findings for either sacroiliac joint dysfunction or asymmetric restriction of lumbar side-bending motion and lumbar segmental hypomobility. Patients with a flexion pattern (preference for

sitting and centralization with lumbar flexion) were given lumbar flexion exercises while those with an extension pattern (preference for standing and centralization with lumbar extension) were given lumbar extension exercises. Trunk strengthening and stabilization exercises were the treatment modalities for patients with frequent previous episodes, a positive response to prior manipulation or bracing as treatment, the presence of an "instability" catch, or lumbar segmental hypermobility. Finally, patients with radicular signs that did not centralize with movement who may have had a lateral shift deformity were given either mechanical traction or autotraction. The findings of this study show that classification-based treatment results in significantly better outcomes for disability (at up to 1 year of follow-up), return to work, and patient satisfaction at 4 weeks compared with the guideline-based group; there was also a trend toward less cost with the more specific treatment.

Several other studies have demonstrated the efficacy of two specific physical therapy regimens, movement therapy based on the results of directional preference testing and core strengthening, for diagnostic subsets of LBP. Directional preference testing is based on the McKenzie technique of repetitive end-range lumbar test movements, which have traditionally been shown to be helpful in evaluating the presence or absence of discogenic pain. With this mechanical assessment, a clinical phenomenon known as centralization commonly occurs where the most distal extent of referred or radicular pain rapidly recedes toward the lumbar midline by a single direction of repeated end-range movement. For example, with a discogenic etiology, the most common direction of lumbar testing that centralizes pain is extension, whereas a smaller group of patients will centralize only with laterally directed movements or even lumbar flexion. The recommended treatment then consists of that specific directional preference of end-range exercises and appropriate symptom-driven posture strategies.

There is strong evidence of good outcomes for centralizers with this directionally driven treatment modality. For example, patients with acute and subacute LBP with or without radicular symptoms who might benefit from an extension-mobilization program based on centralization with extension movements and positive findings from pelvic alignment tests were identified; these patients were then randomized to either an extension-based (with sacroiliac mobilization) or a flexion-based exercise program. The extension group improved more rapidly per the modified Oswestry Low Back Questionnaire, administered at days 3 and 5 of treatment. In addition, one study found that a unidirectional exercise program in extension with an additional focus on posture and ergonomics had superior outcomes at 3 weeks and 1 year compared with education in a "mini back school" in patients with acute LBP with or without radiating pain. In a review of 87 patients with LBP and radiating leg pain, it was reported that centralization occurred in 87% of such patients; the occurrence of this phenomenon during initial mechanical evaluation was an accurate predictor of successful treatment outcome and a reliable determinant of the appropriate direction of treatment exercise. Nonoccurrence of centralization, however, accurately predicted poor treatment outcome. In a multicenter, randomized controlled trial of 312 patients with acute or chronic LBP or sciatica with or without neurologic findings, a standardized mechanical assessment was used to identify two groups of patients, based on the presence or absence of a directional preference. The 230 patients who exhibited a lasting beneficial pain response to one particular movement were then randomized to one of three exercise treatments including directional exercises "matching" the directional preference, exercises directionally "opposite" to the directional preference, and nondirectional exercise. Although all three exercise treatment groups showed improvement in all outcomes including pain intensity and medication usage, there were significantly greater improvements in every outcome in the group treated with matched directional exercises compared with the other treatment groups.

Many studies have reported beneficial outcomes for a core program in the management of lumbar disk herniation, lumbar instability, and acute LBP. In one classic study, a dynamic lumbar stabilization or core strengthening program for patients with lumbar radiculopathy was described. Good or excellent self-reported outcomes were obtained in 50 of 52 patients (96%) with a stabilization and abdominal program, together with flexibility exercises, joint mobilization of the hip and the thoracolumbar spinal segments, gym training, and aerobic activity. Another study then compared a specific core strengthening "stability" protocol for treating patients with chronic LBP secondary to instability from spondylolysis and spondylolisthesis with a standard treatment directed by the treating physician involving supervised exercise programs and modalities. The specific exercise treatment program consisted of 10 weeks of training of the deep abdominal muscles, with co-activation of the lumbar multifidi proximal to the pars defect; this activation was then incorporated into previously aggravating static postures and functional tasks. The core strengthening group showed a statistically significant reduction in pain intensity and functional disability levels, maintained at 30-month follow-up, whereas the control group demonstrated no significant change. In a recent study, patients experiencing a first-time episode of acute LBP were randomly allocated to a control group receiving advice and medications or a specific exercise group performing exercises targeting the multifidus in co-contraction with the transversus ab-

dominis. The core strengthening group had fewer recurrences of LBP in comparison with the nonexercise group at 1 year (30% versus 84%) and at 2 to 3 years (35% versus 75%). It can be concluded from these studies on the McKenzie technique and core strengthening that therapeutic exercise leads to beneficial results for patients with LBP if performed in a specific manner and directed at a specific pain generator.

## A Comprehensive Rehabilitation Program for Low Back Pain

The clinician must have an understanding of the unique biomechanical stresses placed on the lumbar spine and its kinetic chain. A thorough patient history, physical examination, and any appropriate radiologic studies will help facilitate a specific diagnosis including the potential pain generator and any associated musculoskeletal dysfunctions. A specific treatment approach, customized for each patient's unique presentation, can then be used for the most optimum outcomes. A comprehensive rehabilitation program seeks to reduce pain and inflammation, correct soft-tissue inflexibilities, and improve muscle strength deficits and imbalances as well as endurance in the involved spinal segments and the entire kinetic chain. Another important function of LBP rehabilitation is education and training for posture, body mechanics, and proprioception with the goal of maintaining the spine in the most optimal biomechanical position during activity. No single component of the rehabilitation program should be used in isolation, but rather in concert with other appropriate components.

### The Acute Phase of Rehabilitation

Rehabilitation can be conceptualized as occurring in three stages–acute, recovery, and maintenance; however, these phases are not time-dependent and tend to overlap. During the acute stage of rehabilitation, goals are oriented toward decreasing the signs and symptoms of the injury (pain, swelling, stiffness, and other clinical findings). Before initiating a specific physical therapy intervention, the clinician should educate the patient about the proposed etiology of their LBP and the recommended treatment plan. A period of relative rest may also be suggested. Modalities such as ice or low-level heat wrap therapy, as well as medications including acetaminophen, nonsteroidal anti-inflammatory drugs, narcotics, steroids (oral or epidural), or muscle relaxants are frequently prescribed in the acute phase. These agents decrease pain, inflammation, and/or muscle spasm and thereby permit early and more rapid progression of rehabilitation. Corsets are associated with a significant potential for dependence and their use should be gradually discontinued as soon as possible; however, patients with instability may benefit from control of available lumbar range of motion and proprioceptive feedback. Corsets also provide warmth to underlying soft tissue and may decrease intradiskal pressure.

When formal rehabilitation begins, the physical therapist or other appropriate clinician should emphasize education and protection of injured tissues, because this is considered by many to be the most important component of a LBP program. Specific points should include positions of comfort, proper sitting and standing ergonomics, and proper body mechanics for movement including position change, performance of ADLs (dressing, bathing, toileting, driving), and lifting. The clinician also may recommend that the patient avoid early morning flexion, especially during the first hour after awakening, because of the increased fluid content and hydrostatic pressures in the disk during that time. It has been reported that in patients with chronic nonspecific LBP who controlled early morning flexion for 6 months, during the first 6 hours of the day, pain intensity, total days in pain, impairment and disability, and medication usage were decreased. Passive techniques such as manual therapy (see chapter 14) and modalities may also play an important role during the acute phase of rehabilitation. Although such passive treatments may facilitate a patient's progress, if used in a protracted manner they place the patient in a dependent role and become counterproductive to proceeding with participatory function-oriented and ultimately independent care.

## Modalities

Modalities are physical agents used to produce a therapeutic tissue response and to control pain and/or inflammation while the injury is given a period of relative rest. They are most effective when applied in response to a specific diagnosis with close monitoring of the patient's response. Commonly used modalities in the management of LBP include cold, heat, and electricity. The physiologic effects of cryotherapy include vasoconstriction with reflexive vasodilatation and decreased local metabolism, enzymatic activity, and oxygen demand. Because it lessens muscle spindle activity and slows nerve conduction velocity, cryotherapy is often used to decrease muscle spasticity and guarding to improve flexibility and function. On the other hand, cold is associated with increased connective tissue stiffness and muscle viscosity. Indications for cryotherapy in LBP include acute trauma, edema, hemorrhage, pain, and muscle spasm. Cold is preferable to heat for acute spine injury (especially during the first 48 hours after injury) because it controls pain and spasm and also decreases inflammation. To minimize the risk of developing neurapraxia, cold application should not exceed 30 minutes, and efforts should be made to protect peripheral nerves in the region being treated. Contraindications to cryotherapy include ischemia, Raynaud's disease or phenomenon, cold intolerance, skin insensitivity, and inability to report pain.

Heat therapy is also commonly used in the setting of LBP and includes both superficial heat and deep heat or diathermy. In general, heat creates higher metabolic demand, which promotes increased capillary permeability as well as increased blood flow, bringing leukocytes and oxygen to tissue. Deep heat has also been shown to decrease spasm and pain and increase collagen distensibility, thereby improving flexibility. Indications for heat in the treatement of LBP include pain, muscle spasm, and decreased collagen extensibility. Contraindications to heat include inflammation, hemorrhage/bleeding disorder, decreased sensation, poor thermal regulation, malignancy, edema, ischemia, atrophic/scarred skin, and inability to respond to pain. Hydrocollator or heat packs, heating pads, and low-level heat wraps are typically used to provide superficial heat by warming tissue structures via conduction, the transfer of heat directly from one surface to another. Superficial heat typically penetrates greatest at a 0.5- to 2.0-cm depth from the skin surface, depending on the amount of adipose tissue present. Heat packs are heated in stainless steel containers filled with 65° to 90°C water and then applied with towels (to minimize skin trauma and maintain heat insulation) in treatment sessions lasting 20 to 30 minutes. One recent study found that continuous use of low-level heat wrap therapy during sleep by patients with acute nonspecific LBP decreased pain throughout the next day, reduced muscle stiffness and disability, and improved trunk flexibility; these effects were sustained more than 48 hours after treatment was completed.

Ultrasound is the most commonly used form of deep heat therapy and warms tissue via conversion, the transfer of heat via a change in energy. Such heat can penetrate to depths of 5 cm below the skin surface, thereby providing a therapeutic benefit to tendon, ligament, joint capsule, and even bone. Selective heating is greatest when the acoustic impedance is high, such as at the bone-muscle interface. Ultrasound is more typically used for subacute and chronic injuries; other indications for its use in the treatment of LBP include associated tendinopathy and degenerative arthritis. Ultrasound is typically used for periods of 5 to 10 minutes at intensities of 1.0 to 4.0 W/cm$^2$. In addition to general heat precautions, specific contraindications for ultrasound include malignancy, open physeal growth plates, pacemakers, laminectomy sites, regions of acute disk herniation with radiculopathy, fluid-containing cavities (for example, the uterus in a pregnant or menstruating woman, the testicle, or eye), unhealed fractures, joint arthroplasties containing methylmethacrylate or high-density polyethylene, and use near the brain.

Electricity is the third modality used in the treatment of LBP. Although transcutaneous electrical nerve stimulation is the most commonly used form of therapeutic electricity, other types include high-voltage pulsed galvanic stimulation, interferential electrical stimulation, and minimal electrical noninvasive stimulation. Electricity acts physiologically to increase circulation and therefore aids in the removal of inflammatory by-products; it has also been reported to decrease edema, pain, spasm, inflammation, and muscle atrophy. Although typically indicated for chronic pain, transcutaneous electrical nerve stimulation appears to have a role in managing acute pain. Contraindications to electricity to treat LBP include active bleeding sites, cardiac pacemakers and defibrillators, areas with metal close to the skin, anesthetic areas, incompletely healed wounds, and use near the eyes, carotid sinus, or mucous membranes. Cryotherapy, heat therapy, and therapeutic electricity have all been shown to be helpful in relieving the pain and/or inflammation associated with LBP; however, there is little proven benefit when these modalities are used in isolation. Therefore, modalities should be considered an adjunctive treatment and included only as part of a comprehensive rehabilitation program.

During the acute phase of rehabilitation, the clinician should also introduce the concept of neutral spine and determine the patient's initial movement pattern. Neutral spine is an initial training posture, a loose-packed position that decreases tension on the ligaments and joints and allows a more balanced segmental force distribution between the disk and facet joints. It is considered to be the least painful and most biomechanically sound position of power and balance. Because the neutral spine is close to the center of reaction, it provides greater functional stability with axial loading and allows for quick movement into extension or flexion. The clinician should then instruct the patient in performing the first lumbar exercises, either in an extension or flexion bias based on the presumed lumbar pathology and response to repeated end-range movements. An extension bias is most commonly used with discogenic pain where symptoms tend to decrease (or centralize) with repetitive extension on motion pattern testing. In this patient population, extension exercises may reduce intradiskal pressure, allow anterior migration of the nucleus pulposus, and increase mechanoreceptor input, thus activating the pain gate mechanism. Notably, this movement pattern may increase symptoms in patients with large central disk herniations, foraminal herniations, or foraminal stenosis. On the other hand, in the setting of facet joint pathology or spinal stenosis, a flexion bias is typically indicated because symptoms tend to decrease with repetitive flexion movements. Flexion exercises may reduce facet joint compressive forces and provide stretch to the lumbar muscles, ligaments, and myofascial structures; these exercises, however, may also increase intradiskal pressure and thus exacerbate discogenic pain.

Cardiovascular fitness should be initiated in reference to the initial movement pattern. For example, if the disk is the pain generator, aerobic activity that places the spine in a neutral to extension bias such as the treadmill (0° incline) and the cross-country ski machine is typically indicated. Conversely, the stationary bicycle and inclined treadmill, machines that place the spine in a neutral to flexion bias, are usually recommended if LBP originates from the facet joint or spinal stenosis. Although there is a limited amount of literature on the subject, aquatic-based rehabilitation appears to be useful in the acute phase of rehabilitation because it allows early intervention of aerobic conditioning. Advantages of aquatic rehabilitation include eliminating gravitational forces in a graded manner to allow training with comfortable and adjustable axial loads; challenging vertical posture secondary to depth-dependent refractive alterations of proprioceptive cues; controlling velocity through water resistance, viscosity, buoyancy, and training devices; increasing the range of training positions as the result of buoyancy; and improving the margin of error. Aquatic therapy has also been shown to attenuate pain because of hydrostatic pressure, temperature, and turbulence as well as enhance psychological outlook. Criteria for advancement to the next stage of rehabilitation include adequate pain control and tissue healing that allows for normal or near-normal painless range of motion and initial strengthening of the injured tissues.

## The Recovery Phase of Rehabilitation

The recovery phase is the second and typically most lengthy phase of a comprehensive rehabilitation program for LBP. During this stage, treatment emphasis shifts from resolution of clinical signs and symptoms to restoration of function. The goals of this stage are to regain local flexibility, proprioception, and strength at the injured and adjacent motion segments of the lumbar spine. In addition, this focus should be applied to the entire kinetic chain because secondary biomechanical deficits exist at distant sites from the original injury as a result of chronic overload before or as the result of injury. To achieve these objectives, the treatment emphasis in this stage of rehabilitation moves away from passive modalities and manipulation and toward more focused and aggressive active interventions. The focus is on core strengthening. In general, the goals of this type of therapeutic exercise are to improve core muscle activity and endurance; establish neuromuscular control of the core muscles; restore coordination and position sense; increase lumbar mobility; train motor and postural control and balance; and to make exercises functional.

Specifically, the clinician leads the patient through a set of stabilization exercises. The reeducation of the core musculature classically begins with exercises such as the cat and camel (flexing and extending the back in a quadruped position) and the pelvic clock (rotating the pelvis along an imaginary 'clock' in a supine position with the feet on the floor). These movements "turn on" pelvic and hip muscles and help achieve spinal segment and pelvic

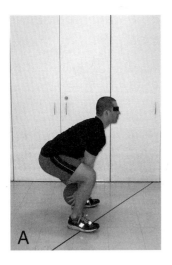 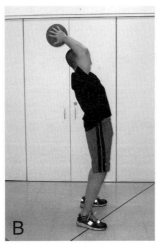 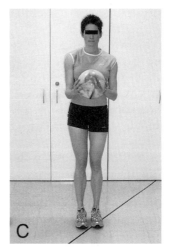 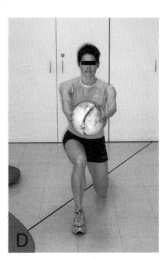

Figure 1  **A** through **D**, Core strengthening exercise in the sagittal plane.

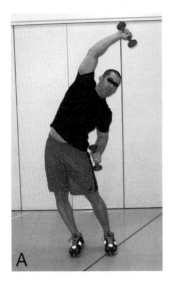 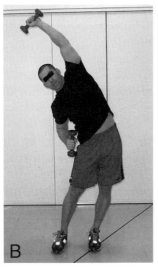

Figure 2  **A** and **B**, Core strengthening exercise in the frontal plane.

accessory motion before more aggressive exercises are attempted. Improving hip range of motion also has been shown to aid in dissipating forces from the lumbar spine. The patient then learns how to maintain the neutral spine in a static position, either supine or prone, which helps initiate awareness of motor patterns. Here, with verbal cues such as "bring the belly button back to the spine" or "squeeze the pelvic floor" and biofeedback, if necessary, the clinician facilitates activation of the core muscles. Once these muscles are "awakened," the exercises progress to functional positions such as sitting and standing and then dynamic activities such as walking, running, and even jumping. In addition, because functional activities move through the neutral position, the exercises are advanced to nonneutral positions. Finally, graded challenges to the neutral spine are created, first

by gravity, and then by the therapist or an assistive device such as the physioball; these challenges should progress from the predictable to the unpredictable.

Activity-specific retraining is then directed based on ADLs and the patient's unique functional activities. Each required motion is broken down into its individual components with the neutral spine trained for each; the parts are then reassembled so that the entire motion uses dynamic stabilization techniques. Finally, if the patient participates regularly in any sports activities, specific training should be included in this set of exercises. Because sports movement occurs in all three cardinal planes, the core should be trained in each of these directions (Figures 1 through 4). Additionally, because proprioception and balance are vital to the performance of sports, exercises should progress to labile surfaces. At the conclusion of this core strengthening program, the patient should have learned how to recruit spinal muscle stabilizers quickly and automatically, thereby controlling pain, optimizing soft-tissue repair and degeneration, gaining dynamic control of the segmental spine and kinetic chain forces, eliminating repetitive motion segment injury, and minimizing the chance of acute dynamic overload.

Other components of the recovery phase of rehabilitation include flexibility and strength programs and cardiovascular training. Flexibility exercises aim to correct muscle tightness, and allow the patient to assume a neutral position so that strength can be developed to help maintain correct neutral positioning during both static and dynamic conditions. Muscular weaknesses and imbalances, total body strength, endurance, and power, specific to the demands of the patient's specific actions, are addressed in the strength program. Cardiovascular training helps provide the necessary aerobic and anaerobic fitness required for activities; when performed in a neutral spine position, such training helps maintain fit-

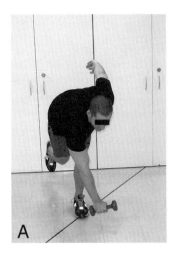 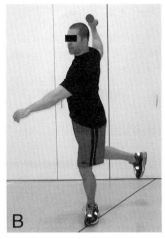 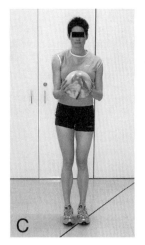 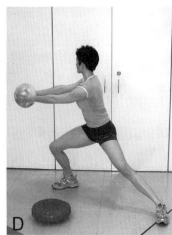

Figure 3   **A** through **D**, Core strengthening exercise in the transverse plane.

ness while protecting the lumbar spine. Criteria for advancement to the third stage of rehabilitation include complete pain control and tissue healing with essentially full painless range of motion and good flexibility. The athlete should be able to demonstrate strength of approximately 75% to 80% or greater compared with the uninjured side; there should also be good strength balance.

### The Maintenance Phase of Rehabilitation

The final stage of a comprehensive rehabilitation program for LBP is the maintenance phase, which forms the basis for the prevention program. The goals of this stage of rehabilitation are to resolve the patient's residual biomechanical deficits and any subclinical adaptations (the substitute motions and/or activities used to compensate for an injury and its associated mechanical problems). This phase is devised as the patient returns to work or sport-specific activity to promote continued cardiovascular fitness and moreover, prevent reinjury. Specific components of the maintenance phase include education about ergonomics, equipment, and assistive devices; eccentric muscular strengthening with work and sport-specific training if applicable; power and endurance exercise; and progression to an independent home exercise program. The patient should also be equipped with the appropriate knowledge to solve problems that occur after discharge from physical therapy. Completion of a rehabilitation program for LBP is indicated by absence of signs and symptoms of the original injury, full pain-free range of motion, normal flexibility, normal strength and strength balance, good general fitness, normal mechanics for work or sport, and the ability to perform job and sport-specific skills. Rehabilitation must progress beyond the absence of symptoms. Because statistics show that 70% to 90% of patients with LBP have recurrent episodes, the absence of symptoms does not

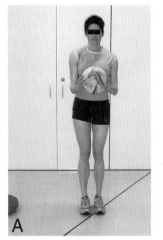 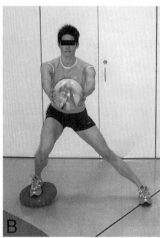

Figure 4   Core strengthening exercise in the frontal plane with labile surface.

necessarily imply normal function. By seeking to resolve the anatomic and functional changes associated with LBP, a comprehensive rehabilitation program may help reduce the incidence of LBP and its related impairments, disabilities, and high treatment costs.

### Annotated Bibliography

Akuthota V, Nadler SF: Core strengthening. *Arch Phys Med Rehabil* 2004;85(suppl 1):S86-S92.
    This review article uses a theoretic framework to describe the available literature on core strengthening in the rehabilitation of patients with LBP.

Fritz JM, Delitto A, Erhard RE: Comparison of classification-based physical therapy with therapy based on clinical practice guidelines for patients with acute low back pain: A randomized clinical trial. *Spine* 2003; 28:1363-1371.

In this study, the effectiveness and medical costs of a classification-based approach to the rehabilitation of patients with acute LBP was compared with an approach based on the Agency for Health Care Policy Research guideline, which indicates a more general approach for the first 4 weeks of rehabilitation. The findings of this study demonstrate that classification-based treatment results in significantly better outcomes for disability (up to 1 year), return to work, and patient satisfaction at 4 weeks compared with the results achieved in the guideline-based group; there was also a trend toward less cost with the more specific treatment regimen.

Hides JA, Jull GA, Richardson CA: Long-term effects of specific stabilizing exercises for first-episode low back pain. *Spine* 2001;26:E243-E248.

LBP patients were randomly allocated to a control group receiving advice and medications or a specific exercise group performing core strengthening exercises targeting the multifidus in co-contraction with the transversus abdominis. The core strengthening group had fewer recurrences of LBP compared with the nonexercise group at 1 year (30% versus 84%) and at 2- to 3-year follow-up (35% versus 75%).

Kavcic N, Grenier S, McGill SM: Determining the stabilizing role of individual torso muscles during rehabilitation exercises. *Spine* 2004;29:1254-1265.

The potential stabilizing role of individual lumbar muscles was evaluated through a systematic biomechanical analysis involving an artificial perturbation. Findings suggested that no single muscle dominated in the enhancement of spine stability, and the muscles' individual roles were continuously changing across tasks. Therefore, it was proposed that global muscle activation by co-contraction of multiple agonist/antagonist muscles was preferable to training primarily "local" muscles.

Long A, Donelson R, Fung T: Does it matter which exercise?: A randomized control trial of exercise for low back pain. *Spine* 2004;29:2593-2602.

In a multicenter, randomized controlled trial of 312 patients with acute or chronic LBP or sciatica with or without neurologic findings, the authors used a standardized mechanical assessment to identify two groups based on the presence or absence of a directional preference. The 230 patients that exhibited a lasting beneficial pain response to one particular movement were then randomized to one of three exercise treatments including directional exercises "matching" the directional preference, exercises directionally "opposite" to the directional preference, and nondirectional exercise. Although all three exercise treatment groups showed improvement in all outcomes including pain intensity and medication usage, there were significantly greater improvements in every outcome in the exercise-matched group compared with the other treatment groups.

Nadler SF, Malanga GA, DePrince M, et al: The relationship between lower extremity injury, low back pain,

and hip muscle strength in male and female collegiate athletes. *Clin J Sport Med* 2000;10:89-97.

In this cohort study of college athletes, a significant difference in side-to-side symmetry of maximum hip extension strength was observed in female athletes who reported lower extremity injury or LBP as compared with those who did not. Side-to-side difference in hip strength, however, did not differ between male athletes, regardless of reported lower extremity injury or LBP status. Female athletes appear to have a differing response of the proximal hip musculature to lower extremity injury or LBP, compared with their male counterparts.

Nadler SF, Steiner DJ, Petty SR, et al: Overnight use of continuous low-level heatwrap therapy for relief of low back pain. *Arch Phys Med Rehabil* 2003;84:335-342.

This study found that 8 hours of continuous low-level heat wrap therapy used during sleep by patients with acute nonspecific LBP decreased pain throughout the next day, reduced muscle stiffness and disability, and improved trunk flexibility. These effects were sustained more than 48 hours after treatment was completed. Adverse events were mild and infrequent.

Panjabi MM: Clinical spinal instability and low back pain. *J Electromyogr Kinesiol* 2003;13:371-379.

This article describes the stabilizing system of the spine which includes the spinal column, spinal muscles, and neural control unit. A hypothesis relating the neutral zone to pain is explained and in vitro experiments and mathematical models showing spinal muscles providing significant stability to the spine are presented. Increased body sway was found in patients with LBP, indicating a less efficient neuromuscular control system with decreased ability to provide the needed spinal stability.

Vad VB, Bhat AL, Basrai D, et al: Low back pain in professional golfers: The role of associated hip and low back range-of-motion deficits. *Am J Sports Med* 2004;32:494-497.

In this study, 42 professional golfers were categorized into group 1 (history of low back pain for more than 2 weeks that affected quality of play) and group 2 (no previous history of pain). A statistically significant correlation ($P < .05$) was observed between the group with a history of low back pain with decreased lead hip internal rotation, Fabere's distance, and lumbar extension.

## Classic Bibliography

Cholewicki J, McGill SM: Mechanical stability of the in vivo lumbar spine: Implications for injury and chronic low back pain. *Clin Biomech (Bristol, Avon)* 1996;11:1-15.

Delitto A, Cibulka MT, Erhard RE, et al: Evidence for use of an extension-mobilization category in acute low back syndrome: A prescriptive validation pilot study. *Phys Ther* 1993;73:216-222.

Deyo RA, Diehl AK, Rosenthal M, et al: How many days of bed rest for acute low back pain?: A randomized clinical trial. *N Engl J Med* 1986;315:1064-1070.

Donelson R, Silva G, Murphy K: Centralization phenomenon: Its usefulness in evaluating and treating referred pain. *Spine* 1990;15:211-213.

Hides JA, Stokes MJ, Saide M, et al: Evidence of lumbar multifidus muscle wasting ipsilateral to symptoms in patients with acute/subacute low back pain. *Spine* 1994;19: 165-172.

Hodges PW, Richardson CA: Inefficient muscular stabilization of the lumbar spine associated with low back pain: A motor control evaluation of transversus abdominis. *Spine* 1996;21:2640-2650.

McGill SM: Low back exercises: Evidence for improving exercise regimens. *Phys Ther* 1998;78:754-765.

Press JM, Livingston BP: The effective use of rehabilitation modalities, in Kibler WB, Herring SA, Press JM (eds): *Functional Rehabilitation of Sports and Musculoskeletal Injuries*. Gaithersburg, MD, Aspen Publishers, 1998.

O'Sullivan PB, Phyty GD, Twomey LT, et al: Evaluation of specific stabilizing exercise in the treatment of chronic low back pain with radiologic diagnosis of spondylolysis or spondylolisthesis. *Spine* 1997;22:2959-2967.

Saal JA, Saal JS: Nonoperative treatment of herniated lumbar intervertebral disc with radiculopathy: An outcome study. *Spine* 1989;14:431-437.

Snook SH, Webster BS, McGorry RW, et al: The reduction of chronic nonspecific low back pain through the control of early morning lumbar flexion: A randomized controlled trial. *Spine* 1998;23:2601-2607.

Stankovic R, Johnell O: Conservative treatment of acute low-back pain: A prospective randomized trial: McKenzie method of treatment versus patient education in "mini back school". *Spine* 1990;15:120-123.

# Chapter 16

# Diagnostic and Therapeutic Spinal Injections

Amy H. Phelan, MD

## Introduction

Spinal injections and percutaneous procedures are used in the assessment and treatment of spinal pain. In recent years, these procedures are being used more often for the diagnosis and treatment of spinal and radicular pain. Diagnostic anesthetic blocks and provocation tests have led to an increased ability to identify specific pain generators and thereby render more targeted, and hopefully more effective, treatment plans. In addition, advances in minimally invasive procedures have added to the treatment options available to address these sources of pain.

## Diagnostics

### Facet Injections/Medial Branch Blocks

The zygapophyseal or facet joints of the posterior column have been defined as a source of axial and somatic referred spine pain. These joints are innervated by the medial branches of the exiting dorsal spinal nerve. Their location in the cervical and lumbar spine has been determined. The referred pain distribution of these joints also has been determined using both intra-articular injections with distention of the joint and medial branch blocks. Previous studies determined that facet joint pain could be diagnosed and localized by intra-articular injection and confirmatory medial branch blocks (Figures 1 and 2). The use of medial branch blocks is considered a diagnostic procedure. Therapeutic intra-articular facet joint injections have been performed using a local anesthetic combined with corticosteroid, although there is

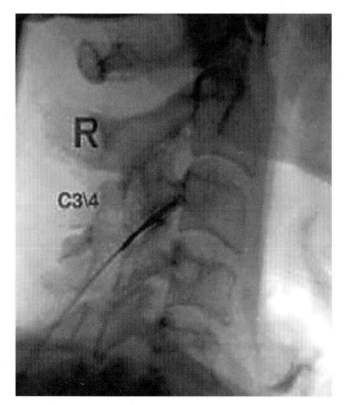

**Figure 1** Lateral fluoroscopic projection of a right C3/4 facet joint injection showing needle and contrast solution within the joint space.

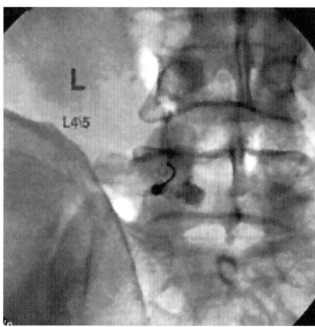

**Figure 2** AP fluoroscopic projection of a left L4/5 facet joint injection showing needle and contrast solution within the joint space.

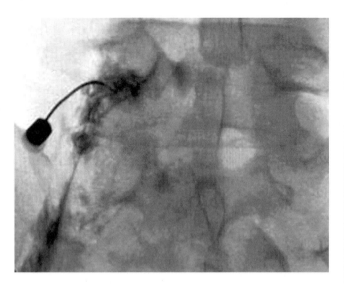

Figure 3 A left L5 selective nerve root block is shown with the needle in the lateral aspect of the neural foramen. Contrast solution outlines the L5 anterior rami with minimal flow of contrast solution within the epidural space.

little evidence of their long-term value. Studies focusing specifically on chronic cervical and lumbar facet joint pain demonstrated no statistically significant benefit from intra-articular injection of corticosteroid for pain relief at 6 months after injection.

### Selective Nerve Root Blocks

Selective nerve root blocks have been used as both a diagnostic and therapeutic intervention (Figure 3). The fluoroscopic technique is the same as that used for transforaminal epidural steroid injections; however, the needle is advanced only to the far lateral aspect of the foramen and a small amount of injectant is used (usually about 1.0 mL). This technique helps to avoid or minimize epidural spread of physiologic solution, which may compromise the selectivity of the block. Selective nerve root blocks are useful when imaging studies and clinical reports do not correlate or when multilevel abnormalities are not corroborated by electromyography and MRI. Results from earlier studies have demonstrated a high positive predictive value between selective nerve root response, nerve root pathology, and surgical outcome; however, no currently published randomized trials are available to clearly establish this positive predictive value. Newer techniques combining electrical stimulation of specific nerve roots followed by nerve block have increased the specificity of this technique.

### Sacroiliac Joint Injection

Diagnostic blocks with intra-articular local anesthetic have also been used to evaluate the sacroiliac (SI) joint as a source of pain (Figure 4). Whether SI joint dysfunction is a source of lumbar and sacral pain is debatable, with some authors claiming it as a common source and

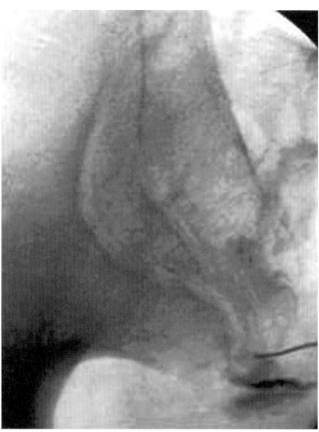

Figure 4 AP fluoroscopic projection of a left SI joint arthrogram showing needle placement in the inferoposterior aspect of the joint. Contrast fills the joint capsule and the joint margins.

others believing it to be a rare entity. Diagnosis of SI joint dysfunction using noninvasive techniques is difficult. Imaging studies such as radiographs, CT, and MRI are generally of limited usefulness because of their low sensitivity and specificity for associated SI joint dysfunction. Studies have shown that radionuclide imaging has a high specificity but too low a sensitivity to be useful.

Various methods of determining SI joint pain by physical examination have been evaluated, but results have been disappointing because of poor specificity and interrater reliability. These methods include provocative tests such as Patrick's and Gaenslen's, and assessment of distraction, compression, sacral sulcus, and posterior superior iliac spine tenderness. A recent study demonstrated the efficacy of combined McKenzie evaluation and SI provocation tests in identifying SI joint pain. The combination of these two techniques, using the centralization and peripheralization phenomena to assess for and rule out discogenic pain and SI joint provocation (distraction, compression, thigh thrust, and Gaenslen's test) to assess for SI joint pain, has increased the predictive value of physical examination in the diagnosis of SI joint-mediated pain. Interrater reliability for this method has not been evaluated, although the McKenzie method showed greater agreement when examiners had completed a formal McKenzie training program.

Fluoroscopically-guided intra-articular SI joint blocks remain the gold standard for the diagnosis of SI joint pain. "Blind" SI joint injections are not acceptable for diagnostic purposes. The injection of corticosteroid and local anesthetic has also been shown to provide a therapeutic benefit in patients with SI joint pain secondary to spondyloarthropathy, but their efficacy in the treatment of SI joint pain secondary to other pain sources has not been proved.

### Diskography

Diskography is used to assess for discogenic pain and intradiskal pathology. It was first developed approximately 60 years ago for evaluation of intervertebral disk herniations. Initially, an interlaminar, transdural approach was used. Techniques have been refined and an oblique, extrapedicular approach is currently used in the lumbar spine (Figure 5). This approach minimized the possibility of dural puncture and the exposure of vulnerable structures, although the exiting segmental nerve root remains at risk for penetration injury. Nerve root puncture or damage can be avoided by keeping the needle close to the superior articular process (as seen on the oblique view) and monitoring the patient's responses in case of transient contact. If the procedure is properly performed, accidental entry into the spinal canal or retroperitoneal space cannot occur.

The cervical disk is accessed from a right anterior approach to avoid the esophagus. The trachea and larynx are pushed to the left of midline. A detailed description of diskography techniques is beyond the scope of this chapter. Organizations such as The International Spinal Injection Society have established guidelines for the appropriate interpretation and performance of diskography. Although its usefulness in assessing discogenic pain is controversial, diskography remains the only selective provocation test available for this purpose.

Imaging studies such as MRI and myelography do not assess for pain, and therefore are inadequate for this purpose if used alone. One MRI finding that is proposed to correlate with disk pain is the annular high intensity zone. Studies have shown that high-intensity zones visualized on T2-weighted images of lumbar disks are indicators of inflamed symptomatic annular tears in patients with low back pain. This correlation has been confirmed by other investigators and disputed by some. Although not considered pathognomonic for diagnosing discogenic pain (high-intensity zones may be found on the MRI scans of asymptomatic patients), the high-intensity zone remains a useful predictive imaging finding in the assessment of patients with low back pain.

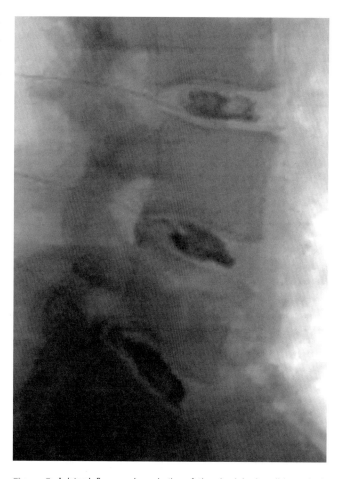

Figure 5  A lateral fluoroscopic projection of three-level lumbar diskography is shown. The L3/4 disk (top) is normal. The L4/5 disk (middle) and L5/S1 disk (bottom) demonstrate posterior fissures.

The role of provocation diskography in the assessment of disk pain and its usefulness in planning potential levels of fusion surgery has been debated extensively. The literature supports both sides of the argument. Critics of diskography believe that the test is not objective enough and is subject to numerous confounding factors. Proponents contend that, when performed by skilled practitioners and interpreted under strict scientific guidelines, diskography provides valuable diagnostic information regarding discogenic pain and intradiskal pathology that cannot be obtained by other means. Multiple studies have examined outcomes of lumbar surgery using a presurgical diskography evaluation (Table 1). The overall correlations are positive, although randomized trials are lacking. With the advent of percutaneous intradiskal therapies such as intradiskal electrothermal annuloplasty and nucleoplasty, diskography has gained effectiveness in the assessment of the disk before these procedures.

Intradiskal electrothermal therapy (IDET) using annuloplasty was developed to treat annular disk pathology. The technique involves inserting an electrode into the outer annulus and heating it. Heating of the outer

**Table 1 | Discogenic Pain: Surgical Outcome**

| Source | Number of Patients | Duration of Follow-up (months) | Criteria for Successful Outcome | | | Success Rate % |
| | | | > 75% Pain Relief | No Opioids or Pain Medicines | Return to work or Normal ADLs | |
|---|---|---|---|---|---|---|
| Lee et al (1995) | 62 | > 18 | + | + | + | 87 |
| Blumenthal et al (1988) | 34 | 29 | | + | + | 74 |
| Kozak and O'Brien (1990) | 69 | > 19 | + | + | + | 74 |
| Gill and Blumenthal (1993) | 53 | > 24 | + | + | + | 66 |
| Loguidice et al (1988) | 85 | > 15 | | + | | 61 |
| Knox and Chapman (1993) | 22 | NS | + | + | | 35 |

ADLs = activities of daily living, NS = not specified

Data from 17th Annual Scientific Session and Business Meeting American Academy of Disability Evaluation Physicians, Hotel InterContinental, November 13-15, 2003 New Orleans, Louisiana. Lecture title: Discograms: Pros and Cons by Charles N. Aprill, MD.

annulus is believed to relieve pain by an as yet unknown mechanism. IDET demonstrated initial promise in early studies; however, inconsistent therapeutic responses have resulted in decreased enthusiasm for this treatment. Two randomized, placebo-controlled trials were performed in 2004, with conflicting results. One study demonstrated a modest, but significant benefit in treated patients compared with a group of patients treated with a placebo. An Australian study demonstrated no benefit from IDET. Although not consistently successful, intradiskal electrothermal annuloplasty remains a treatment option for specific, highly selected patients; varying levels of improvement can be expected. In both studies, none of the treated patients had any adverse effects from the treatment.

## Therapeutics
### Epidural Steroid Injections
Epidural steroid injections have long been used to address spinal axial pain and radicular pain. Their efficacy in the treatment of radicular pain has been documented in multiple studies. Prospective, randomized, controlled, double-blind studies are few; however, epidural steroid injections are endorsed by professional and health care organizations for the treatment of radicular pain. They are known to produce both short- and long-term benefits, and in some instances obviate the need for surgical intervention. The use of epidural steroid injections to treat lumbar spinal stenosis and axial spinal pain is less encouraging, although studies have shown this treatment to be beneficial in some patients.

Epidural steroids are used to reduce inflammation associated with disk herniation. Increased levels of phospholipase A2 are present in the tissues surrounding the disk and nerve root in acute disk injuries. Phospholipase A2 is known to stimulate precursors in the prostaglandin and leukotriene pathways. Corticosteroids are known to decrease prostaglandin synthesis and reduce

both the cell-mediated and humoral immune responses. Corticosteroids have also been shown to block nociceptive C fiber conduction, which may constitute a direct analgesic effect. This neural blockade is believed to be chemically mediated by polyethylene glycol and benzyl alcohol preservatives contained in steroid formulations.

The injection of epidural steroid solutions is an invasive procedure that has risks and complications. Known complications include adverse reactions to the solutions, inadvertent injection in locations and structures other than the epidural space, and hematoma or abscess formation. Meningitis and arachnoiditis have been reported following epidural steroid injection. Preservatives found in all commercially available corticosteroid solutions are known to be neurotoxic. Corticosteroid solutions are also known to have a higher osmolarity than the cerebrospinal fluid and nerve tissue, which may add to their neurotoxicity. Although epidural injection of corticosteroid solutions is often used in the treatment of spinal pain, it should be noted that this is considered an off-label use and is not included in the Food and Drug Administration-approved uses of these suspensions.

The use of fluoroscopy and contrast in administration of epidural steroid has greatly increased the accuracy of delivery and decreased the incidence of inadvertent injection into potentially dangerous structures; however, epidural injections, specifically cervical transforaminal injections, continue to be associated with the risk of adverse reactions and injury (Figure 6). Recent catastrophic outcomes associated specifically with cervical transforaminal epidural injections have caused some clinicians to rethink the use of this approach and consider alternative approaches. The incidence of neurologic injury and death associated with cervical epidural steroid injections currently is not known and further investigation is required.

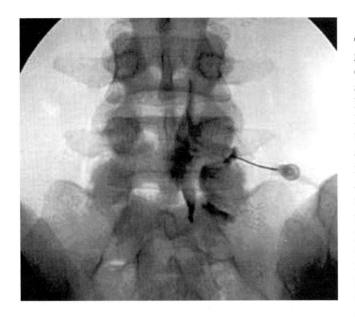

Figure 6 A right L5 transforaminal epidural steroid injection is shown. The needle is placed in the L5/S1 neural foramen. Contrast solution is shown within the right epidural space. The contrast solution does not cross midline and there is no subarachnoid filling. There is filling of the right L5/S1 facet joint with contrast solution noted in the ventral joint capsule.

## Radiofrequency Neurotomy

There has been increasing interest in the use of radiofrequency (RF) neurotomy in the management of chronic pain. RF-mediated heat lesions of the medial branches have been used with success in the cervical and lumbar spine for denervation of painful facet joints. The technique requires careful patient selection with at least two sets of diagnostic blocks to identify and localize the painful joints. It also requires knowledge of fluoroscopic procedures and the use of meticulous technique in locating and adequately heating the medial branches.

RF neurotomy of the cervical medial branches has resulted in significant pain relief for as long as 422 days. The response to this intervention is not considered permanent, but the procedure may be repeated. RF neurotomy of the lumbar medial branches demonstrates similar results.

RF neurotomy using a heat lesion applies a high-frequency alternating current through a percutaneous probe to heat the adjacent tissues. Temperatures of 85°C to 90°C are used to create irreversible thermocoagulation of the medial branches. This increase in temperature also causes denervation of the adjacent multifidus muscle in the lumbar spine. Complications are rare and include local procedure pain that is associated with probe placement and heat lesions, neuritic pain lasting less than 2 weeks, and potential deafferent pain. Complications specific to the cervical spine and third occipital nerve procedures include cutaneous numbness, dysesthesia, and ataxia; these conditions are usually self-limiting.

The use of RF neurotomy has been expanded to include lesions of the dorsal root ganglion, sympathetic ganglia, and peripheral nerves. RF has been used to address an increasing number of chronic pain conditions and syndromes, including trigeminal neuralgia, occipital headache and neuralgia, cervicobrachialgia, cervical and lumbar radiculitis, complex regional pain disorders, intrathoracic visceral pain, SI joint pain, coccygodynia, and perineal pain. Controlled clinical trials are lacking in many of these applications; however, initial reports and case series have demonstrated promising results in the expanded use of RF. In one randomized controlled trial, RF was used to treat patients with cervicobrachial pain, with a significant positive response. A recent randomized, double-blind, controlled study, using RF neurotomy for chronic lumbosacral pain, demonstrated no advantage over treatment with local anesthetics. More trials are needed to confirm the usefulness of RF treatments in these other applications.

The need for thermocoagulation to achieve therapeutic benefit was questioned in a 1997 study comparing 40°C and 67°C RF lesions of the dorsal root ganglion; both applications were equally effective. Pulsed RF was developed as a means of applying a high-frequency current to neuronal structures while avoiding the potential complications of heat lesions. Interest in the use of pulsed RF has increased because of its presumed safety and clinical benefit; pulsed mode RF at lower temperatures has led to the advent of many of the newer applications. Pulsed RF does not produce thermocoagulation and therefore the risk of side effects, specifically deafferent pain, is decreased. Pulsed RF delivers high-frequency current in pulses of 20 ms, with pauses of 480 ms. Temperatures do not exceed 42°C, which significantly decreases the destruction of neuronal tissue. Results from studies using pulsed RF lesions of the dorsal root ganglion of rats, showed increased *c-fos* gene expression in the superficial laminae of the spinal cord gray matter. Continuous RF did not produce this effect. It is proposed that the induced *c-fos* expression is a response to the electrical forces and not a thermal effect. *c-fos* expression is believed to be related to the clinical improvement seen with pulsed RF. No controlled clinical trials of pulsed RF have been published to date and additional studies in animal models and clinical trials are warranted to further define the mechanism and clinical use of pulsed RF neurotomy.

## Summary

Spinal injection procedures can be used for both diagnostic and therapeutic purposes. The use of diagnostic blocks has greatly increased understanding of pain generators such as intervertebral disks, facet joints, and nerve roots and has led to more targeted treatments. The efficacy of epidural steroid injections in the treatment of radicular pain and RF neurotomy of the medial branches for facet joint mediated axial spine pain has been demonstrated in clinical trials. Pulsed RF neurotomy also shows promise for use in other clinical applications. Nonsurgical treatment of disk herniations and discogenic pain has led to an increased use of diskography in the assessment of axial spine pain. To obtain the most precise diagnostic information and optimal clinical benefit, these procedures should be performed by physicians with a detailed knowledge of spinal anatomy and skill in the use of fluoroscopy and proper injection techniques.

## Annotated Bibliography
### Diagnostics

DePalma MJ, Bhargava A, Slipman CW: A critical appraisal of the evidence for selective nerve root injection in the treatment of lumbosacral radiculopathy. *Arch Phys Med Rehabil* 2005;86:1477-1483.

This article presents a literature review of six randomized clinical trials showing level III (moderate) evidence in support of transforaminal epidural steroid injections for lumbar radicular symptoms.

Derby R, Howard MW, Grant JM, Lettice JJ, Van Peteghem PK, Ryan DP: The ability of pressure-controlled discography to predict surgical and nonsurgical outcomes. *Spine* 1999;24:364-372.

This article presents a review of a multicenter, retrospective study of long-term surgical and nonsurgical patient outcomes after lumbar diskography. Results demonstrated that patients with chemically sensitive disks on diskography had significantly better outcomes following interbody/combined fusion.

Dreyfuss P, Dreyer SJ, Cole A, Mayo K: Sacroiliac joint pain. *J Am Acad Orthop Surg* 2004;12:255-265.

This review article discusses the incidence, diagnosis, and treatment of SI joint pain. A diagnosis using imaging, laboratory tests, and physical examination is unreliable in identifying SI joint pain. Controlled analgesic injection of the SI joint is the most important diagnostic tool.

Endres S, Bogduk N: Lumbar disc stimulation, *in International Spinal Intervention Society Practice Guidelines and Protocols*. Kentfield, CA, International Spinal Intervention Society, 2005, p 20.

This chapter on lumbar disk stimulation includes a review of the historical background, principles, techniques, and interpretation of lumbar diskography. Specific guidelines for the interpretation and validity of disk provocation as a diagnostic evaluation tool are also included. References are provided for each section.

Gajraj NM: Selective nerve root blocks for low back pain and radiculopathy. *Reg Anesth Pain Med* 2004;29:243-256.

A literature review of available studies, relevant anatomy, pathology, technical considerations and complication associated with the use of selective nerve root blocks in the management of patients with low back pain and radiculopathy is presented.

Huston CW, Slipman CW: Diagnostic selective nerve root blocks: Indications and usefulness. *Phys Med Rehabil Clin N Am* 2002;13:545-565.

This review article discusses the use of selective nerve root blocks as a diagnostic technique for determining specific nerve root involvement. These blocks can be useful in patients in whom imaging studies and clinical presentation do not correlate or when other diagnostic tests (MRI, electromyograms) are equivocal as well as to evaluate for anomalous innervations. Selective nerve root blocks do not provide information regarding etiology or prognosis for patients with nerve root pain.

Laslett M, Young S, Aprill C, McDonald B: Diagnosing painful sacroiliac joints: A validity study of a McKenzie evaluation and sacroiliac provocation tests. *Aust J Physiother* 2003;49:89-97.

This clinical trial evaluated 48 patients with chronic lumbopelvic pain for outcomes after SI joint injections. The evaluation used clinical reasoning involving assessment of the centralization/peripheralisation phenomena and SI joint provocation tests to predict primary SI joint pain. Fluoroscopic intra-articular SI joint injections were used to validate the clinical reasoning. The results indicated improved sensitivity, specificity, and positive likelihood ratio compared with the use of SI joint provocation tests alone

Narozny M, Zanetti M, Boos N: Therapeutic efficacy of selective nerve root blocks in the treatment of lumbar radicular pain. *Swiss Med Wkly* 2001;131:75-80.

A review of a retrospective study of 30 patients with monoradiculopathy and minor sensory/motor deficits and unequivocal MRI findings of disk herniation and/or foraminal stenosis is presented. Rapid and substantial regression of pain was reported in 87% of patients and 60% had permanent resolution of pain. Follow-up results showed that surgery was avoided for an average of more than 16 months. It was concluded that nerve root blocks are very effective in the nonsurgical treatment of minor monoradiculopathy and should be recommended as the initial treatment of choice for this condition.

Riddle DL, Freburger JK: Evaluation of the presence of sacroiliac joint region dysfunction using a combination of tests: A multicenter intertester reliability study. *Phys Ther* 2002;82:772-781.

This clinical trial evaluated the use of four tests of pelvic symmetry or SI joint movement that are advocated in the literature for diagnosing SI joint region dysfunction. Sixty-five patients were paired randomly with 34 therapists for evaluation. Results indicated that the reliability of measurements obtained with the four tests were too low for clinical use.

Slipman CW, Lipetz JS, DePalma MJ, Jackson HB: Therapeutic selective nerve root block in the nonsurgical treatment of traumatically induced cervical spondylotic radicular pain. *Am J Phys Med Rehabil* 2004;83:446-454.

This retrospective study of 15 patients investigated the results of using fluoroscopically-guided therapeutic selective nerve block for the treatment of cervical spondylotic radicular pain that resulted from trauma. The patients were treated with the nerve root block and with physical therapy. Good or excellent results were found in three patients (20%). The authors concluded that these early findings did not support the use of therapeutic selective nerve block for the studied patient population.

Slipman CW, Lipetz JS, Plastaras CT, et al: Fluoroscopically guided therapeutic sacroiliac joint injections for sacroiliac joint syndrome. *Am J Phys Med Rehabil* 2001; 80:425-432.

In this retrospective clinical review, patients diagnosed with SI joint dysfunction using fluoroscopically-guided diagnostic SI joint injection, received therapeutic injections in conjunction with physical therapy. Findings suggest that therapeutic SI joint injections are clinically effective in the treatment of patients with SI joint syndrome.

Slipman CW, Patel RK, Zhang L, et al: Side of symptomatic annular tear and site of low back pain: Is there a correlation? *Spine* 2001;26:E165-E169.

This study used a retrospective chart review consisting of the evaluation of CT scans of patients after diskography. Patients in the study had single-level, concordantly painful and fissured disks identified during diskography. Radiographs were reviewed by the lead author and a spine radiologist to determine a correlation between the side of the annular tear and the side of clinical pain. Results indicated a random correlation with no clear predictive value.

## Therapeutics

Botwin KP, Gruber RD, Bouchlas CG, et al: Fluoroscopically guided lumbar transforaminal epidural steroid injections in degenerative lumbar spinal stenosis: An outcome study. *Am J Phys Med Rehabil* 2002;81:898-905.

A prospective cohort study to identify the short- and long-term therapeutic benefit of fluoroscopically-guided lumbar transforaminal epidural steroid injections in patients with lumbar spinal stenosis resulting in radicular pain is presented. Of the 34 patients meeting selection criteria (the presence of unilateral radicular pain), 75% reported at least a 50% reduction in pain, 64% had improved walking tolerance, and 57% had improved standing tolerance at 1-year follow-up.

Ferrante FM, King LF, Roche EA, et al: Radiofrequency sacroiliac joint denervation for sacroiliac sendrome. *Reg Anesth Pain Med* 2001;26:137-142.

This article presents the results of a prospective study of 50 SI joint RF denervations on 33 patients diagnosed with SI syndrome by diagnostic SI injections with local anesthetic. A reduction in pain of at least 50% for approximately 12 months duration was reported by 33.6% of patients. A positive response was associated with an atraumatic etiology. Failure of denervation was associated with disability determination and pain on lateral flexion to the affected side.

Freeman BJ, Fraser RD, Tain CM, Hall DJ: A randomized double-blind controlled efficacy study: Intradiscal electrothermal therapy (IDET) versus placebo. *Eur Spine J* 2003;12:S23.

This prospective, placebo-controlled clinical trial compared IDET heating with sham procedure. In all cases, the IDET catheter was inserted into the disk. Outcome was assessed by pain and disability using the Low Back Outcome Scale, Oswestry Disability Index, Medical Outcomes Study 36-Item Short Form, Zung Depression Index, and Modified Somatic Perception Questionnaire. Results showed no significant change in outcome measures in either group at 6 months.

Geurts JW, van Wiljk RM, Wynne HJ, et al: Radiofrequency lesioning of the dorsal root ganglia for chronic lumbosacral radicular pain: A randomized, double-blind, controlled trial. *Lancet* 2003;361:21-26.

A randomized, double-blind clinical trial involving patients with chronic lumbosacral radicular pain is presented. Sixteen percent of the patients receiving RF lesioning of the dorsal root ganglion and 25% of the control group were successfully treated based on visual analog scores, physical impairment, and the use of analgesics. The results did not indicate a significant difference in benefit for the treatment group.

Govind J, King W, Bailey B, Bogduk N: Radiofrequency neurotomy for the treatment of third occipital headache. *J Neurol Neurosurg Psychiatry* 2003;74:88-93.

A prospective clinical trial of a revised technique for RF neurotomy of the third occipital nerve is presented. Changes in technique included using a large gauge electrode with minimum separation between placement of the three electrodes and using the hand to hold the electrode in place. Results indicated that 88% of patients had a successful outcome, defined as complete relief of pain for 90 days, restoration of normal activities of daily living, and no use of medication. The median duration of relief was 217 days with six patients demonstrating ongoing relief. Of 14 patients undergoing repeat neurotomy, 86% had similar positive responses. Results indicate that this is a successful treatment for third occipital headache.

Huang RC, Shapiro GS, Lim M, Sandhu HS, Lutz GE, Herzog RJ: Cervical epidural abscess after epidural steroid injection. *Spine* 2004;29:E7-E9.

This article describes a case report of a patient with cervical epidural abscess with neurologic deficits following cervical epidural steroid injection. A discussion including diagnosis, treatment, and outcome of this complication is presented. Cervical epidural abscess is a rare but serious complication after epidural steroid injection. Rapid diagnosis and treatment may result in good clinical outcomes.

Kawaguchi M, Hashizume K, Iwata T, Furuya H: Percutaneous radiofrequency lesioning of sensory branches of the obturator and femoral nerves for the treatment of hip joint pain. *Reg Anesth Pain Med* 2001;26:576-581.

A retrospective evaluation of 14 patients with hip joint pain who were treated with percutaneous RF lesioning of the sensory branches of the obturator and/or femoral nerves is presented. Results showed 86% of patients reported at least 50% relief of pain for 1 to 11 months with no motor weakness or other side effects.

Kornick C, Kramarich S, Lamer T, Sitzman BT: Complications of lumbar facet radiofrequency denervation. *Spine* 2004;29:1352-1354.

A study using a chart review of lumbar RF denervation procedures performed over a 5-year period at a single location (Mayo Clinic in Jacksonville) is presented. Results indicate a 1% incidence of minor complications consisting of localized pain and neuritic pain lasting less than 2 weeks. No patients had infection or new neurologic deficits.

Kwan O, Friel J: Critical appraisal of facet joints injections for chronic whiplash. *Med Sci Monit* 2002;8: RA191-RA195.

This article presents a literature review of studies identifying facet joint pain in patients with whiplash that was diagnosis via facet joint blocks and treated with RF neurotomy. The authors concluded that there is a paucity of research to support this theory and treatment. It was recommended that RF treatment not be used pending further study.

Larkin TM, Carragee E, Cohen S: A novel technique for delivery of epidural steroids and diagnosing the level of nerve root pathology. *J Spinal Disord Tech* 2003;16:186-192.

This article presents a description of an alternative technique for transforaminal injection to avoid complications of intravascular injection of steroid.

Leclaire R, Fortin L, Lambert R, Bergeron YM, Rossignol M: Radiofrequency facet joint denervation in the treatment of low back pain: A placebo-controlled clinical trial to assess efficacy. *Spine* 2001;26:1411-1416.

This article presents a review of a trial to assess the efficacy of using percutaneous RF articular facet denervation to treat low back pain. The study included 70 patients with low back pain lasting for more than 3 months. The patients received either percutaneous RF articular facet denervation using fluoroscopic guidance or a sham procedure. The Roland-Morris and Oswestry scales were used to assess functional disability and the visual analog scale was used to assess pain. At 12 week follow-up, results did not show any treatment effect. The authors concluded that the efficacy of this treatment had not been established.

Lew HL, Coelho P, Chou LH: Preganglionic approach to transforaminal epidural steroid injections. *Am J Phys Med Rehabil* 2004;83:378.

A description of an alternative technique for transforaminal injection which may avoid complications is presented.

Lord SM, Bogduk, N: Radiofrequency procedures in chronic pain. *Best Pract Res Clin Anesthesiol* 2002;16: 597-617.

This review article assesses the evidence for efficacy and safety of RF procedures in the management of trigeminal neuralgia, nerve root avulsion, and spinal pain.

Nelson DA, Landau WM: Intraspinal steroids: History, efficacy, accidentality and controversy with review of United States Food and Drug Administration reports. *J Neurol Neurosurg Psychiatry* 2001;70:433-443.

The authors of this literature review made the following conclusions: (1) intraspinal steroid therapy is not effective for back pain or radicular syndromes because steroid formulations, placebos, and sham injections have similar outcomes; (2) when injected, epidural medication may not remain confined to the epidural space and inaccuracies of placement can be as high as 40%; (3) the additives of steroid formulations can be neurotoxic when injected intrathecally; (4) epidural steroid infusion may result in increased pain, which may occur early or late and serious complications of arachnoiditis, spinal infection, or permanent neurologic deficits may also occur; (5) patients should be informed that there is no evidence that epidural steroid injections provide permanent relief of pain and that serious permanent complications to the spinal cord, nerve roots, or peripheral nerves are a rare but certain risk.

Pauza KJ, Howell S, Dreyfuss P, Peloza J, Dawson K, Bogduk N: A randomized placebo-controlled trial of intradiscal electrothermal therapy for the treatment of discogenic low back pain. *Spine J* 2004;4:27-35.

This prospective clinical trial compared IDET with sham procedure. Outcomes were assessed using pain and disability as measured by the visual analog scale, Medical Outcomes Study 36-Item Short, and the Oswestry Disability Scale. Results showed that the group treated with IDET showed significant improvement in pain and disability, compared with the group receiving the sham treatment. Approximately 40% of the patients had pain relief greater than 50% with approximately 50% reporting no benefit. The mechanism by which IDET relieves pain is currently unknown, but cannot be attributed solely to the placebo effect.

Peters G, Nurmikko TJ: Peripheral and gasserian ganglion-level procedures for the treatment of trigeminal neuralgia. *Clin J Pain* 2002;18:28-34.

This article presents a literature review of various techniques for managing trigeminal neuralgia including RF thermocoagulation, balloon compression, and glycerolysis. All techniques are more effective than peripheral procedures but do not reliably result in long-term pain relief and may cause sensory loss and dysesthesia.

Rathmell JP, Aprill C, Bogduk N: Cervical transforaminal injection of steroids. *Anesthesiology* 2004;100:1595-1600.

This article presents a review of the rationale, relevant anatomy, recommended technique, indications, efficacy, and complications associated with cervical transforaminal steroid injections. No controlled studies of cervical transforaminal steroid injections have been performed. Observational studies indicated some clinical benefit. It was concluded that understanding the anatomy of the cervical intervertebral foramina and contents is critical to the safety of the procedure.

Samanta A, Samanta J: Is epidural injection of steroids effective for low back pain? *BMJ* 2004;328:1509-1510.

The authors of this review article conclude that epidural injection of steroids for low back pain has not been shown to be effective; however, this treatment has not been shown to be ineffective either. Observational studies and the authors' clinical experience indicate that the injections have a role in certain clinical situations. The authors recommend consideration the use of epidural steroid injections in patients with low back pain lasting longer than 3 months and in patients with radicular symptoms.

Schofferman J, Kine G: Effectiveness of repeated radiofrequency neurotomy for lumbar facet pain. *Spine* 2004;29:2471-2473.

A retrospective chart review of 20 patients undergoing repeat RF neurotomy denervation for lumbar facet joint pain is presented. Results indicate that the frequency of success and duration of relief remain consistent after each subsequent RF treatment.

Van Wijk RM, Geurts JW, Wynne HJ: Long-lasting analgesic effect of radiofrequency treatment of the lumbosacral dorsal root ganglion. *J Neurosurg Spine* 2001; 94:227-231.

The results of a prospective open clinical trial assessing the efficacy and safety of RF treatment of the dorsal root ganglion of patients with chronic lumbosacral pain radiating into the leg is presented. Satisfactory pain reduction at 2 months with no serious side effects was reported by 59% of patients. Mean duration of pain was approximately 3.7 years. The mechanism of action remains unclear.

Yin W, Willard F, Carreiro J, Dreyfuss P: Sensory stimulation-guided sacroiliac joint radiofrequency neurotomy: Technique based on neuroanatomy of the dorsal sacral plexus. *Spine* 2003;28:2419-2425.

This article presents a retrospective chart review of patients undergoing sensory stimulation-guided sacral lateral branch RF neurotomy. The outcomes of 14 patients were reviewed, with 64% of patients reporting 60% subjective relief of pain and a decrease in the visual integer pain score of more than 50% for at least 6 months. No improvement was reported in 14% of patients. No patients reported complications or worsening pain following the procedure.

## Classic Bibliography

Aprill C: Diagnostic disc injection, in Frymoyer JW (ed): *The Adult Spine: Principles and Practices*. New York, NY, Lippincott-Raven, 1997, pp 523-562.

Aprill C, Bogduk N: High intensity zone. *Br J Radiol* 1992;65:361-369.

Barnsley L, Bogduk N: Medial branch blocks are specific for the diagnosis of cervical zygopophyseal joint pain. *Reg Anesth* 1993;18:343-350.

Barnsley L, Lord S, Wallis B, Bogduk N: Lack of effect of intraarticular corticosteroids for chronic pain in the cervical zygopophyseal joints. *N Engl J Med* 1994;330: 1047-1050.

Blumenthal SL, Baker J, Dossett A, Selby DK: The role of anterior lumbar fusion for internal disc disruption. *Spine* 1988;13:566-569.

Bogduk N, Modic M: Lumbar discography. *Spine* 1996; 21:402-404.

Bush K, Hillier S: Outcome of cervical radiculopathy treated with periradicular/epidural corticosteroid injections: A prospective study with independent clinical review. *Eur Spine J* 1996;5:319-325.

Carette S, Marcoux S, Truchon R, et al: A controlled trial of corticosteroid injections into facet joints for chronic low back pain. *N Engl J Med* 1991;325:1002-1007.

Carragee EJ, Paragioudakis SJ, Khurana S: Lumbar high intensity zone and discography in subjects without low back problems. *Spine* 2000;25:2987-2992.

Derby R, Howard M, Grant J, et al: The ability of pressure controlled discography to predict surgical and non-surgical outcome. *Spine* 1999;24:364-371.

Dreyfuss P, Halbrook B, Pauza K, Joshi A, McLarty J, Bogduk N: Efficacy and validity of radiofrequency neurotomy for chronic lumbar zygapophysial joint pain. *Spine* 2000;25:1270-1277.

Forouzanfar T, van Kleef M, Weber WE: Radiofrequency lesions of the stellate ganglion in chronic pain syndromes: Retrospective analysis of clinical efficacy in 86 patients. *Clin J Pain* 2000;16:164-168.

Gill K, Blumenthal SL: Posterior lumbar interbdy fusion: A 2-year follow up of 238 patients. *Acta Orthop Scand Suppl* 1993;251:108-110.

Knox BD, Chapman TM: Anterior lumbar interbody fusion for discogram concordant pain. *J Spinal Disord* 1993;6:242-244.

Kozak JA, O'Brien JP: Simultaneous combined anterior and posterior fusion: An independent analysis of a treatment for the disabled low back pain patient. *Spine* 1990; 15:322-328.

Lee CK, Vessa P, Lee JK: Chronic disabling low back pain syndrome caused by internal disc derangements: The result of disc excision and posterior interbody fusion. *Spine* 1995;20:356-361.

Loguidice VA, Johnson RG, Guyer RD, et al: Anterior lumbar interbody fusion. *Spine* 1988;13:366-369.

Lord S, Barnsley L, Wallis B, et al: Chronic cervical zygopophyseal joint pain after whiplash: A placebo-controlled prevalence study. *Spine* 1996;21:1737-1745.

Lord S, Barnsley L, Wallis B, McDonald G, Bogduk N: Percutaneous radio-frequency neurotomy for chronic cervical zygopophyseal-joint pain. *N Engl J Med* 1996; 335:1721-1726.

Lutz GE, Vad VB, Wisneski RJ: Fluoroscopic transforaminal lumbar epidural steroids: An outcome study. *Arch Phys Med Rehabil* 1998;79:1362-1366.

Rosenberg JM, Quint TJ, de Rosayro AM: Computerized tomographic localization of clinically-guided sacroiliac joint injections. *Clin J Pain* 2000;16:18-21.

Schellhas KP, Pollei SR, Gundry CR, Heithoff KB: Lumbar disc high intensity zone: Correlation of magnetic resonance imaging and discography. *Spine* 1996;21:79-86.

Slappendel R, Crul BJ, Braak GJ, et al: The efficacy of radiofrequency lesioning of the cervical spine dorsal root ganglion in a double blinded randomized study: No difference between 40 degrees C and 67 degrees C treatments. *Pain* 1997;73:159-163.

Whitecloud TS, Seago RA: Cervical discogenic syndrome: Results of operative intervention in patients with positive discography. *Spine* 1987;12:313-316.

# Chapter 17

# Advanced Pain Therapies for Failed Back Surgery Syndrome

James B. Billys, MD

## Introduction

Failed back surgery syndrome (FBSS) is especially common in the United States where more surgery for back and leg pain is done, perhaps more than any other country in the world. FBSS is defined as the outcome of surgery in which the established expectations of the surgeon and patient are not met. The patient's expectation may be unrealistic, especially after multiple surgeries. Success is generally 50% or greater pain reduction or improvement in visual analog scale scores of 3 or more. It is important to ascertain a diagnosis by obtaining a patient history supplemented with physical examination, radiographic studies, and diagnostic injections. Objective or structural causes can be isolated in more than 90% of patients with FBSS. Table 1 shows comparative data identifying objective causes of FBSS.

If a nociceptive (structural) abnormality is identified and is correctable, surgical reconstruction should be considered. Otherwise, chronic pain can be treated nonsurgically with modalities such as opioid medications or spinal injection blocks. Chronic neuropathic (nonstructural) pain is usually not responsive to surgical correction and can be treated with medications and spinal cord stimulation (SCS). Mixed nociceptive and neuropathic syndromes may require combined treatments such as surgery first to correct ongoing neural compression (nociceptive component) and then nonopioid medications and SCS for the neuropathic component (Table 2).

## Neuropathic Pain Treatment With Spinal Cord Stimulation

SCS modulates afferent input into the spinal cord and central nervous system and is useful in the treatment of neuropathic pain. The technique has been used since 1967 for treatment of chronic pain. Since the 1990s, results using this technique have significantly improved because of technologic advancements such as the use of multichannel devices, dual lead systems, and improved programming. The use of monitored anesthesia care allows for interaction between the physician and patient during implantation.

In a 1993 study, sensory responses were mapped to neurostimulation, leading to better coverage of lower and upper extremity neuropathic pain and outcomes. It was shown that lead placement in the T8-T9 area allows for excellent coverage of the low back and lower extremities.

### Mechanisms of Action

The gate control theory is the theoretic basis for SCS, which is the balance of small (c fibers) and large (a β) fiber activity in the peripheral nervous system that governs central transmission of pain. When pain occurs, an excess of small fiber activity at the dorsal horn opens the gate leading to pain perception. Preferential stimulation of larger fibers occurs during SCS because these fibers are myelinated and have a lower threshold to depolarization than small fibers. As a result, increased large fiber activity occurs that rebalances the input to the dorsal horn and closes the gate, resulting in pain inhibition.

It has also been noted that patients using SCS will have 2 to 3 hours of pain relief with the stimulator turned off. This prolonged effect has been supported by biochemical data gathered in rat model studies. SCS increases the levels of gamma amino butyric acid (GABA) and activation of GABA receptors. Because GABA is a major inhibitory spinal transmitter at the level of the dorsal horn, it may contribute to this effect. GABA also seems to decrease levels of excitatory amino acids, which are the prime excitatory neurotransmitters mediating nociception.

Changes in brain activity in response to SCS also have been noted. In eight patients with chronic occipital headaches who were treated with neurostimulation, positron emission tomography scans showed activation of the dorsal rostral pons with stimulation.

A SCS electrode placed in the epidural space produces an electrical field that stimulates the spinal cord. This scenario is illustrated by the Holsheimer model. If a neuron is depolarized or made more electrically positive, an action potential will be produced. SCS uses a

## Table 1 | Comparative Data Identifying Objective Causes

|  | Burton | Waguespack | Slipman |
|---|---|---|---|
| **Diagnosis** | | | |
| Lateral stenosis | 58% | 29% | 25% |
| Herniated nucleus pulposus | 12% to 16% | 7% | 12% |
| Painful disk(s) | | 20% | 22% |
| Neuropathic | 6% to 16% | 10% | 10% |

## Table 2 | Failed Back Surgery Syndrome: Pain Types and Potential Treatments

| Types of Pain | Potential Treatments |
|---|---|
| Nociceptive | Opioid medications (intrathecal drug delivery system) |
| | Corrective surgery |
| Neuropathic | Nonopioid medications |
| | Spinal cord stimulation |
| Mixed | Corrective surgery |
| Nociceptive-Neuropathic | Medications (intrathecal drug delivery system) |
| | Spinal cord stimulation |

negatively charged electrode (cathode) to produce a positively charged neuron. These activated large fiber myelinated neurons are then able to block pain at the level of the dorsal horn.

### Patient Selection

The main indication for the use of SCS in the United States is FBSS, which occurs each year in 20% to 40% of 200,000 Americans who undergo lumbosacral spine surgery. Other indications include peripheral nerve injury, chronic regional pain syndrome, phantom limb pain, and spinal cord injury. Patient selection is key to success. The patients must undergo a complete evaluation including history, physical examination, and review of imaging studies. It is important to establish an observable pathology that is concordant with pain and to ensure that other conservative treatments have failed and that no further surgeries are indicated. The patients must undergo psychologic screening to evaluate for secondary pain issues, inappropriate drug habituation, borderline personality disorder, and depression. It is also important that patients understand and be committed to the procedure. For example, patients with monoradicular leg pain have a better prognosis than patients with bilateral radicular pain or axial back pain because monoradicular leg pain is easier to treat.

### Implant Technique

A patient deemed a candidate for SCS must undergo a trial screening for 3 to 7 days. Trial screenings can be accomplished by implantation of a percutaneous lead or laminectomy lead (Figure 1). With both techniques, trial stimulation is performed with an external pulse generator. It is important that paresthesia is felt in the area where the patient has pain. If located in the proper position, the lead is anchored and brought out through the skin with temporary lead extensions. If the trial is successful, the permanent pulse generator is placed. A successful trial is defined as a 50% reduction in pain.

Lead implantation is performed under monitored anesthesia care with local anesthesia (1% lidocaine with epinephrine and 0.5% bupivacaine hydrochloride with epinephrine). Fluoroscopy is used to mark the interspinous intervals. For percutaneous lead placement, a Tuohy needle is inserted into the epidural space using the loss of resistance technique. A percutaneous lead is then introduced through the needle into the epidural space and directed to the appropriate level; generally the T8-T10 level in FBSS. If a laminectomy lead is used, an incision is made at the T10-T11 level and a laminectomy is performed. The lead is then placed in the epidural space and guided cephalad to the T8-T10 level.

In comparing the use of percutaneous leads with laminectomy leads, percutaneous leads are less expensive and are less invasive; however, they have lower coverage of the area of neuropathic pain and higher rates of lead migration. Laminectomy leads are more expensive and are more invasive; however, they have better coverage and lower rates of lead migration.

In 2002, a randomized prospective study compared percutaneous leads with laminectomy leads in 24 patients. It was concluded that laminectomy leads provide better coverage, lower amplitudes (double battery life), and better pain relief. Results of a nonrandomized prospective study on 41 patients showed that the use of laminectomy leads decreased Visual Analog Scale (VAS) scores by 4.6, compared with a 3.1 decrease in VAS scores with the use of percutaneous leads. Overall, laminectomy lead results were better (90% excellent and 10% good versus 60% excellent and 25% fair results for percutaneous leads).

Complications related to the use of SCS include lead migration in 13.2% of patients, infection in 3.4%, lead breakage in 9.1%, hardware malfunction in 2.9%, unwanted stimulation in 2.4%, and cerebrospinal fluid leak in 0.3%.

### SCS Efficacy and Outcomes

A review of the literature reveals two prospective randomized study trials comparing SCS with repeat surgery. In one study, 50 patients (all revision candidates) were randomized to have repeat surgery or SCS. The

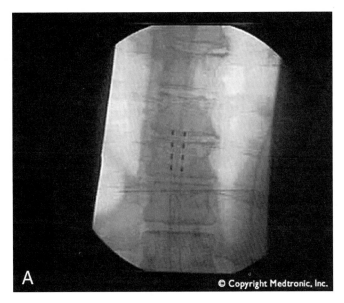
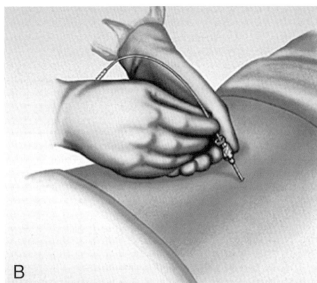

Figure 1   **A** and **B,** Percutaneous lead placement. (Copyright © Medtronic, Inc.)

## Table 3 | Spinal Cord Stimulation: Reduction in Pain

| Reference | Number of Patients | Mean Follow-up | Results |
|---|---|---|---|
| North, 1993 | 171 | 7 years | 52% with ≥ 50% relief |
| Turner, 1995 | 39 study<br>meta-analysis | 16 months | 59% with ≥ 50% relief |
| De La Porte, 1993 | 64 | 4 years | 55% good to excellent relief |
| Segal, 1998 | 24 | 19 months | 78% good to very good effect |
| Kumar, 1991 | 111 | 5.6 years | 59% good to excellent results |
| Burchiel, 1996 | 70 multicenter | 1 year | 55% with ≥ 50% relief |
| Kay, 2001 | 17 | > 5 years | 65% ≥ 50% relief |
|  | 12 | < 5 years | 54% ≥ 50% relief |
| Van Buyten, 2001 | 153 | 4 years | 68% good/excellent |
| Cameron, 2004 | 747 | 24 months | 62% > 50% pain relief |
| Dario, 2001 | 20 medical treatment<br>23 SCS (previously failing<br>medical treatment) | 42 months | Pain score 0-100:<br>VAS decreased from 76 to 25<br>VAS decreased from 85 to 22 |
| Ohnmeiss, 1996 | 40 | 12 months | VAS decreased from 7.4 to 5.6 |

frequency of crossover was the primary measure of outcome. At 6 months, 10 of 15 patients (67%) who underwent repeat surgery opted for crossover to SCS, and 2 of 12 patients (17%) who underwent SCS opted for crossover to repeat surgery. A 3-year follow-up study concluded that SCS is more effective than revision surgery; 90% of patients had better outcome, decreased opioid use, and lower crossover rates.

In the second study, SCS and physical therapy were compared with physical therapy alone. At 1-year follow-up, VAS scores in patients receiving SCS and physical therapy decreased an average of 7.1 to 4.4. VAS scores

of patients receiving only physical therapy increased from 6.7 to 7.1 ($P < 0.001$).

A review of class III and IV data in the literature revealed that 52% to 79% of patients with chronic pain treated with SCS demonstrated greater than 50% pain relief (Table 3). Long-term reduction or elimination of analgesics was seen in 58% to 90% of patients (Table 4). The ability to perform activities of daily living was improved in 61% to 66% of patients (Table 5). According to published statistics comparing time off work versus return to work, in more than 2 years fewer than 2% of patients returned to work, whereas 20% to 31% of

### Table 4 | Spinal Cord Stimulation: Reduction in Opioids

| Reference | Number of Patients | Mean Follow-up | Results |
|---|---|---|---|
| Ohnmeiss, 1996 | 40 | 2 years | 66% decreased/ eliminated |
| North, 1995 | 171 | 7 years | 58% reduced/ eliminated |
| De La Porte, 1993 | 64 | 4 years | 90% reduced medication |
| Kumar, 1991 | 111 | 5.6 years | 59% satisfactory relief |
| Racz, 1989 | 26 | 1.8 years | 81% reduced/ eliminated |

### Table 5 | Spinal Cord Stimulation: Enhanced Activities of Daily Living (ADLs)

| Reference | Number of Patients | Mean Follow-up | Results |
|---|---|---|---|
| De La Porte, 1993 | 64 | 4 years | 61% improved ADLs |
| Racz, 1989 | 26 | 1.8 years | 66% improved ADLs |
| Ohnmeiss, 1996 | 40 | 2 years | Statistically significant improvement in "pain effect on lifestyle" |

### Table 6 | Spinal Cord Stimulation: Return to Work

| Reference | Number of Patients | Mean Follow-up | % of Those Disabled Who Return to Work |
|---|---|---|---|
| De La Porte, 1993 | 64 | 4 years | 22% |
| North, 1993 | 171 | 7 years | 24% (of those patients under age 65) |
| Burchiel, 1996 | 70 | 1 year | 20% |
| Van Buyten, 2001 | 153 | 4 years | 31% |
| Kumar, 2002 | 60 | 5 years | 15% SCS 0% non SCS |
| Ohnmeiss, 1996 | 40 | 1 year | 10% |

patients return to work following treatment with SCS (Table 6).

Even though the literature lacks long-term prospective randomized controlled studies, SCS appears to have a positive effect, particularly when it is taken into account that in this group of patients almost all conventional therapies have failed.

## Nociceptive Pain Treatment With Intrathecal Drug Delivery

In patients with chronic, persistent pain, there are two groups of patients: surgical/revision candidates and patients who are candidates for long-term pain management when surgery is not indicated. Patients with nociceptive or structural pain may be treated with intensive rehabilitation, oral narcotics, or intrathecal drug delivery.

Intrathecal drug delivery allows for drugs to directly affect the opioid receptors with fewer side effects, improved pain relief at lower dosages, reduced consumption of systemic medication, and an improved ability to perform activities of daily living with long-term cost effectiveness.

### Mechanism of Action

When a drug is introduced into the intrathecal space it is distributed through convection and diffusion. Convective flow is secondary to the natural flow of cerebrospinal fluid, resulting in the mixing of cerebrospinal fluid in the intrathecal space. As a result, a steady state of concentration of fluid from the lumbar to cervical area is achieved. Diffusion is the movement of drug molecules through the intrathecal space and is determined by solubility and concentration gradient. Opioids are water soluble and not subject to rapid metabolic breakdown. They have a very slow diffusion rate, which leads to slow onset and slow diminution, in effect making them especially useful for treating pain. Opioids also do not cross the blood-brain barrier, further prolonging their effect. This central action on opioid receptors allows the more effective treatment of pain with lower doses of pain medication.

### Patient Selection

Prior to a trial of intrathecal drug delivery, it is important to perform a full diagnostic evaluation and establish an objective pathology for the patient's chronic pain. If no objective pathology is established, prolonged pain relief with intrathecal drug delivery is less likely. The workup includes a detailed patient history, physical examination, and review of medical imaging studies.

A trial of transdermal or oral narcotics may provide satisfactory pain relief, making intrathecal drug delivery unnecessary. Patients usually are treated with opioids along with antidepressants, anticonvulsants, nonsteroidal anti-inflammatory drugs, and/or nonnarcotic analgesic agents. Patients can be treated with antiemetics for nausea, laxatives for constipation, and stimulants for lethargy. If oral or transdermal narcotics do not provide adequate pain relief and/or if there are unacceptable or uncontrollable adverse effects, intrathecal drug delivery is indicated.

The procedure's true benefits are lower dosing with improved efficacy and fewer systemic side effects.

A psychologic evaluation is also essential. Patients with severe depression or acute psychotic illness should undergo treatment before the procedure is begun. A social support system should be in place to aid in maintenance of intrathecal drug delivery and in the event of an emergency.

A trial procedure is the final step in patient selection. Several methods can be used. Numerous screening protocols exist and include single bolus, multiple boluses, or continuous infusion. The length of the trial varies from 24 hours to 1 week. Current literature does not support one protocol over another. A successful trial is one in which a patient's pain is reduced at least 50% without significant adverse effects.

### Surgical Technique

The surgery is performed in the operating suite with the patient under general or monitored anesthesia care. A catheter is placed into the lumbar intrathecal space, generally between L2 and L4, using a paramedian approach. Fluoroscopic guidance is essential to document the level of insertion and final catheter position. Catheter tips are generally positioned between T10 and T12. An anchor is placed in the lumbar spinal fascia at the point of the insertion, and the free end of the catheter is threaded anteriorly in a subcutaneous fashion. A second incision is generally made in the abdomen and the end of the catheter is attached to the pump and placed subcutaneously. There are two types of infusion pumps. One type of pump infuses at a fixed rate, allowing for changes in medication dosage by emptying the pump and refilling it with a different concentration of medication. The second type of pump is programmable, using noninvasive telemetry that controls flow rate. Pumps are refilled percutaneously every 2 to 3 months (Figure 2).

### Drugs

Morphine and baclofen are the only two drugs the Food and Drug Administration has approved for intrathecal infusion. However, other opioids, including hydromorphine, fentanyl, sufentanil, and meperidine, are being used in patients who cannot tolerate morphine. Although these opioids work well in the treatment of nociceptive pain, they do not provide significant relief for chronic peripheral neuropathic pain. Most experienced physicians using intrathecal drug delivery will combine an opioid with clonidine, bupivacaine, or baclofen and create a synergistic effect, allowing for treatment of both nociceptive and neuropathic components of pain. It also has been noted that the use of combination therapy not only provides better pain relief, but also slows the development of tolerance to medication over time. An algorithm detailing the use of various medications is

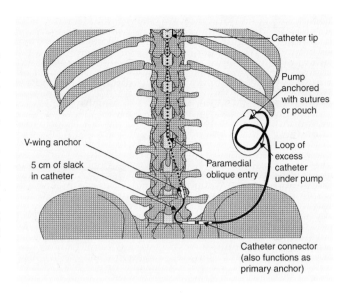

**Figure 2**   Intrathecal drug delivery pump and catheter placement.

shown in Figure 3. The polyanalgesic survey represents current thoughts and recommendations on dosing regimens and drug combinations.

### Complications

Complications occur in three categories. Medical complications include pruritus, nausea and vomiting, urinary retention, constipation, decreased libido, edema, and respiratory depression. These adverse effects generally resolve with symptomatic management and time. If they do not, a change in medication is indicated.

Surgical complications include infection, neurologic changes, and cerebrospinal fluid leakage. Most pump infections lead to explantation. Neurologic changes and bleeding are rare. Device-related complications occur in 20% to 25% of patients and include migration of the catheter, occlusion, cerebrospinal fluid leakage, disconnection from the pump, catheter tip granuloma, and pump failure. Catheter tip granuloma is an extremely rare complication. The mass generally is seen after 2 years of therapy and has been associated with the administration of high doses of morphine. Signs and symptoms of catheter tip granuloma include neurologic changes or loss of pain relief. MRI confirms the diagnosis. The condition is often treated by changing the catheter and, in rare instances, surgical removal of the mass.

### Outcomes

One randomized prospective study evaluated 202 cancer patients randomized to medical treatment versus intrathecal drug delivery. Outcomes demonstrated improved pain relief in both groups; 70.8% in the medical treatment group versus 87.5% in those treated with intrathecal drug delivery. Fewer patients receiving intrathecal drug delivery had fatigue and toxicity (1 in 10 pa-

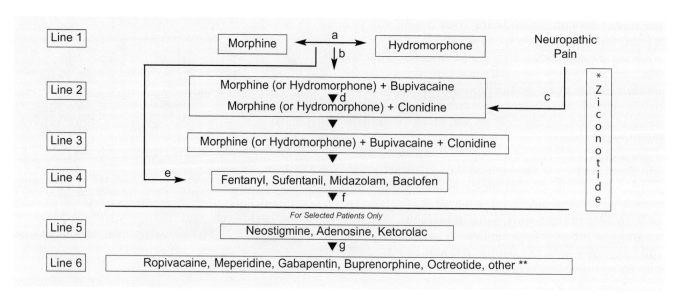

**Figure 3** Update of clinical guidelines for the use of intraspinal drug infusion in pain management.
*The specific line to be determined after FDA review.
.**Potential spinal analgesics: Methadone, Oxymorphone, NMDA opioid antagonists.
a. If side effects occur, switch to other opioid.
b. If maximum dosage is reached without adequate analgesia, add adjuvant medication (Line 2).
c. If patient has neuropathic pain, consider starting with opioid monotherapy (morphine or hydromorphone) or, in selected patients with pure or predominant neuropathic pain, consider opioid plus adjuvant medication (bupivacaine or clonidine) (Line 2).
d. Some of the panel advocated the use of bupivacaine first because of concern about clonidine-induced hypotension.
e. If side effects or lack of analgesia on second first-line opioid, may switch to fentanyl (Line 4).
f. There are limited preclinical data and limited clinical experience; therefore, caution in the use of these agents should be considered.
g. There are insufficient preclinical data and limited clinical experience; therefore, extreme caution in the use of these agents should be considered.

## Table 7 | Intrathecal Drug Delivery System: Pain Reduction

| Reference | Number of Patients | Mean Follow-up | Results |
|---|---|---|---|
| Paice, 1996 | 425 (133 cancer patients) | 15 months | 88% satisfaction |
| Winkelmuller, 1996 | 120 | 3.4 years | 67% decrease in pain intensity |
| | | | 92% satisfied with therapy |
| Kumar, 2001 | 16 | 2 years, 5 months | 57% decrease pain |
| Deer, 2004 | 136 | 12 months | 87% satisfied |
| Roberts, 2001 | 88 | 3 years | 60% reduction in pain |
| | | | 88% satisfied |
| Angel, 1998 | 11 | 3 years | 67% good to excellent |
| Likar, 1999 | 10 | 9.5 months | 90% satisfactory pain relief |
| | | | 90% would redo procedure |

## Table 8 | Intrathecal Drug Delivery System: Activities of Daily Living (ADLs)

| Reference | Number of Patients | Mean Follow-up | Results |
|---|---|---|---|
| Paice, 1996 | 425 (133 cancer patients) | 15 months | ADLs increased 80% |
| Roberts, 2001 | 88 | 36.2 months | 74% increased ADLs |

## Table 9 | Intrathecal Drug Delivery System: Changes in Medication Dosages (Tolerance)

| Reference | Number of Patients | Mean Follow-up | Results (Dose Increase in mg/day) |
|---|---|---|---|
| Paice, 1996 | 425 (133 cancer patients) | 15 months | 5 to 9.2 |
| Rainov, 2001 | 26 (nonmalignant low back pain) | 24 months | 1.2 to 5.1 |
| Kumar, 2001 | 16 | 29 months | 1.1 to 10 |
| Roberts, 2001 | 88 | 36.2 months | 9.95 to 15.26 |

tients), compared with medically treated patients (1 in 4 patients). It was also noted that patients receiving intrathecal drug delivery seemed to live longer than the medically treated group. The summary of the pain reduction studies detailed in Table 7 shows improvement in 57% to 90% of patients treated with intrathecal drug delivery, a treatment method that also demonstrates improvement in the ability to perform activities of daily living and acceptable development of tolerance to medications over time (Tables 8 and 9).

## Summary

In reviewing the literature, more prospective randomized controlled studies are needed. The current literature does demonstrate significant benefits of SCS and intrathecal drug delivery for patients with chronic neuropathic/nociceptive pain. These modalities represent viable methods to treat many FBSS patients in whom other treatment modalities have failed.

## Annotated Bibliography

### General

Farrar JT, Young JP Jr, LaMoreaux L, Werth JL, Poole RM: Clinical importance of changes in chronic pain intensity measured on an 11-point numerical pain rating scale. *Pain* 2001;94:149-158.
  This study discusses methods of quantitating levels of pain and clinical trials of chronic pain modalities.

Slipman CW, Shin CH, Patal RK, et al: Etiologies of failed back surgery syndrome. *Pain Med* 2002;3:200-214.
  Different etiologies of FBSS are described in this review. The study found that 95% of patients can be provided with a specific diagnosis.

Waguespack A, Schoffeuman J, Slosar P, Reynolds J: Etiology of long-term failures of lumbar spine surgery. *Pain Med* 2002;3:18-22.
  This article discusses the study evaluation percentage of patients with objective cause for FBSS. In 181 patients studied, a specific diagnosis was established in 94%.

### Neuropathic Pain Treatment With Spinal Cord Stimulation

Cameron T: Safety and efficacy of spinal cord stimulation for the treatment of chronic pain: A 20-year literature review. *J Neurosurg* 2004;100(suppl 3):254-267.
  This article provides a literature review and discusses outcomes in 3,679 patients treated with SCS over a 20-year period. SCS had a positive long-term effect. The need for prospective controlled randomized studies was stressed.

Dario A, Fortini G, Bertollo D, Bacuzzi A, Grizetti C: Treatment of failed back syndrome. *Neuromodulation* 2001;4:105-110.

In this study, 49 patients were treated for FBSS; 24 underwent SCS and 21 received medical treatment. SCS was found to be effective for relief of leg pain but was not effective in relieving back pain.

Deer TR: Current and future trends in spinal cord stimulation for chronic pain. *Curr Pain Headache Rep* 2001; 5:503-509.
  This review article outlines current trends in SCS.

Kay AD, McIntyre MD, Macrae WA, Varma TR: Spinal cord stimulation: A long-term evaluation in patients with chronic pain. *Br J Neurosurg* 2001;15:335-341.
  This article discusses patient selection, indications, new techniques, complications, and outcomes.

Kemler MA, Burendse GA, VanKleef M, et al: Spinal cord stimulation in patients with chronic reflex dystrophy. *N Engl J Med* 2000;343:618-624.
  In this prospective randomized study, results were compared in patients receiving SCS and physical therapy versus physical therapy alone. In the group receiving SCS and physical therapy, there was a 2.4-cm decrease in pain intensity at 6 months. In the group receiving physical therapy alone, there was a 0.2-cm increase in pain intensity.

Kumar K, Malik S, Demeria P: Treatment of chronic pain with spinal cord stimulation versus alternative therapy: Cost effectiveness analysis. *Neurosurgery* 2002;51: 106-116.
  The cost effectiveness of SCS versus medical therapy was assessed. Over a 5-year period, SCS-related costs were approximately $29,000 per patient versus $38,000 for medical therapy.

Linderoth B, Meyerson BA: Spinal cord stimulation: Mechanisms of action, in Barchiel KL (ed): *Surgical Management of Pain*. New York, NY, Theime, 2002, pp 505-526.
  This chapter outlines the mechanism of action of SCS.

Matharu MS, Burtsch T, Ward N, Frackowiak RS, Weiner R, Goadsby PJ: Central neuromodulation in chronic migraine patients with suboccipital stimulators: A PET study. *Brain* 2004;127:220-230.
  Each patient underwent a PET scan with the stimulator on and off. Increased activity in the dorsal rostral pons was noted with the stimulator activated.

North RB, Kidds DH, Olin PA, Sieracki JM: Spinal cord stimulation electrode design: Prospective, randomized controlled trial comparing percutaneous and laminectomy electrodes: Part I. Technical outcomes. *Neurosurgery* 2002;51:381-390.
  The authors compared the use of percutaneous and laminectomy electrodes, correlating them with patient outcomes.

North RB, Wetzel FT: Spinal cord stimulation for chronic pain of spinal origin. *Spine* 2002;27:2584-2591.

This prospective, randomized study comparing SCS and revision surgery found that SCS was more effective than revision surgery in 90% of patients, with better outcomes, decreased use of opioids, and lower crossover rates.

Oakley JC: Spinal cord stimulation: Patient selection, technique and outcomes. *Neurosurg Clin North Am* 2003;14:365-380.

Patient selection and recent outcomes are reviewed in this article.

Oakley JC, Prager JP: Spinal cord stimulation: Mechanisms of action. *Spine* 2002;27:2574-2583.

This article discusses current understanding of the mechanisms of SCS in relation to the physiology of pain.

Turner JA, Loeser JD, Deyo RA, Sanders SB: Spinal cord stimulation for patients with failed back surgery syndrome or complex regional pain syndrome: A systematic review of effectiveness and complications. *Pain* 2004;108:137-147.

This review article covers all recent studies on SCS outcomes and complications.

Van Buyten JP, Van Zundert JV, Vueghs D, Vanduffel L: Efficacy of spinal cord stimulation: 10 years of experience in pain center in Belgium. *Eur J Pain* 2001;5:299-307.

Of 153 patients studied (average follow-up of 4 years), 68% rated results of SCS as excellent to good, with 31% of patients resuming work.

Villavicencio AT, Leveque J, Rabin L, Bubara K, Gorecki JP: Laminectomy versus percutaneous electrode placement for spinal cord stimulation. *Neurosurgery* 2000;46:399-406.

The long-term effectiveness of SCS using percutaneous leads versus laminectomy electrodes was compared in this study.

*Nociceptive Pain Treatment With Intrathecal Drug Delivery*

Ackerman LL, Follett KA: Long-term outcomes during treatment of chronic pain with intrathecal clonidine or clonidine/opioid combinations. *J Pain Symptom Manage* 2003;26:668-677.

In this retrospective study/chart audit of 15 patients, the rate of initial pain relief was greater than 50%; these results were short lived (less than 11 months). Intrathecal clonidine should be used in combination with an opioid for long-term pain relief.

Coffey RJ, Burchiel K: Inflammatory mass lesions associated with intrathecal drug infusion catheters: Report and observation on 41 patients. *Neurosurgery* 2002;50:78-87.

This article presents a review of the diagnosis of granulomas and treatment with intrathecal drug therapy. In 41 patients with granulomas, the mean duration of intrathecal drug therapy was 24.5 months. Intrathecal drugs included morphine or hydromorphone in 39 of 41 patients. Thirty patients underwent surgery to relieve spinal cord compression; 11 patients were ambulatory at follow-up.

Deer TR, Caraway DL, Kim CK, Dempsey CD, Stewart CD, McWerl KI: Clinical experience with intrathecal bupivacaine in combination with opioid for the treatment of chronic pain related to failed back surgery and metastatic cancer pain of the spine. *Spine J* 2002;2:274-278.

In this retrospective outcome study, the efficacy of intrathecal bupivacaine and opioid was evaluated. When used in combination with opioids, bupivacaine treatment results in improved patient satisfaction and reduction in the amount of opioid necessary for pain relief.

Deer T, Chupple I, Clussen A, et al: Intrathecal drug delivery for treatment of chronic low back pain: Report from the national outcome registry for low back pain. *Pain Med* 2004;5:6-13.

In this multicenter outcome study, 166 patients using intrathecal drug delivery for treatment of low back pain were studied; 136 patients were identified at 12-month follow-up. More than 65% of patients had reduced Oswestry scores by at least one level, and 80% were satisfied with treatment.

Follett KA, Bootz-Marx RL, Drake JM, et al: Prevention and management of intrathecal drug delivery and spinal cord stimulation system infections. *Anesthesiology* 2004;100:1582-1594.

Treatment of infection with intravenous antibiotics is discussed.

Follett KA, Naumann CP: A prospective study of catheters: Related complications of intrathecal delivery systems. *J Pain Symptom Manage* 2000;19:209-215.

The complications associated with intrathecal drug delivery are described.

Hassenbusch SJ, Portenoy RK, Cousins M, et al: An update on the management of pain by intraspinal drug delivery: Report of an expert panel. *J Pain Symptom Manage* 2004;27:540-563.

The drugs and dosage recommendation for intrathecal drug delivery are outlined.

Kumar K, Kelly M, Pirlot T: Continuous intrathecal morphine treatment for chronic pain of nonmalignant etiology: Long-term benefits and efficacy. *Surg Neurol* 2001; 55:79-88.

In this prospective study, 12 of 16 patients had a 67.5% reduction in pain at 6 months and a 57.5% reduction in pain at 29 months on the visual analog scale. Ten patients were satisfied with results and 11 patients reported an improvement in quality of life.

Penn RD: Intrathecal medication delivery. *Neurosurg Clin North Am* 2003;14:381-387.

This review article discusses the mechanism of action, response, and complications related to intrathecal delivery of medication.

Prager JP: Neuraxial medication delivery: The development and maturity of a concept for treating chronic pain of spinal origin. *Spine* 2002;27:2593-2605.

This review article discusses the history of and indications for intrathecal drug delivery.

Rainov NG, Heidecke V, Burkett W: Long-term intrathecal infusion of drug combinations for chronic back and leg pain. *J Pain Symptom Manage* 2001;22:862-871.

This study discusses the use of combination drug therapy in a pump. Fifty-six patients were studied; results were good to excellent in 49, sufficient in 6, and poor in 1. There were no long-term clinical adverse effects.

Roberts LJ, Finch PM, Goucke CR, Price LM: Outcome of intrathecal opioids in chronic noncancer pain. *Eur J Pain* 2001;5:353-361.

Eighty-eight patients were studied for an average of 36.2 months. At follow-up, mean pain relief was 60%, with 74% of patients reporting increased activity levels. There was no change in work status; patient satisfaction was 88%.

Simpson RK: Mechanism of action of intrathecal medications. *Neurosurg Clin N Am* 2003;14:353-364.

Patient selection, mechanism of action, and technique are described.

## Classic Bibliography

Barolat G: Experience with 509 plate electrodes implanted epidurally from C1-L1. *Stereotact Funct Neurosurg* 1993;61:60-79.

Barolat G, Massaro F, He J, Zeme S, Keteik B: Mapping of sensory responses to epidural stimulation of the intraspinal neural structures of man. *J Neurosurg* 1993;78: 233-239.

Burton CV, Kirkaldy-Willis WH, Yong-Hing K, Heithoff KB: Cause of failure of surgery of the lumbar spine. *Clin Orthop Relat Res* 1981;157:191-199.

Burchiel KJ, Anderson VC, Brown FD, et al: Prospective multicenter study of spinal cord stimulation for relief of chronic back and extremity pain. *Spine* 1996;21:2786-2794.

Cabbell KL, Turner JA, Sygher O: Spinal cord compression by catheter granulomas in high-dose intrathecal morphine therapy: Case report. *Neurosurgery* 1998;42: 1176-1180.

Cherkin DC, Deyo RA, Locser JD, Bush T, Waddell G: An international comparison of back surgery rates. *Spine* 1994;19:1201-1206.

Doleys D, Murray J, Coleton M: Behavioral medicine/ psychological assessment of the pain patient, in Ashburn M, Rice L (eds): *The Management of Pain*. NewYork, NY, Churchill Livingstone, 1996, 56-98.

Holsheimer J, Struijk JJ: How do geometric factors influence epidural spinal cord stimulation?: A quantitative analysis by computer modeling. *Stereotact Funct Neurosurg* 1991;56:234-249.

Kumar K, Toth C, Nath RK, Loring P: Epidural spinal cord stimulation for treatment of chronic pain: Some predictors of success. A five-year experience. *Surg Neurol* 1998;50:110-120.

Likar R, Spendel MG, Amberger W, Kepplinger B, Supanz S, Sadjak A: Long-term intraspinal infusions opioids with a new implantable medication pump. *Arzneimittelforschung* 1999;49:489-493.

Linderoth B, Stiller CO, Gunasekera L, O'Connor WT, Undersedt U, Brodin E: Gamma-aminobutyric acid is released in the dorsal horn by electrical spinal cord stimulation: An in vivo study in the rat. *Neurosurgery* 1994;34:484-489.

Long D: Failed back surgery syndrome. *Neurosurg Clin North Am* 1991;2:899-919.

Melzack R, Wall PD (eds): *Textbook of Pain*. New York, NY, Churchill Livingstone, 1989.

Melzack R, Wall PD: Pain mechanisms: A new theory. *Science* 1965;150:971-979.

Merskey H, Bogduk N (eds): *Classification of Chronic Pain: Descriptions of Chronic Pain Syndromes and Definitions of Pain Terms*, ed 2. Seattle, WA, IASP Press, 1994.

Nelson D: Psychological selection criteria for implantable spinal cord stimulators. *PRN Forum* 1996;5:93-103.

North RB, Kidds DH, Lee MS, Piantadosi S: A prospective randomized study of spinal cord stimulation versus reoperation for failed back surgery syndrome. *Stereotact Funct Neurosurg* 1994;62:267-272.

North RB, Kidds DH, Zahurak M, James CS, Long DM: Spinal cord stimulation for chronic intractable pain experience over two decades. *Neurosurgery* 1993;32:384-394.

Ohnmeiss DD, Rasbaum RF, Bugdanffy GM: Prospective outcome evaluation of spinal cord stimulation in patients with intractable leg pain. *Spine* 1996;21:1344-1351.

Paice J, Penn R, Shott S: Intraspinal morphine for chronic pain: A retrospective, multicenter study. *J Pain Symptom Manage* 1996;11:71-80.

Racz GB, McCarron RF, Tulboys P: Percutaneous dorsal column stimulator for chronic pain control. *Spine* 1989; 14:1-4.

Schofferman J: Long term opioid therapy for severe refractory lumbar spine pain. *Clin J Pain* 1999;15:136-140.

Segal R, Stacey BR, Rudy TE, Basen S, Markham J: Spinal cord stimulation revisited. *Neurol Res* 1998;20:391-396.

Shealy C, Mortimer J, Reswik J: Electrical inhibitors of pain by stimulation of the dorsal column: Preliminary clinical reports. *Anesth Analg* 1967;46:489-491.

Slavin KV, Burchie KJ, Anderson VC, Cooke B: Efficacy of transverse tripolar stimulation for relief of chronic low back pain. *Stereotact Funct Neurosurg* 1999;73:126-130.

Turner JA, Loeser JA, Bell KG: Spinal cord stimulation for chronic low back pain: A systemic literature review. *Neurosurgery* 1995;37:1088-1095.

Wilkinson HA (ed): *The Failed Back Syndrome: Etiology and Therapy*, ed 2. Philadelphia, PA, Harper and Row, 1991.

Winkelmuller M, Winkelmuller W: Long-term effects of continuous intrathecal opioid treatment in chronic pain of nonmalignant etiology. *J Neurosurg* 1996;85:458-467.

# Chapter 18

# Psychosocial Care

Daniel M. Doleys, PhD

## Psychosocial Factors and Pain

Any discussion of psychosocial care in pain treatment and rehabilitation requires an understanding and appreciation of the role of psychosocial factors in chronic noncancer pain. The International Association for the Study of Pain specifically noted that "pain" is a product of physical and emotional factors. The central nervous system mechanisms involved, especially those of the brain, and the manner in which psychosocial factors exert their influence also have been examined. All too often psychosocial factors are addressed only after physiologically based therapies (interventional and invasive) have been undertaken, particularly if unsuccessful, or if a reason is needed to avoid a given therapy or procedure.

Psychosocial care begins with identification of the factors involved. These psychosocial factors can include mood states, personality variables, and/or the individual patient's approach to the pain and its management. Depression and anxiety are common mood states; however, anger, frustration, and irritability can also play a significant role. When these mood states are combined with unrealistic expectations, insufficient education on pain, repeated inadequate outcomes, or questions about one's authenticity, patients can become despondent, depressed, or suicidal, with a profound sense of helplessness and/or hopelessness. Sometimes these patients are discounted as being too impaired to profit from additional treatment.

Certain personality traits or disorders can influence the patient's experience of and reaction to pain and suitability for certain therapies. Focusing on some presumed "pain generator" in the absence of a biopsychosocial approach that recognizes the potential contribution of these other factors will only exacerbate the situation. Several of these personality traits can be associated with drug addiction or abuse, adding to an already complicated situation. A partial list of these personality traits is provided in Table 1.

Patients develop or acquire ways of coping with pain; some strategies are adaptive, others are not. Several common coping strategies have been identified (Table 2). Particular attention has been given to the role of catastrophizing (exaggerated negative orientation toward a noxious stimulus) in the perception of pain, response to treatment, and degree of pain-oriented disability. More recently, awareness has been raised as to the importance of acceptance, a term that refers to an adaptive and functional response to pain rather than helpless resignation. It is argued that coping strategies are more likely to have a significant impact on improved quality of life in the presence of adaptive acceptance.

Readiness for change is a long-standing concept in the literature on addiction that has received more attention in discussions of pain. Although it is often assumed that any patient reporting pain would be willing and prepared to do whatever is recommended to resolve the pain, many do not comply with treatment recommendations. There are several stages of readiness for change, including precontemplation, contemplation, action, and maintenance. Anyone who has committed to making a behavioral change such as weight loss, increased exercise, or smoking cessation can appreciate the importance and the impact of readiness stages. Unfortunately, patients are often encouraged, if not compelled, to comply with therapeutic recommendations, regardless of how invasive they may be and independent of their readiness to comply. Sometimes the physician's zeal to do, and contentment over having done all that can be done, appears to supersede the patient's readiness. On the other hand, treatment is often delayed by the physician or insurance company because of questions about the authenticity of the patient's reported pain to the point where a patient, once ready to get better and return to work, now wonders if it is the best strategy. Although factors associated with poor outcomes from surgery performed on patients with pain have been identified, relatively little time has been devoted to developing the patient into a better candidate for surgery. Cognitive behavior therapy, behavioral modification, or altering environmental contingencies and consequences, such as the willingness of an employer to accommodate

**Table 1 | Personality Traits That Influence Pain**

Somatoform pain disorder
Schizoid affective disorder
Borderline personality disorder
Hysterical personality
Hypochondriasis
Depressive/anxious personality

**Table 2 | Examples of Coping Strategies**

Distraction
Prayer
Activity avoidance
Relaxation
Request for support from family and peers
Reinterpretation (eg, "The pain is not going to kill me")
Venting of emotions

a patient's physical restrictions, could be beneficial. The relative lack of emphasis on how to assist a patient in becoming a better candidate for treatment can unwittingly encourage the assumption that psychosocial factors are irrelevant and/or their influence cannot be altered, or that it is someone else's concern.

The emphasis placed on psychosocial care is, in part, related to the outcome measures considered to be important. The various measures used include numerical pain rating, visual analog scale, function, quality of life, percent improvement in pain, and overall patient satisfaction. The more sensory oriented the outcome (for example, reduction in pain intensity), the greater the emphasis on physiologic therapies as they are often mistakenly assumed to address the ineffable pain generator. This unfortunate cascade of misplaced confidence and logic may not be beneficial to patient care.

Caution must be exercised when interpreting the outcome of acute diagnostic or therapeutic measures as they relate to chronic pain. It is not uncommon to assume that because a provocative test such as diskography successfully reproduced some aspect of the patient's pain that the pain generator has been found. This interpretation ignores not only the psychosocial factors involved in the testing process, but also the influences previously outlined. It should not be surprising when the destruction or removal of the so-called pain generator does not resolve the pain or restore the patient to improved function. It may be more appropriate to describe the structure under examination as a nociceptive generator. This term clearly identifies the offending structure as a contributing factor but leaves room for inclusion of other components.

The role of psychosocial care should be correlated with the role of psychosocial factors. These factors may function in several ways. One scheme noted that these factors may function as mediators, modulators, and/or maintainers of pain. As mediators, psychosocial factors are judged to be causally related, either directly or indirectly, to the experience of pain. As such, they must be addressed if the pain is expected to resolve. In most situations, psychosocial factors modulate pain, suggesting that physiologically oriented therapies may be effective but to a lesser degree than if these psychosocial factors were also addressed. The importance of psychosocial factors as maintainers of pain highlights the role of social reinforcement and has been discussed in the literature.

## Therapy

A broad range of psychologically oriented therapies exists; these therapies have been applied to patients of all ages for treatment of noncancer-related and cancer-related pain. These therapies can be done with individual patients, in groups, or with family/support persons and have been performed in outpatient, inpatient, or day-treatment/residential settings. Such treatments may be implemented before, during, after, or, sometimes, in place of interventional or invasive treatments. The goals may involve changes in overt pain behavior, cognition/thought, physiologic response, and/or interaction patterns.

Behavioral therapies, among the most researched and commonly used psychological therapies, are based on principles of learning theory and conditioning. Contrary to popular opinion, the changes in behavior are not just superficial or mental but can be mediated via rather profound changes in neurochemistry, physiology, and gene expression. Any patient-physician interaction is potentially some form of psychologic therapy and, therefore, can be either positive or negative.

Behavior modification is perhaps the most recognized of the behavioral therapies. It makes use of behavioral principles such as reinforcement, punishment, and extinction (the withdrawal of positive reinforcement). Contingencies are arranged in such a fashion so as to enhance adaptive and well behavior while decreasing maladaptive or pain behavior. Increasing positive reinforcing behavior can mitigate depression and enhance quality of life. Establishing rule or contingency-governed behavior versus pain-contingent behavior can minimize the development of chronic pain behavior characterized by activity avoidance and anticipatory pain that can lead to depression and anxiety. The simple use of exercise goals/quotas versus the "do what you can" concept, combined with reinforcement, can pay big dividends. Even the use of time-contingent versus pain-contingent medications has been shown to have certain advantages. Many health care professionals, especially physicians, overlook and underestimate their ability to modify pain beyond the procedures they perform.

Operant and classic conditioning principles have been applied to alter cortical responses to nociceptive and nonnociceptive stimuli, producing what appears to be conditioned nociception. At least one study suggested that this conditioned pain response was relatively resistant to extinction in patients with low back pain. This line of research may help in the understanding of why pain persists even after the apparent cause is addressed.

Cognitive behavior therapy is based, in part, on the observation that some aspects of pain, pain-related disability, and mood states are mediated by thoughts, self-statements, appraisal, attributions, and expectations. Such cognitions can be acquired with or without the patient's awareness, directly or indirectly via role models. They may be maladaptive and self-defeating or positive and self-reinforcing. In brief, cognitive behavior therapy involves educating the patient on the role of these cognitions, identifying those that are negative and inappropriate, and replacing them with adaptive ones.

In essence, almost any significant verbal exchange between a physician and patient can be viewed in the context of cognitive behavior therapy. Explaining the results of tests can establish causal attributions and appraisals. For example, in a patient with nerve damage, if the patient perceives the damage as permanent and pain as inevitable, subsequent treatments such as antiepileptic drugs, which may be physiologically or psychologically beneficial, may fail. Patients may not benefit from functional restoration programs for the same reason. A positive exchange between the physician and patient, however, could also set the foundation for positive expectations, a well-known component of the placebo response (a generally positive nonspecific response to treatment). Most physicians appreciate the power and omnipresence of the placebo effect, and every effort should be made to maximize its use to the patient's advantage.

Relaxation therapy, imagery, self-hypnosis, desensitization, and in vivo exposure (gradual exposure to the anxiety-provoking stimulus) are treatments that play a role in decreasing anxiety, phobias, and avoidance behavior. Preprocedure anxiety, generalized anxiety states, muscle tension headaches, fear of reinjury, and pain-based activity avoidance have responded to one or more of these treatments.

Psychologic and physical traumas, whether before, during, or after a pain-producing event, can have a profound effect on pain. Posttraumatic stress disorder refers to a constellation of symptoms including hypervigilance, avoidance, nightmares/flashbacks, autonomic overactivity, and depression. Although normally associated with wartime experiences or sexual or physical assault/molestation, posttraumatic stress disorder can also be a result of the trauma of injury or surgery. Eye movement desensitization and reprocessing has been used separately and in combination with other relaxation/desensitization procedures to alter pain-enhancing recurrent images and emotional responses. If unrecognized and left untreated, posttraumatic stress disorders can remarkably impede recovery and negatively affect pain-oriented therapies.

Biofeedback involves providing real-time information about one or more physiologic responses in an effort to assist in the development of self-management skills. Muscle activity, hand or foot temperature, skin conductance (galvanic skin conductance response) and electroencephalographic responses are the most common measures used. Standard relaxation therapy, with a clinician or by audiotape or CD, is often incorrectly referred to as biofeedback. Reduction in abnormal muscle activity in patients with headache and low back pain, alteration in autonomic, especially sympathetic, activity in patients with Raynaud's disease and complex regional pain syndrome, and increased efficacy of distraction via altered electroencephalographic response have been shown to be effective in altering the pain response.

Comprehensive multidisciplinary day-treatment and/ or residential programs are effective but are underfunded. These programs combine the above mentioned behavioral therapies emphasizing functional restoration and adaptive pain coping strategies. The goal of some of these programs has been the elimination of opioid use whereas others have been more flexible. Patients are involved in treatment several hours a day, 5 to 7 days a week for up to 4 weeks. Outcomes have been generally impressive, yet many third party insurance companies do not provide sufficient reimbursement, leading to a substantial attrition of such programs. Ironically, the cost of these comprehensive programs is significantly less than with many surgical approaches, and obviously do not carry the same risk of complications. One novel use of this model has been in conjunction with the placement of an intrathecal catheter or spinal cord stimulator as a way to provide a trial for prospective candidates for neuroaugmentation therapies. This type of functional-based trial may help to eliminate the false positive and false negative responders so frequently found in shorter and less functionally oriented trials.

## Annotated Bibliography

### Psychosocial Factors and Pain

Block AR, Gatchel RJ, Deardorff WW, Guyer RD (eds): *The Psychology of Spine Surgery*. Washington, DC, American Psychological Association Press, 2003.

This book provides a detailed overview and current state of the knowledge regarding presurgical psychological evaluations. Chapters on the use of psychometric testing, conceptual models, and preparing patients for surgery are particularly informative.

Doleys DM: Outcomes. *Southern Pain Society Newsletter*. June 2004, pp 4-7.

This brief article summarizes several of the issues regarding outcome measures in chronic pain therapy and research. The "disconnect" between these measures, especially reduction in pain and increased functioning, is noted.

Doleys DM, Dinoff B: Psychological aspects of interventional therapy. *Anesthesiol Clin North Am* 2003;21:767-783.

The role of psychological factors in procedures such as differential blocks, diskography, sympathetic blocks, and lumbar epidural blocks is given. The difference in nociceptive generators versus pain generators is discussed.

Keefe FJ, Rumble ME, Scipio CD, Giordano LA, Perri LM: Psychological aspects of persistent pain: Current state of the science. *J Pain* 2004;5:195-211.

This article presents a concise overview of many of the psychologic factors associated with chronic pain. Among those discussed are expectations, readiness for change, appraisals, and attributions. The role of coping strategies and acceptance is reviewed.

Kerns RD, Habib S: A critical review of the pain readiness to change model. *J Pain* 2004;5:357-367.

This article summarizes the adaptation of the readiness for change model from the addiction to the chronic pain setting. The authors highlight the research on the validity of the concept and existing questionnaires.

McCracken LM: Learning to live with pain: Acceptance of pain predicts adjustment in persons with chronic pain. *Pain* 1998;74:21-27.

The definition, reliability, and validity of the concept of acceptance and a questionnaire designed to assess it in the treatment of chronic pain are reviewed. Acceptance is considered as adaptive coping and not helpless resignation.

McCracken LM, Eccleston C: Coping or acceptance: What to do about chronic pain. *Pain* 2003;105:197-204.

The relationship between coping and acceptance is debated. There is some suggestion that the development and execution of coping strategies may be relatively ineffective unless the patient with chronic pain has accepted the situation.

Price DD (ed): *Psychological Mechanisms of Pain and Analgesia*. Seattle, WA, IASP Press, 1999.

This book describes the various psychological states and phenomena related to the experience of pain and analgesia. The author expertly ties basic research to clinical observations,

and emphasizes the importance of negative emotions and perceived threat as part of the definition of pain.

Price DD, Bushnell MC (eds): *Psychological Methods of Pain Control: Basic Science and Clinical Perspectives*. Seattle, WA, IASP Press, 2004.

A detailed discussion and brain imaging data relevant to the modulation of pain by attention, cognitive factors, emotions, placebos, and hypnosis is presented. An appreciation of the relation between the sensory/discriminative, affective/motivational, and cognitive/evaluative components of pain becomes essential to understanding its treatment.

Sullivan MJ, Thorn B, Rodgers W, Ward LC: Path model of psychological antecedents to pain experience: Experimental and clinical findings. *Clin J Pain* 2004;20:164-173.

This article ties together some otherwise independent lines of research regarding the role of various psychological factors, especially catastrophizing (exaggerated negative orientation toward a noxious stimulus), in the development and maintenance of chronic pain.

### Therapy

Doleys DM, Kraus T: Psychological and addiction issues in intraspinal therapy. *Semin Pain Med* 2004;2:46-52.

The definition and characteristics of addiction are summarized. Considerations in treating the chronic pain patient with a history of addiction, especially as it relates to the use of intraspinal medicine, are reviewed.

Flor H, Herman C: Biopsychosocial models of pain, in Dworkin RH, Breitbart WS (eds): *Psychosocial Aspects of Pain: A Handbook for Heath Care Providers*. Seattle, WA, IASP Press, 2004, pp 139-178.

This chapter highlights the role of conditioning and learning in the development and treatment of chronic pain. The concept of conditioned nociception, rarely alluded to in the literature, must be given consideration.

Rome HP Jr, Rome JD: Limbically augmented pain syndrome (LAPS): Kindling, corticallimbic sensitization, and the convergence of affective and sensory symptoms in chronic pain disorders. *Pain Med* 2000;1:7-23.

The authors provide a very detailed analysis of the mechanism by which previous physical and psychological trauma, such as childhood sexual molestation, can influence chronic pain and its treatment.

Turk DC, Gatchel RJ (eds): *Psychological Approaches to Pain Management: A Practitioner's Handbook*. New York, NY, The Guilford Press, 2002.

This book provides a comprehensive overview of the commonly used psychological/behavioral therapies. Chapters are organized by technique and specific disorder/population.

# Chapter 19

# Functional Restoration

James Rainville, MD

Reilly Keffer, DO

## Introduction

Functional restoration is a treatment approach to chronic back pain and other musculoskeletal disorders that is based on the premise that it is generally safe for people with chronic pain to function despite the presence of symptoms. Functional restoration uses exercise performed in a quota-based manner to deliver and reinforce this message to patients. This chapter will review the history and basic principles that support the functional restoration approach, with updates from recent relevant studies of this approach.

## History of Functional Restoration and Recent Randomized Controlled Studies

Decades ago, it was recognized that for workers disabled with chronic low back pain for more than 1 year, the likelihood of returning to work was only 25%; after 2 years, the likelihood of these individuals returning to work decreased to almost zero. It was also observed that many of these disabled workers had coexistent issues that contributed to their pain, including unresolved work conflicts, ongoing litigation, financial disincentives, depression, anxiety, and behavioral issues. These patients were often considered untreatable using available medical treatments. In 1985, a landmark study by Mayer and associates used an aggressive interdisciplinary program known as functional restoration that yielded extremely high return-to-work rates in workers with chronic disability. The program ignored the traditional medical goals of reduction or eradication of pain, and focused on improving physical function and reducing disability.

To produce successful results, a time-proven medical principle was incorporated into the treatment program: measurements of the parameters that were to be treated. A series of objective measurements of back function and physical activities that were often affected by chronic back pain were developed. These included measurement of trunk flexibility, trunk strength, lifting ability, and endurance. Patient performance on these tests was documented at the time of evaluation,

throughout treatment, and at discharge. The impairment in physical ability documented by these tests drove the physical aspect of treatment, which was exercise-focused to improve physical ability. Exercise was done in an aggressive, quota-based format under the supervision of physical and occupational therapists; that is, exercises were performed despite the occurrence of pain during exercise. According to Mayer, the guiding force of functional restoration was to restore joint mobility, muscle strength, endurance, and conditioning, as well as cardiovascular fitness. As a result, the ability to perform specific tasks such as lifting, bending, twisting, and tolerance of prolonged static positioning (sitting and standing) would be restored. Treatment lasted 6 to 8 weeks, with a 3-week intensive phase of treatment; patients attended the program for a time compatible with a typical full workweek.

Recognizing the importance of vocational, medicolegal, and psychosocial issues, the functional restoration program advocated by Mayer included vocational and psychological evaluations and used the services of appropriate professionals to explore, manage, and resolve identified problems in these areas that were barriers to recovery. At the completion of treatment, the patients' physical abilities were quantified, and these data were used to develop a work release plan with physical capacities. A workable plan for returning to vocational activities and resolving the workers' compensation claim was also put into place by occupational therapists, vocational counselors, and the treating physician who validated this plan with medically documented physical capacities and maximal medical improvement.

The original prospective trial in 1985 and the 2-year follow-up study from 1987 documented extraordinary success, with 87% of the workers completing treatment and returning to work, versus a 41% return-to-work rate in the control subjects, who were denied treatment by their insurance companies. Physical capacities, self-reported disability, depression, and pain scores improved substantially in the treated group. Additionally, the frequency of office visits to health care providers was five times higher and the subsequent spine surgery rates twice as high in the comparison group than in the treatment group.

In 1989, a functional restoration program was carefully designed to duplicate Mayer's program and similar results were observed. At 1-year follow-up, 81% of the graduates from the functional restoration program had returned to work compared with 29% of the comparison group.

These studies caused the medical community to take a closer look at this treatment approach and to explore the components of treatment that lead to successful return to work and function. It appeared that the social and disability system (workers' compensation versus socialized disability systems) in which the program is administered influenced success. In several randomized controlled studies of functional restoration in the setting of socialized disability systems, less favorable results for return to work were noted. Recently, a study of functional restoration versus physical therapy three times weekly revealed a reduction in the mean number of sick days in the functional restoration group and slightly better physical capacities, although no differences were noted for other outcomes, including pain, self-reported disability, or utilization of medical care at 6-month follow-up.

These differences in outcomes in different settings may be partially attributed to the ability of medical documentation of work capacities to alter or terminate disability benefits. In workers' compensation systems commonly used in some jurisdictions of the United States, medical documentation of work capacity and medical end point usually triggers an administrative phase during which the employer offers the claimant a job opportunity within their capacities, or the case is settled and weekly salary replacements are reduced or terminated by the insured or insurance company. These actions eliminate many of the financial incentives for continued disability and reinforce work as a means to maintain financial viability. In socialized disability systems, the documentation of physical capacities by a treatment program in the presence of continued symptoms may have less impact on the administrative decisions of the government agencies overseeing disability benefits, allowing disability benefits to continue.

A recent Cochrane review concluded that there is evidence that intensive physical conditioning with a cognitive-behavioral approach reduces work absence when compared with usual care; however, no evidence was found to support the efficacy of specific exercises without a cognitive-behavioral approach.

## Impact of Functional Restoration

Despite conclusions made about the effectiveness of functional restoration, this treatment has not become part of the mainstream of medical care for chronic back pain. Two decades after Mayer's original study, few functional restoration programs have been implemented in either the United States or worldwide, resulting in limited access to this comprehensive treatment approach for most patients with chronic low back pain. The reasons for this occurrence have not been researched, but probably result from a combination of factors including the complexity of the organization of these programs, the required levels of expertise for the providers involved with this treatment approach, the time requirement, and cost.

Although functional restoration programs are not in widespread use, much medical knowledge has been gained from the research associated with these programs. Perhaps the greatest contribution of functional restoration is the insight given into chronic low back pain and its treatment (Table 1).

### It is Safe to Function With Chronic Back Pain

An important lesson from functional restoration is that improving function, and not pain relief, can be a primary goal of treatment. The results from functional restoration programs demonstrate that exercise and activities are well tolerated by most participants, and result in a decrease in symptoms over time. These results suggest that intensive exercise is safe and not harmful for patients with chronic back pain. Several epidemiologic and long-term exercise studies have shown that exercise does not increase the risk of back pain or sciatica or accelerate spinal degeneration, and may in fact have a protective function against back pain.

It has been observed that health care providers who use functional restoration strongly endorse the notion that exercise and activities are safe. This characteristic of these health care providers may be essential to their effectiveness, as it allows them to encourage their patients to work through pain symptoms during treatment to accomplish their exercise and functional goals. In contrast, most community health care providers, including physical therapists, do not strongly endorse the notion that it is safe to work through pain. This belief often leads to a reluctance to encourage exercise in the presence of pain and limits the effectiveness of most health care providers for improving function without first improving pain symptoms.

### Cognitive and Psychological Factors Influence Disability

Evidence from functional restoration programs and pain research suggests that patients with chronic back pain often have cognitive and psychological factors that strongly influence their levels of disability. One relevant factor is that these patients often have strong pain beliefs, and associate activities that produce pain with the fear that these activities are harmful. Through what has

## Table 1 | Principles of Functional Restoration

| Outcome of Interest | Objective Measurement | Treatment |
|---|---|---|
| **Impaired Back Function** | | |
| Flexibility | Inclinometer measurements of trunk flexion, extension, side flexion and straight-leg raising | Daily stretching of the trunk and lower extremities to physiologic end range |
| Back strength | Timed isometric hold of extended trunk over end of table, exercise ball, or Roman chair | Back strengthening on exercise equipment done 2 to 5 times per week using quota-based exercise protocol |
| | Maximum weight lifted on back exercise machine | Back exercise on floor, exercise ball, or Roman chair |
| | Measured strength on computerized back strength testing equipment | |
| Lifting ability | Progressive Isoinertial Lifting Evaluation to waist and shoulder height shelves using adjustable weight in a milk crate | Quota-based training lifting weights in milk crates to shelves at waist and shoulder heights |
| | Dead lifts using free weights | Dead lifts with free weights |
| Endurance | Work performed over a fixed time period on isokinetic exercise bicycle | Endurance training at 75% maximum heart rate for at least 15 minutes, 3 to 5 times per week |
| | Treadmill test | |
| | Timed shuttle run/walk | |
| **Psychological and Psychosocial Issues** | | |
| Pain attitudes and beliefs | Fear Avoidance Beliefs questionnaire | Education and counseling |
| | Tampa Scale of Kinesiophobia: Pain and Impairment Relationship Scale | Reassurance by health care providers |
| | | Successful exercise experience |
| Depression, anxiety, somatization | Structured psychological interview | Education and counseling |
| | Minnesota Multiphasic Personality Inventory test | Medical management |
| | Beck Depression Inventory | Successful exercise experience |
| | Zung Depression Scale | |
| | Modified Somatic Perception Questionnaire | |
| **Functional Disability** | | |
| Disability for daily activities | Oswestry Disability Scale: Roland Morris Disability Scale | Education addressing the safety of exercise and activities in the presence of pain |
| | Medical Outcomes Study 36-Item Short Form | Consistent encouragement to function by health care providers |
| | | Successful exercise in the presence of pain |
| Work disability | Work status | Defined physical capacities based on exercise performance |
| | Physical work requirements | Defined maximum medical recovery at completion of functional restoration |
| | Unresolved work-related issues | Vocational counseling |
| | | Communication between medical provider, injured worker and employer |
| | | Establishment of vocational retraining if needed |
| Pain | Pain scales | Exercise |
| | | Self-applied cold |
| | | Over-the-counter analgesics |
| | | Nonsteroidal anti-inflammatory drugs |
| | | Discontinue narcotics |

been described as operant conditioning, activities that are perceived as harmful are avoided, resulting in considerable disability. With time, this fear-avoidance behavior may result in significant deconditioning and limited use of the back.

When pain reduction does not occur after medical intervention, psychosocial issues and patients' beliefs about pain and function must be addressed to improve disability. To accomplish this goal, it is essential that the treating physician possess attitudes and beliefs about pain that lead the patient in the desired direction of greater function despite the pain. The physician's treatment and advice should reflect those beliefs. It has been demonstrated that educational efforts by physicians to lessen fears and concerns about pain and endorse the safety of function despite pain have a powerful ability to lessen disability.

Physician expertise in managing depression and other concurrent psychological problems can be helpful in the treatment of patients with chronic disability. Re-

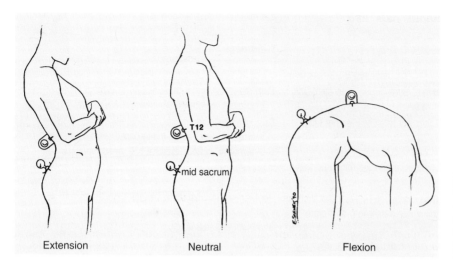

**Figure 1** Assessment of back flexibility. With the single inclinometer technique, the subject stands in the neutral position, and the inclinometer is placed over T12 and zeroed. The inclinometer readings are recorded as the subject bends forward and backward at maximum range. With the dual inclinometer technique, a second inclinometer is placed on the sacrum, and its readings recorded during flexion and extension. The sacral readings are subtracted from the T12 readings, which results in a calculation of true lumbar motion during flexion and extension.

search has shown that appropriately addressing these issues through counseling and medications can neutralize the negative influence of these factors on the outcomes from rehabilitation.

## Impairments in Physical Functional Abilities Are Common and Can Be Identified

The literature on functional restoration bases much of its validity on its ability to document improvements in impaired back function. This approach requires the validation of objective means of measuring flexibility, strength, and endurance. Using several devices, ranging from inexpensive hand held inclinometers to sophisticated computerized strength testing equipment, relevant components of back function can be assessed, compared with normative data, and impairments identified. Treatment plans are then devised to improve those impairments, and the success of treatment is assessed by requantification of back function. This dependence on numbers is essential to the success of treatment, as it keeps the patient and treatment staff focused on verifiable goals and eliminates the focus on soft or nonquantifiable goals common to outpatient therapy.

To be accessible to the medical community, the ability to measure back function should be simple and inexpensive but also remain reliable and valid. These methods of assessing back flexibility include either single or dual inclinometer techniques. These inexpensive handheld devices use gravity as a reference to measure trunk flexion, extension, side flexions, and straight-leg-raising (Figure 1).

Mayer developed the Progressive Isoinertial Lifting Evaluation as an inexpensive protocol for assessing lifting ability. A suggested setup is to place weights into a milk crate; the crate is then lifted onto shelves positioned at tabletop and shoulder height. A four-repetition to maximum weight lifted protocol is used to assess floor to tabletop, and tabletop to shoulder-height lifting abilities.

Testing back strength can be more challenging. Timed vertical hold of the unsupported upper body over an exercise ball or off the end of an examining table can be used to measure back endurance, which is relevant to back strength. Other methods require the use of back exercise equipment. Sobel and associates described back strength testing on back exercise equipment common to fitness facilities, using a four-repetition to maximum weight lifted protocol. Others have used computerized testing of back strength, although these devices are expensive.

Measured physical function for patients with chronic low back pain often does not reflect true physical abilities, but instead the patient's willingness to perform the test based on their fears and self-efficacy (termed psychophysical performance level). Regardless of the lack of measurement of true physiologic ability, the validity of functional measures is that they reflect the impact of low back pain on physical function as demonstrated by the willingness of the patient to use their body to perform a given function.

## Exercise Improves Impaired Functional Abilities

The basic principles of exercise support the notion that physiologic function can be improved with consistent exercise. The amount of exercise required to induce changes depends on the physiologic goals of exercise. Three sessions of stretching per week improve flexibility, but even greater gains in flexibility are made when stretching is performed five times per week. The frequency of strength training has been studied, and with efficacy demonstrated for once, twice, and three times per week. Functional restoration programs often use strength training five or six days per week. Although this high frequency of strength training is not supported by physiologic research, it may have an advantage in rapidly resolving fears and concerns about pain and function. Training frequencies of three times per week, for at least 15 minutes at 75% of maximal heart rate have been demonstrated to improve endurance. A greater frequency of endurance training may have additional physiologic benefits.

In addition to the frequency of exercise, the intensity of exercise must be adequate to induce changes in exercise performance, including improving physiologic abilities and diminishing fears and concerns about disability. The functional restoration approach of quota-based exercise is especially well suited to accomplish these goals, as exercise intensity is established independent of variations in pain symptoms that occur at or near the patients' true physiologic limits. Surprisingly, exercising in the presence of pain is well tolerated and acceptable to most patients, with reported dropout rates of only 15% according to most studies. The setting for delivery of this type of exercise need not be complex. With adequate staff training to ensure appropriate attitudes and beliefs about pain, and following the principles as previously outlined, physical therapy delivered twice a week for an average of 6 weeks can produce clinically relevant improvements in flexibility and strength and reduction of disability.

## Exercise Improves Chronic Back Pain

A 10% to 50% reduction in pain has been observed in most studies of exercise as treatment for patients with chronic low back pain. This pain reduction is documented in the presence of improved back function and increased participation in daily activities, thus countering the concern that use of the back is harmful for those with chronic back pain. The mechanism through which pain is reduced by exercise is not well understood, although some data suggest that exercise may desensitize the pain-producing process either in the pain-producing tissues or within the central nervous system. In addition, although the stated goal of functional restoration is to improve back function and disability, it is encouraging that patients who undergo this treatment usually feel substantial relief of pain.

## Summary

The use of functional restoration has shown that patients with chronic pain have great potential for leading normal and productive lives despite the persistence of pain. Physicians must be willing to accept the belief that it is safe for patients with pain to function in order to direct these patients toward improved function. Exercise is a powerful therapeutic modality that can be used to improve physiologic function, lessen disability, and reduce pain.

## Annotated Bibliography

*History of Functional Restoration and Recent Randomized Controlled Studies*

Joussett N, Fanello S, Bontoux L, et al: Effects of functional restoration versus 3 hours per week physical therapy: A randomized controlled study. *Spine* 2004;29:487-493.

This study randomly assigned patients with chronic low back pain and work disability to either functional restoration or physical therapy. The functional restoration group had less work absence in the follow-up period, and slightly better physical capacities, but other outcomes were similar.

Schonstein E, Kenny DT, Keating J, Koes BW: Work conditioning, work hardening and functional restoration for workers with back and neck pain. *Cochrane Database Syst Rev* 2003;1:CD001822.

This systematic review of 18 studies found evidence that physical conditioning that included a cognitive behavioral approach can reduce the number of sick days for workers with chronic low back pain, but noted no evidence of efficacy for exercise without a cognitive behavioral approach.

*Impact of Functional Restoration*

Houben RM, Vlaeyen JW, Peters M, Ostelo RW, Wolters PM, Stomp-van den Berg SG: Healthcare providers' attitudes and beliefs toward common low back pain: Factor structure and psychometric properties of the HC-PAIRS. *Clin J Pain* 2004;20:37-44.

This study of 156 therapists who treated back pain found that therapists' attitudes and beliefs about pain were the only significant predictors of recommendation for work and physical activities for vignettes describing patients with chronic low back pain.

Miranda H, Vikari-Juntura E, Martikainen R, Takala EP, Rihimaki H: Individual factors, occupational loading, and physical exercise as predictors of sciatic pain. *Spine* 2002;27:1102-1109.

This survey of 2,404 forestry workers with and without sciatica found no association between overall physical exercise and participation in most sports activities with the incidence of sciatic pain.

Rainville J, Hartigan C, Jouve C, Martinez E: The influence of intense exercise based physical therapy program on back pain anticipated before and induced by physical activities. *Spine J* 2004;4:176-183.

For a cohort of 70 subjects with chronic low back pain, intense exercise with a cognitive-behavioral approach resulted in a reduction of pain anticipated before and induced by a series of physical activities. These results suggest that exercise may desensitize the pain-producing process.

Rainville J, Jouve CA, Hartigan C, Martinez E, Hipona M: Comparison of short- and long-term outcomes for

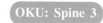

aggressive spine rehabilitation delivered two versus three times per week. *Spine J* 2002;2:402-407.

This study compared the outcomes of intensive physical therapy with a cognitive-behavioral approach delivered either two or three times per week and found no differences in any outcomes.

## Classic Bibliography

Bendix T, Bendix A, Labriola M, Haestrup C, Ebbehoj N: Functional Restoration versus outpatient physical therapy training in chronic low back pain: A randomized comparative study. *Spine* 2000;25:2494-2500.

Croft PR, Papageorgiou AC, Thomas E, Macfarlane GJ, Silman AJ: Short-term physical risk factors for new episodes of low back pain: Prospective evidence from the South Manchester Back Pain Study. *Spine* 1999;24:1556-1561.

Gatchel RJ, Polatin PB, Mayer TG: The dominant role of psychosocial risk factors in the development of chronic low back pain disability. *Spine* 1995; 20:2702-2709.

Gatchel RJ, Polatin PB, Mayer TG, Garcy PD: Psychopathology and the rehabilitation of patients with chronic low back pain disability. *Arch Phys Med Rehabil* 1994; 75:666-670.

Hazard RG, Fenwick JW, Kalisch SM, et al: Functional restoration with behavioral support: A one-year prospective study of patients with chronic low-back pain. *Spine* 1989;14:157-161.

Keeley J, Mayer TG, Cox R, Gatchel RJ, Smith J, Mooney V: Quantification of lumbar function: Part V. Reliability of range-of-motion measures in the sagittal plane and an in vivo torso rotation measurement technique. *Spine* 1986;11:31-35.

Mayer TG, Barnes D, Kishino ND, et al: Progressive isoinertional lifting evaluation: Part 1. A standard protocol and normative database. *Spine* 1988;13:993-997.

Mayer TG, Gatchel RJ, Mayer H, Kishino ND, Keeley J, Mooney V: A prospective two-year study of functional restoration in industrial low back injury. *JAMA* 1987; 258:1763-1767.

Mayer TG, Smith S, Keeley J, Mooney V: Quantification of lumbar function: Part 2. Saggital plane trunk strength in chronic low back pain patients. *Spine* 1985;10:765-772.

Rainville J, Ahern DK, Phalen L: Altering beliefs about pain and impairment in a functionally oriented treatment program for chronic back pain. *Clin J Pain* 1993; 9:196-201.

Rainville J, Carlson N, Polatin P, et al: Exploration of physicians' recommendations for activities in chronic low back pain. *Spine* 2000;25:2210-2220.

Sobel JB, Hartigan C, Rainville J, Wright A: Rehabilitation of the post spinal arthrodesis patient, in Margulies JY, Floman Y, Farcy JPC, Neuwirth MG (eds): *Lumbosacral and Spinopelvic Fixation Arthrodesis.* Philadelphia, PA, Lippincott-Raven, 1996.

Videman T, Sarna S, Battie MC, et al: The long term effects of physical loading and exercise lifestyles on back related symptoms, disability, and spinal pathology among men. *Spine* 1995;20:699-709.

Waddell G, Newton M, Henderson I, Somerville D, Main CJ: A fear-avoidance beliefs questionnaire and the role of fear avoidance beliefs in chronic low back pain and disability. *Pain* 1993;52:157-168.

# Chapter 20

# Rehabilitation of Spinal Cord Injury

David Chen, MD

## Demographics

Despite greater public awareness and efforts toward injury prevention, the incidence of spinal cord injuries (SCIs) in the United States has remained relatively constant over time. Changes in population demographics appear to have contributed to recent trends in age at injury, gender of persons injured, racial distribution, and etiology of injuries. Although younger adults continue to make up the largest group of patients with SCI, the average age at injury has steadily increased over time. Since 2000, the average age of a patient with a new SCI has been 38 years. As the median age of the US population has continued to rise, the percentage of patients with SCI who are older than 60 years of age also has increased. The implications of older age at time of injury include the greater likelihood of coexisting medical conditions (for example, cardiovascular disease and diabetes) that may complicate the initial acute care and rehabilitation of the SCI, and an increase in the risk of secondary complications. Although SCI continues to occur predominantly in males, there has been a gradual increase in the percentage of new injuries in females (21.8% since 2000). In terms of racial distribution, it has been previously reported that an increasing percentage of injuries are occurring in African Americans and Hispanics. Among those injured since 2000, 19% were African Americans, 10.4% were Hispanic, and 3.1% were from other racial, non-Caucasian groups. The etiology of injury has shown some variation over time. Motor vehicle crashes continue to account for the greatest number of new SCIs, but interestingly, the percentage of new injuries resulting from falls continues to increase, mirroring the increased percentage of injuries occurring in older adults.

Greater awareness of the potential of SCI at the injury scene and improved trauma care has led to an increase in survival rate, which underscores the importance of providing care to minimize secondary medical conditions/complications and rehabilitation to maximize patients' functional abilities.

## Spasticity

Spasticity, a common sequela of upper motor neuron SCI, is characterized by a velocity-dependent resistance to passive joint movement. Other characteristics of spasticity include increased muscle tone, exaggerated tendon jerks, involuntary movements (spasms), and clonus. Some or all of these symptoms may begin to emerge as spinal shock resolves. It has been reported that up to 80% of patients experience symptoms of spasticity during the first year after injury; however, not all patients require treatment. Factors that influence the decision to treat spasticity include the risk of developing contractures and skin breakdown, development of pain, and interference with self-care activities, hygiene activities, wheelchair positioning or transfer, and gait. In patients with chronic SCI, an increase in any of the symptoms of spasticity may be caused by other medical complications such as bowel impaction, hemorrhoids, urinary tract infection, kidney or bladder stones, pressure ulcers, ingrown toenails, deep venous thrombosis, or syringomyelia. For these patients, treatment of the spasticity is primarily focused on appropriate management of the underlying medical complication.

Nonpharmacologic treatment of spasticity includes regular stretching activities, attention to proper posture and positioning of patients with SCI when in bed and in wheelchairs, and the use of inhibitive casting, splinting, and orthotic devices. Other therapeutic modalities that have been shown to have short-term effectiveness in reducing spasticity include cryotherapy and electrical stimulation.

Pharmacologic treatment of spasticity includes oral and intrathecal medications and nerve/motor point blocks. Oral medications commonly used for managing spasticity include baclofen, diazepam, clonazepam, clonidine, tizanidine and dantrolene sodium. No single medication has been found to be universally effective in all patients with SCI; therefore, a trial with any of these agents is often necessary to ascertain effectiveness and to monitor for any individual side effects. Although frequently prescribed, muscle relaxants such as cyclobenza-

| Table 1 | Factors That Increase the Likelihood of Pressure Ulcers |
|---|

Poor hygiene
Poor nutrition
Uncontrolled spasticity
Development of contractures
Recurrent urinary tract infections
Bladder or bowel incontinence
Substance abuse
Cigarette smoking

| Table 2 | Staging of Pressure Ulcers | |
|---|---|
| Stage I | An area of nonblanchable erythema involving intact skin |
| Stage II | An area of partial-thickness skin loss, including the epidermis and down to, but not through, the dermis |
| Stage III | An area of full-thickness skin loss that involves subcutaneous tissue and down to the fascial layers |
| Stage IV | An area of full-thickness tissue injury involving the loss of muscle, connective tissue, joint, or bone |

prine and carisoprodol usually are not effective in treating spasticity in patients with SCI, and there is no evidence to support their efficacy in treating spasticity of spinal origin. The use of intrathecal baclofen has been studied extensively in patients with SCI; it is effective in those with intractable spasticity who do not tolerate or respond well to oral medications. Administration of intrathecal baclofen via an implanted programmable pump is advantageous over an overall lower dosage of baclofen, allowing the ability to program different doses at different times of the day to most effectively manage the spasticity. Disadvantages of this system include the need to surgically implant the pump in an abdominal pocket and to tunnel the catheter from the pump to the L3-4 or L4-5 disk space, the need for regular pump refills, and the occasional occurrence of mechanical pump malfunctions and catheter dislodgment, kinking, or leakage. Nerve or motor point blocks are not widely used in patients with SCI because spasticity is generally widespread and affects multiple extremities and muscle groups. However, in instances where isolated muscles affected by spasticity are causing particular difficulties with functional activities, positioning, or ambulation, the use of phenol or botulinum toxin for nerve/motor point blocks can be very effective.

## Pressure Ulcers

Pressure ulcers continue to be one of the most common and frequent medical complications in patients with SCI. Pressure ulcers not only have significant detrimental effects on the health and function of these patients, but on a larger scale, the costs of treatment weigh heavily on the health care system. It has been estimated that up to 80% of patients with SCI will experience a pressure ulcer during their lifetime, and 30% will have recurrent ulcers. Because of the significant health, functional, and economic implications, prevention of pressure ulcers is clearly desirable.

Several well-recognized factors contribute to the development of pressure ulcers in this patient population. External factors include excessive/prolonged pressure,

shearing, friction, and maceration of the skin. Pressure sores most frequently occur over bony prominences such as the sacrum, greater trochanter, heel, ischial tuberosity, scapula, and occiput. Measures to minimize excessive pressure over these areas, including a regular turning schedule when in bed, proper positioning in the bed or wheelchair, padding/protection of bony prominences, a properly fitting wheelchair and appropriate seat cushion, and performing regular pressure relief activities when sitting in a wheelchair, will greatly reduce the risk of pressure ulcer development. Shear and friction are forces across susceptible skin that can greatly increase the risk of skin breakdown that should be minimized or avoided if possible. Inadequately controlled spasticity and poorly performed transfers in and out of the wheelchair or bed can create significant shearing and friction. Conditions that affect skin integrity and create maceration, such as bowel and bladder incontinence or excessive perspiration, may increase the risk of pressure ulcers and therefore should be minimized.

In addition, individual factors also can contribute to or increase the likelihood of pressure ulcers in the patient with SCI, and attention to these factors can significantly reduce risk. Some of these factors are listed in Table 1.

The management and treatment of pressure ulcers should always include accurate staging and documentation to objectively assess any improvement or worsening of the ulcer so that changes can be made in treatment if necessary. A staging system advocated by the National Pressure Ulcer Advisory Panel is one of the most frequently used to describe pressure ulcers (Table 2). Other objective data that should be documented include the diameter and depth of the ulcer, tissue color, odor, and drainage color.

Active treatment of pressure ulcers generally focuses on providing an optimal environment for wound healing. Treatment may include the use of mechanical or chemical débridement to remove necrotic or devitalized tissue, the use of any number of commercially available dressings that keep the wound bed moist, control exudates, eliminate dead space, and keep the surrounding skin dry, and on occasion, the use of topical or systemic antibiotics if there is clinical suspicion of wound infection (not including osteomyelitis). For more extensive and severe pressure ulcers, surgical treatment may be required, involving procedures such as skin grafts or musculocutaneous flaps.

## Osteoporosis

Osteoporosis and increased risk for fractures are well-known complications of chronic SCI. Although several investigators have documented the significant reduction in bone mineral content and bone mineral density (BMD) in persons with chronic SCI, there are fewer studies documenting changes in BMD in the early, acute stage of SCI, which makes it less clear as to when preventive measures should be initiated. It is well known that urinary excretion of calcium and hydroxyproline is increased immediately after injury, a process that is a general marker of bone resorption. Most of the serum and urinary markers of bone response to SCI return to normal levels within 1 year after injury, which appears to indicate an adaptation to a new skeletal steady state.

The reduction in bone mass contributes to an elevated fracture risk in persons with SCI. Most fractures occur in the lower extremities and commonly are spiral fractures of the diaphysis and simple, bending fractures of the distal femur and/or proximal tibia. Fractures are infrequently caused by trauma, but usually occur as a result of minor falls from wheelchairs, during transfer activities, and during low strain activities such as dressing and bathing, and range-of-motion exercises.

It is generally accepted that the primary etiology for osteoporosis in persons with SCI is the immobilization, disuse, and absence of weight bearing that accompanies the paralysis. However, it is possible that a nutritional deficiency component contributes to the bone loss. Persons with chronic SCI tend to restrict their intake of dairy products because of the tendency to develop kidney and bladder stones. This dietary restriction results in reduced intake of calcium and vitamin D and consequently, reduced serum calcium concentration. This reduction stimulates the release of parathyroid hormone, resulting in increased bone resorption.

Measures to prevent or minimize osteoporosis have included weight bearing and assisted ambulation activities, electrical stimulation to increase muscle activity, and pharmacologic treatments. Weight-bearing activities have included standing activities using lower extremity orthotic and assistive devices, tilt tables and other standing frames, and body-weight support equipment. Unfortunately, no studies have shown any significant effect on reversal of bone loss. Functional electrical stimulation is used to reintroduce mechanical loading on the paralyzed extremities through muscular contraction, but similar to weight-bearing activities, there has been little consistent evidence to show that this modality limits or

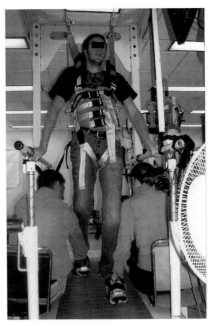

**Figure 1** Manual-assisted body-weight support treadmill training.

reverses bone loss following SCI. Pharmacologic treatments are focused on limiting the metabolic process that takes place following SCI. Studies have shown little benefit from the use of calcitonin, clondronate, etidronate, and toludronate in reversing bone loss in patients with SCI; however, according to one study, the use of intravenous pamidronate has been effective in reducing bone mass loss after acute SCI. Another more recent study has also shown evidence of a positive effect of alendronate in reducing bone loss after acute SCI. Despite these recent findings, the role of bisphosphonates in the treatment of bone loss in patients with acute and chronic SCI has not been clearly established, and additional studies are necessary.

## Rehabilitation: Advances in Ambulation Training

Recently, there has been a great deal of attention focused on new and innovative treatment strategies for ambulation training in persons with SCI. Several investigators have suggested that recovery of the ability to walk in specific SCI populations may be enhanced using manual assistance and body-weight support treadmill (BWST) training. This type of training may have several advantages over conventional gait training. BWST training uses a harness system to assist the patient with SCI in maintaining an upright position, and allows step training without any dependence on upper extremity loading on an assistive device (such as a walker) or parallel bars (Figure 1). The ability to initiate standing and stepping activities earlier after SCI appears to activate the trunk musculature and facilitate earlier independence in holding an upright posture. BWST training also is advantageous for patients with incomplete injuries because loading on the lower extrem-

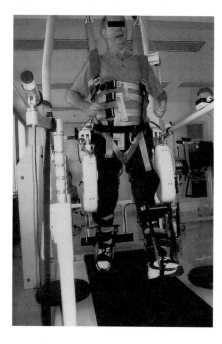

**Figure 2** Robotic-assisted body-weight support treadmill training.

ities can be adjusted to allow step training for those who may have less than antigravity strength in the hip flexors and knee extensors. The theory underlying BWST training is that the repetitive activity of the segmental sensory-motor pathways generated during the normal gait cycle improves the probability of generating more effective stepping. With this type of training, a therapist has better control over the kinematics and temporal patterns of stepping than when using parallel bars or overground with assistive devices.

More recently, an advanced version of BWST training, robotic-assisted BWST training, has become available and is under clinical study in several SCI rehabilitation centers in the United States. This version of BWST training involves the use of an exoskeletal, computer-controlled orthostic device that moves the legs of the SCI patient, who is supported by a harness over the treadmill, in a more physiologic gait pattern (Figure 2). Actuators are located at each knee and hip joint, and are controlled and move independently. One advantage of robotic-assisted BWST training over manual assistance is that separate therapists are not required to move each of the patient's legs. Because the work and effort by the therapists to move the legs on the treadmill can be physically demanding, the use of robotic assistance allows training sessions of longer duration and more repeatable, normal gait patterns. A small clinical study on patients with chronic, incomplete SCI has shown improvement in gait speed and muscle strength, but no change in need for any bracing, assistive device, or physical assistance that may have been necessary for ambulation before training. Several clinical studies examining the benefits of robotic-assisted BWST training in acute and chronic SCI are currently underway.

## Annotated Bibliography

### Demographics

Jackson AB, Dijkers M, DeVivo MJ, Poczatek RB: A demographic profile of new traumatic spinal cord injuries: Change and stability over 30 years. *Arch Phys Med Rehabil* 2004;85:1740-1748.

This is a report of an analysis of the National Spinal Cord Injury Database, which is a collection of demographic variables on 30,532 individuals who were admitted to Model Spinal Cord Injury System facilities between 1973 and 2003. The paper reports epidemiologic trends in new SCIs in the United States over three decades.

Spinal cord injury facts and figures at a glance. *J Spinal Cord Med* 2004;27(suppl 1):S139-140.

This is the most recent publications of the National Spinal Cord Injury Statistical Center summarizing specific demographic data collected by the Model Spinal Cord Injury System program. This information represents the largest single collection of data pertaining to SCIs in the United States.

### Spasticity

Nance PW: Management of spasticity, in Lin VW (ed): *Spinal Cord Medicine: Principles and Practice*. New York, NY, Demos Medical Publishing, 2003, pp 461-476.

This chapter provides a comprehensive review of the pathophysiology, evaluation, and management of spasticity in spinal cord disorders.

### Osteoporosis

Luethi M, Zehnder Y, Michel D, et al: Alendronate in the treatment of bone loss after spinal cord injury (SCI): Preliminary data of a 2-year randomized controlled trial in 60 paraplegic men. *J Bone Miner Res* 2001;16:s219.

A randomized control trial of 51 patients with acute SCIs showed a reduction in bone loss after 18 months of treatment using alendronate and calcium.

### Rehabilitation: Advances in Ambulation Training

Hornby TG, Zemon DH, Campbell D: Robotic-assisted, body-weight supported treadmill training in individuals following motor incomplete spinal cord injury. *Phys Ther* 2005;85:52-66.

A case report describing the use of a robotic device to enhance motor recovery and ambulation in three patients with motor incomplete SCI is presented. Two patients recovered independent over-ground ambulation and the third patient showed improvement in gait speed and endurance.

## Classic Bibliography

Barbeau H, Ladouceur M, Norman KE, Pepin A, Leroux A: Walking after spinal cord injury: Evaluation, treatment and functional recovery. *Arch Phys Med Rehabil* 1999;80:225-235.

Colombo G, Joery M, Schreier R, Dietz V: Treadmill training of paraplegic patients using a robotic orthosis. *J Rehabil Res Dev* 2000;37:693-700.

Consortium for Spinal Cord Medicine: *Pressure Ulcer Prevention and Treatment Following Spinal Cord Injury: A Clinical Practice Guideline for Health-Care Professionals.* Washington, DC, Paralyzed Veterans of America, 2000.

Nance P, Schryvers O, Leslie W, et al: Intravenous pamidronate attenuates bone density loss after acute spinal cord injury. *Arch Phys Med Rehabil* 1999;80:243-251.

Wernig A, Nanassy A, Muller S: Laufband (treadmill) therapy in incomplete paraplegia and tetraplegia. *J Neurotrauma* 1999;16:719-726.

# Section 3

# Adult Topics

Section Editors:
Sanford E. Emery, MD
Henry Claude Sagi, MD

# Chapter 21

# Initial Evaluation and Management of Spinal Trauma

Joji Inamasu, MD, PhD

Bernard H. Guiot, MD, FRCSC

## Introduction

Spinal trauma is estimated to affect more than 1 million people in the United States each year. Because of the diversity of injury patterns and the potential neurologic deficits, the evaluation and treatment of spinal trauma remains complex. In an effort to gain insight into the scope of issues involved with this complex injury, the National Spinal Cord Injury Statistical Center was established at the University of Alabama in Birmingham. This center supervises and directs the collection, management, and analysis of all spinal cord injury (SCI) data from a network of 16 federally sponsored regional facilities located at major medical centers throughout the United States. The data have been compiled into the largest database on SCIs and forms the basis of much of the epidemiologic information provided in this chapter. The information presented is based on the most recently updated version (August 2004) of the National Spinal Cord Injury Statistical Center database.

## Epidemiology

### Incidence and Prevalence

The annual incidence of SCI is approximately 40 cases per 1 million people in the United States, or 11,000 new cases each year. Additionally, there are approximately 50,000 fractures to the bony spinal column each year. The number of people living with an SCI in the United States in 2004 is estimated to be 247,000 persons.

### Age at Injury

SCI primarily affects young adults. From 1973 to 1979, the average age of a patient at the time of injury was 28.6 years; most injuries occurred between the ages of 16 and 30 years. Recently, as the median age of the general population has risen (an increase of 8 years since the mid 1970s), the average age at the time of SCI has also increased and is now estimated at 38 years. The percentage of patients older than 60 years at the time of injury also has increased from 4.7% prior to 1980 to 10.9% since 2000.

### Gender

Most SCIs occur in males. Prior to 1980, 81.8% of new SCIs occurred in males. Since 2000, that number has decreased slightly to 78.2%.

### Ethnic Groups

Between 1973 and 1979, 76.9% of SCI patients were Caucasians, 14.1% were African Americans, 6% were Hispanics, and 3% were from other racial/ethnic groups. More recently, there has been a decreasing incidence of SCIs in Caucasians. In 2000, 67.5% of SCI patients were Caucasians, whereas 19% were African Americans, 10.4% were Hispanics, and 3.1% were from other racial/ethnic groups. The changing incidence of this injury among racial groups probably has multifactorial reasons and may be related to changing demographics and population shifts.

### Etiology

Motor vehicle crashes accounted for 50.4% of reported SCIs in 2000. Rollover motor vehicle crashes are the most common mechanism resulting in SCI and account for 70% of these injuries. Thirty-nine percent of those injured were ejected from the vehicle and only 25% of patients reported using seat belts. Seat belts and air bags have been shown to be effective in decreasing the extent of neurologic deficit in patients involved in motor vehicle crashes. However, the use of air bags alone does not confer the same protection and may cause hyperextension-type injuries to the cervical spine.

Falls, acts of violence (primarily gunshot wounds), and recreational sports injuries are responsible for most of the remaining SCIs. The proportion of injuries that are the result of participation in sport activities has decreased over time, possibly as a result of improvements in equipment, medical care, and athletic education. The incidence of SCI resulting from sports-related injuries has dropped from 20 cases per year during the period from 1971 to 1975, to 7.2 cases per year during the past 10 years. The number of SCIs occurring as a result of violent acts has fluctuated. Prior to 1980, the incidence was 13.3%. Between 1990 and 1999, the incidence rose to 21.8%, but has decreased to 11.2% since 2000. SCIs resulting from falls have increased in number.

### Neurologic Status

Fifty-five percent of SCIs occur in the cervical spine. The remaining injuries are equally distributed throughout the thoracic, thoracolumbar, and lumbosacral spine with an incidence of 15% in each region. Neurologically, most patients sustain incomplete tetraplegia (34.3%), followed by complete paraplegia (25.1%), complete tetraplegia (22.1%), and incomplete paraplegia (17.5%). It should be noted that the frequency of incomplete tetraplegia is increasing slightly compared with the frequency of complete paraplegia and complete tetraplegia. Only 1% of patients have complete neurologic recovery at the time of hospital discharge.

## Field Evaluation and Stabilization

The field evaluation of a patient with an SCI is made up of the primary and secondary surveys. The primary survey consists of evaluation of the airway, breathing, and circulation (the ABCs of basic trauma life support). Maintenance of oxygenation and hemodynamic stability are paramount in attenuating secondary injury to the damaged spinal cord; therefore, all patients with suspected SCI should be given supplemental oxygen during transport to the hospital. Securing an airway in the field may be necessary. The utmost care is required during intubation to prevent hyperextension of the neck. The use of an Intubating Laryngeal Mask Airway (LMA North America, San Diego, CA) at the scene of the injury has been shown to facilitate blind orotracheal intubation in patients wearing a rigid Philadelphia collar. Vascular access is mandatory and is detailed in the literature on both advanced and basic trauma life support. In a patient with an SCI, the administration of fluids must be undertaken with caution. Circulatory collapse may occur as a result of neurogenic or hemorrhagic shock. The former is distinguished by bradycardia and a slow regular pulse in the presence of hypotension. In contrast, hemorrhagic shock is characterized by tachycardia and a rapid irregular pulse. The administration of a large volume of fluid in patients with neurogenic shock may result in fluid overload, pulmonary edema, and heart failure. The maintenance of hemodynamic stability in patients with neurogenic shock may require the use of inotropic and chronotropic agents.

The secondary survey consists of a thorough evaluation of the patient from head to toe, with attention directed to all organ systems. From a neurologic standpoint, loss of sensory and motor function indicates the presence of SCI. Patients also may have signs of bowel and bladder sphincter dysfunction. Unconscious patients or those whose mental status is altered by alcohol or drugs should be considered to have an SCI until proved otherwise.

Spinal immobilization is recommended for all trauma patients with a suspected cervical spinal column injury or with a mechanism of injury having the potential to cause cervical spine injury. Immobilization of the cervical spine is best accomplished using a rigid cervical collar and supportive blocks on a backboard with straps. The longstanding practice of attempting cervical spine immobilization using sandbags and tape alone is no longer recommended. The thoracic and lumbar spines are immobilized with a backboard at the scene of the injury. Because of potential drawbacks, concerns have been raised regarding the uniform practice of applying spine immobilization to all trauma patients. Spine immobilization can cause airway obstruction and can increase intracranial pressure; vigorous immobilization can cause neurologic deterioration in patients with some conditions. For example, patients with ankylosing spondylitis cannot tolerate the flat supine position. Furthermore, immobilization may not be necessary in certain types of penetrating injuries such as gunshot wounds to the torso.

When spinal immobilization is indicated for the transportation of children, the type of immobilization should take into account the child's age and physical maturity. The relatively large head size of a child compared with the size of the torso force the neck into a position of flexion when the head and torso are supine on a flat surface. Mild elevation of the torso against the head or the use of a cutout board to accommodate the occiput has been recommended to maintain the airway and neutral position of the cervical spine in children.

## Transport

Transfer of SCI patients to centers with the resources and expertise to treat these injuries must occur as soon as possible. Early transfer has been shown to decrease the incidence of complications and is associated with improved neurologic outcomes. SCI patients who are hemodynamically stable should be transported from the field to the nearest hospital where definitive spine care can be provided. However, if the patient is unstable, or a level I trauma center is too distant, transfer should be made to the nearest hospital. After the patient has been stabilized, transfer to an appropriate facility should be undertaken as quickly as possible. The means of transporting patients to facilities offering definitive care does not appear to affect the ultimate clinical outcome. Patients with acute SCI transferred to the University of Michigan Medical Center were reviewed to determine the effect on impairment and neurologic improvement of ground versus air transportation. The authors concluded that outcome was not affected by the mode of transportation and that standard precautions should be used in moving patients to sites of definitive care.

## Emergency Department Evaluation

When the patient arrives in the emergency department, the ABCs of resuscitation are once again performed. The airway must be secured to ensure adequate oxygenation. Observing the respiratory pattern of the patient with cervical SCI provides crucial information regarding the level of the SCI and the need for ventilatory assistance. SCI above C5 is more likely to require intubation (87.5% of patients) than injury from C5-C8 (61% of patients). Similarly, patients with complete quadriplegia are more likely to require intubation (90%) than those with incomplete quadriplegia or paraplegia (48.5%). Routine and early intubation in patients with cervical SCI above C5 and complete quadriplegia is recommended. Evaluation of the circulatory system should proceed concomitantly with airway management. Heart rate and blood pressure must be continuously monitored to permit early detection of shock. Patients with SCI are at risk for hemodynamic and neurogenic shock because of systemic injuries as well as spinal cord trauma. Neurogenic shock, defined as circulatory collapse resulting from neurologic injury, is caused by an interruption of sympathetic output to the heart and peripheral vasculature. This collapse gives rise to bradycardia (because of the unopposed parasympathetic input to the heart) and loss of vascular and muscular tone (relative hypovolemia) below the level of injury. One study found neurogenic shock present in 19 of 62 patients (31%) with high cervical SCI, and in 5 of 21 patients (24%) with lower cervical SCI. Patients with a high cervical SCI had a significantly greater requirement for a cardiovascular intervention, including use of pressors, chronotropic agents, and pacemakers, compared with patients with lower injuries.

After the initial survey and resuscitation have been completed, patients are examined for signs of obvious injuries to the head, torso, and abdomen. A thorough neurologic assessment should be performed. Details of the injury and the patient's history should be obtained from the patient, family members, bystanders, or paramedics because understanding the mechanism of injury is important. The past medical history provides information regarding the patient's general state of health, but also may reveal systemic processes that may predispose the patient to SCI after minor trauma. These processes include rheumatoid arthritis, ankylosing spondylitis, severe osteoporosis, primary or metastatic spinal tumor, and ossification of the posterior longitudinal ligament.

The neurologic examination should establish the level of SCI. When motor function is absent, sacral sensation must be carefully tested to distinguish between complete and incomplete lesions. The examination should be repeated frequently to detect any deterioration or improvement in neurologic function. Early neurologic findings may be confounded by spinal shock, which is usually a transient acute neurologic syndrome of sensorimotor dysfunction that develops with SCI at any level; this shock is characterized by flaccid areflexic paralysis and anesthesia. The duration of spinal shock varies from hours to weeks; however, resolution in most patients occurs within 48 hours. The termination of spinal shock marks the onset of spasticity below the level of the SCI.

The recognition of particular patterns of neurologic deficits, such as anterior cord syndrome, central cord syndrome, or Brown-Séquard syndrome, also may help to determine a prognosis. Anterior spinal artery syndrome is characterized by paraplegia or quadriplegia (depending on the level of injury) and a dissociated sensory deficit below the level of injury. The sensory deficit is caused by injury to the spinothalamic tracts, which mediate pain and temperature sensation and are supplied by the anterior spinal artery, and by preservation of the posterior columns, which mediate two-point discrimination, position sense, and vibration, and are supplied by the posterior spinal arteries. In general, anterior spinal artery syndrome carries the worst prognosis of the incomplete injuries, with only 10% to 20% of patients recovering functional motor control.

Central cord syndrome is the most common type of incomplete SCI and is usually caused by hyperextension forces applied to a spine in which stenosis and ligamentous hypertrophy are present. It is characterized by weakness affecting the upper extremities more than the lower extremities, with deficits typically worse distally than proximally. Sensory deficits are variable but often include hyperpathia (severe burning dysesthetic pains in the distal upper extremity).

Brown-Séquard syndrome, also known as spinal cord hemisection, occurs most frequently as a result of penetrating trauma. The classic presentation of this syndrome involves ipsilateral paralysis and loss of posterior column function (position sense and vibration) and contralateral loss of spinothalamic function (pain and temperature). The anterior spinothalamic tract that mediates crude touch is preserved. This incomplete SCI syndrome carries the best prognosis for recovery of functional motor activity and sphincter control.

The American Spine Injury Association (ASIA) International Standards for Neurologic and Functional Classification of Spinal Cord Injury have been recommended as the preferred neurologic examination tool. The ASIA Impairment Scale provides a method to characterize any residual function below the level of the SCI. A recent multicenter survey showed that the initial ASIA Impairment Scale score was a reliable predictor of long-term outcome of patients with cervical and thoracic SCI.

## Associated Injuries

SCI is associated with extraspinal fractures. A consecutive sample of 5,711 SCI patients who were admitted to the National Spinal Cord Injury Statistical Center database from 1986 to 1995 showed that 1,585 (28%) had extraspinal fractures, with 1,005 (63%) occurring at a single anatomic site and 580 (37%) occurring at multiple sites. Categorized by anatomic regions, fractures most frequently involve the chest (52%), the lower extremity (25%), the upper extremity (24%), the head (17%), the pelvis (9%), and other locations (11%). The five most common anatomic sites for fractures were rib and/or sternum (43%), clavicle and/or scapula (17%), radius and/or ulna (14%), face and/or mandible (12%), and tibia and/or fibula (12%).

SCI may also occur with other types of injuries such as closed head injuries. In one study of 447 patients with moderate to severe closed head injuries, 24 (5.4%) had cervical spine injury (fracture/subluxation), and 14 of the 24 (58.3%) sustained SCI. Noncontiguous spinal fractures occur with an incidence ranging from 3% to 23.8%. Etiologies associated with noncontiguous fractures include falls from heights and motor vehicle crashes. Combinations of spinal fractures include cervical plus cervical (28.4%), thoracic plus lumbar (24.7%), cervical plus thoracic (17.3%), thoracic plus thoracic (11.1%), and cervical plus lumbar (9.9%). Approximately 81% of patients in this study had a stable noncontiguous fracture.

SCI in the cervical region may be associated with vertebral artery injury. Most patients remain asymptomatic after unilateral vertebral artery occlusion because of the rich collateral blood flow, and as such, this entity may be underdiagnosed. In contrast, bilateral vertebral artery injury is potentially fatal. Basilar artery embolism from an occluded vertebral artery has caused acute deterioration of SCI patients who were previously conscious. A large, prospective angiographic study in blunt trauma patients showed that 36 of 109 patients (33%) with cervical SCI were found to have vertebral artery injury. Injuries that are more commonly associated with vertebral artery injury include high cervical fractures, fractures extending into the transverse foramen, and unilateral or bilateral facet subluxations. The current literature does not provide absolute recommendations for evaluation or treatment of these injuries. Most are asymptomatic intimal tears. Magnetic resonance angiography is a noninvasive method of evaluation; however, the only patients for whom evaluation and treatment is currently recommended are those with cervical injuries associated with a neurologic deficit attributable to basilar or vertebral artery perfusion. Treatment often consists of stent application.

## Initial Radiographic Assessment

A significant quantity of work has been done by Eastern Association for Surgery of Trauma, the American Association of Neurological Surgeons, and the Congress of Neurological Surgeons to synthesize the literature and formulate scientific recommendations for radiographic clearance algorithms. Plain radiographs of the cervical spine are not indicated in fully oriented asymptomatic patients without distracting injuries. Any patient suspected of cervical SCI and/or spinal fracture based on the mechanism of injury and/or symptoms requires, at a minimum, three views of the cervical spine screening series (AP, lateral, and open mouth odontoid views). In a patient with neck pain or tenderness who is awake, alert, and oriented, and whose initial radiographic studies are normal, cervical spine immobilization can be discontinued after obtaining normal and adequate dynamic flexion/extension radiographs and a normal CT or MRI study within 48 hours of injury.

In an obtunded patient, clearing the cervical spine is more difficult. If the initial plain radiographs are normal, the cervical spine can be cleared by CT and/or MRI (if the study is obtained within 48 hours of injury). After 48 hours, MRI is not reliable in clearing the cervical spine and other methods must be used in the obtunded patient. The incidence of missing a cervical SCI when using this algorithm is less than 0.25%. Fluoroscopic flexion/extension radiographs have been used to clear the cervical spine, but should not be performed without initial MRI to rule out spinal cord compression. It should be noted that the normal excursion of the cervical spine has not been documented in the sedated obtunded patient.

The potential for missing a significant cervical SCI with radiographic-based protocols is well recognized and has been estimated at 10% to 20%. The accuracy of flexion/extension radiographs in the diagnosis of SCI in patients with blunt cervical trauma also has been questioned. With the advent of high-speed and high-resolution CT, it has been proposed that CT be used as the primary screening examination in polytrauma patients and specifically in patients with altered mental status, inadequate radiographic studies, abnormal or equivocal radiographic findings, and in patients with neurologic deficits.

As discussed, MRI is indicated in trauma patients. In addition, MRI should be obtained for patients with radiculopathy, myelopathy, and progressive neurologic deficits. MRI is essential in patients in whom the neurologic deficits fail to correspond to the level of radiographic abnormality. Magnetic resonance angiography may be an important adjunctive test if deficits are progressive or are not adequately explained on the basis of the findings of other imaging studies. MRI is contraindicated in patients with SCI from gunshot wounds because of the potential risk of metal fragment migration.

Radiographic protocols have not been well defined for patients with suspected thoracic, lumbar, and sacral spine injuries. Typically, AP and lateral radiographs of the spine are obtained. However, CT has been gaining popularity as the initial imaging tool. In a recent study, 222 patients who sustained high-risk trauma had a prospective follow-up. These patients required thoracolumbar screening because of clinical findings or altered mentation. All patients had CT scans of the chest, abdomen, and pelvis in addition to radiographs of the thoracolumbar spine. Thirty-six of 222 patients (17%) were known to have fractures. CT scans identified 99% of the fractures, whereas radiographs identified only 87%. Sensitivity, specificity, as well as positive and negative predictive values were better for CT than for radiography, leading the authors to conclude that CT was more accurate and should replace plain radiography in the evaluation of high-risk trauma patients.

## Initial Closed Reduction

Current guidelines suggest that early closed reduction of cervical spine fracture-dislocations is safe and effective in conscious patients. Reduction of the fracture should be performed in the intensive care unit using bedside fluoroscopy, while monitoring the clinical and neurologic status of the patient. When appropriate, traction can be started using 3 lb for each vertebral segment above the injury site. Weight may be added every 10 to 15 minutes, provided there is close clinical, neurologic, and radiographic monitoring. Traction should cease immediately if the patient's neurologic state worsens or if overdistraction is noted on fluoroscopy. If the deformity has been successfully reduced, or if a determination has been made that closed reduction has failed, the patient is immobilized until definitive treatment is initiated. Using this technique, closed reduction will be achieved in approximately 80% of patients.

Closed reduction of traumatic cervical SCI is the subject of considerable discussion. The possible presence of a herniated disk fragment at the injury site raises concern that the fragment could cause compression of the spinal cord during reduction of the deformity. It is estimated that such a disk fragment occurs in one third to one half of patients. The possible presence of such a fragment has led to the controversy concerning the necessity of performing routine MRI in patients with facet dislocation before undertaking closed reduction. The overall permanent neurologic complication rate of closed reduction is approximately 1%, whereas the risk of a transient injury is approximately 2% to 4%. Because of these risk factors, it is generally accepted that closed reduction can be undertaken before MRI for the detection of a disk herniation in an awake patient who is able to communicate or demonstrate a worsening neurologic deficit. Contraindications for closed reduction of fracture-dislocations include most skull fractures, severe local soft-tissue trauma, and distractive ligamentous injury.

The role of closed reduction in patients with acute thoracic and lumbar spine fractures is less clear. In a recent retrospective study, 41 neurologically intact patients with thoracolumbar or lumbar burst fractures were treated with closed reduction. Reduction was achieved using a Cotrel traction frame with fluoroscopic visualization at a mean of 3 days (range, 1 to 10 days) after the injury. Following reduction, the patients were immobilized in a thoracolumbar plaster cast. Significant pain relief and marked correction of vertebral wedging was achieved in most patients; no complications resulted from the fracture reduction procedure.

## Medical Management

Patients with acute SCI should be treated in the intensive care unit. Respiratory, cardiac, and hemodynamic monitoring is necessary and beneficial for SCI patients. Hypotension (systolic blood pressure < 90 mm Hg) should be avoided and corrected as soon as possible to maintain mean arterial blood pressure at 85 to 90 mm Hg for the first 7 days after acute injury.

Potential pitfalls in the treatment of patients with SCI include electrolyte abnormalities (specifically hyponatremia), which commonly occur. Sympathetic dysfunction is believed to be involved in the etiology of the hyponatremia and, although usually mild and self-limiting, altered mental status also has been reported. Cardiac monitoring to diagnose cardiac dysrhythmias is essential in patients with cervical SCI.

Deep venous thrombosis and pulmonary embolism must be avoided. In the absence of coagulopathy and intracranial hemorrhage, prophylactic use of low-molecular-weight heparins, rotating beds, adjusted-dose heparin, or a combination of modalities is recommended. Pneumatic compression stockings or electrical stimulation also may be used. Routine prophylactic vena cava filtration is not indicated. In patients suspected of having deep venous thrombosis and/or pulmonary embolism, duplex Doppler ultrasound, impedance plethysmography, and venography are useful diagnostic tests. Aggressive pulmonary hygiene protocols, including frequent changes in position, incentive spirometry, chest percussion, assisted coughing, and tracheal suctioning, are important tools in preventing other pulmonary complications. Infection including pneumonia, urinary tract infection, and skin (decubitus) ulcers are common in SCI patients and must be detected and treated promptly. Coordinated activity by the nursing staff and physical and respiratory therapists has been proved effective in reducing these complications.

## Pathophysiology and Pharmacotherapy

Injury to the nervous tissue consists of primary and secondary processes. The mechanical forces that affect the spinal column during the traumatic event are imparted to the neural tissue resulting in the primary injury to the spinal cord. The spectrum of the primary injury ranges from local axonal depolarization to axonal and neuronal damage. The injury resulting from the primary event is generally understood to be irreversible and can be mitigated only through preventive measures. Tissue adjacent to the primary injury is not damaged at the time of the trauma but is vulnerable to secondary pathophysiologic processes, which may bring about a propagation of the injury. These secondary processes include alterations in microvascular perfusion, elaboration of free radicals, lipid peroxidation, necrosis and apoptosis of the cell, and ionic imbalance. The first step in this process appears to consist of mechanical disruption of the spinal cord microvasculature, leading to petechial hemorrhages and intravascular thrombosis. These changes, in combination with vasospasm and spinal cord edema, results in hypoperfusion and ischemia within the spinal cord. The effects of hypoperfusion and ischemia are compounded by the loss of autoregulation, which under normal conditions is a physiologic mechanism that maintains tight control of the microvasculature hemodynamics within the spinal cord during systolic blood pressure fluctuations between 50 and 100 mm Hg. The loss of autoregulation renders the spinal cord vulnerable to fluctuations in blood pressure, which unfortunately is common in trauma settings.

During the hypoperfusion phase and the subsequent reperfusion phase, free radicals are formed. These highly reactive molecules interact with lipids, proteins, and DNA. Progressive oxidation of the lipids in the cell membrane by free radicals (lipid peroxidation) leads to the formation of more free radicals in a chain reaction that ultimately propagates along the cell. If uncontrolled, lipid peroxidation and free radical formation lead to metabolic collapse and to the subsequent death or apoptosis of the cell. During hypoperfusion and reperfusion of the spinal cord, glutamate release occurs. Glutamate acts on specific cell membrane receptors (N-methyl-D-aspartate receptor), which when activated allow entry of massive amounts of calcium into the intracellular space. N-methyl-D-aspartate receptor activation may also cause the release of calcium from intracellular stores. The elevated calcium triggers the activation of lytic enzymes, the generation of free radicals, and the dysregulation of mitochondrial function leading to apoptotic cell death.

Current treatment protocols attempt to attenuate these secondary pathophysiologic events. Many chemical compounds have proved beneficial in experimental SCI models, but most failed to show efficacy in clinical trials and were abandoned. Methylprednisolone is one of the few drugs commercially available for treatment of acute SCI and is indicated for patients with acute, non-penetrating SCIs who are admitted for treatment within 24 hours of injury. The effective neuroprotective mechanisms of methylprednisolone are not completely understood but may include inhibition of lipid peroxidation and inflammatory cytokines, modulation of inflammatory cells, improved vascular perfusion, and prevention of calcium influx and accumulation.

Several trials have studied the effects of methylprednisolone in the clinical setting; however, the National Acute Spinal Cord Injury Studies (NASCIS) II and III have made the use of methylprednisolone the standard treatment in clinical practice for patients with acute SCI. Criticism has recently been directed at the interpretation and conclusions of these studies, leading some centers to discontinue the use of methylprednisolone. The validity of these studies has been questioned because of the fact that in NASCIS II, the primary outcome analysis of motor and sensory recovery in all randomized patients was in fact negative, and only after a post hoc analysis was an arguably small yet statistically significant benefit found in patients in whom treatment was started within 8 hours of injury. Similarly, the primary outcome measures of NASCIS III were negative, but a post hoc analysis determined a benefit of 48 hours of methylprednisolone treatment in patients in whom treatment was initiated 3 to 8 hours after injury.

Systemic administration of monosialotetrahexosyl-ganglioside (GM-1) has been shown to be neuroprotective in a variety of experimental models of central nervous system injury. Promising results from a single-center, prospective double-blinded randomized study of 37 patients with SCI prompted a large-scale multicenter randomized trial. This study, however, did not find that the use of GM-1 yielded better neurologic outcome. Patients treated with GM-1 did appear to have a more rapid rate of recovery. Many parameters, including motor and sensory scores and bowel and bladder function, showed trends of improvement in those treated with GM-1 (particularly in patients with incomplete injuries) compared with patients receiving a placebo.

Induced hypothermia has been used on many patients with neurotrauma, including SCIs, for more than 40 years. Although efficacy of hypothermia in mitigating secondary injury is well known, its application to SCI has not yielded satisfactory results, both clinically and experimentally. Hyperthermia is detrimental to patients with neurotrauma, including SCI, and should be avoided.

## Summary

The treatment of SCI continues to evolve as the understanding of the mechanisms of injury grows. Patient tracking is critical to improving clinical outcome, and ongoing research into the pathophysiology of cord injury results in new treatment modalities. Despite progress in these areas, the best treatment of SCI remains prevention.

## Annotated Bibliography

*Epidemiology*

Cantu RC, Mueller FO: Catastrophic spine injuries in American football, 1977-2001. *Neurosurgery* 2003;53: 358-362.

This article discusses how teaching the fundamental techniques of the game, instituting equipment standards, and improving medical care, both on and off the playing field, have led to a significant reduction in permanent SCI in athletes participating in American football.

National Spinal Cord Injury Statistical Center: Spinal cord injury: Facts and figures at a glance. Available at: http://www.spinalcord.uab.edu/show.asp?durki=21446. Accessed August, 2004.

This Web site is operated jointly by the National Spinal Cord Injury Statistical Center and the University of Alabama at Birmingham. Most epidemiologic data on SCIs in the United States are available online. The Web site and data are updated regularly.

Sekhon LH, Fehlings MG: Epidemiology, demographics, and pathophysiology of acute spinal cord injury. *Spine* 2001;26(24 suppl):S2-12.

This is a concise yet comprehensive review on the epidemiology, demographics, and pathophysiology of acute SCI. Detailed information on the biologic aspect of acute SCI is available.

Vaccaro AR, Silber JS: Post-traumatic spinal deformity. *Spine* 2001;26(24 suppl):S111-S118.

Epidemiologic data and the natural history of acute spine fracture are provided in this review article. The pathogenesis of posttraumatic spinal deformity is also described.

Wesner ML: An evaluation of Think First Saskatchewan: A head and spinal cord injury prevention program. *Can J Public Health* 2003;94:115-120.

This article discusses the importance of educating children in preventing sports-related SCIs. The self-reported knowledge of the children receiving the Think First message statistically improved.

*Field Evaluation and Stabilization*

Cornwell EE III, Chang DC, Bonar JP, et al: Thoracolumbar immobilization for trauma patients with torso gunshot wounds: Is it necessary? *Arch Surg* 2001;136: 324-327.

The results of this study showed little benefit of spinal immobilization in patients with a gunshot wound to the torso. The authors suggest reexamination of the role of formal spinal immobilization for patients with gunshot wounds to the torso.

Guidelines for management of acute cervical spinal injuries: Introduction. *Neurosurgery* 2002;50(3 suppl):S1.

This is a collection of evidence-based guidelines on virtually every aspect of acute cervical spinal cord/spine injury management. It was edited by an expert panel of spine neurosurgeons and is based on a thorough, critical review of the data available by 2001.

Komatsu R, Nagata O, Kamata K, Yamagata K, Sessler DI, Ozaki M: Intubating laryngeal mask airway allows tracheal intubation when the cervical spine is immobilized by a rigid collar. *Br J Anaesth* 2004;93:655-659.

An intubating laryngeal mask airway may be a good alternative to an endotracheal tube for stabilizing patients in the field. The authors investigated whether an intubating laryngeal mask airway would allow tracheal intubation even in patients wearing a rigid cervical collar. They found that blind intubation through such a mask was a reasonable strategy for controlling the airway in patients who were immobilized with a cervical collar.

Kwan I, Bunn F, Roberts I: Spinal immobilisation for trauma patients. *Cochrane Database Syst Rev* 2001;2: CD002803.

A meta-analysis of the literature was conducted to evaluate the efficacy of spinal immobilization. Although spinal immobilization seems to be beneficial in most instances, no conclusion could be drawn because of the lack of randomized control trials. The possibility that immobilization could increase mortality and morbidity could not be excluded.

Tins BJ, Cassar-Pullicino VN: Imaging of acute cervical spine injuries: Review and outlook. *Clin Radiol* 2004;59: 865-880.

This review summarized the recent trend in the use of imaging modalities in patients suspected of having acute cervical spine injury.

Ummenhofer W, Scheidegger D: Role of the physician in prehospital management of trauma: European perspective. *Curr Opin Crit Care* 2002;8:559-565.

The importance of prehospital treatment of patients with spinal injuries is described in this review. The authors suggest that the role of both the physician and paramedic should be redefined in treating patients with spinal injuries prior to hospitalization.

*Emergency Department Evaluation*

Bilello JF, Davis JW, Cunningham MA, Groom TF, Lemaster D, Sue LP: Cervical spinal cord injury and the need for cardiovascular intervention. *Arch Surg* 2003; 138:1127-1129.

The authors of this study investigated whether the level of cervical SCI can be used to predict the need for a cardiovascular intervention. They found that patients with a high cervical SCI (level C1-C5) had a significantly greater requirement for a cardiovascular intervention compared with patients with lower SCIs (level C6-C7).

Coleman WP, Geisler FH: Injury severity as primary predictor of outcome in acute spinal cord injury: Retrospective results from a large multicenter clinical trial. *Spine J* 2004;4:373-378.

This article presents the results of a retrospective analysis to identify predictors of outcome in 760 patients with acute SCI. The ASIA Impairment Scale was found to be the strongest predictor of outcome. Anatomic region was also a strong predictor, but was confounded by the severity effect.

Nockels RP: Nonoperative management of acute spinal cord injury. *Spine* 2001;26(24 suppl):S31-S37.

This article presented a discussion of prehospital and preoperative management of patients with acute SCI.

Stevens RD, Bhardwaj A, Kirsch JR, Mirski MA: Critical care and perioperative management in traumatic spinal cord injury. *J Neurosurg Anesthesiol* 2003;15:215-229.

This is a review article on critical care management of patients with an acute SCI from the point of view of an anesthesiologist. Pulmonary and cardiovascular management are emphasized. The distinction between neurogenic and spinal shock was described in detail.

Velmahos GC, Toutouzas K, Chan L, et al: Intubation after cervical spinal cord injury: To be done selectively or routinely. *Am Surg* 2003;69:891-894.

The timing of intubation in patients with SCI is often difficult. The authors of this study suggest that intubation needs to be offered routinely and early in patients with cervical SCI above C5 and complete quadriplegia.

### Associated Injuries

Holly LT, Kelly DF, Counelis GJ, Blinman T, McArthur DL, Cryer HG: Cervical spine trauma associated with moderate and severe head injury: Incidence, risk factors, and injury characteristics. *J Neurosurg* 2002;96:285-291.

The incidence of cervical spine trauma is relatively high in patients with closed head injury. Twenty-four of the 447 patients (5.4%) with moderate and severe head injury treated by the authors of this article had a cervical spine injury. Fourteen of the 24 patients (58.3%) had SCI.

Korres DS, Boscainos PJ, Papagelopoulos PJ, Psycharis I, Goudelis G, Nikolopoulos K: Multiple level noncontiguous fractures of the spine. *Clin Orthop* 2003;411:95-102.

The authors of this article report on the treatment of 81 patients with noncontiguous fractures of the spine. Diagnostic pitfalls for this uncommon type of fractures are described.

Miller PR, Fabian TC, Croce MA, et al. Prospective screening for blunt cerebrovascular injuries: Analysis of diagnostic modalities and outcomes. *Ann Surg* 2002;236:386-393.

This large, prospective angiographic study showed that vertebral artery injury was common in patients with a cervical spine injury. Results showed that 36 of 109 patients (33%) with major cervical spine injury had a vertebral artery injury.

Wang CM, Chen Y, DeVivo MJ, Huang CT: Epidemiology of extraspinal fractures associated with acute spinal cord injury. *Spinal Cord* 2001;39:589-594.

The incidence of extraspinal fractures associated with acute SCI was calculated using the National SCI Database and was stratified by anatomic sites, demographics, and injury-related characteristics. Of 5,711 patients, 1,585 (28%) of patients had extraspinal fractures and 580 (37%) had more than one fracture site.

### Initial Radiographic Assessment

Hauser CJ, Visvikis G, Hinrichs C, et al: Prospective validation of computed tomographic screening of the thoracolumbar spine in trauma. *J Trauma* 2003;55:228-235.

The sensitivity of standard PA and lateral radiographs of the thoracolumbar spine to diagnose a fracture may not be satisfactory. The authors prospectively studied 222 consecutive patients sustaining high-risk trauma requiring screening of the thoracolumbar spine with a helical CT. Screening the thoracolumbar spine with helical CT was more accurate than with standard radiography.

Insko EK, Gracias VH, Gupta R, Goettler CE, Gaieski DF, Dalinka MK: Utility of flexion and extension radiographs of the cervical spine in the acute evaluation of blunt trauma. *J Trauma* 2002;53:426-429.

The authors of this study investigated the usefulness of dynamic radiographs of the cervical spine for the acute evaluation of ligamentous injury. In 30% of patients, the dynamic examinations were interpreted as inadequate because of limited motion. In 12.5% of patients with inadequate dynamic examinations, injuries were missed and were later detected by CT or MRI.

Van Goethem JW, Maes M, Ozsarlak O, van den Hauwe L, Parizel PM: Imaging in spinal trauma. *Eur Radiol* 2005;15:582-590.

This article presents a review of the initial radiographic evaluation of patients with an acute SCI. The authors emphasize that rapid progress in medical imaging technology, represented by multidetector row helical CT, will change the sequence of imaging studies in patients with acute SCI.

### Initial Closed Reduction

Harrop JS, Vaccaro A, Przybylski GJ: Acute respiratory compromise associated with flexed cervical traction after C2 fractures. *Spine* 2001;26:E50-E54.

In this article, the authors report that respiratory deterioration occurred frequently after reduction of posteriorly displaced type II odontoid fractures. They also suggest that cervical flexion during and after reduction may significantly

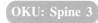 

increase the risk of airway obstruction because of the presence of acute retropharyngeal swelling.

Tropiano P, Huang RC, Louis CA, Poitout DG, Louis RP: Functional and radiographic outcome of thoracolumbar and lumbar burst fractures managed by closed orthopaedic reduction and casting. *Spine* 2003;28:2459-2465.

This retrospective review of 45 patients with stable thoracolumbar and lumbar burst fractures treated conservatively showed that closed reduction and casting of burst fractures is a safe treatment method that yields acceptable functional and radiographic results.

Vaccaro AR, Nachwalter RS: Is magnetic resonance imaging indicated before reduction of a unilateral cervical facet dislocation. *Spine* 2002;27:117-118.

The need for MRI before reduction of a cervical facet dislocation is controversial because an unrecognized disk herniation may produce SCI if reduction is performed before decompression. This article presents arguments both pro and con regarding whether MRI is necessary before reduction.

### Medical Management

Urdaneta F, Layon AJ: Respiratory complications in patients with traumatic cervical spine injuries: Case report and review of the literature. *J Clin Anesth* 2003;15:398-405.

Patients with cervical spine injury are vulnerable to various respiratory complications. The mechanism and management of each respiratory complication is described in this article.

### Pathophysiology and Pharmacology

Geisler FH, Coleman WP, Grieco G, Poonian D, Sygen Study Group: The Sygen multicenter acute spinal cord injury study. *Spine* 2001;26(suppl 24):S87-S98.

This article presents the results of a randomized, double-blind, multicenter clinical trial of GM-1 ganglioside for human SCI. Although the study did not find that the use of GM-1 yielded better neurological outcome, patients treated with GM-1 did appear to have a more rapid rate of recovery.

Inamasu J, Nakamura Y, Ichikizaki K: Induced hypothermia in experimental traumatic spinal cord injury: An update. *J Neurol Sci* 2003;209:55-60.

This article presents a review of the use of therapeutic hypothermia to treat patients with acute SCI. Although hypothermia is beneficial in patients with mild to moderate SCI, it may not be protective against severe SCI. At present, induced hypothermia has yet to be recognized or approved as a potential treatment having therapeutic value for SCI in humans.

Kwon BK, Tetzlaff W, Grauer JN, Beiner J, Vaccaro AR: Pathophysiology and pharmacologic treatment of acute spinal cord injury. *Spine J* 2004;4:451-464.

This is an excellent review which covers the pathophysiology and pharmacologic treatment of an acute SCI. Detailed account on the recent "methylprednisolone controversy" for acute SCI was also provided.

## Classic Bibliography

Askins V, Eismont FJ: Efficacy of five cervical orthoses in restricting cervical motion: A comparison study. *Spine* 1997;22:1193-1198.

Burney RE, Waggoner R, Maynard FM: Stabilization of spinal injury for early transfer. *J Trauma* 1989;29:1497-1499.

Dyson-Hhudson TA, Stein AB: Acute management of traumatic cervical spinal cord injuries. *Mt Sinai J Med* 1999;66:170-178.

Hart RA, Mayberry JC, Herzberg AM: Acute cervical spinal cord injury secondary to air bag deployment without proper use of lap or shoulder harnesses. *J Spinal Disord* 2000;13:36-38.

Heary RF, Vaccaro AR, Mesa JJ, et al: Steroids and gunshot wounds to the spine. *Neurosurgery* 1997;41:576-584.

Thurman DJ, Burnett CL, Beaudoin DE, Jeppson L, Sniezek JE: Risk factors and mechanisms of occurrence in motor vehicle-related spinal cord injuries: Utah. *Accid Anal Prev* 1995;27:411-415.

# Chapter 22

# Fractures of the Cervical Spine

John C. France, MD

## Introduction

Cervical spine injury remains one of the focal points in treating trauma patients because of the potential for devastating spinal cord injury. Young adult men make up most of this patient population. However, as the baby-boom generation ages and patients remain healthy and active at an older age, there has been an increase in the number of elderly patients with cervical fractures. This trend appears to exist worldwide. Data from Sweden from 1987 to 1999 indicate that, although the overall number of cervical fractures has decreased, there has been an increase in the prevalence of this injury in the older adult population. As might be expected, the mechanism of motor vehicle crashes plays a lesser role in cervical injuries in older adults, whereas falls as the mechanism of injury play a greater role. The unique diagnostic and treatment issues posed by elderly patients will likely present a great challenge to spine surgeons over the next decade.

Improvements in imaging capabilities have enhanced the ability to detect and more fully characterize cervical spine injuries; however, controversy remains on how and when to use some imaging modalities as well as how to apply the acquired information. Improvements in surgical techniques have aided in restoring anatomic alignment and achieving stability, but many questions remain about which technique or approach to use for any given fracture. Thus, cervical spinal fractures require a comprehensive understanding of injury biomechanics and adaptability on the part of the treating physician to apply these modern tools in a manner that suits the individual needs of each patient.

## Imaging

The continued growth in imaging capabilities is probably one of the fastest-changing areas of spine trauma. With improved visualization, physicians are better able to identify and define injuries, but are also presented with new questions concerning the significance of many radiographic findings. Some long-accepted principles in the initial trauma evaluation of the spine are now being questioned. It is likely that trauma evaluation will continue to evolve over the next few years. In a very specific subset of patients, no radiographs are necessary. These patients are alert, cooperative, have no pain, no neurologic findings, no distracting injuries, and have sustained a low-risk mechanism of injury. All other trauma patients require clearance of the cervical spine. The new helical CT scanners can rapidly obtain complete data in a spiral fashion rather than using axial slices; this process allows more accurate sagittal and coronal reconstructions. The sensitivity of these scanners to detect bony injury approaches 100%. In select patients, such as those who have sustained high-energy trauma in which there is an increased risk for spinal injury, the difficulty in obtaining the necessary plain radiographs may become obsolete. The issues of cost and radiation exposure remain a concern, and the criteria for using plain radiographs (supplemented with CT scans when needed) compared with using a helical scan are yet to be determined.

The technique to use when assessing patients for occult isolated ligamentous injury remains controversial. Because these injuries can realign into an anatomic position when the patient is lying immobilized and supine, they can go undetected on plain radiographs or CT scans (Figure 1). In addition, there is a real potential for instability and late neurologic deterioration. Any patient who continues to report neck pain, has an unexplained neurologic deficit, or is unable to cooperate with an examination must be considered to have a potentially unstable ligamentous injury until it is proved otherwise. In treating occult injury, patients can be divided into two groups: the alert patient who is able to cooperate with the evaluation and the impaired patient whose mental status significantly impedes cooperation. If the impairment in mental status is expected to be temporary, such as in an intoxicated patient, the ligamentous assessment can be delayed as long as proper immobilization and spinal precautions are maintained. In the cooperative patient, flexion-extension radiographs are the most common method used to clear the spine. If these radiographs are obtained immediately, the flexion-extension excursion is often limited and the study would be con-

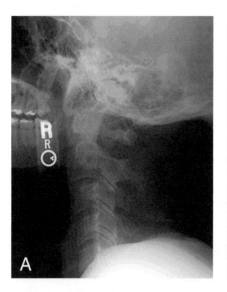 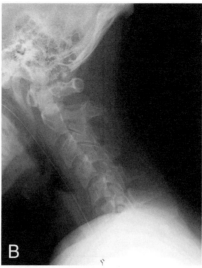 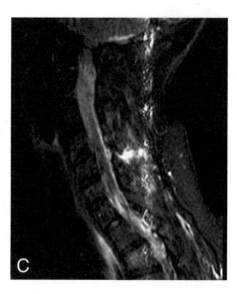

**Figure 1**   **A,** A neutral lateral radiograph shows normal alignment. The CT scan was negative for fracture. **B,** Because of persistent neck pain, a flexion-extension series of radiographs was performed and clearly revealed instability at C4-5. **C,** An inversion recovery MRI scan verified the ligamentous injury that created the instability.

sidered inadequate to clear the spine. Early flexion-extension radiographs are only useful if the degree of excursion indicates an injury or if no injury is detected with a full excursion. In the latter situation, the spine can be considered clear. In the cooperative patient, the collar often is maintained until pain subsides enough to allow full excursion or until the 2-week follow-up reassessment. In the patient with impaired mental status in whom prolonged impairment is expected (such as the intubated patient or patient with a head injury), other means are necessary to rule out ligamentous injury. Protocols for spinal clearance in these patients can vary between hospitals and even among physicians within the same hospital. It is recommended that each hospital involved in the treatment of trauma patients have a protocol in place that can be reliably and consistently executed for clearing the spine in patients who are unable to cooperate. The two basic means of evaluation would be stress testing with fluoroscopic control, or MRI. Fluoroscopic evaluation can be difficult to use because of limited visualization of the cervicothoracic junction; it also requires the presence of a physician. A distraction test before manually flexing or extending the neck may detect an injury without risking dislocation that could occur during flexion.

MRI offers visualization of the soft tissues without the need to manipulate the neck. MRI is capable of revealing disruption of the ligamentous structures, particularly in the posterior complex, and showing edema that may be indicative of acute injury to the soft tissues. The addition of gradient echo and inversion recovery sagittal images greatly enhances the visualization of edema and thus should be included in the trauma protocol. The potential for overdiagnosis exists with MRI, because the significance of many of the shadows seen is not fully un-

derstood. Also, it can be quite cumbersome to move a patient requiring intensive care to the scanner, to continue intensive care monitoring during scanning, and to achieve adequate patient cooperation to obtain quality images.

In recent years more attention has been given to the potential for vertebral artery injury associated with cervical trauma. This attention may be related to the increased use of MRI for cervical trauma patients and the improved technology provided by magnetic resonance angiography (MRA) that has made visualization of the vertebral arteries relatively easy without the need for standard angiography. These improved imaging methods have created controversy because it is unclear how the information obtained from such studies should be used. The incidence of vertebral artery pathology has been reported to be as high as 46% in facet dislocations and 16% in fractures that enter the transverse foramen. The injuries noted are typically intimal flaps or occlusions rather than lacerations. However, symptoms or clinical manifestations resulting from arterial injury are rare. Because anticoagulation treatment is often used, caution must be exercised in any decision to treat this component of injury in a patient with a cervical fracture who has the potential for epidural hematoma and who also may have other nonspinal injuries with bleeding potential. It has also been shown that after traumatic vertebral artery occlusion, reconstitution of blood flow seldom occurs even after 2 years. If a patient has clinical manifestations that could be attributed to vertebral artery occlusion, evaluation with MRA is warranted. In a fracture pattern that has a high risk for underlying vertebral artery injury and in which surgical treatment, such as screw placement, will present a significant injury risk to the vertebral artery, a preoperative MRA should

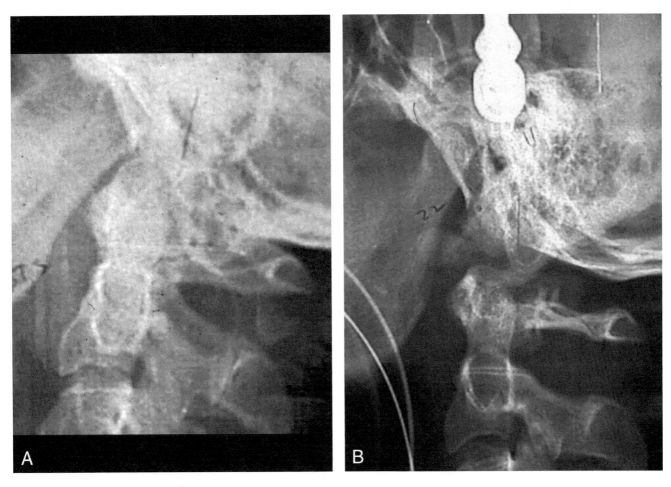

Figure 2  Pretraction radiograph **(A)** and posttraction radiograph **(B)** show overdistraction at the occipital cervical junction.

be considered to avoid bilateral vertebral artery injury. At the present time, the routine use of MRA assessment in cervical trauma patients cannot be recommended; however, it is an area that justifies further study.

## Specific Injury Patterns
### Upper Cervical Fractures

#### Occipitocervical
Although occipitocervical injuries rarely occur in the surviving patient, the increased use and understanding of MRI has dramatically improved the early recognition of this injury. It is also likely that advances in car safety devices (such as airbags) and better prehospital treatment has increased the likelihood of surviving an occipitocervical injury. It is critical that such injuries be identified early because they cause significant instability and the potential dire neurologic consequences of displacement. Noncontiguous fracture is found in approximately 15% of cervical fractures. If a patient has another cervical fracture that would benefit from traction, particular attention should be paid to the occipitocervical area before using traction because traction is contraindicated for patients with occipitocervical dissociations. If no ob-

vious injury is identified, traction should be initiated at low weights of 10 to 15 lb followed by a repeat lateral radiograph and reassessment of this area to avoid overdistraction of an occult injury (Figure 2).

Power's ratio has long been considered a means of identifying occipitocervical injuries, but it has shortcomings. The ratio is the distance from the basion to the posterior arch of C1 divided by the distance from the anterior arch of C1 to the opisthion. A ratio of greater than 1.0 indicates an anterior occipitoatlantal dislocation. Only an anterior occipitocervical dislocation can be identified using Power's ratio; however, these injuries can occur posteriorly or in pure distraction. In fact, the direction of displacement can vary at any given time depending on head position. Harris lines may prove to be more sensitive in screening for this injury (Figure 3). Also, any soft-tissue swelling anterior to the spine noted on plain lateral radiographs or CT should be an indication for more careful consideration of the occipitocervical junction. If suspicion for this injury remains, MRI can be used.

After an occipitocervical injury has been identified, rigid immobilization should be maintained until defini-

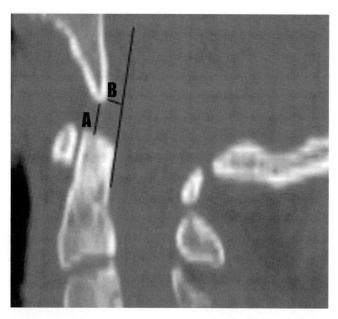

Figure 3 Harris lines for assessing occipital cervical alignment. A line drawn from the basion to the tip of the dens should not exceed 12 mm (A). A line is drawn parallel to the posterior border of the dens and a measurement is then taken from that line to the tip of the basion (B). That measurement should not be more than 12 mm or less than -4 mm.

tive surgical stabilization can be performed. If a significant delay is anticipated before surgical stabilization, temporary halo vest immobilization is warranted. Ultimately, the treatment of choice is a posterior occipitocervical fusion (Occ-C2).

If an occipital condyle fracture is identified, care must be taken to determine if a more severe occipitocervical dissociation is present. An avulsion-type fracture would cause more concern than a crush-type fracture. CT and MRI are useful diagnostic tools for evaluating these fractures.

### C1 Ring Fractures
Most C1 ring fractures can be treated nonsurgically with external immobilization ranging from a rigid collar to a halo vest depending on the degree of instability. A simple posterior ring fracture is generally treated in a rigid collar for 6 to 12 weeks; however, these fractures often occur in association with another upper cervical fracture that may be considered more significant and may dictate the method of treatment. In fractures involving the anterior and posterior ring, the degree of displacement is used to determine the method of treatment. Nondisplaced fractures can be treated in a Minerva or four-poster brace whereas a halo vest should be considered for patients with mild or moderately displaced fractures. If both lateral masses are significantly displaced (Jefferson fracture) and greater than 7 mm of combined lateral overhang is present, it is likely that the transverse ligament has been disrupted, creating greater potential for long-term instability. Under these circumstances more

aggressive treatment is instituted. Traction can often reduce the amount of lateral displacement but must be maintained for approximately 6 weeks to avoid redisplacement when traction is released. Because a halo vest cannot effectively maintain traction, patients would require 6 weeks of bed rest, which is poorly tolerated. One treatment option is to surgically span the fracture with an occipitocervical fusion; however, the use of C1 lateral mass screws has become more widely accepted and can be used as a technique of direct osteosynthesis at C1 avoiding immobilization of the Occ-C1 and C1-2 levels. This technique also can be used for a unilateral lateral mass fracture that is displaced enough to allow the occipital condyle to settle down onto C2, creating a cock-robin deformity.

### Odontoid Fractures
Odontoid fractures are challenging to treat. Anderson-D'Alonzo type I fractures (avulsion fractures at the tip of the odontoid process) rarely occur and if present should raise suspicion for occipitocervical dissociation. As an isolated injury, type I fractures can be treated with rigid collar immobilization. There is general consensus that type III fractures can be treated nonsurgically; however, the exact nature of immobilization can vary from rigid collar to halo vest depending on displacement, patient age, associated injuries, and other factors.

The treatment of type II fractures (fracture at the base of the odontoid process) remains controversial because they tend to be more difficult to control and have a propensity for nonunion. In addition to the fracture pattern itself, the amount of initial displacement (greater than 5 mm), quality of reduction achieved, and comorbidities such as smoking and a patient age older than 65 years are additional risk factors for nonunion. Two groups of patients are usually affected by this injury: younger patients with high-energy trauma and elderly patients that undergo low-energy trauma. These two groups are distinct and should be considered separately. The main treatment goal for both groups is achieving union without excessive morbidity from the treatment. Four basic treatment options exist: minimal external immobilization (such as a rigid collar), more aggressive external immobilization (such as a halo vest), anterior screw fixation for direct osteosynthesis, or posterior C1-C2 fusion.

Minimal immobilization with a rigid collar is seldom the treatment of choice in the younger patient in whom achieving bony union is the principal goal. It can be considered a more viable option in elderly patients with minimally or nondisplaced fractures and has been advocated by some authors as the preferred treatment choice in this patient population. The morbidity of treatment is minimal; however, there is a higher rate of nonunion. It has been proposed that a stable fibrous union would be acceptable in elderly patients, but no study exists that clearly defines the long-term potential for pain, neurologic symptoms, or even sudden death resulting from a fibrous union. Anecdotal reports exist of patients presenting with progressive myelopathy years after such treatment. In an elderly patient population, it is likely that a sudden death event occurring distant to the time of the fracture would be attributed to a cardiopulmonary event rather than to a long-term complication of fracture treatment. In addition, an unstable nonunion may not be deemed an acceptable outcome. Simple collar immobilization may not be an adequate treatment for some elderly patients and should be reserved for older patients who are less functional, have significant medical comorbidities, and lower outcome expectations.

The most traditional method of treatment is the halo vest, which, although nonsurgical, still has significant associated morbidity. Younger patients are more likely to tolerate halo immobilization; however, a halo vest may be less tolerable if associated injuries, such as a chest wall injury, are present. Cosmetically, the typical transverse anterior scar left by anterior screw fixation is better accepted than that from the halo pins. Although this issue is relatively minor in comparison with other complications of odontoid fractures, it is nonetheless of concern, particularly to young female patients. Over time the scars can be revised to a more cosmetic incision if desired. In recent years, attention has been focused on halo morbidity in elderly patients resulting from skull penetration, imbalance with ambulation, dysphagia, and respiratory difficulty. Some of these complications can be overcome with time, speech therapy, and the use of a walker; however, many patients fail to thrive despite such efforts. Some elderly patients tolerate halo immobilization with little difficulty and should be considered for this treatment option. If the patient cannot tolerate this form of immobilization, other treatment options must be considered.

Anterior screw fixation has gained increasing support as a more effective means of maintaining reduction, adding compression across the fracture, and allowing minimal to no external immobilization while improving the rate of union. The union rates of anterior screw fixation for type II odontoid fractures reported in the literature varies from 81% to 100% (the combined average of several studies is 89%) in comparison with union rates of approximately 30% with traditional halo immobilization. However, screw fixation also has associated morbidities including infection, dysphagia from the dissection, and loss of fixation. Loss of fixation is particularly problematic in elderly patients in whom the fracture was initially displaced, especially posterior, from an extension injury. The anterior C2 body is relatively hollow and the screw threads can remain attached to the odontoid, but the shaft and head of the screw are cut out of the anterior body as the fracture redisplaces (Figure 4). By taking care to place the screw entry point

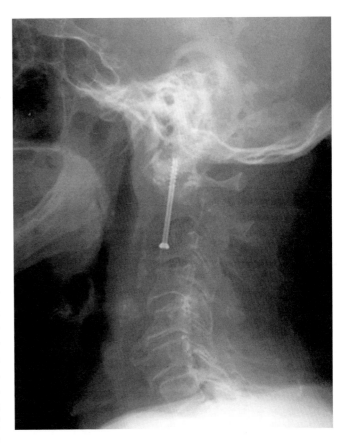

**Figure 4** An odontoid fracture in an elderly patient that initially was anatomically reduced and fixed with an odontoid screw, but was noted to be significantly displaced at 2-week follow-up. The threads remain fixed within the tip of the odontoid but the shaft and head of the screw have lost fixation in the vertebral body.

within the C2-3 disk along the inferior end plate of C2, this complication can be minimized but not eliminated. Better quality bone can be found posteriorly in elderly patients, making posterior C1-2 fusion more attractive.

Posterior C1-2 fusion is the treatment of choice for odontoid nonunion and in those elderly patients or osteopenic patients who are deemed appropriate candidates for surgical stabilization. The union rate of this procedure has improved and the postoperative immobilization requirements have decreased with the use of transarticular screws. Unfortunately, this treatment has the potential for vertebral artery injury. More recently, C1 lateral mass screws have become popular and may allow posterior fixation to be done using a combination of a C1 lateral mass screw and a C2 pars or pedicle screw or intralaminar screws, without the need to cross the C1-2 joint (Figure 5). This technique could potentially minimize the risk of vertebral artery injury while maintaining stability and high rates of union; however, this benefit is yet to be determined.

### C2 Traumatic Spondylolisthesis (Hangman's Fracture)
Treatment options for C2 traumatic spondylolisthesis injuries have changed little in the past several years. Type

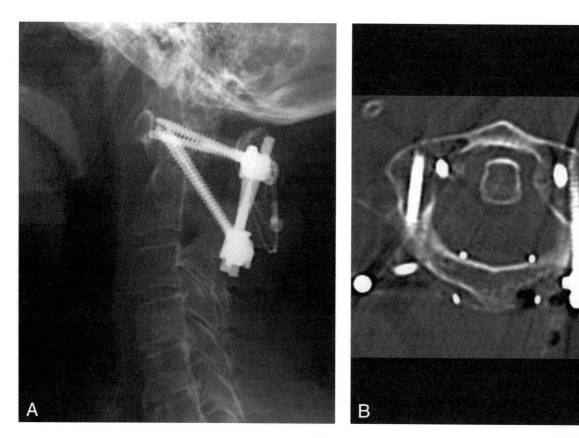

Figure 5  C1 lateral mass screws shown on plain lateral radiograph **(A)** and axial CT scan **(B)**.

I or nondisplaced fractures are treated by rigid external immobilization using a rigid collar, sternal occipital mandibular immobilization brace, or a Minerva brace. Type II injuries are divided into types II and IIA. These displaced fractures are distinguished by the propensity of the type IIA injuries to overdistract if placed in traction. These fractures are managed by gentle extension and placement directly into a halo vest. Type IIA injuries are distinguished radiographically because there is angulation at the C2-3 disk space but no translation, and the fracture line through the pars tends to be more horizontal. Despite the distinguishing characteristics of these fractures, traction should begin with only 10 to 15 lb followed immediately by a cross-table lateral radiograph to rule out overdistraction not only at the C2-3 level, but at other levels. The type II injury can be reduced with traction then held in a halo vest for 12 weeks. If there are contraindications to using a halo vest or if the patient has multiple trauma, direct osteosynthesis with a screw across the fracture may be used. The mainstay of treatment of type III (associated with dislocation of the C2-3 facets) injury is open reduction of the facets, a C2-3 posterior fusion, and treatment of the pars fracture in a halo vest. Using screw fixation of the pars for type III fractures may be indicated because the area is already surgically exposed to perform the facet reduction, thus avoiding the need for a halo vest.

## Lower Cervical Fractures

### Facet Fracture-Dislocations

The treatment of facet fracture-dislocations has generated the most controversy during recent years. There is currently a general consensus that, regardless of neurologic deficit, even unilateral facet dislocations should be reduced to minimize late pain. The controversy centers on the timing of that reduction relative to MRI. For the facets to dislocate, there must be enough distraction/flexion to disengage the superior from the inferior facet, and the cephalad vertebral body must translate anteriorly, which uniformly injures the corresponding disk. There is concern that if some of the disk material has herniated posteriorly, reduction of the dislocation will force material further posteriorly and cause cord compression and a potential neurologic deficit. This phenomenon has been reported during reductions performed with the patient under anesthesia, which prevented an active neurologic examination. There is concern that this phenomenon can occur during a reduction in an awake patient. Prereduction MRI offers the potential to better define soft-tissue injury, including disk herniation (Figure 6). Findings from that study could help the surgeon to determine if an anterior diskectomy should be performed before reduction to fully evacuate the disk material from the canal to diminish the likelihood of increasing the deficit during the course

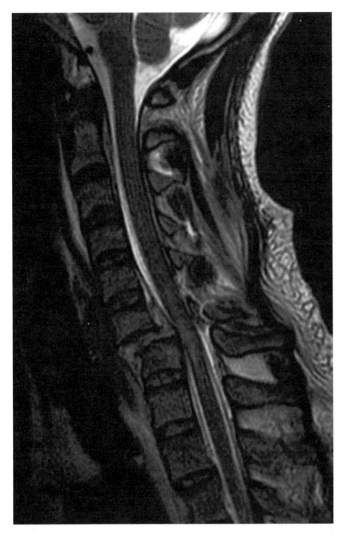

Figure 6 A sagittal T-2 weighted MRI scan of a patient with a facet dislocation and associated disk herniation extending up behind the cephalad vertebral body.

of reduction. However, the true meaning of the MRI signal posteriorly within the canal is not well understood and the implications of the presence of these changes have not been defined. In one study of awake patients, an MRI scan was obtained before reduction, followed by closed traction reduction using serial neurologic examinations, followed by a postreduction MRI scan. In 18% of patients, an associated disk herniation was diagnosed before reduction; this percentage increased to 45% after reduction without a change in neurologic status. Many patients undergoing similar reductions have been reviewed without identifying patients who had neurologic deterioration; some improvement in deficit has been reported. Based on this evidence, it appears to be safe, perhaps even prudent, to proceed with an immediate closed reduction using serial increases in traction weight and neurologic examinations if the patient is alert and able to cooperate. This treatment option would be widely accepted in those patients who

have complete or incomplete spinal cord deficits because they are most likely to benefit from a successful reduction for effective decompression of the canal. More controversy concerning this treatment plan exists in those patients who remain neurologically intact. In those patients, this treatment choice would depend on institutional issues such as access to the MRI scanner. Prior to performing an open reduction under anesthesia or in the obtunded patient, MRI is recommended before reduction. The awake patient who undergoes a closed reduction should also undergo MRI before surgical stabilization to document that the canal has been decompressed by the reduction and to verify that no disk material or hematoma remains within the canal that would warrant removal at the time of stabilization. Even if the patient is neurologically intact after completion of the reduction, MRI should be done if a posterior stabilization will be performed because disk material can be displaced into the canal during tightening of the posterior tension band.

After reduction, the next step is stabilization. Although unilateral facet dislocations can at times be stable in the reduced position, and may even automatically fuse, this stability is not reliable. Surgical stabilization of bilateral facet dislocations is universally accepted as the treatment of choice. Traditionally, posterior fusion has been preferred because it biomechanically and anatomically best addresses the injured tissue. More recently, anterior approaches have gained favor. The anterior approach has been shown to achieve adequate clinical stability if good technical principles are followed such as avoiding overdistraction of the posterior elements and assuring that any facet fracture is not too excessive (such that it would create significant translational instability). Using the anterior approach, any disk material in the canal can be directly addressed, kyphosis can be avoided, and wound complications are less frequent. At this time, both anterior and posterior approaches are considered viable alternatives.

### Axial Load Injuries

Axial load injuries include compression fractures, burst fractures, and "teardrop" fractures. In these injury patterns, the ability of the anterior column to resist compression loads is lost and canal decompression, if necessary, must be achieved by directly removing bone from the canal rather than simple realigning the vertebrae as with facet dislocations. The term "teardrop" fracture can be confusing because there also is a teardrop avulsion fracture, which usually represents a relatively minor extension injury with a small fleck of bone off the anterior end plate by the annular attachment (Figure 7). This benign injury is treated with wearing of a rigid collar for 6 weeks. In contrast, the term teardrop fracture is used to signify a flexion axial load injury (such as injury resulting from a diving accident) characterized by a large

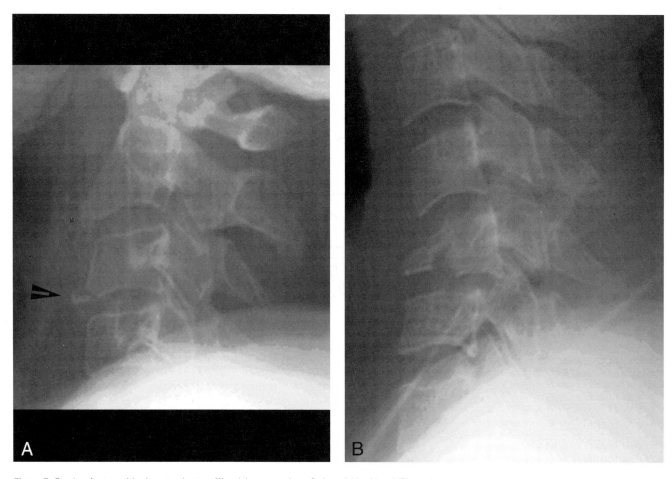

Figure 7   Teardrop fractures. A benign extension type **(A)** and the more ominous flexion axial load type I **(B)** are shown.

chunk of bone knocked off the anteroinferior end of a vertebral body as it is driven caudally and into flexion causing retrolisthesis of the remaining vertebral body into the spinal canal. A sagittal split on the axial CT scan is a common finding (Figure 8). This injury is frequently associated with neurologic deficit and is usually considered to be sufficiently unstable to mandate surgical treatment.

The type of treatment required in axial load injuries is determined by neurologic status and stability. If a spinal cord injury exists, significant instability can generally be implied, which warrants surgical stabilization. The mode of instability is the loss of the anterior column's ability to resist compressive loads. In this type of injury, patients often have retropulsed bone or posteriorly subluxated vertebral bodies compromising the canal and requiring surgical decompression. In the neurologically impaired patient, an anterior decompression via corpectomy and strut graft fusion is recommended. If a severe degree of posterior ligament or facet injury is present, the addition of a posterior fusion should be considered.

In the neurologically intact patient, treatment decisions are based solely on the degree of instability, which can be difficult to define. The degree of kyphosis, amount

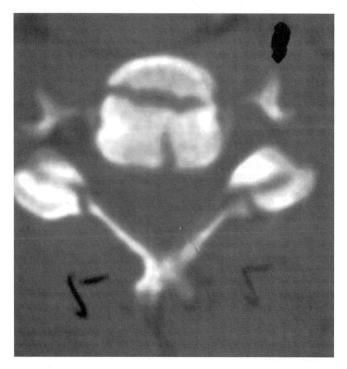

Figure 8   Classic sagittal split on the axial CT image seen with flexion teardrop fractures.

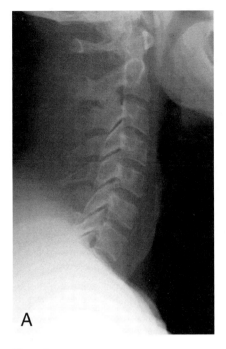 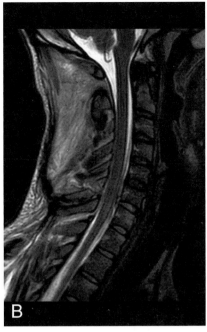 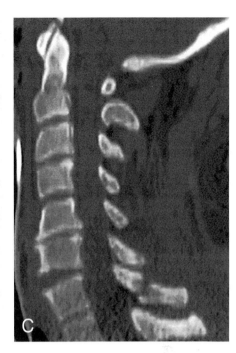

**Figure 9**  Spinous process fractures represent more severe injury than the typical benign type clay shoveler's fracture. A flexion injury **(A)** at the base of the process with the corresponding MRI scan **(B)** showing disruption through the posterior anulus fibrosus of the disk and cord edema. An extension injury **(C)** with disruption of the anterior anulus fibrosus of the disk.

of vertebral body height loss, and posterior injury must all be taken into account. Treatment can range from the use of a rigid collar, halo vest, or anterior fusion. Relative kyphosis of 11° has been defined by some authors as a measure of cervical instability; however, this is only one measure in a series of criteria used to determine instability as defined by White and Panjabi. To date there are no universally accepted specific criteria to determine instability in axial load injuries. The more general assessment of deciding whether the spine has lost its ability to resist physiologic loads and protect the underlying neurologic structures must be used to determine instability.

### Spinous Process Fractures

Spinous process fractures can occur through various mechanisms and represent degrees of instability at both ends of the spectrum (Figure 9). The most commonly described spinous process fracture is the classic "clay shoveler's" fracture, which is believed to result from sudden hyperextension of the neck such as would occur when a shovel becomes lodged in clay. This fracture is generally noted at or near the tip of the spinous process, usually C7, and is considered a benign injury that is treated using a collar for comfort for approximately 6 weeks. Conversely, other spinous process fractures are part of more unstable patterns and care must be taken to identify injuries that may warrant surgical treatment. These injuries can occur via an extension or flexion mechanism and are often located at the base of the spinous process. Sometimes an associated deformity will

indicate that this is a more severe injury; however, flexion-extension radiographs may be needed to properly identify it as an unstable pattern. Flexion-extension radiographs should be obtained for spinous process fractures before determining a final treatment plan.

## Special Circumstances
### Sports Injuries

Fractures and dislocations that occur during participation in sports activities are treated the same as those that occur via other mechanisms. Transient spinal neurapraxia is a unique condition that affects athletes participating in contact sports (such as football), which have the risk for sudden impact that places an excessive load on the neck. The impact is followed by a brief episode of quadriparesis that can last from seconds to hours. There is no radiographic evidence of acute fracture or dislocation. Controversy exists on whether the athlete should return to participation in contact sports. Evaluation should consist of a thorough neurologic examination. The athlete should not return to sports activities until examination findings have completely normalized, which is similar to treatment for patients with a cerebral concussion. All patients should be evaluated radiographically with standard trauma studies such as plain radiographs and CT to eliminate the possibility of a fracture or dislocation. MRI should be used to assess for occult ligamentous injury or underlying pathology such as congenital stenosis, disk herniation, or spondylosis that compromise the canal dimensions. MRI can also identify cord contusions and edema if present. Several studies have shown that patients with normal canal dimensions or congenital stenosis do not have a greater risk for catastrophic spinal cord injury and can resume participation in sports activities. Greater caution must be exerted in clearing patients with significant radiographic pathology such as herniation, cord edema, gliosis, and advanced spondylosis. Patient factors also play a role in the decision to return to sports activities. Patients who have recurrent episodes of transient spinal neurapraxia or who are subjected to repetitive spear tackling should also be cautioned concerning the risk of returning to sports participation. If a patient subjected to spear tackling also has radiographic changes, participation in contact sports that put them at risk should be discontinued. It has been shown that people with smaller canals are more likely to suffer a catastrophic neurologic injury with a fracture or dislocation of the cervical spine.

## Ankylosing Spondylitis

Patients with ankylosing spondylitis are more vulnerable to fractures from low-energy mechanisms such as falls from a standing height because of the rigidity of the spine, which acts more like a long bone. Any patient with ankylosing spondylitis who experiences even a minor traumatic event who reports neck pain should be considered to have a fracture until proved otherwise. The most common location of the fracture is the cervicothoracic junction. This area can be very difficult to visualize because of osteopenia, exaggerated thoracic kyphosis, rigidity, and obstruction by the patient's shoulders. CT is the best imaging modality. If fractured, the rigid, ankylosed spine acts like a long bone. If surgical treatment is necessary, fixation should extend over multiple levels cephalad and caudal to the fracture to provide adequate lever arms as in fixation of a long-bone fracture such as the femur. Progressive neurologic deficit can occur because of the propensity for epidural hematoma.

## Summary

The treatment of patients with cervical spine trauma is an area of spine care that is in a slow state of evolution relative to other areas of spine care. Most recent changes have occurred in imaging technology and techniques of spinal fixation. How to best use these advances in the interest of patients and in a cost-effective manner remains to be determined.

## Annotated Bibliography

### General

Brolin K, von Holst H: Cervical injuries in Sweden: A national survey of patient data from 1987 to 1999. *Inj Control Saf Promot* 2002;9:40-52.

The Swedish injury surveillance national database from 1987 to 1999 was analyzed to determine the incidence and cause of cervical injury. The incidence of fracture was found to be on the increase only in elderly patients with falls overtaking motor vehicle crashes as the mechanism of injury. Fifty percent of the falls occur in elderly patients, implying that the incidence of cervical fractures may continue to rise as the population ages and remains more active at an older age.

### Imaging

Bolinger B, Shartz M, Marion D: Bedside fluoroscopic flexion and extension cervical spine radiographs for clearance of the cervical spine in comatose trauma patients. *J Trauma* 2004;56:132-136.

This article presents a review of 56 comatose trauma patients in whom an attempt at cervical clearance was made using fluoroscopically assisted, flexion-extension radiographs. Because adequate visualization of C7-T1 was achieved in only 4% of patients, this technique was no longer considered an option at the institution that conducted the study.

Geck MJ, Yoo S, Wang JC: Assessment of cervical ligamentous injury in trauma patients using MRI. *J Spinal Disord* 2001;14:371-377.

A retrospective review of 89 trauma patients with suspected occult ligamentous injury but negative plain radiographs and CT imaging is presented. Ligamentous injury was identified in 2 of 89 patients and there were no apparent false negatives. No time frame for obtaining the MRI scan was given.

### Specific Injury Patterns

Fisher CG, Dvorak MF, Leith J, Wing PC: Comparison of outcomes for unstable lower cervical flexion teardrop fractures managed with halo thoracic vest versus anterior corpectomy and plating. *Spine* 2002;27:160-166.

This retrospective cohort study of the treatment of cervical flexion teardrop fractures compared treatment with a halo vest with anterior cervical plating. Anterior plating was found to be more effective in restoring and maintaining sagittal alignment as well as minimizing treatment failures, but did not show a benefit in quality of life outcome measures (perhaps because the study was underpowered for secondary outcomes).

Johnson MG, Fisher CG, Boyd M, Pitzen T, Oxland TR, Dvorak MF: The radiographic failure of single segment anterior cervical plate fixation in traumatic cervical flexion distraction injuries. *Spine* 2004;29:2815-2820.

A retrospective radiographic review of 87 patients with unilateral or bilateral facet fractures treated with single-level anterior cervical plate fusion is presented. A 13% failure rate was noted as defined by more than 4 mm translation and/or an 11° angulation change between the immediate postoperative film and the most recent radiographic follow-up. Failure correlated with facet fractures and end-plate fractures on the injury radiographs. Overdistraction of the facets at the time of fixation was not mentioned.

Koivikko MP, Kiuru MJ, Koskinen SK, Myllynen P, Santavirta S, Kivisaari L: Factors associated with nonunion in conservatively-treated type-II fractures of the odontoid process. *J Bone Joint Surg Br* 2004;86:1146-1151.

Halo vest treatment of type II odontoid fractures was reviewed in 69 patients. An overall union rate of 46% was found. Factors associated with nonunion included a fracture gap of more than 1 mm, posterior displacement of more than 5 mm, a delayed start of treatment of more than 4 days, and posterior redisplacement of more than 2 mm. Nonunion was not correlated with age, gender, or anterior displacement.

Muller EJ, Schwinnen I, Fischer K, Wick M, Muhr G: Non-rigid immobilisation of odontoid fractures. *Eur Spine J* 2003;12:522-525.

A series of 26 patients with stable type II or type III odontoid fractures treated with nonrigid external immobilization (no halo) demonstrated fusion rates comparable with those of patients undergoing historic halo treatment.

Vaccaro AR, Madigan L, Bauerle WB, Blescia A, Cotler JM: Early halo immobilization of displaced traumatic spondylolisthesis of the axis. *Spine* 2002;27:2229-2233.

Twenty-seven type II and four type IIA hangman's fractures were retrospectively reviewed. All of the patients were treated with early halo vest immobilization. All of the patients with type IIA fractures had uneventful fracture union. Patients with the type II fractures also had fracture union; however, 6 of 27 required re-reduction with halo vest traction because of fracture displacement. The tendency to redisplace was noted in those fractures with greater than 12° of initial angulation.

## Classic Bibliography

Anderson LD, D'Alonzo RT: Fractures of the odontoid process of the axis. *J Bone Joint Surg Am* 1974;56:1663-1674.

Andersson S, Rodrigues M, Olerud C: Odontoid fractures: High complication rate associated with anterior screw fixation in the elderly. *Eur Spine J* 2000;9:56-60.

Hadley MN, Browner CM, Liu SS, Sonntag VK: New subtype of acute odontoid fractures (type IIA). *Neurosurgery* 1988;22:67-71.

Harris JH Jr, Carons GC, Wagner LK, Kerr N: Radiographic diagnosis of traumatic occipitovertebral dissociation: 2. Comparison of three methods of detecting occiptiovertebral relationships on lateral radiographs of supine subjects. *AJR Am J Roentgenol* 1994;162:887-892.

Harris MB, Kronlage SC, Carboni PA, et al: Evaluation of the cervical spine in the polytrauma patient. *Spine* 2000;25:2884-2891.

Hoffman JR, Mower WR, Wolfson AB, Todd KH, Zucker MI: Validity of a set of clinical criteria to rule out injury to the cervical spine in patients with blunt trauma: National Emergency X-Radiography Utilization Study Group. *N Engl J Med* 2000;343:94-99.

Kang JD, Figgie MP, Bohlman HH: Sagittal measurements of the cervical spine in subaxial fractures and dislocations: An analysis of two hundred and eighty-eight patients with and without neurological deficits. *J Bone Joint Surg Am* 1994;76:1617-1628.

Sasso R, Doherty BJ, Crawford MJ, Heggeness MH: Biomechanics of odontoid fracture fixation: Comparison of the one- and two-screw technique. *Spine* 1993;18:1950-1953.

Spence KF Jr, Decker S, Sell KW: Bursting atlantal fractures associated with rupture of the transverse ligament. *J Bone Joint Surg Am* 1970;52:543-549.

Torg JS, Sennett B, Pavlov H, Leventhal MR, Glasgow SG: Spear tackler's spine: An entity precluding participation in tackle football and collision activities that expose the cervical spine to axial energy inputs. *Am J Sports Med* 1993;21:640-649.

Vaccaro AR, Falatyn SP, Flanders AE, Balderston RA, Northrup BE, Cotler JM: Magnetic resonance evaluation of the intervertebral disc, spinal ligaments, and spinal cord before and after closed traction reduction of cervical spine dislocations. *Spine* 1999;24:1210-1217.

Vaccaro AR, Klein GR, Flanders AE, Albert TJ, Balderson RA, Cotler JM: Long-term evaluation of vertebral artery injuries following cervical spine trauma using magnetic resonance angiography. *Spine* 1998;23:789-794.

# Chapter 23

# Thoracolumbar Trauma

Christopher M. Bono, MD

Marie D. Rinaldi, BA

## Introduction

The thoracolumbar junction (T11-L2) is the most common site of injury following trauma to the thoracic and lumbar spines. It is the biomechanical transition zone between the relatively rigid thoracic spine and the highly flexible lumbar region. Stability is provided by factors such as facet morphology and lamina overlap. A large proportion of this additional stability is provided by the rib cage through the costovertebral junctions along the posterolateral disk space that each span two vertebrae. Additional ligaments link the medial portion of the rib to the anterior aspect of the thoracic transverse processes. The thoracolumbar junction is an alignment transition zone between the kyphotic thoracic spine and lordotic lumbar region.

Trauma, such as during a motor vehicle collision, causes abrupt changes in acceleration that can focus large forces at the thoracolumbar spine. Both osseous and ligamentous components can fail. Resultant injuries can range from isolated, minor vertebral body compression fractures to highly unstable circumferential osteoligamentous disruption. The likelihood of neurologic injury increases with lesions resulting from higher energy forces.

Approximately 90% of all thoracic and lumbar injuries occur at the thoracolumbar junction. In a recent study of injuries in Austrian mountain climbers, thoracolumbar fractures accounted for more than 80% of all spine injuries. Men between the ages of 15 and 35 years are the most frequently affected. The likelihood of severe and multiple level spinal injuries are higher in motorcycle crashes compared with automobile crashes. The incidence of thoracolumbar fractures in Army pilots has been shown to be approximately 13%; helicopter crashes and parachuting accidents were the most common cause, accounting for 73% of injuries.

## Diagnostic Considerations
### Plain Radiographs

Plain radiographs should be obtained if injury is suspected. Although spinal fractures are often first detected using CT of the chest or abdomen, this does not obviate the need for high-quality plain radiographs. Once a thoracolumbar injury is detected, complete radiographs of the entire spine should be obtained. The rate of concomitant, noncontiguous spinal injury can be as high as 12%. AP and lateral thoracic and lumbar views should be obtained. Additional views centered at the T12-L1 junction are needed in any patient with a suspected thoracolumbar injury.

### Lateral Views
Sagittal alignment, which is normally neutral (flat or straight) at the thoracolumbar junction, can be assessed using a lateral radiograph. Kyphosis can be measured using the Cobb method, which has been shown to be more consistent than the posterior vertebral body tangent method. The Cobb method is performed by measuring the angle between the superior end plate of the nearest uninjured cranial vertebra and the inferior end plate of the nearest uninjured caudal vertebra (Figure 1). The percentage of height loss of the injured vertebral body is another useful calculation. This percentage is determined by comparing values of the injured segment

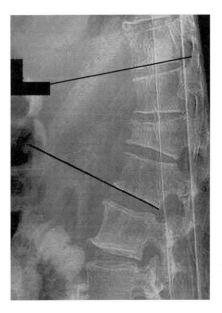

Figure 1 The loss of vertebral body height can be seen on a lateral radiograph of the thoracolumbar junction. Kyphosis can be measured using the Cobb technique. The angle between the superior end plate of the nearest uninjured cranial vertebra and the inferior end plate of the nearest uninjured caudal vertebra are measured (black lines).

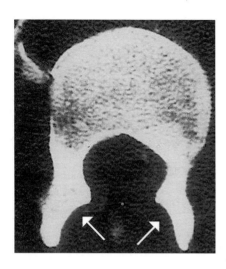

Figure 2 The empty or naked facet sign (arrows) is a sign of facet dislocation.

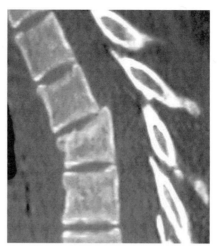

Figure 3 Coronal CT reconstructions can show translation, which would otherwise be difficult to see using axial images alone.

with those of adjacent cranial and caudal uninjured vertebrae. Anterior and posterior vertebral body height should be measured separately to more accurately detect compression of one or both regions. A loss of height of greater than 50% is suggestive of posterior ligamentous complex (PLC) disruption, although this value has never been clinically validated. Although a CT scan is more sensitive, posterior vertebral body fragment retropulsion can often be seen on a lateral radiograph.

### AP View

Coronal and rotational alignment of the spine can be assessed using an AP radiograph. The relative distance between the spinous process and its corresponding pedicles is a reflection of rotation. Coronal translation suggests high-energy trauma and osteoligamentous instability. Interpedicular width should successively increase from caudal to cranial. Abnormal interpedicular widening suggests lateral displacement of the pedicles, and therefore separation of the posterolateral vertebral body fragments; this finding is a radiographic hallmark of burst fractures.

### Computed Tomography

Thin cut (2 mm) CT slices should be obtained through the level of injury, as well as through the normal adjacent levels. Fracture lines extending into the posterior vertebral body distinguish burst fractures from compression fractures. Canal compromise from burst fractures is usually best appreciated on axial CT images. Posterior column injuries such as facet dislocations, facet fractures, and pedicle fractures also can be clearly seen. A concomitant lamina fracture at the level of a burst fracture is often associated with a dural tear and nerve root entrapment. The so-called naked or empty facet is an indication of facet dislocation (Figure 2). In the absence of this sign, however, most other translational deformities can be easily overlooked because they are in the plane of axial CT images. High-quality sagittal and coro-

nal CT reconstructions can facilitate the diagnosis of distraction or translational injuries (Figure 3).

Canal compromise can be quantified by several methods. The superiority or reproducibility of one method versus another has not been clearly demonstrated. Midsagittal canal diameter is among the more simple measurements because it represents the distance between the posterior aspect of the most posteriorly displaced wall fragment to the anterior aspect of the lamina. This value is compared with the sagittal diameters of uninjured levels above and below the fracture to arrive at a percentage of canal compromise. Those who believe that this method can underestimate the amount of neural compression are advocates of cross-sectional area measurement. Area measurements, however, are cumbersome and difficult to perform using commonly available CT software. Canal compromise from translation (as occurs with fracture-dislocations) can be underestimated by axial CT images and may be better assessed by coronal or sagittal image reconstructions. Rotational deformity is best detected by overlaying consecutive axial CT images.

### Magnetic Resonance Imaging

MRI is superior for evaluating the neural elements, the intervertebral disks, and the spinal ligaments. It can be instrumental in evaluating patients with neurologic injuries that are anatomically incongruous with the skeletal level of injury. Spinal cord, cauda equina, or nerve root compression is readily visualized. Edema within the spinal cord can be noted as bright signal on T2-weighted images; this finding may portend a poor neurologic prognosis. Although less common with thoracolumbar than cervical injuries, intervertebral disk herniations can lead to canal compromise that is not easily seen on CT scans.

MRI can be used to assess the integrity of the posterior longitudinal ligament (PLL). In one study, an intact PLL as visualized on MRI scans was associated with better canal clearance through posterior distraction in-

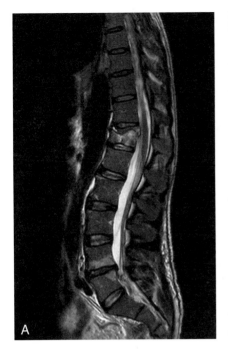
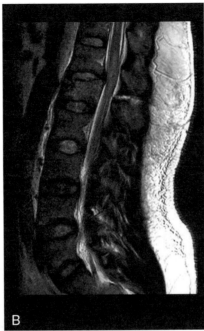
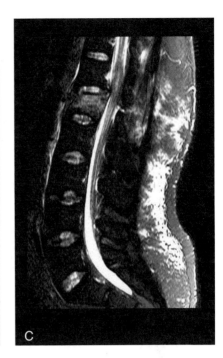

**Figure 4** **A,** A mild increased signal within the posterior ligaments after a T12 burst fracture most likely represents a sprain. The mechanical competence of the PLC is not compromised. **B,** A T2-weighted image shows increased signal within the PLC at the level of a burst fracture. Note that continuity of the ligamentum flavum as well as the supraspinous ligament has been disrupted. **C,** Short-tau inversion recovery images more clearly show the increased soft-tissue edema within the disrupted posterior ligaments, which was confirmed during posterior surgery.

strumentation than in patients in whom the PLL was disrupted.

With the recent rediscovery of nonsurgical treatment of thoracolumbar burst fractures, the use of MRI to assess the PLC has become more common. PLC integrity is an important determinant of burst and compression fracture management. T2-weighted images are more useful than T1-weighted images. Short-tau inversion recovery images may be the most sensitive in detecting edema within the soft-tissues, albeit at the expense of decreased image clarity.

MRI findings may vary from mild increased signal between spinous processes on T2-weighted images (indicative of benign ligament sprain) (Figure 4, *A*) to a bright and expansive signal extending from the tip of the spinous process to the interlaminar interval (indicative of gross PLC disruption) (Figure 4, *B* and *C*). Although the extremes of this spectrum are easily discerned, the varying gradations between them are more difficult to interpret. An MRI grading system has been developed to help differentiate the varying degrees of ligamentous injury. Using this system, PLC disruption was predictive of the recurrence of kyphosis in surgically treated patients at final follow-up.

## Classification of Thoracolumbar Injuries

Many classification systems for thoracolumbar injuries, each with unique advantages and disadvantages, have been proposed. Although an ideal system would be clin-

ically useful, prognostic, and aid in treatment decision making, no universally accepted system currently exists. Complex systems have led to poor interobserver and intraobserver reproducibility, whereas simpler systems have better reproducibility but are useful for only one or two injury patterns. Two of the more commonly used systems are the McAfee and the Magerl systems.

### McAfee Classification System

The McAfee classification system is an adaptation of the Denis system, which divides the spine into three columns (Figure 5). The McAfee system was based on the analysis of multiplanar CT images and plain radiographs of 100 consecutive thoracolumbar injuries. The goal was to determine or, more accurately, to postulate the mechanism of failure of the middle column (posterior vertebral body, posterior disk, and PLL). The researchers concluded that the middle column could fail by axial compression, axial distraction, or translation. Sagittal CT reconstruction was then used to determine if the posterior column had failed, specifically by noting facet joint distraction.

The McAfee classification system was an important reactive step to the limited options then available for stabilization of thoracolumbar injures. These options were limited to sublaminar wiring and hook devices. Although effective in maintaining sagittal alignment, wires could not be used to provide compression or distraction. Early nonsegmental hook constructs could be placed in

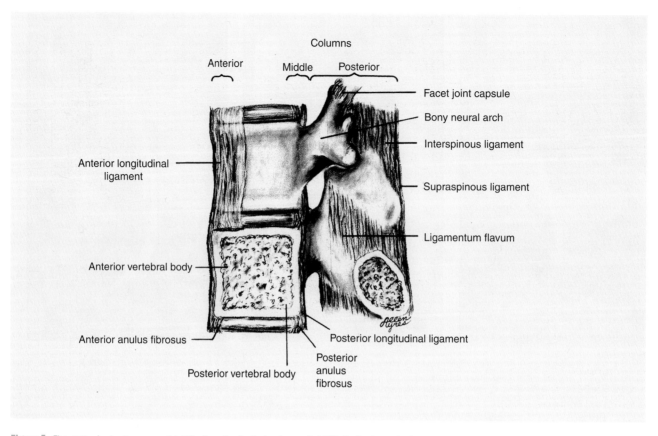

Columns

Anterior    Middle    Posterior

Facet joint capsule

Bony neural arch

Interspinous ligament

Anterior longitudinal ligament

Supraspinous ligament

Ligamentum flavum

Anterior vertebral body

Posterior longitudinal ligament

Anterior anulus fibrosus

Posterior anulus fibrosus

Posterior vertebral body

**Figure 5** The anatomic structures comprising the three longitudinal columns of stability in the thoracolumbar spine: the anterior column (anterior two thirds of the vertebral body, anterior part of the anulus fibrosus, and anterior longitudinal ligament), middle column (posterior one third of the vertebral body, posterior part of the anulus fibrosus, and posterior longitudinal ligament), and posterior column (facet joint capsules, ligamentum flavum, osseous neural arch, supraspinous ligament, interspinous ligament, and articular processes). *(Adapted with permission from McAfee P, Yuan H, Fredrickson BE, Lubicky JP: The value of computed tomography in thoracolumbar fractures: An analysis of one hundred consecutive cases and a new classification. J Bone Joint Surg Am 1983;65:461-473.)*

either compression or distraction. Recognizing that some injuries could be worsened, displaced, or exaggerated with compression or distraction, McAfee and associates distinguished injuries caused by primarily distractive forces from injuries resulting from primarily compressive forces. Although understanding of these concepts is crucial to effectively reduce thoracolumbar injures, the subsequent development of modern multiple (claw) hook systems and pedicle screw constructs enabled segmental fixation that does not rely on distractive or compressive forces for fixation.

The McAfee system played an important role in understanding and treating thoracolumbar fractures; however, it is not an all-inclusive classification system. Despite its widespread use, its prognostic value has not been assessed since its development, nor has its interobserver and intraobserver reproducibility been assessed.

### AO or Magerl Classification System

With the support of the AO group, Magerl and associates introduced a comprehensive classification system for thoracolumbar spinal fractures that divided these fractures into three general groups: A (compression),

B (distraction), and C (torsion) injuries. Fractures are further subdivided based on fracture morphology, distinguishing between primarily bone or ligamentous failure, and the direction of displacement (Figure 6). The system was based on CT and plain radiographic examinations of over 1,400 consecutive injuries.

The AO/Magerl system is more inclusive than the McAfee system, but is more complex. Its interobserver reliability has been found to be inversely proportional to its complexity. Given the task of classifying injuries as only A, B, or C, the mean interobserver agreement among participants of a recent study averaged 67%. The kappa statistic was as low as 0.33 (perfect is 1.0) for some of the injuries assessed. As subgroups were added to the decision process, the interobserver reliability precipitously declined. Interestingly, the authors found injury classification to be improved if MRI findings were used.

### Suggested Injury Nomenclature

It is useful to establish terminology when referring to specific injuries. Although not an all-inclusive list, the most common injuries are compression fractures, burst

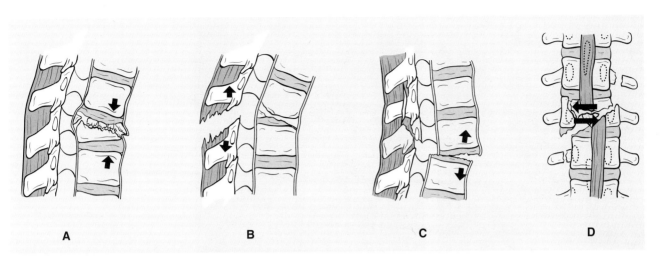

fractures, bending injuries (such as flexion-distraction and chance injuries), and fracture-dislocations.

Compression fractures lead to some degree of vertebral body height loss without involvement of the posterior vertebral body or middle column. Burst fractures extend into the posterior wall of the vertebral body without translation or dislocation. Pure dislocations at the thoracolumbar junction are rare and usually occur from a flexion-distraction–type mechanism. The classic example of such a mechanism is an automotive lap-belt injury in which the facet joints can be subluxated, perched, or jumped. However, these injuries are usually associated with some degree of vertebral body compression depending on the position of the axis of rotation. In pure flexion-distraction injuries, the axis of flexion or fulcrum is anterior to the vertebral body. If the axis of rotation is in the vertebral body, some part of the body will be compressed. Fracture-dislocation injuries refer to those injuries with a translational component in addition to varying fracture patterns.

It should be noted that fracture-dislocation injuries can exhibit posterior vertebral body fractures that, on CT scans alone, may appear to have a burst pattern. However, translation on plain radiographs or CT reconstructions distinguishes a burst fracture from a fracture-dislocation.

## Burst and Compression Fractures
### Nonsurgical Treatment

#### Options
Most thoracolumbar fractures can be treated nonsurgically. The clinical challenge is predicting, based on injury characteristics, which fractures can be successfully and safely treated in this manner. Despite extensive published literature on this topic, specific treatment recommendations do not exist.

Nonsurgical treatment can range from observation with external immobilization to extended bed rest. Progressive mobilization and observation without an external support device may be used for patients with some minor injuries. External orthotic devices are commonly used for more substantial fractures. Hyperextension braces (such as a Jewett device) can counteract sagittal flexion moments but offer minimal resistance to rotation or lateral flexion; these braces may be most appropriate for compression fractures. Custom-fit, clam-shell devices, such as a thoracolumbosacral orthosis, provide multiplanar support and may be used to treat burst fractures.

In rare circumstances in which surgery poses an extremely high risk, patients with mechanically unstable fractures are treated nonsurgically by extended bed rest and the continued use of spinal precautions. Some complications of prolonged recumbency, such as decubitus ulcers and pulmonary compromise, can be mitigated with the use of a specially designed rotating bed that continuously oscillates from side to side. Trap-door devices allow inspection and care of the posterior skin and integument without moving the patient. Chemical thromboprophylaxis should be considered in these patients. Notwithstanding other factors (such as other sites of continued bleeding), anticoagulation should be delayed 72 hours from the time of injury to avoid the formation of epidural hematoma at the fracture site.

#### Suggested Treatment Guidelines
Compression fractures can usually be treated nonsurgically. An intact PLC is considered a prerequisite for nonsurgical care. Plain radiographic findings that are suggestive of PLC disruption include substantial anterior height loss (greater than 50%), interspinous process gapping, or more than 30° to 35° of kyphosis. In patients

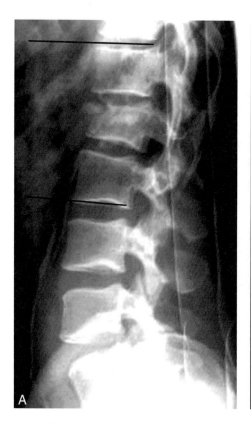 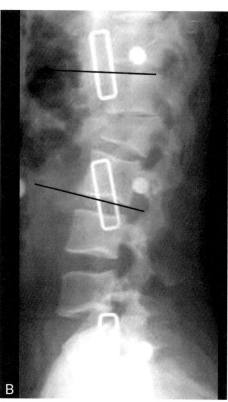

Figure 7 Initial supine lateral **(A)** and weight-bearing in-brace lateral **(B)** radiographs of a patient with a thoracolumbar burst fracture. There is a dramatic increase in the kyphotic angle with weight bearing. The angle can be measured from the lines shown (2° on supine view and 11° on weight-bearing lateral view). A subsequent MRI scan was highly suggestive of PLC disruption, which was later confirmed at the time of posterior surgery.

with such conditions, surgical treatment may be considered. MRI is often useful to confirm (or rule out) posterior ligament injury in equivocal cases. For mild compression fractures (particularly in the thoracic spine where the rib cage offers intrinsic support) with minimal height loss (less than 10%), the patient can be mobilized as tolerated without an external immobilization device. For more substantial fractures, a Jewett hyperextension brace can be used for 6 to 8 weeks to maintain alignment until healing. Weight-bearing radiographs should be obtained with the patient in the brace to confirm adequate control of the fracture (no progression of kyphosis) after the initial fitting (Figure 7). Follow-up radiographs should be made at regular intervals until bony healing occurs (usually at 3 months).

Burst fractures result from higher energy injuries than do compression fractures. The classic primary mechanism of injury for burst fractures was believed to be an axial load applied to a flexed spine. However, recent in vitro evidence suggests that extension moments may be necessary to cause characteristic lateral pedicle (vertebral body) splaying.

As is the case with compression fractures, an intact PLC should be considered a prerequisite for nonsurgical care. Some physicians believe that canal compromise of more than 50% is an indication for surgical decompression and/or stabilization; however, there are few data to support this treatment option in patients who are neurologically intact and have an intact PLC. Kyphosis of more than 25° to 30° and/or loss of anterior height of more than 50% are highly suggestive indications of posterior ligament injury.

Patients with burst fractures are usually immobilized with a custom-made, form-fitting, thoracolumbosacral orthosis or hyperextension cast. The patient should remain on log-roll precautions until the brace is applied. Before ambulation is begun, weight-bearing radiographs in the brace should be obtained. The kyphotic angle and height loss should be measured and compared with initial values. The integrity of the posterior ligaments should be more closely evaluated if kyphosis or height loss increases. The brace is worn for 3 months, with the theoretic goal of eventuating fracture healing with minimal additional height loss or kyphosis. Follow-up radiographs should be obtained at regular intervals. Patients should be advised of the clinical signs of conus medullaris compression and cauda equina syndrome.

In general, the indications to proceed with surgical treatment (stabilization and/or decompression) include unacceptable alignment or instability, incomplete neurologic deficit or cauda equina syndrome, and intractable pain and/or nonunion of the fracture. Although some reports in the literature describe nonsurgical care for some patients with neurologic deficits, the decision to surgically treat thoracolumbar fractures is multifactorial; nonsurgical care for patients with neurologic deficit is often reserved for patients who are medically unfit for surgery.

## Outcomes

**Compression Fractures** A recent study reported on 85 patients with thoracolumbar wedge (compression) fractures who were treated nonsurgically and had a minimum 3-year follow-up. Although the exact treatment regimen was not detailed, some patients received physiotherapy and/or braces. The authors reported a 69% incidence of nonspecific chronic low back pain of varying severity. The degree of kyphosis correlated with pain intensity, although a critical value of kyphosis was not reported. Vertebral body height loss was not correlative. The use of either bracing or physiotherapy did not influence outcomes.

**Burst Fractures** The long-term results of nonsurgical treatment of stable thoracolumbar burst fractures in 42 patients without neurologic deficit who were followed for 11 to 55 years have been recently published. The average kyphosis in flexion was 26° and in extension 17°; however, kyphosis did not correlate with the degree of pain or function at final follow-up. No patients had neurologic deterioration. Low pain scores (average, 3.5 on the visual analog scale) were documented, with no patient using narcotics for pain control. Eighty-eight percent of patients returned to work in their preinjury occupation.

In another recent retrospective study, the outcomes of nonsurgical treatment of 38 patients with thoracolumbar burst fractures without neurologic deficit were reported. Patients with posterior arch fractures or dislocations, or with kyphosis of more than 35°, were excluded from the study. All patients were permitted early ambulation. Nine patients were treated in a brace. The average kyphosis increased from 20° to 24° (average follow-up, 4 years). Thirty-two patients had no pain or mild pain, and four had moderate pain. Two patients had severe pain and both underwent surgery more than 1 year after injury. No correlation between kyphosis or canal compromise and clinical outcome was found. Seventy-six percent of patients returned to their preinjury occupation. Complications included transient hematuria (three patients) and urinary retention (six patients).

Another study reported on the results of 60 consecutive neurologically intact patients with thoracolumbar burst fractures treated with an orthosis and followed for an average of 42 months. Initial and final kyphosis averaged 6° and 8°, respectively. Satisfactory functional outcome was found in 91% of these patients, and 83% reported slight or no pain and returned to their preinjury activity level. Three patients with urinary tract infections were successfully treated with antibiotics.

Another group reported the results of 24 neurologically intact patients with burst fractures who were treated with a thoracolumbosacral orthosis, a Jewett hyperextension brace, or a hyperextension cast and early

ambulation. No patient developed a neurologic deficit. A statistically insignificant increase in kyphosis was observed.

**Patients With Neurologic Deficit** Nonsurgical care is rarely used to treat patients with neurologic compromise. This treatment option would usually be indicated for patients with a complete neurologic injury who are medically unfit for surgery. One study found that no patient with a thoracolumbar burst fracture associated with a complete injury (Frankel A) demonstrated neurologic recovery, regardless of the use of surgical or nonsurgical treatment. Other studies have found comparable recovery rates in patients with neurologic deficits. In an early review of the results of 89 patients, neurologic recovery was documented in 35% of nonsurgically treated patients and 38% of surgically treated patients. The general medical benefits of surgical stabilization in patients with complete neurologic injury, such as improved patient mobilization, pulmonary toilet, and pain relief, although intuitive, should be considered on an individual patient basis.

### Comparison: Nonsurgical Versus Surgical Treatment

The results of surgical and nonsurgical treatment have been compared in select groups of patients with clearly defined thoracolumbar injuries. A classic report compared the results of surgical versus nonsurgical treatment of unstable thoracolumbar fractures in a group of neurologically intact patients. Significantly longer hospital stays were noted in the nonsurgical group (80 days) compared with the surgical group (30 days); the duration of immobilization was also longer in the nonsurgical group (67 days compared with 18 days). Final kyphosis was greater in the nonsurgical group, but the degree of deformity did not affect functional outcomes. No patient had neurologic deterioration, and there was no difference in pain scores or rates of return to work. From these data, the main benefit of surgical treatment appears to be earlier mobilization in patients with unstable fractures; however, the potential risk for secondary neurologic compromise, despite the low incidence reported, remains a concern for most practitioners.

A more recent prospective study compared the outcomes of patients without neurologic deficit who were treated with either posterior surgery or nonsurgical management for thoracolumbar burst fractures. Patients with injuries that involved the posterior arch, such as facet dislocations, were excluded. A hyperextension brace and early ambulation was used to treat 47 of the nonsurgically managed patients. Short-segment pedicle screw fixation was used to treat the surgical group consisting of 33 patients. Although outcome scores were better in the surgical group at 3-month follow-up, the scores at 6-month and 2-year follow-ups were not statistically different. Correction of kyphosis was also initially better in the surgical group, but this benefit was not demonstrable at final follow-up. Pain scores followed a similar pattern.

In a 2003 well-designed randomized prospective study, surgical and nonsurgical treatment of stable thoracolumbar burst fractures were compared in patients without neurologic deficit. Patients with suspected or confirmed posterior ligamentous disruption were excluded from this study. Nonsurgical care included a brace or cast followed by early mobilization. Surgical treatment consisted of either anterior or posterior surgery. Results showed no statistical differences in kyphosis, functional outcome, or pain scores between the two groups. However, surgically treated patients tended to have higher pain scores and more complications.

These data strongly suggest that nonsurgical management, consisting of bracing and early mobilization, is an effective treatment method for patients with thoracolumbar burst fractures without posterior ligamentous injury. These studies, however, do not provide clear recommendations of a method for determining the integrity of the PLC.

## Surgical Treatment

Surgical treatment includes stabilization with or without decompression. Surgical goals are to restore and maintain spinal alignment and stability until solid bony fusion is achieved. In patients with neurologic deficit and canal compromise, decompression is targeted at maximizing the space available for the neural elements. Anterior and posterior procedures can be used for both stabilization and decompression.

### Compression Fractures

In the infrequent instance in which a compression fracture is associated with a posterior ligament injury, posterior stabilization is the preferred treatment method. The surgical goal is to realign the spine (for example, to correct kyphosis) until solid fusion is achieved. Posterior pedicle screw or hook constructs can both be useful. Compressive forces placed along posterior constructs can be corrective; however, this treatment method is not recommended in the presence of posterior vertebral body comminution (such as burst fracture) because of the risk of causing intrusion of bony fragments into the canal. An anterior procedure is rarely indicated to stabilize a compression fracture.

### Burst Fractures

Controversy exists regarding the indications and optimal method of surgical treatment of thoracolumbar burst fractures, particularly for patients without neurologic deficit. Some physicians advocate posterior surgery alone, whereas others believe that anterior or combined anterior and posterior surgery is preferable. In patients with neurologic deficit (in particular those with incomplete deficits), most physicians agree that a decompressive maneuver is warranted. Indirect reduction of displaced vertebral body fragments can be achieved through distraction and realignment with posterior instrumentation; however, this approach appears to be more effective if the PLL is intact and if surgery is performed early (less than 2 to 4 days after injury). Direct fragment removal through an anterior approach offers better anatomic decompression, although the neurologic benefits have not been conclusively established. Other techniques have been developed to remove vertebral body fragments and perform interbody fusion through a posterior approach; however, these techniques are not widely used. Various anterior and posterior instrumentation options are available.

### Suggested Surgical Indications

A progressive neurologic deficit is an indication for urgent decompression. Patients with neurologic deficit associated with at least 25% canal compromise can benefit from surgical decompression. Progressive kyphotic deformity as a result of mechanical instability also warrants surgical stabilization. Injury characteristics that are highly suggestive of PLC disruption are progressive kyphotic deformity, kyphosis greater than 25° to 30°, and a loss of vertebral body height greater than 50%. Patients who have continued pain after 3 to 6 months and have documented nonunion on bone scans and/or MRI scans may also require surgical stabilization.

### Posterior Surgery

**Stabilization** Posterior surgery is mainly used for the stabilization of burst fractures in neurologically intact patients. Stabilization can be effected using a variety of constructs. Pedicle screws are among the more popular methods of fixation and allow short-segment fusion with a theoretic advantage of three-column stability over hook constructs. At a minimum, the level above and below the fracture should be included in the fusion (short-segment instrumentation), with some authors advocating fusion two levels above and below the fracture (Figure 8). Short-segment instrumentation can lead to pedicle screw breakage or failure rates as high as 50%. This complication is believed to be the result of continued cyclic loading amplified by anterior column deficiency. Transpedicular intracorporeal bone grafting had been introduced in an attempt to reconstitute the vertebral body height, but this technique has not diminished the rate of hardware failure with short-segment pedicle screw stabilization. Although a useful option, posterior stabilization using hooks and rods has declined in popularity because it requires inclusion of at least two to three segments above and below the injury. Sublaminar

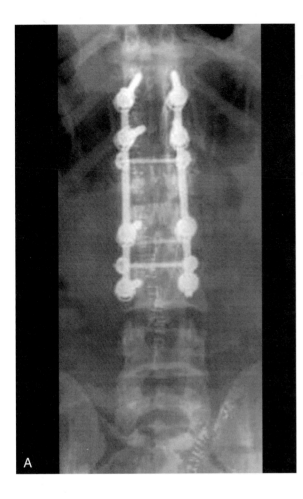

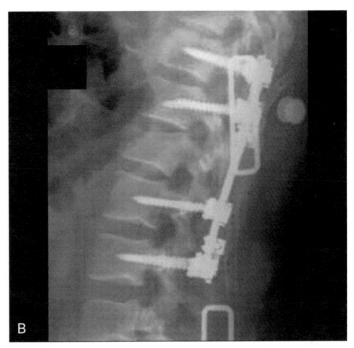

Figure 8 AP **(A)** and lateral **(B)** radiographs of a patient who underwent long-segment posterior instrumentation for an unstable thoracolumbar burst fracture. Long constructs may be more effective in maintaining kyphotic correction when used to stabilize thoracolumbar burst fractures. Hardware failure is more likely with short-segment constructs.

wire constructs have played only a small role in the stabilization of unstable burst fractures.

**Indirect Decompression** Several posterior methods of decompressing the spinal canal have been advocated. Simple decompressive laminectomy is no longer favored because it causes further posterior destabilization and can lead to a progressive kyphotic deformity. Indirect decompression, a concept that relies on longitudinal distraction along the fractured segment, works through ligamentotaxis of the displaced posterior vertebral fragments. With distraction, an intact PLL and/or posterior anulus are believed to pull the fragments back into place. In one study, this technique was used in 22 junctional (T11 to L2) burst fractures with a reported average 28% improvement in canal compromise. Although patients with an incomplete neurologic injury improved an average of 1.8 Frankel grades, the rate of neurologic recovery or injury could not be predicted based on the amount of canal clearance. A cadaveric study found a relationship between measured vertebral height loss/kyphosis and spinal canal compromise with simulated burst fractures. Interestingly, extension of the motion segment (a commonly performed maneuver to reduce burst fractures) did not affect canal clearance.

Indirect reduction has not been uniformly endorsed because disruption of the PLL appears to compromise its effectiveness. One study of 30 patients documented an average improvement in canal compromise of only 19% (from 57% preoperatively to 38% postoperatively) after posterior distractive instrumentation. Independent of canal clearance, incomplete (Frankel grades B through D) injuries improved one or more grades. Although the authors believed that disruption of the PLL was a contributing factor to the modest effects on canal clearance, MRI was not used to assess the PLL. From these findings, it was inferred that canal compromise of more than 50% may be indicative of PLL disruption, and that decompression should be performed through an anterior approach in such cases.

A longer delay from injury to surgery is believed to compromise the efficacy of indirect canal clearance. One surgeon found that surgery performed within 1 week of injury resulted in an average 33% improvement of canal compromise. Surgery performed more than 1 or 2 weeks after injury resulted in only a 24% improvement and in no improvement of canal compromise. As was the case with other reports, all incomplete injuries improved by one or more Frankel grade regardless of canal clearance. Other researchers have found modest improvement in canal clearance in patients stabilized within 4 days of injury (56% to 38% improvement) compared with those stabilized more than 4 days after injury (52% to 44%).

**Direct Canal Decompression Using a Posterior Approach** Methods of anterior canal decompression using an all-posterior approach have been developed. In one study of 31 patients, a posterolateral approach was used to reduce the displaced vertebral body segments to clear the spinal canal. The technique included removal of the facet joint and/or pedicle to gain access to the posterior vertebral body. Statistically significant decreases in canal compromise were achieved, as measured by CT, with neurologic improvement in 96% of patients. Supplementation with a pedicle screw construct was used.

**Special Circumstance: Concomitant Lamina Fracture**
The combination of a concomitant lamina fracture with a burst fracture can be associated with a dural tear or entrapped nerve roots. One group of investigators showed a high rate of dural lacerations in patients with this injury pattern and subsequently recommended posterior laminectomy for exploration and dural repair before any planned anterior procedure. Another group reported on a variation of this injury pattern in which nerve roots were entrapped in the laminar fractures. These authors also recommended freeing the roots through a posterior approach before any planned anterior decompression and stabilization.

*Anterior Surgery*
Anterior decompression is the most direct and efficacious method of clearing the spinal canal after a burst fracture. Most of the injured vertebral body along with the adjacent cephalad and caudal disks can be removed. Retropulsed fragments are carefully removed to relieve pressure on the spinal cord or cauda equina. The highest rates of neurologic recovery have been reported after anterior decompressive surgery for burst fractures in patients with incomplete neural injuries. One report documented a median improvement of two Frankel grades in patients undergoing anterior decompression within 48 hours of injury.

Because this maneuver destabilizes the spine, the vertebral body defect must be replaced with a supportive strut that will also result in bony fusion. Structural bone graft can be used, such as autograft rib, fibula, iliac crest, or allograft struts. More recently, titanium mesh cages have become popular. These devices can be filled with harvested morcellized cancellous autograft iliac crest or salvaged bone from the corpectomy. Anterior column reconstruction (strut grafting) should be stabilized by anterior or posterior instrumentation, or both. Numerous constructs can be used for anterior stabilization. In vitro biomechanical studies have compared vari-

ous anterior devices. Among the more rigid devices are plates with fixed-angle vertebral body screws and cross-linked, rod-screw-staple designs such as the Kaneda system (DePuy Spine, Raynham, MA). In general, anterior instrumentation and fusion leads to better maintenance of alignment compared with stand-alone procedures.

In an early study, anterior surgery was performed for thoracolumbar burst fractures in 35 patients with neurologic injury. Iliac crest autograft struts were used to reconstruct the anterior column. A modified Harrington rod-screw system spanning from the vertebral bodies above and below the fractured segment were used. High rates of neurologic recovery were shown in patients with incomplete injuries, whereas those with complete neural damage showed no improvement. Of 21 patients who initially had incomplete loss of bowel or bladder function, 19 showed some improvement. Twelve of 13 patients who were treated early (within 10 days of injury) recovered useful bladder function. Five of eight patients who were treated late (more than 10 days after injury) gained useful bladder function without incontinence. Similarly, another group of surgeons used anterior plating techniques in conjunction with anterior decompression and strut grafting for a variety of thoracolumbar fractures and documented excellent maintenance of alignment and rates of neural recovery.

The use of stand-alone instrumentation with a plate in 12 patients with thoracolumbar burst fractures has been reported. In 10 patients, postoperative correction of kyphosis was maintained at 1-year follow-up. The other two patients had 10° to 20° loss of correction. Both of these patients had preoperative kyphotic angles greater than 50°, suggesting that anterior surgery alone may not be sufficiently rigid to stabilize patients with significant posterior ligamentous injury. However, this loss of correction may have been related to the type of implant used (the Z-plate, Medtronic-Sofamor Danek, Memphis, TN), which has shown a high rate of fatigue failure as a stand-alone implant.

In a 1997 study, 150 consecutive patients with thoracolumbar burst fractures were treated with a single-stage anterior decompression, strut grafting, and instrumentation using the Kaneda rod-sleeve-staple device. Canal clearance was nearly 100%. A 93% fusion rate was reported. Patients with pseudarthroses were successfully treated by posterior instrumentation and fusion. Improvement of at least one Frankel grade was reported in 142 of 150 patients (93%).

**Influence of Timing on Neurologic Outcomes** It has been suggested that the timing of surgery will influence the rate of neurologic recovery. In a study of 22 patients with thoracolumbar burst fractures, anterior decompressive surgery performed within 48 hours of injury resulted in a mean improvement of two Frankel grades and complete resolution of bowel and bladder function in 44% of patients. Surgery after 48 hours improved Frankel scoring by only one grade, with no patient recovering complete bowel or bladder function. Although the study was not randomized, these data provide some evidence that early anterior decompressive surgery may benefit neurologic outcome.

**Delayed Decompression** For a variety of reasons, not all patients undergo early decompressive surgery. Residual canal stenosis can be present for long periods (weeks to years) in some patients. One study examined the effects of late decompression after a burst fracture. In 49 patients with conus medullaris or cauda equina level injuries, neurologic improvement (Frankel grade and bladder control) was statistically better if patients underwent decompressive surgery within 2 years after injury. The overall rate of bladder improvement was 50% for patients with fractures at or below T12. These data suggest that substantial improvements in Frankel grade and bladder/bowel function can be expected even with long periods of compression after burst fracture.

### Combined Anterior and Posterior Surgery
In some patients, combined anterior and posterior surgery can be performed. The specific indications and benefits of this maneuver remain unclear. Theoretic advantages include maximization of canal clearance, maximal stability, and improved fusion rates. However, the added morbidity of the combined procedures is a potential disadvantage.

In a recent retrospective review, the results of combined anterior/posterior surgery were compared with those of posterior surgery alone for the treatment of thoracolumbar burst fractures. Although the method of treatment did not affect neurologic recovery, combined anterior/posterior surgery resulted in better maintenance of kyphotic correction. Interestingly, loss of correction was not associated with a higher rate of back pain. Some surgeons advocate combined anterior and posterior techniques to maximize canal decompression and overall construct stability. For some surgeons, PLC disruption is an important factor to consider.

### Comparing Anterior Versus Posterior Methods
Few studies have compared anterior to posterior methods. An early comparison of these methods was reported for patients with incomplete neurologic injury. Although not all of the 59 patients in the study had burst fractures, neurologic recovery was related to the adequacy of canal clearance. Motor, sensory, and bladder improvement was statistically better in the group receiving anterior decompression compared with the group receiving posterior surgery. Interestingly, posterior surgery included posterolateral decompression through a transpedicular approach and stabilization, whereas anterior surgery entailed a full corpectomy at

that level of injury. Bladder function for patients with conus level lesions improved in 70% of patients in the anterior surgery group, whereas improvement was found in only 12% of patients in the posterior surgery group. The posterior group was treated an average of 6.4 days from injury, whereas no patients in the anterior group had surgery sooner than 1 month after injury. In contrast, motor recovery was not statistically affected by the choice of approach. More recently, the results of these approaches have been analyzed in patients with mechanically unstable thoracolumbar burst fractures without neurologic deficit. Although anterior and posterior procedures resulted in equivalent clinical results, less blood loss and shorter surgical times were documented in patients undergoing posterior surgery.

### Less Invasive Methods
Less invasive methods of surgery for thoracolumbar burst fractures have been developed; however, few reports on these methods exist in the literature. In 2001, a study examined the results of using a thoracoscopic approach to perform corpectomy, anterior column reconstructions, and anterior instrumentation. Although the complication rate was considered low by the study authors, calculable rates of vascular injury and neurologic deterioration were reported. Such complications rarely occur with open surgery. Recognizing the slow learning curve required for using the thoracoscopic approach, the efficacy and advantages of this approach to spinal fractures must still be determined, particularly in light of the increasing number of reports of equivalent results using nonsurgical treatment.

### Neurologic Outcomes and Canal Compromise
The relationship between canal compromise as measured on CT scans and neurologic injury has been extensively investigated. The severity of the deficit does not appear to be predictable based on the amount of residual canal stenosis. The degree of deficit is probably more influenced by the instantaneous canal compromise that occurs at the time of impact, which is substantially more than can be detected on initial imaging. Also, there is no consensus regarding the optimal method of measuring canal compromise.

In a 2001 study, canal remodeling was determined in 115 patients treated with posterior distraction instrumentation (two levels above and below the injured vertebra) by measuring the midsagittal diameter and the cross-sectional area of the spinal canal. An immediate postoperative mean canal clearance from 49% to 72% of normal was found. At final follow-up, the mean canal measurements were 87% of normal. Importantly, canals with greater initial compromise showed greater clearance. These findings strongly suggest that direct decompression (anterior or posterior) may not be necessary in neurologically intact patients with varying degrees of canal compromise. Despite its importance, canal clearance was not statistically different in patients who had surgery early (less than 3 days after injury) or late (more than 3 days after injury). In another 2001 study, the CT scans and plain radiographs of 83 patients with thoracolumbar burst fractures treated surgically or nonsurgically with a minimum follow-up of 12 months were retrospectively reviewed. It was determined that the spinal canal underwent substantial remodeling, regardless of the type of treatment. None of the patients worsened neurologically over the follow-up period. The authors concluded that, in neurologically intact patients, the spinal canal can undergo natural resorption and clearance.

In a 1999 review, the amount of canal compromise was found to be greater in patients with neural deficit (mean, 52%) compared with patients who were neurologically intact (mean, 35%). However, the average amount of canal clearance was not different for those who showed neural recovery (20%) compared with those who did not (23%). A more important predictor of neurologic deficit was the presence of posterior ligamentous disruption (61% versus 25% for patients with and without neurologic deficit, respectively). Unfortunately, the study did not specify the method by which the integrity of the PLC was determined, which can be challenging in some injuries. In an analysis of various radiologic canal measurements in patients with burst fractures and neural deficit, the only measurement that correlated with neural status was the sagittal-to-transverse ratio. The absolute cross-sectional area, sagittal canal diameter, and transverse diameter by themselves were not correlative. Another group of researchers found that a 25%, 50%, and 75% canal compromise corresponded to a 0.29, 0.51, and 0.71 predictive value, respectively, for the presence (but not severity) of a neural deficit. In a similar study, 45% canal compromise and posterior column injury was predictive of the presence of neurologic injury at the L1 level. Again, the severity of deficit could not be correlated. By measuring the cross-sectional area of the canal, one study found that 1.0 cm$^2$ was the critical level below which all patients had some degree of neurologic deficit, whereas patients with 1.0 cm$^2$ to 1.25 cm$^2$ canal area had incomplete or no neurologic injuries.

## Bending Injuries: Flexion-Distraction and Chance Injuries

In contrast to dislocations of the cervical spine, pure dislocations at the thoracolumbar level are rare. The most common mechanism of such dislocations is believed to be flexion-distraction forces, which are often associated with wearing automobile lap seat-belts. In head-on collisions, improperly worn, high-riding lap belts can concentrate high-energy forces along an apex that is anterior to the thoracolumbar junction, which potentiates distractive forces along the entire vertebral segment. These injuries are distinguished, mechanically, from flexion-compression injuries in which the axis of flexion is about the spinal canal, resulting in anterior compressive and posterior tensile forces.

Flexion-distraction injuries can cause varying fracture patterns of the vertebral body and posterior elements. By convention, these injuries are distinguished from fracture-dislocation injuries by the absence of translation, although these injuries are often confused in the literature. Flexion-distraction injuries can be purely ligamentous, osteoligamentous, or purely osseous. Fractures are typically transverse. In some patients, a fracture line can be noted from the tip of the spinous process, through the laminae, and exiting the middle anterior aspect of the vertebral body. In pure ligamentous injuries, the facet joints can be subluxated or, in some instances, frankly dislocated (perched or locked) (Figure 9).

Nearly two thirds of patients with flexion-distraction injuries have a neurologic deficit, presumably from distraction of the neural elements. A commonly associated nonspinal injury is a perforated viscus, which is believed to be secondary to the sudden increases of pressure within the intestines from abdominal compression. In some patients, the abdominal injury is discovered first and the spinal injury may be missed. An ecchymotic region along the abdomen is suggestive of this injury pattern.

Thoracolumbar flexion-distraction dislocations are rarely treated nonsurgically. In purely bony flexion-distraction injuries, hyperextension casting or bracing may be an option. This treatment should be continued until bony union is radiographically and clinically confirmed, usually at about 3 to 4 months. Most other flexion-distraction injuries should be treated surgically. Because the spine flexes about an anterior axis of rotation, the anterior longitudinal ligament is usually intact and there is little, if any, vertebral body comminution. In most patients, anterior surgery (which necessitates resection of the anterior longitudinal ligament) would further destabilize the spine. Therefore, posterior compressive instrumentation and fusion is the most common treatment. Because the intervertebral disk can be ruptured with severe injuries, care must be taken to prevent overcompression of the construct that could result in the expulsion of loose disk fragments into the spinal canal. Short-segment pedicle screw or hook constructs are an effective means of stabilizing these injuries.

## Fracture-Dislocations

Thoracolumbar fracture-dislocations are high-energy injuries that cause a high rate of complete neurologic deficit. In patients with complete neurologic deficits, surgery is indicated to stabilize the spine, which can facilitate patient transfers, mobilization, and pulmonary care. Injuries

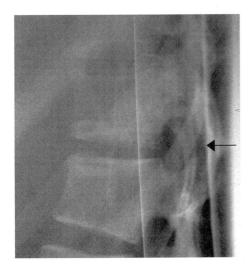

Figure 9 Flexion-distraction injury of the thoracolumbar junction. Mild compression of the vertebral body is noted. However, the more significant finding is the perched facets (arrow).

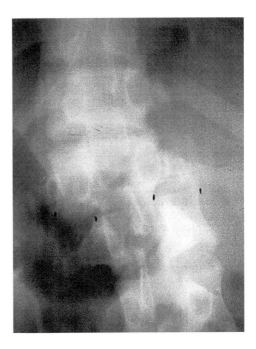

Figure 10 Fracture dislocations can demonstrate various bony fracture patterns. They are distinguished from other injuries by the presence of translational deformity, a sign of high-energy trauma.

can occur from a variety of mechanisms, including flexion, shear, and extension forces (Figure 10). Fractures can be realigned in the operating room through postural reduction with the patient prone. In some patients, misalignment requires open reduction through direct manipulation. In the neurologically intact or incompletely injured patient, this procedure must be performed carefully to prevent additional neurologic injury.

In most patients, posterior instrumentation and fusion is adequate treatment for fracture-dislocations. In patients with extensive vertebral body comminution, compression, or fragments displaced into the spinal canal, a combined anterior and posterior approach may be used; however, anterior stand-alone procedures should be avoided. A recent report showed excellent maintenance of alignment in 15 patients stabilized by short-segment pedicle screw instrumentation.

## Complications

The timing of surgery is an important consideration, particularly when dealing with polytraumatized patients. In a retrospective chart review of patients with spinal fractures (including cervical, thoracic, and lumbar injuries), patients with injuries that were surgically treated within 3 days of injury had a lower rate of pneumonia and shorter hospital stays compared with those who were surgically treated more than 3 days after injury. Although the two groups were not randomized, and it is possible that the patients receiving late fixation may have included patients who were more severely injured, the injury severity scores did not show a significant statistical difference. The average age, Glasgow Coma Scale score, and chest injury score were significantly higher in the group receiving late fixation.

In a prospective study of 75 consecutive patients with polytrauma including spine fractures, anterior surgery performed within 24 hours of injury (urgent group) was associated with significantly greater blood loss com-

pared with surgery performed between 24 and 72 hours (early group) after injury. In contrast, patients treated with posterior surgery showed comparable blood loss regardless of the timing of the surgery. There were no reports of thromboembolism, neurologic deterioration, pressure sores, deep wound infections, or systemic sepsis in either the early or urgent groups.

Results of another study showed a 10% incidence of wound infections after surgery for patients with thoracolumbar fractures. Although this retrospective study did not include a control group, the authors believed that this rate of infection was higher than that reported in the literature for elective thoracolumbar procedures. A complete neurologic deficit was a statistically significance risk factor for infection. Other possible risk factors, which include concomitant distant site infections or potential bacteremic sources (such as open fractures), were not included in the analysis.

## Summary

Many challenges remain in the treatment of patients with thoracolumbar spinal injuries. Agreement on a uniform method of injury description and fracture classification has yet to be achieved. Future goals will be to more clearly identify patients who would maximally benefit from surgery and will likely include more methods of minimally invasive stabilization and decompression.

## Annotated Bibliography
### General

Belmont PJ, Taylor KF, Mason KT, Shawen SB, Polly DW, Klemme WR: Incidence, epidemiology, and occupational outcomes of thoracolumbar fractures among U.S. Army Aviators. *J Trauma* 2001;50:855-861.

Using a prospective database, the authors found that 12.8 thoracolumbar fractures occurred for every 100,000 aviators in the United States army. This group was identified as a high-risk subgroup of military personnel.

Hohlrieder M, Eschertzhuber S, Schubert H, Zinnecker R, Mair P: Severity and pattern of injury in survivors of alpine fall accidents. *High Alt Med Biol* 2004;5:349-354.

The results of this study showed that 81% of spine fractures sustained in Alpine climbers occurred at the thoracolumbar junction. From an analysis of the patterns of injury, the authors concluded that direct impact was a more likely mechanism than indirect deceleration.

Robertson A, Branfoot T, Barlow IF, Giannoudis PV: Spinal injury patterns resulting from car and motorcycle accidents. *Spine* 2002;27:2825-2830.

This retrospective study showed that patients involved in motorcycle crashes were more severely injured and had thoracic spine injuries that were more likely caused by forced hyperflexion compared with patients injured in car crashes.

## Diagnostic Considerations

Oner FC, van Gils APG, Faber JAJ, Dhert WJA, Verbout AJ: Some complications of common treatment schemes of thoracolumbar spine fractues can be predicted with magnetic resonance imaging. *Spine* 2002;27:629-636.

In this prospective study, the authors found that MRI indicating posterior ligamentous disruption was predictive of recurrent kyphotic deformity following treatment of thoracolumbar spine fractures.

## Classification of Thoracolumbar Injuries

Mirza SK, Mirza AJ, Chapman JR, Anderson PA: Classifications of thoracic and lumbar fractures: Rationale and supporting data. *J Am Acad Orthop Surg* 2002;10: 364-377.

This article offers a basic overview of the most commonly used systems for classifying thoracolumbar spine fractures. The rationale, key components, and advantages and disadvantages of each system are discussed.

Oner FC, Ramos LM, Simmermacher RK, et al: Classification of thoracic and lumbar spine fractures: Problems of reproducibility: A study of 53 patients using CT and MRI. *Eur Spine J* 2002;11:235-245.

In this study, the interobserver and intraobserver reliability of the AO and Denis classification systems were assessed. The Denis system had somewhat better kappa values.

## Burst and Compression Fractures

Alanay A, Acaroglu E, Yazici M, Oznur A, Surat A: Short-segment pedicle instrumentation of thoracolumbar burst fractures: Does transpedicular intracorporeal grafting prevent early failure. *Spine* 2001;26:213-217.

In this prospective randomized study of 20 patients, the progression of kyphosis and the incidence of screw failure was similar for fractures treated with and without transpedicular bone grafting (50% and 40%, respectively).

Aligizakis A, Katonis P, Stergiopoulos K, Galanakis I, Karabekios S, Hadjipavlou A: Functional outcome of burst fractures of the thoracolumbar spine managed non-operatively with early ambulation, evaluated using the load sharing classification. *Acta Orthop Belg* 2002; 68:279-287.

This study was a prospective evaluation of the use of the load sharing classification (originally developed to guide surgical management) in 60 consecutive patients with thoracolumbar injuries who were treated nonsurgically. The authors found the system to be reliable and easy to use in this patient population.

Dai LY: Remodeling of the spinal canal after thoracolumbar burst fractures. *Clin Orthop Relat Res* 2001; 382:119-123.

This study showed the remarkable remodeling potential of the spinal canal following thoracolumbar burst fractures. Importantly, no difference was found in the percentage of remodeling between patients treated surgically compared with those treated nonsurgically.

Folman Y, Gepstein R: Late outcome of nonoperative management of thoracolumbar vertebral wedge fractures. *J Orthop Trauma* 2003;17:190-192.

In this study of patients with thoracolumbar wedge (compression) fractures without neurologic involvement, nonsurgical treatment resulted in adequate clinical and radiographic outcomes. Importantly, 69.4% of patients had reported chronic pain in the low lumbar region.

Knop C, Fabian HF, Bastian L, Blauth M: Late results of thoracolumbar fractures after posterior instrumentation and transpedicular bone grafting. *Spine* 2001;26:88-99.

Results of this retrospective study showed no advantage of transpedicular grafting performed in conjunction with posterior pedicle screw stabilization for patients with thoracolumbar burst fractures.

Shen WJ, Liu TJ, Shen YS: Nonoperative treatment versus posterior fixation for thoracolumbar junction burst fractures without neurologic deficit. *Spine* 2001;26:1038-1045.

In this prospective nonrandomized study, outcome scores for nonsurgical treatment compared with posterior fixation for patients with thoracolumbar junction burst fractures without neurologic deficit were better in the surgical group at 3 months; however, the 6-month and 2-year scores were not statistically different. Kyphosis correction was initially better in the surgical group, but not at final follow-up. Pain scores followed a similar pattern.

Stancic MF, Gregorovic E, Nozica E, Penezic L: Anterior decompression and fixation versus posterior reposition and semirigid fixation in the treatment of unstable burst thoracolumbar fracture: Prospective clinical trial. *Croat Med J* 2001;42:49-53.

In this study, anterior decompression and stabilization was compared with posterior stabilization and indirect decompression for the treatment of thoracolumbar burst fractures. With the limited number of patients in the study, no difference in neurologic or functional outcomes was found.

Wessberg P, Wang Y, Irstam L, Nordwall A: The effect of surgery and remodelling on spinal canal measurements after thoracolumbar burst fractures. *Eur Spine J* 2001; 10:55-63.

In this study, treatment of thoracolumbar burst fractures with posterior distractive instrumentation resulted in spinal canal clearance from 49% to 72% of normal values following surgery. At final follow-up of a minimum of 5 years, this percentage improved to 87%.

Wood K, Butterman G, Mehbod A, Garvey T, Jhanjee R, Sechriest V: Operative compared with nonoperative treatment of a thoracolumbar burst fracture without neurological deficit. *J Bone Joint Surg Am* 2003;85-A: 773-781.

This randomized prospective study of neurologically intact patients with stable burst fractures showed no statistical differences in kyphosis, functional outcome, or pain scores between groups receiving surgical and nonsurgical treatment. Surgically treated patients tended to have higher pain scores and more complications.

## Complications

Croce MA, Bee TK, Pritchard E, Miller PR, Fabian TC: Does optimal timing for spine fracture fixation exist. *Ann Surg* 2001;233:851-858.

In this review of the surgical literature, early fixation (within 3 days of injury) of spine fractures was found to be safe in patients with multiple injuries. The study also found a lower incidence of pneumonia, a shorter stay in the intensive care unit, and lower hospital charges in the group receiving early compared with late fixation.

## Classic Bibliography

Been HD, Bouma GJ: Comparison of two types of surgery for thoraco-lumbar burst fractures: Combined anterior and posterior stabilisation vs. posterior instrumentation only. *Acta Neurochir (Wien)* 1999;141:349-357.

Bradford D, McBride G: Surgical management of thoracolumbar spine fractures with incomplete neurologic deficits. *Clin Orthop Relat Res* 1987;218:201-215.

Brightman R, Miller C, Rea G, et al: Magnetic resonance imaging of trauma to the thoracic and lumbar spine: The importance of the posterior longitudinal ligament. *Spine* 1992;17:541-550.

Burke DC, Murray DD: The management of thoracic and thoracolumbar injuries of the spine with neurological involvement. *J Bone Joint Surg Br* 1976;58:72-78.

Cammisa F, Eismont F, Green B: Dural laceration occurring with burst fractures and associated laminar fractures. *J Bone Joint Surg Am* 1989;71:1044-1052.

Chow GH, Nelson BJ, Beghard JS, Brugman JL, Brown CW, Donaldson DH: Functional outcome of thoracolumbar burst fractures managed with hyperextension casting or bracing and early mobilization. *Spine* 1996;21: 2170-2175.

Clohisy J, Akbarnia B, Bucholz R, et al: Neurologic recovery associated with anterior decompression of spine fractures at the thoracolumbar junction (T12-L1). *Spine* 1992;17:S325-S330.

Dendrinos GK, Halikias JG, Krallis PN, Asimakopoulos A: Factors influencing neurological recovery in burst thoracolumbar fractures. *Acta Orthop Belg* 1995;61:226-234.

Denis F, Burkus J: Shear fracture-dislocation of the thoracic and lumbar spine associated with forceful hyperextension (lumberjack paraplegia). *Spine* 1992;17:156-161.

Fontijne W, deKlerk L, Braakman R, et al: CT scan prediction of neurological deficit in thoracolumbar burst fractures. *J Bone Joint Surg Br* 1992;74:683-685.

Gertzbein S, Crowe P, Fazl M, et al: Canal clearance in burst fractures using the AO internal fixator. *Spine* 1992; 17:558-560.

Ghanayem AJ, Zdeblick TA: Anterior instrumentation in the management of thoracolumbar burst fractures. *Clin Orthop Relat Res* 1997;335:89-100.

Haas N, Blauth M, Tscherne H: Anterior plating in thoracolumbar spine injuries: Indication, technique, and results. *Spine* 1991;16:S100-S111.

Hashimoto T, Kaneda K, Abumi K: Relationship between traumatic spinal canal stenosis and neurological deficits in thoracolumbar burst fractures. *Spine* 1988;13: 1268-1272.

Isomi T, Panjabi MM, Kato Y, Wang JL: Radiographic parameters for evaluating the neurological spaces in experimental thoracolumbar burst fractures. *J Spinal Disord* 2000;13:404-411.

Kaneda K, Taneichi H, Abumi K, Hashimoto T, Satoh S, Fujiya M: Anterior decompression and stabilization with the Kaneda device for thoracolumbar burst fractures associated with neurological deficits. *J Bone Joint Surg Am* 1997;79:69-73.

Katonis P, Kontakis G, Loupasis G, Aligizakas A, Christoforakis J, Velivassakis E: Treatment of unstable thoracolumbar and lumbar spine injuries using Cotrel-Dubousset instrumnetation. *Spine* 1999;24:2352-2357.

Kim NH, Lee HM, Chun IM: Neurologic injury and recovery in patients with burst fracture of the thoracolumbar spine. *Spine* 1999;24:290-294.

Kostuik J: Anterior fixation for fractures of the thoracic and lumbar spine with or without neurologic involvement. *Clin Orthop Relat Res* 1984;189:103-115.

McLain RF, Benson DR: Urgent surgical stabilization of spinal fractures in polytrauma patients. *Spine* 1999;24: 1646-1654.

Rasmussen P, Rabin M, Mann D, et al: Reduced transverse spinal area secondary to burst fractures: Is there a relationship to neurologic injury? *J Neurotrauma* 1994; 11:711-720.

Razak M, Mahmud MM, Hyzan MY, Omar A: Short segment posterior instrumentation, reduction and fusion of unstable thoracolumbar burst fractures: A review of 26 cases. *Med J Malaysia* 2000;55:9-13.

Rechtine GR, Cahill D, Chrin AM: Treatment of thoracolumbar trauma: comparison of complications of operative versus nonoperative treatment. *J Spinal Disord* 1999;12:406-409.

Shen WJ, Shen YS: Nonsurgical treatment of three-column thoracolumbar junction burst fractures without neurologic deficit. *Spine* 1999;24:412-415.

Silvestro C, Francaviglia N, Bragazzi R, et al: Near-anatomical reduction and stabilization of burst fractures of the lower thoracic or lumbar spine. *Acta Neurochir (Wien)* 1992;116:53-59.

Starr J, Hanley E: Junctional burst fractures. *Spine* 1992; 17:551-557.

Transfeldt E, White D, Bradford D, Roche R: Delayed anterior decompression inpatients with spinal cord and cauda equina injuries of the thoracolumbar spine. *Spine* 1990;15:953-957.

Vaccaro AR: Combined anterior and posterior surgery for fractures of the thoracolumbar spine. *Instr Course Lect* 1999;48:443-449.

Vaccaro AR, Nachwalter RS, Klein GR, et al: The significance of thoracolumbar spinal canal size in spinal cord injury patients. *Spine* 2001;26:371-376.

Weinstein JN, Collalto P, Lehmann TR: Thoracolumbar "burst" fractures treated conservatively: A long-term follow-up. *Spine* 1988;13:33-38.

Willen J, Lindahl S, Nordwall A: Unstable thoracolumbar fractures: A comparative clinical study of conservative treatment and Harrington instrumentation. *Spine* 1985;10:111-122.

# Chapter 24

# Sacral Fractures

Henry Claude Sagi, MD

## Introduction

Sacral fractures are unique because they occur in a region of the anatomy that bridges two very different disciplines: spinal surgery and orthopaedic traumatology (pelvic fracture surgery). The sacrum is the most caudal spinal segment that contains neurologic structures and forms the lumbosacral spinal junction, which is the last mobile vertebral column articulation. The sacrum also serves as the keystone structure for the posterior pelvic ring, joining the two hemipelves and lower appendicular skeleton to the trunk via the strong sacroiliac (SI) joints. Injuries and pathology in this area of the body are not yet completely understood, in part because spinal surgeons view the sacrum as a vertebral segment in terms of spinal mechanics, function, and alignment, whereas orthopaedic traumatologists view the sacrum as the central element of the posterior aspect of the pelvic ring. Orthopaedic traumatologists treat pathology of the sacrum with respect to pelvic and hip joint mechanics, function, and alignment. Because each subspecialty focuses on its own biomechanical and physiologic principles, the principles of the other discipline are often ignored.

This chapter outlines injuries to the sacrum in a manner that will integrate the philosophies of both disciplines. A useful approach to diagnosing and treating sacral fractures is presented.

## Anatomy

Although the anatomy of the sacrum has been well described in the literature, a few important points merit review. The sacrum is an inverted triangular-shaped bone that is not planar, but is rather concave when viewed from the lateral projection. It articulates with each ilium via the SI joints. The SI joints are inherently unstable by virtue of their bony anatomy and rely completely on their ligamentous structures (the anterior, posterior, and intra-articular SI ligaments) for stability. The posterior SI ligaments are the primary stabilizers of this joint and the strongest in the body, resisting the tendency for cephalad and posterior displacement of the

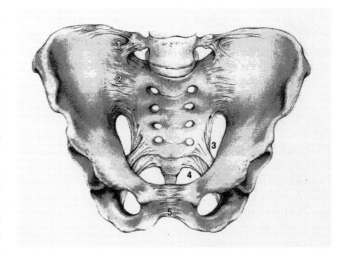

Figure 1 Diagram of pelvic bones and supporting ligaments: (1) iliolumbar ligaments, (2) SI ligaments, (3) sacrospinous ligaments, (4) sacrotuberous ligaments, and (5) symphyseal ligaments.

ilia with weight bearing. The sacrotuberous and sacrospinous ligaments act as secondary stabilizers (Figure 1).

The sacrum also articulates with the fifth lumbar vertebra via the L5-S1 disk anteriorly and the paired L5-S1 facet joints posteriorly. Unlike the other vertebral articulations, the L5-S1 motion segment is inclined at approximately 30° to the horizontal plane secondary to the anterior pelvic tilt (forward sagittal rotation or extension of the pelvis). The L5 vertebra also is tethered to the pelvis via the strong iliolumbar ligaments which pass from the transverse processes of L5 to the iliac crest just above the posterior superior iliac spine.

Because the lumbosacral junction is transitional, segmentation defects and dysmorphism frequently occur and must be recognized before surgical reduction and instrumentation procedures. Failure of segmentation often occurs with L5 being partially or completely attached to S1, with or without a vestigial disk space. At times the transverse process of L5 is enlarged and unilaterally articulates with the ilium or the sacral ala. In other instances, S1 is completely segmented from S2 and

| Table 1 | Innervation From the Lumbosacral Plexus | |
|---|---|---|
| **Nerve Root** | **Motor Function** | **Sensory Function** |
| L5 | Extensor hallucis longus, extensor digitorum longus | Lateral calf, dorsum of foot, medial sole of foot |
| S1 | Lateral hamstrings, gastrocnemius-soleus complex | Lateral posterior thigh and calf, lateral sole of foot |
| S2 | Flexor hallucis longus, flexor digitorum longus, sphincters | Medial posterior thigh and calf, lateral sole of foot |
| S3 | Flexor hallucis longus, flexor digitorum longus, sphincters | Buttocks. perineum |
| S4 | Sphincters | Perineum, perianal |
| S5 | Coccygeus | Perineum, perianal |

appears as a "sixth" lumbar vertebra. Clues to segmentation anomalies can be deduced from several other radiologic landmarks. The L4-5 disk space is usually found at the level of the iliac crest. If a chest radiograph is available, one can count down from T1 (the first vertebra at the cervicothoracic junction to have transverse processes that are directed cephalad).

Anatomically, the spinal cord terminates at L1-2; therefore, spinal cord injury does not occur with sacral fractures. The thecal sac at this level contains the cauda equina and sacral nerve roots. The L5 nerve root lies directly on the sacral ala as it courses from the L5 foramen to join the lumbosacral plexus within the pelvis. Neurologic injury at this level depends on the pattern and location of the fracture. Innervation from the lumbosacral plexus is described in Table 1.

## Classification and Diagnosis

Sacral fractures result from a wide variety of factors. These fractures can be divided into three broad groups based on the patient population involved and the energy imparted to the sacrum: (1) insufficiency fractures resulting from low-energy injury in osteoporotic bone; (2) fatigue/stress fractures resulting from cyclic low-energy injury in normal bone; and (3) traumatic fractures resulting from high-energy injury in any type of bone.

Insufficiency fractures in osteoporotic bone occur in three patient populations: elderly patients (those who are senile or have postmenopausal osteoporosis); patients with drug-induced (corticosteroids, heparin, and phenytoin) or irradiation-induced osteoporosis; and in women who are pregnant or who are in the postpartum period. Osteoporosis is a rapidly growing clinical problem in the United States with 44 million people at risk for developing the condition. The annual occurrence of insufficiency fractures is 1.5 million with most of these fractures occurring in the hip, wrist, and spine.

Although vertebral compression, hip, and wrist fractures are easily diagnosed radiographically, the diagnosis of a sacral insufficiency fracture is much more elusive. This diagnostic entity did not exist in the literature until a report in 1982 which described three patients with

"spontaneous osteoporotic fracture of the sacrum." The diagnosis of a sacral insufficiency fracture is difficult. Patients usually do not relate a history of trauma. They report activity-related (weight-bearing) low back and buttocks pain. Patients have localized tenderness to the sacrum. If the fracture is unilateral, weight bearing with a single-leg stance is painful; pain is relieved by transferring weight to the unaffected extremity. SI joint stress maneuvers (such as the Patrick's or Gaenslen's tests) may be positive. Neurologic deficit, which occurs rarely (in 2% of patients), is most commonly associated with sphincter dysfunction (urinary and or fecal incontinence) followed by leg paresthesias and weakness. Some patients report radicular symptoms secondary to irritation of the L5 or S1 nerve roots from periosteal callus on the ala, or from compression within the sacral foramina.

Diagnosing a sacral insufficiency fracture is further complicated by normal findings on plain radiographs of the pelvis and spine. In patients with severe sacral insufficiency, impaction, anterior displacement, and kyphotic deformity may be seen on the lateral projection; however, this is not the rule. CT may disclose callus or periosteal reaction in the anterior aspect of the ala, but again, this is not the rule.

An MRI scan and/or a bone scan is required to make the diagnosis. A classic sign of a sacral insufficiency fracture is increased signal or uptake in the sacral ala (at times bilaterally), showing the shape of an "H" (Figure 2). Although not all patients exhibit this sign, some variation of the sign without increased uptake in other body areas is highly suggestive of a sacral insufficiency fracture. Bone scans require significant radiation exposure (approximately equivalent to 200 chest radiographs); therefore, MRI is considered the superior imaging modality. In an elderly patient with a history of cancer, the presence of pain and increased uptake or signal on MRI or bone scans often leads to an extensive metastatic workup and biopsy. However, isolated metastases to the sacrum are rare. The use of fat suppression MRI helps to rule out the diagnosis of neoplasia.

Stress or fatigue fractures of the sacrum occur in young patients with normal bone that is subjected to abnormal cyclic stress. The typical patient is a young, elite or high-level athlete or a military recruit. The clinical presentation is similar to that of patients with sacral insufficiency fractures, with the patient reporting activity-related low back and buttocks pain. The patient's history usually involves a report of pain that initially occurs following activity. As the condition progresses, pain with strenuous activities and then with normal activities is common. Neurologic deficit is rare, and, if present, usually represents irritation of the L5 or S1 nerve root from callus.

These fractures differ from sacral insufficiency fractures in that repetitive subthreshold stresses placed on the bone cause microfractures or damage that does not heal. A high degree of clinical suspicion of the condition and a confirmation of the diagnosis using MRI and/or bone scans is needed as in patients with insufficiency fractures.

Traumatic high-energy sacral fractures can be subdivided into groups based on the fracture pattern or location. The Denis classification system is the most commonly used and categorizes fractures based on fracture line orientation and location (Figure 3). Traumatic sacral fractures occur in approximately 30% of all pelvic ring injuries. Zone 1 fractures, which represent 50% of sacral fractures and result in neurologic deficits in 6% of patients, are vertical or oblique and pass lateral to the sacral foramina. Zone 2 fractures are vertical or oblique and traverse one or more of the sacral foramina. These fractures make up 36% of sacral factures and result in neurologic deficit in 30% of patients. Zone 3 fractures are a more heterogeneous group. They can be horizontal or vertical, but are all medial to the sacral foramina and enter the sacral spinal canal. Zone 3 fractures comprise 16% of sacral fractures and carry a 60% risk of neuro-

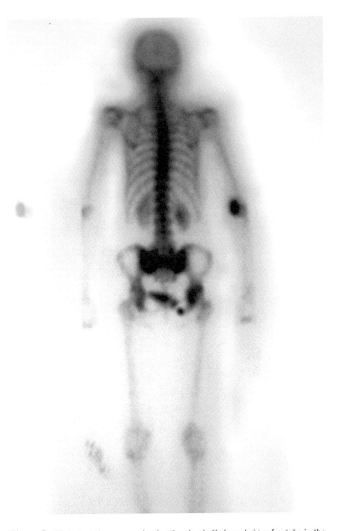

Figure 2  Whole body bone scan showing the classic H-shaped sign of uptake in the sacrum.

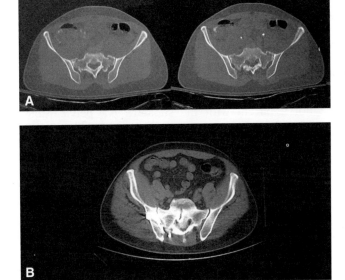

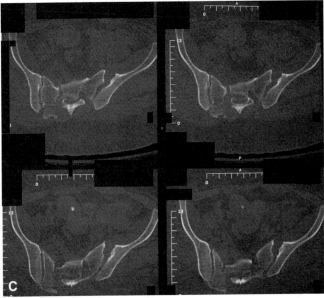

Figure 3  **A,** Axial CT scan of zone 1 sacral fracture. **B,** Axial CT scan of zone 2 sacral fracture. **C,** Axial CT scan of zone 3 sacral fracture.

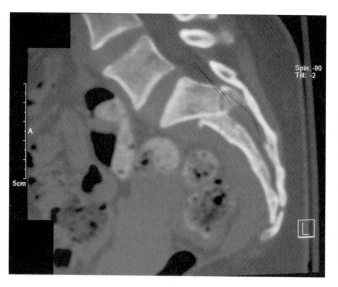

Figure 4  Sagittal CT reconstruction of U-shaped sacral fracture-dislocation.

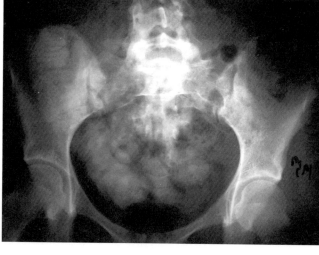

Figure 5  AP pelvic radiograph of a patient with a U-shaped sacral fracture. Note the subtle inlet view of proximal sacrum and the outlet view of distal sacrum.

logic injury both to nerve roots and the cauda equina.

Zone 1 and 2 sacral fractures compromise pelvic ring stability but do not affect spinal stability unless the fracture line extends proximally to disrupt the L5-S1 articulation. Zone 3 fractures can disrupt both the pelvic ring and spinal stability depending on the fracture pattern.

Vertical midline splits are associated with anteroposterior compression-type instabilities of the pelvic ring. Horizontal fracture patterns do not affect pelvic ring stability, but may affect spinal stability depending on their location relative to the SI joints. Horizontal fractures below the level of the SI joints are stable injuries that present a risk for injury to the spinal nerves and cauda equina secondary to canal occlusion from fracture fragments.

Horizontal fractures at the level of the SI joints are always associated with bilateral vertical splits (usually transforaminal) creating a U-shaped or H-shaped fracture pattern. The various fracture configurations have been described in the literature. Unlike other sacral fractures (zone 1 and 2), which are the result of vertical shear and/or internal and external rotation injury to the pelvic ring, these injuries are the result of rapid, acute hyperflexion of the pelvis and lumbosacral junction. This unstable injury pattern results in spinal-pelvic dissociation (no mechanical continuity between the spine and pelvis). These injuries lead to kyphotic deformation and impaction with compromise of the sacral spinal canal (Figure 4). Diagnosis at presentation can be difficult, particularly with zone 3 injuries. Patients usually report a history of significant trauma such as a fall from a height or motor vehicle collision and also report low back pain.

Patients with zone 1 or 2 fractures have injuries of the pelvic ring. Depending on the amount of energy absorbed and direction of the force, these patients may have injuries involving lateral compression, anteroposterior compression, vertical shear, or any combination of these injury types with little displacement or with wide-open pelvic instability. Minimally displaced or impacted fractures of the sacrum can be difficult to detect on plain radiographs (AP pelvis), but should be suspected in any trauma patient with low back or buttocks pain. Because the pelvis is a ring structure, minimally displaced fractures in the anterior aspect of the pelvic ring should provide a clue to secondary posterior ring disruption. CT scanning of the pelvis with 3 mm cuts should disclose an occult posterior sacral fracture.

Patients with higher-energy fractures and disruptions can have limb-length inequality in vertical shear-type injuries of the unstable hemipelvis, and scrotal/labial ecchymosis with externally rotated lower extremities in open-book type injuries. Rectal and vaginal examinations are necessary to rule out mucosal perforation from fracture spikes, and cystography is mandatory to rule out bladder and urethral injury.

A delay in diagnosis is common in patients with zone 3 injuries unless there is a high index of suspicion for the injury. Transverse and U-shaped sacral fractures are not apparent with the standard AP pelvic radiograph used in the trauma series (Figure 5). The classic radiographic finding is an inlet view of the proximal sacrum and an outlet view of the distal sacrum. The lateral radiograph of the pelvis or sacrum which shows the acute angulation between sacral elements with or without AP translation is the key to diagnosis. This injury may be missed with axial cut CT scanning because the cuts are in the same plane as the fracture; sagittal reconstructions are helpful and should be obtained at the same time. The CT images are helpful in assessing foraminal and canal stenosis secondary to fracture fragments and deformity.

A rectal examination is mandatory in any patient with a suspected sacral fracture to rule out cauda equina syndrome. Patients with pelvic ring injuries are often given a cursory lower extremity neurologic examination that, at best, assesses L4 to S1. Although this examination may reveal no abnormalities, the patient may have complete loss of sensation at S2-4 because of cauda equina compression or sacral nerve root entrapment. The neurologic rectal examination should focus on perianal sensory deficits, loss of rectal tone, inability to voluntarily contract the anal sphincter, and loss of the bulbocavernosus reflex. The bulbocavernosus reflex can be elicited by squeezing the glans penis in a male or by gently tugging on a urinary catheter in a female.

## Treatment

### Sacral Insufficiency Fractures

Sacral insufficiency fractures have been treated with variable amounts of relative bed rest and the administration of analgesics for 3 to 5 weeks, followed by mobilization and physical therapy. Treatment for osteoporosis is initiated if needed. However, concerns remain regarding the complications associated with prolonged bed rest in elderly patients. Some physicians have found favorable results with immediate mobilization, the administration of appropriate analgesics, and the initiation of osteoporosis management when needed. Nonsurgical management with variable periods of bed rest and mobilization yields resolution of symptoms in most patients within 3 months. In a small subset of patients, symptoms are not resolved and continued pain with activity impairs their ability to perform activities of daily living. In this group of patient, sacroplasty is recommended by some authors.

Sacroplasty involves augmentation of the fractured region with polymethylmethacrylate (bone cement) injected percutaneously. This procedure is akin to cement augmentation of vertebral compression fractures (vertebroplasty or kyphoplasty). In 2002, sacroplasty was first described as a treatment for sacral insufficiency fractures after its use achieved notable success in treating metastatic lesions to the sacrum. Numerous reports in the past few years have reported the nearly immediate relief or substantial reduction of symptoms that occurs following treatment with sacroplasty.

### Sacral Stress or Fatigue Fractures

Sacral stress or fatigue fractures can be more difficult to treat because these fractures usually occur in young, active, athletic patients who do not respond well or who are not compliant with immobilization or activity restrictions. As a general rule, most sacral fatigue fractures will heal if the patient avoids the stress producing activity for approximately 6 weeks and then participates in an additional 6-week program of gradual physical re-

conditioning, strengthening, and reintroduction of the stress producing activity. Aquatic activities and cycling are permissible to maintain aerobic conditioning.

If the patient's symptoms are chronic and occur with regular daily activities, immobilization is then required. Fatigue fractures tend to be unilateral in young patients as opposed to the bilateral fractures usually found in older patients with osteoporosis. In patients who have protracted symptoms, a period of touch-down weight bearing with crutches is indicated to allow sufficient healing before initiating a gradual reintroduction of physical activity and weight bearing. Radicular symptoms can be expected to dissipate spontaneously with healing of the fracture and diminution of the callus. Sacroplasty is not recommended for young patients with fatigue fractures of the sacrum.

### Traumatic Sacral Fractures

Appropriate treatment of traumatic sacral fractures depends on the location and pattern of the fracture, the presence of impaction, the integrity of the L5-S1 facet joint, and the presence of neurologic deficit (radiculopathy or cauda equina syndrome). Any longitudinal sacral fracture that is impacted without vertical shift or limb-length discrepancy can be treated with a trial of nonsurgical care because impaction provides some stability to the fracture and pelvic ring. Bed rest for 3 to 5 days followed by mobilization with protected weight bearing is safe. Repeat inlet, outlet, and AP pelvic radiographs are performed within the first week of mobilization. If no shift in the fracture occurs, then continuation of protected weight bearing for 12 weeks with close radiographic follow-up is indicated.

The presentation of the patient while in bed is often a good indicator of whether nonsurgical care will be possible for a nondisplaced fracture. Patients that are unable to roll over and use a bed pan effectively without severe low back pain tend to have unstable injuries and may require evaluation of pelvic stability using general anesthesia and fluoroscopy. If gross instability is apparent on evaluation under anesthesia, surgical stabilization to allow early mobilization is recommended. Delaying surgery for 3 to 5 days to allow stabilization of pelvic hematoma and clotting is recommended to help minimize intraoperative bleeding. The patient should be kept on bed rest with skeletal traction to minimize further limb-length inequality.

### *Type 1 Sacral Fractures: Nonimpacted With Displacement*

In type 1 sacral fractures with minimal displacement, open reduction and internal fixation (ORIF) of the anterior ring (symphysis pubis or rami fractures) helps to align the hemipelvis and indirectly reduces the sacral fracture to allow the placement of percutaneous iliosac-

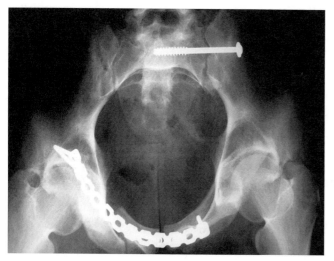

Figure 6    Iliosacral screw used for treatment of a zone 1 sacral fracture.

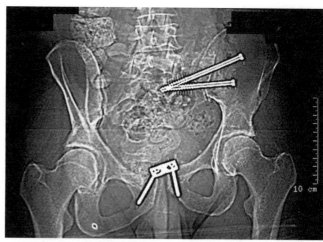

Figure 7    Failure of the iliosacral screws used for an unstable comminuted zone 2 sacral fracture. Note the loose screws and vertical displacement of the hemipelvis.

ral screws. This surgery can be done with the patient supine. If, however, the sacral fracture is widely displaced, ORIF of the sacrum should be done through a posterior approach to allow anatomic reduction of the posterior pelvic ring. Again, iliosacral screws are used. The patient can then be repositioned supine for ORIF of the anterior pelvic ring if necessary (Figure 6).

### Type 2 Sacral Fractures: Nonimpacted With Displacement

By definition type 2 sacral fractures traverse the sacral foramina. Treatment and fixation of these injuries must take into account the potential for iatrogenic injury to the L5 and sacral nerve roots. Careful preoperative neurologic assessment must document function of the sacral nerve roots as previously discussed. The CT scan must be carefully assessed to rule out residual compression of the sacral nerve roots by fracture fragments as well as any injury and potential instability of the L5-S1 facet joint. If residual nerve root compression is observed and the patient exhibits a neurologic deficit attributable to that compression, the patient should have a sacral nerve root decompressive laminectomy in addition to reduction and stabilization.

In fractures in which there is minimal or no comminution with an intact L5-S1 facet joint (such that there is only a small chance of vertical displacement), iliosacral screw fixation with supplemental anterior stabilization is adequate if the patient can maintain touch-down weight bearing on the affected side for 10 to 12 weeks. In fractures in which there is significant comminution and displacement, or if the L5-S1 facet joint is disrupted, iliosacral screw fixation is less reliable with a reported high failure rate both clinically and biomechanically (Figure 7). The use of these screws for this particular sacral fracture pattern results in poor resistance to vertical shear deforming forces.

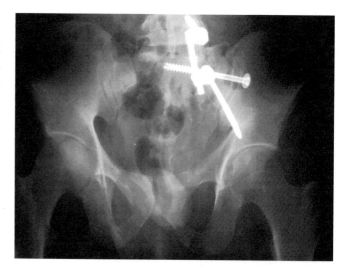

Figure 8    Spinal pelvic fixation used for a zone 2 fracture with vertical shear.

Spinal-pelvic fixation (also known as lumbopelvic fixation or triangular osteosynthesis) has been used to address these concerns for this particular clinical scenario. A lumbar pedicle screw is connected to an iliac screw positioned at the posterior superior iliac spine. This connection uses clamps that have a fixed angle, which allows vertical alignment of the fixation to resist vertical shear forces. The fixation is often supplemented with a "position" iliosacral screw (not placed under compression) to resist rotation around the iliac screw. Biomechanical and clinical studies have confirmed the superiority of this fixation technique compared with the use of iliosacral screws for this particular injury pattern (Figure 8).

### Pros and Cons of Spinal-Pelvic Fixation

Because spinal-pelvic fixation is rigid and fixed-angled, early (immediate to 6 weeks) weight bearing is permit-

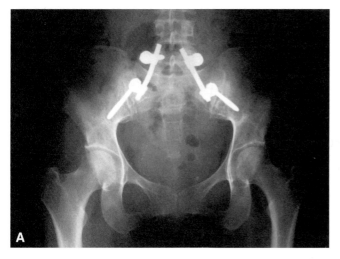

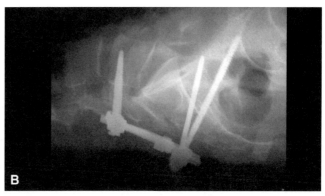

Figure 9  AP pelvis **(A)** and lateral **(B)** postoperative radiographs of the sacrum of a patients treated with surgical decompression, reduction, and fixation for a U-shaped sacral fracture.

ted. Little to no postoperative loss of reduction is observed compared with traditional iliosacral screw fixation. However, the fixation can be quite prominent at the posterior superior iliac spine in thin patients. This fixation crosses two potentially normal articulations (the SI joint and L5-S1 joint) and limits their normal motion that occurs with normal activities at these articulations. Most patients report activity-related low back pain or discomfort from the implant that almost invariably necessitates removal of the fixation after the fracture has healed. Fracture healing is confirmed by a CT scan taken 6 months after fixation.

### Type 3 Sacral Fractures
These injuries usually involve an open-book type pattern with diastasis anteriorly and gapping of the sacral fracture posteriorly, secondary to external rotation of the hemipelvis. Vertical shear/displacement usually does not occur secondary to the buttressing effect of the L5 vertebra and L5-S1 facet joint above. With significant energy and disruption of the L5-S1 facet joint however, vertical shear can occur. These injuries can be treated by closing the pelvic ring anteriorly. If a residual fracture gap exists in the sacrum, a long iliosacral screw can be placed across into the contralateral ala to compress the fracture and prevent fibrous nonunion. If vertical shear is present with comminution and facet disruption, consideration should be given to spinal-pelvic fixation.

### Transverse and U-Shaped Sacral Fractures
Transverse and U-shaped sacral fractures do not disrupt the integrity of the pelvic ring, but may result in discontinuity of the spine and pelvis (spinal-pelvic dissociation) and/or compression of the sacral spinal canal and cauda equina syndrome. Transverse fractures below the level of the SI joints do not compromise pelvic ring or spinal-pelvic stability. Consideration of surgical treatment, therefore, is predicated on the presence of cauda

equina syndrome. If cauda equina syndrome is present, a sacral laminectomy should be performed as soon as the patient's condition permits; this procedure will help prevent long-term bowel, bladder, and sexual dysfunction.

Transverse fractures at the level of the SI joints are associated with bilateral longitudinal fractures, usually having a zone 2 pattern. These fractures are highly unstable at the spinal-pelvic junction with resultant kyphotic and/or translational deformity. Surgical stabilization is required for mobilization and/or sacral canal decompression if indicated. Treatment consists of decompressing the spinal canal, reducing the deformity, and stabilizing the fracture. Often, placing the patient prone and extending the hips will affect some reduction and canal decompression. If the patient has signs of cauda equina syndrome, a sacral laminectomy should be performed.

Stabilization involves controlling the sagittal plane deformation (increased kyphosis and anterior translation). To effectively control the sagittal plane deforming forces, the posterior tension band must be restored. Spinal-pelvic fixation or standard lumbosacral instrumentation has the ability to lock into the lumbar spine and reestablish a stable connection to the pelvis while resisting anterior rotation and translation (Figure 9). However, there are reports in the literature that advocate the application of bilateral iliosacral screws alone for stabilization of this injury pattern.

## Summary
Sacral fractures encompass a large spectrum of injuries. They can result from low-energy or high-energy trauma in osteoporotic or healthy bone. Sacral fractures can destabilize the lumbosacral junction and/or the pelvic ring. Because of these varied presentations, diagnosis and treatment can be complex.

## Annotated Bibliography

### Anatomy

Zinghi GF, Briccoli A, Bungaro P, et al: Principles of anatomy, in *Fractures of the Pelvis and Acetabulum*. Thieme, 2004, p 20.

This chapter describes general principles of anatomy.

### Classification and Diagnosis

Aylwin A, Saifuddin A, Tucker S: L5 radiculopathy due to sacral stress fracture. *Skeletal Radiol* 2003;32:590-593.

A clinical case of L5 radioculopathy secondary to callus from a sacral alar fracture is described.

Finiels PJ, Finiels H, Strubel D, Jaquot JM: Spontaneous osteoporotic fractures of the sacrum causing neurological damage: Report of three cases. *J Neurosurg* 2002; 97(suppl 3):380-385.

This report outlines the pathoanatomic mechanisms by which radiculopathy can be generated by neural irritation from fracture callus.

Fujii M, Abe K, Hayashi K, et al: Honda sign and variants in patients suspected of having a sacral insufficiency fracture. *Clin Nucl Med* 2005;30:165-169.

Bone scan appearances for sacral/stress/insufficiency fractures are reviewed.

Lin JT, Lutz GE: Post-partum sacral fracture presenting as lumbar radiculopathy: A case report. *Arch Phys Med Rehabil* 2004;85:1358-1361.

This case report discusses postpartum sacral fracture in a patient who presented with low back pain and radicular symptoms.

National Osteoporosis Foundation. Available at http://www.nof.org/osteoporosis/diseasefacts.htm. Accessed January 2006.

This website provides demographic/epidemiologic statistics on osteoporosis in the United States.

Slipman CW, Gilchrist RV, Isaac Z, Lenrow DA, Chou LH: Sacral stress fracture in a female field-hockey player. *Am J Phys Med Rehabil* 2003;82:893-896.

This article describes the first reported case of a sacral stress fracture in a field hockey player.

Wild A, Jaeger M, Haak H, Mehdian SH: Sacral insufficiency fracture: An unsuspected cause of low-back pain in elderly women. *Arch Orthop Trauma Surg* 2002;122:58-60.

In a 72-year-old woman with severe low back pain, MRI revealed edema on both sides of the sacrum and CT confirmed the presence of an insufficiency fracture.

### Treatment

Butler CL, Given CA II, Michel SJ, Tibbs PA: Percutaneous sacroplasty for the treatment of sacral insufficiency fractures. *AJR Am J Roentgenol* 2005;184:1956-1959.

Deen HG, Nottmeier EW: Balloon kyphoplasty for treatment of sacral insufficiency fractures: Report of three cases. *Neurosurg Focus* 2005;18:e7.

Garant M: Sacroplasty: A new treatment for sacral insufficiency fracture. *J Vasc Interv Radiol* 2002;13:1265-1267.

These three articles present an excellent review of the current literature regarding techniques, indications, and pitfalls of the most recent treatments for sacral insufficiency fractures.

Griffin DR, Starr AJ, Reinert CM, Jones AL, Whitlock S: Vertically unstable pelvic fractures fixed with percutaneous ilio-sacral screws: Does posterior injury pattern predict fixation failure. *J Orthop Trauma* 2003;17:399-405.

This article discusses the high incidence of failure/reoperation when iliosacral screws alone are used to treat comminuted zone 2 sacral fractures.

Nork SE, Jones CB, Harding SP, Mirza SK, Routt ML Jr: Percutaneous stabilization of U-shaped sacral fractures using iliosacral screws: Technique and early results. *J Orthop Trauma* 2001;15:238-246.

The technique and results (including decompression and postoperative mobilization) for treating spinal pelvic dissociation with iliosacral screws alone is described in this article.

Schildhauer TA, Ledoux WR, Chapman JR, Henley MB, Tencer AF, Routt ML Jr: Triangular osteosynthesis and iliosacral screw fixation for unstable sacral fractures: A cadaveric and biomechanical evaluation under cyclic loads. *J Orthop Trauma* 2003;17:22-31.

This article introduces the technique and compares triangular osteosynthesis to iliosacral screw fixation for zone 2 sacral fractures.

## Classic Bibliography

Babayev M, Lachmann E, Nagler W: The controversy surrounding sacral insufficiency fractures: To ambulate or not to ambulate. *Am J Phys Med Rehabil* 2000;79:404-409.

Carter SR: Stress fracture of the sacrum: Brief report. *J Bone Joint Surg Br* 1987;69:843-844.

Crockett HC, Wright JM, Madsen MW, Bates JE, Potter HG, Warren RF: Sacral stress fracture in an elite college basketball player after the use of a jumping machine. *Am J Sports Med* 1999;27:526-528.

Denis F, Davis S, Comfort T: Sacral fractures: An important problem: Retrospective analysis of 236 cases. *Clin Orthop Relat Res* 1988;227:67-81.

Featherstone T: Magnetic resonance imaging in the diagnosis of sacral stress fracture. *Br J Sports Med* 1999; 33:276-277.

Fyhrie DP, Milgrom C, Hoshaw SJ, et al: Effect of fatiguing exercise on longitudinal bone strain as related to stress fractures in humans. *Ann Biomed Eng* 1988;26: 660-665.

Grasland A, Pouchot J, Mathieu A, Paycha F, Vinceneux P: Sacral insufficiency fractures: An easily overlooked cause of back pain in elderly women. *Arch Intern Med* 1996;156:668-674.

Isler B: Lumbosacral lesions associated with pelvic ring injuries. *J Orthop Trauma* 1990;4:1-6.

Jones DN, Wycherley AG: Bone scan demonstration of progression of sacral insufficiency stress fracture. *Australas Radiol* 1994;38:148-150.

Kach K, Trentz O: Distraction spondylodesis of the sacrum in "vertical shear lesions" of the pelvis. *Unfallchirurg* 1994;97:28-38.

Lechevalier D, Magnin J, Eulry F: Truncated sciatica as the first manifestation of fatigue fracture of the sacrum in a young male. *Rev Rhum Engl Ed* 1996;63:505.

Lourie H: Spontaneous osteoporotic fracture of the sacrum: An unrecognized syndrome of the elderly. *JAMA* 1982;248:715-717.

McFarland EG, Giangarra C: Sacral stress fractures in athletes. *Clin Orthop Relat Res* 1996;329:240-243.

Moed BR, Morawa LG: Displaced midline longitudinal fracture of the sacrum. *J Trauma* 1984;24:435-437.

Orava S, Hulkko A: Delayed unions and nonunions of stress fractures in athletes. *Am J Sports Med* 1988;16: 378-382.

Roy-Camille R, Saillant G, Gagna G, Mazel C: Transverse fracture of the upper sacrum: Suicidal jumper's fracture. *Spine* 1984;10:838-845.

Savolaine ER, Ebrahim NA, Rusin JJ, Jackson WT: Limitations of radiography and computed tomography in the diagnosis of transverse sacral fracture from a high fall. *Clin Orthop* 1991;272:122-126.

Schildhauer TA, Josten C, Muhr G: Triangular osteosynthesis of vertically unstable sacrum fractures: A new concept allowing early weight-bearing. *J Orthop Trauma* 1998;12:307-314.

Simonain PT, Routt C Jr, Harrington RM, Tencer AF: Internal fixation of the transforaminal sacral fracture. *Clin Orthop* 1996;323:202-209.

Strange-Vognsen HH, Lebech A: An unusual type of fracture in the upper sacrum. *J Orthop Trauma* 1991;5: 200-203.

Thienpont E, Simon JP, Fabry G: Sacral stress fracture during pregnancy: A case report. *Acta Orthop Scand* 1999;70:525-526.

Volpin G, Milgrom C, Goldsher D, Stein H: Stress fractures of the sacrum following strenuous activity. *Clin Orthop Relat Res* 1989;243:184-188.

Young JW, Burgess AR, Brumback RJ, Poka A: Pelvic fractures: Value of plain radiography in early assessment and management. *Radiology* 1986;160:445-451.

# Chapter 25

# Acute Neck Pain and Cervical Disk Herniation

Michael J. Bolesta, MD

Kevin Gill, MD

## Introduction

Acute neck pain has a diverse differential diagnosis. When high-energy trauma is involved, the physician must assess the patient for fracture, dislocation, instability, and neural compression. In the absence of significant trauma, acute pain warrants immediate assessment if there is a reasonable possibility of neoplasm or infection. Attendant significant neurologic deficit will also prompt early testing. In the absence of these conditions, acute neck pain can usually be treated expectantly and symptomatically. Testing is reserved for patients who do not respond to standard nonsurgical treatment.

The cervical disk is an important component of the vertebral column, providing support and facilitating movement. Although the cells of the disk are capable of homeostasis and repair, many disks will show some degeneration as individuals reach midlife. Almost all individuals who are age 70 years and older have degeneration of the cervical spinal column. This degeneration is strongly influenced by genetic and lifestyle factors; furthermore, the lower cervical levels are more susceptible to this process. Whereas a normal disk can sustain greater loads than the adjoining bone, a degenerative disk may fail with physiologic loading. Depending on the pattern of stress, the anulus fibrosus may tear with or without herniation of the nucleus.

Most herniations occur in a paramedian location but also may occur centrally, foraminally, or anteriorly. The most common level for a herniation is C5-6. Herniations also commonly occur at C4-5 and C6-7; however, they may occur at any level. The size and location of the herniation coupled with the degree of inflammation determine the symptoms. Other important factors are the native size of the canal and foramina (which vary between individuals); the presence of other degenerative pathology such as uncovertebral hypertrophy, facet arthropathy, ligamentum flavum hypertrophy and ossification; and ossification of the posterior longitudinal ligament. Some patients with disk herniations are asymptomatic, whereas other patients may have pure axial neck pain. Disk herniations may incite radiculopathy, with or without neurologic deficit, may precipitate cervical myelopathy, or may manifest in some patients as a combination of myelopathy, radiculopathy, and cervicalgia.

## Diagnosis

The diagnosis of cervical disk herniation can usually be made based on the patient's history when attended by radiculopathy or myelopathy. The physical examination will often corroborate the history or suggest a different pathology. Further testing is prompted by severe, persistent, or worsening pain, or significant neurologic deficit. MRI is highly sensitive and specific and will often be sufficient to make a diagnosis. Both hardware and software improvements have yielded better imaging in less time. Scanners allowing the patient to sit upright and to assume different positions (such as flexion and extension) may enhance the ability to characterize pathologic anatomy. When MRI is equivocal or contraindicated, cervical myelography followed by CT or CT with intrathecal contrast (and no formal myelogram) will precisely define the nature, location, and extent of the herniation, as well as other attendant pathology.

The visualized pathology should be correlated to symptoms and signs. If this correlation is not acceptable (the observed deficit does not correspond to the myotome or dermatome of the involved root), nerve conduction velocity studies and electromyography may be useful. Other indications for electrical studies are a history of neuropathy or peripheral nerve entrapment, a history of surgery for entrapment or upper extremity trauma, and previous cervical surgery. Individual deviations from expected dermatomal and myotomal patterns occur and should be considered as part of the assessment.

Disk degeneration and herniation can produce axial pain without cord or nerve root involvement. Unless the herniation is an isolated abnormality, there is poor correlation between cervical disk disease and symptoms in the absence of radiculopathy or myelopathy. Some clinicians use diskography to plan surgical intervention for cervicalgia; however, the literature offers few data to support this technique. It is important to remember that disk degeneration is common in asymptomatic individuals.

## Nonsurgical Treatment

The natural history of disk herniation is usually favorable. Cervical radiculopathy caused by disk herniation will resolve spontaneously in approximately 95% of patients. Symptomatic treatment will suffice unless symptoms persist, worsen, or are attended by a significant loss of motor or sensory function. Myelopathy also may be treated without surgery if it is mild and not progressive. Because symptoms are nonspecific, disk herniation as a cause of axial neck pain is seldom identified based on clinical findings alone. When the condition is diagnosed, most practitioners prefer nonsurgical management.

Nonsurgical treatment has remained unchanged for many years and includes physical therapy, cervical collars, traction, and medications. Breakthroughs in nonsurgical care are probably decades away from use in clinical practice. Several investigators have conceptually proven that it is possible to repopulate the cellular component of the disk or to introduce the cells that could reconstitute a more normal structure. Although such developments are exciting, much more research is needed.

## Surgical Treatment
### Indications for Surgery

Absolute indications for surgery in patients with acute neck pain include progressive neurologic deficit caused by treatable pathology and significant instability. With cervical disk herniation, absolute indications are progressive or significant myelopathy, and radiculopathy with progressive or significant motor deficit that is not improving. Relative indications are radicular symptoms that are not resolving with appropriate nonsurgical management. Axial pain without neurologic symptoms or signs is generally not amenable to surgery unless there is discrete pathology such as infection, neoplasm, fracture, or instability.

Posterior approaches are useful for lateral (intraforaminal) disk herniations, foraminal stenosis, and posterior element pathology. Anterior approaches can address canal or foraminal neural compression (Figure 1).

### Minimally Invasive Surgery

The concept of minimally invasive surgery is very popular with the general public, who often attribute too much importance to the size of the external scar. The size or type of incision is important, but should not compromise the success of the procedure.

Anterior cervical disk surgery can often be accomplished through a short, oblique incision using standard equipment, which results in a cosmetically acceptable

scar. Diskectomy without fusion is well described but has not achieved the popularity of diskectomy combined with fusion. Diskectomy without fusion may result in persistent cervicalgia and recurrent radiculopathy from settling and foraminal narrowing. There have been reports of the use of limited anterior diskectomy (dissecting only enough anterior disk to remove the herniated portion while preserving the remaining disk). This procedure is technically demanding and may result in inadequate decompression. Furthermore, the residual disk is degenerate. No convincing data show that limited diskectomy is superior to conventional anterior cervical diskectomy and fusion (ACDF).

Foraminal disk herniations are amenable to laminoforaminotomy. This procedure can also be performed through small incisions. Some surgeons have used paramedian muscle-splitting approaches to further minimize the dissection. This approach has been facilitated by the use of serial dilation and tube retractors originally developed for lumbar microdiskectomy.

### Surgical Technique

Most disk herniations may be treated with an anterior approach. Many orthopaedic spine surgeons prefer ACDF because it is predictable and achieves almost uniformly good results in the management of both radiculopathy and myelopathy. Although autogenous iliac crest bone has been used for decades as the standard graft material, donor site morbidity has prompted the search for alternative materials.

Anterior diskectomy and fusion is performed through an oblique incision in a skin crease at the level of interest. Although many surgeons favor the left side because of the more predictable course of the recurrent laryngeal nerve, recent studies indicate that iatrogenic palsies of that nerve are of equal incidence on the right and the left. After dividing the platysma and superficial layer of the deep cervical fascia, the trachea and esophagus are mobilized medially. The sternocleidomastoid and carotid bundle are gently retracted laterally. The pretracheal and prevertebral fasciae are split longitudinally. After confirming the level radiographically, the longus colli is reflected laterally. The anterior longitudinal ligament and anterior anulus fibrosus are incised, and diskectomy is performed with magnification and illumination (operating microscope or loupes with headlight). Osteophytes and the posterior longitudinal ligament are removed as necessary. Decompression is facilitated by traction or distraction of the interspace. Foraminotomy may be performed by removing part of the uncinate process. End plates are prepared and the graft of choice inserted. Restoration of segmental height will enlarge the foramina, decompressing the nerve roots, even without formal foraminotomy. An anterior plate is often used, and some surgeons will not immobi-

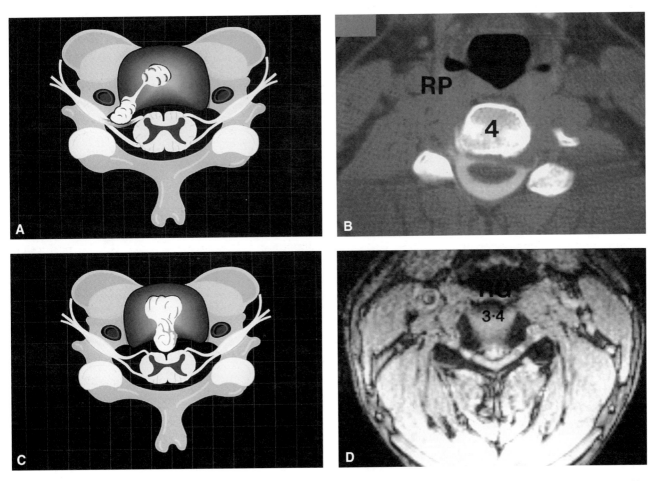

Figure 1  An axial schematic representation of a right posterolateral soft disk herniation **(A)** with a corresponding CT/myelogram image **(B)** from a patient with a left C4-5 disk herniation causing a C5 radiculopathy. This pathology could be effectively treated with either an anterior cervical diskectomy and fusion or a posterior keyhole lamino-foraminotomy. In contrast, **C** and **D** illustrate a central cervical disk herniation with severe cord compression and advanced myelopathy that should be treated with an anterior excision to avoid manipulation of the spinal cord. Indirect decompression via a laminoplasty might also be considered. Attempts to remove the disk fragment via a posterior exposure would risk further spinal cord injury. *(Reproduced from Heller JG: Surgical treatment of degenerative cervical disc disease, in Fardon DF, Garfin SR (eds): Orthopaedic Knowledge Update Spine 2. Rosemont, IL, American Academy of Orthopaedic Surgeons, 2002, p 299-309.)*

lize the patient. Without a plate most surgeons have the patient use a cervical orthosis for a period of time (for example, 6 weeks). A drain is usually used. The platysma, subcutaneous tissue, and skin are closed, and the wound is dressed. Diet is advanced as tolerated, observing the patient for dysphagia, dysphonia, and dyspnea. Absent significant airway or swallowing difficulties, patients generally mobilize quickly. Those patients with significant myelopathy may benefit from inpatient rehabilitation. Patients with radiculopathy generally enjoy relief of pain and improvement of motor function; sensory recovery is not always complete, nor is motor function always normal if the preoperative deficit was severe. Prognosis of myelopathy depends on the severity and duration of the cord compression. Most of the time, progression can be arrested. Milder myelopathy of short duration will often resolve.

Posterior diskectomy or foraminotomy can be done in the prone, lateral, or sitting position. Either a midline muscle stripping or paramedian muscle splitting approach may be used. The latter approach provides unilateral exposure, and may be less painful. The medial third of the facet joint (overlap of the inferior and superior articular processes) are removed with a burr. The underlying root is carefully mobilized and hemostasis achieved. The soft disk herniation is removed. Accessible osteophytes may also be removed. The wound is closed in layers. A collar may be used for a short period of time for comfort. In carefully selected patients, relief of radiculopathy is rapid, equivalent to anterior diskectomy, and fusion is avoided. Visualization and adequate decompression are essential to a good outcome. A soft foraminal disk herniation is the best indication for a posterior approach. If the herniation is not removed or there is inadequate decompression of the foraminal stenosis, the procedure will fail.

### Graft for Fusion

Various forms of allograft have been used and are still popular. Clinical outcomes for neurologic symptoms are

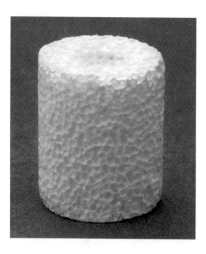

Figure 2 This ceramic of tricalcium phosphate resembles cancellous bone, providing a lattice for osteoprogenitor cells to populate. It is osteoconductive, but not osteoinductive (Chronos, Synthes Spine).

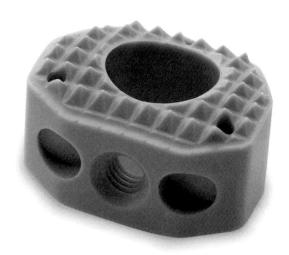

Figure 3 A spacer fabricated of polyethyletherketone resembles a tricortical iliac crest graft for a Smith-Robinson type fusion. The central cavity may be filled with cancellous autograft, synthetic matrix (with or without marrow aspirate), or BMP and carrier. There are metal markers to determine implant position, but the bulk of the implant is radiolucent, allowing the physician to assess the fusion (Vertebral Spacer, Synthes Spine).

similar to those achieved using autograft, which is not surprising because decompression is identical. Fusion rates seem to be comparable for single-level fusions. With multiple-level fusions, the use of allograft results in a high rate of fibrous nonunion when no instrumentation is used. Anterior plating seems to partially mitigate this complication. However, the current literature is inconclusive concerning the efficacy of anterior plating in multilevel allografting and is limited by the relatively small number of studies that have been done. The Cervical Spine Research Society sponsored a multicenter prospective (but not randomized) study examining cervical spine fusions (anterior initially, and later expanded to include the posterior approach) with and without instrumentation. To date, the data have not been published. Such studies are difficult to perform but provide very valuable information.

Many surgeons use allograft bone as a structural support and supplement it in some manner to stimulate fusion. Techniques include the use of releasing hormone bone morphogenetic protein (rhBMP)-2 and rhBMP-7 (osteogenic protein-1). This off-label use of these proteins is being studied at some centers with an investigational device exemption. The safety and efficacy of this strategy has yet to be determined. rhBMP-2 that is not well contained has been associated with massive anterior swelling during the early postoperative period. Other researchers have advocated the use of platelet-derived growth factors. Although basic science principles suggest that this technique is feasible, clinical data concerning the use of platelet-derived growth factors in the cervical spine is lacking. BMP is osteoinductive, whereas platelet-derived growth factors are not; however, they are said to be osteopromotive. In the lumbar spine, one of the autogenous platelet preparations has been associated with a decreased rate of fusion when combined with autogenous iliac crest. Such observations, although a cause for concern, are critical in the application of new technologies.

Another strategy to stimulate fusion is the use of a synthetic matrix, usually a combination of collagen and a mineral such as hydroxyapatite. Several formulations are commercially available. Synthetic matrices are said to be osteoconductive and are usually combined with autogenous bone marrow to provide osteoprogenitor cells. Although this process is based on sound theory and supportive animal studies, confirmation based on studies in the cervical spine are not yet available. These implants are probably safe; however, their efficacy relative to autograft or allograft alone has not been proven. Ceramic matrices have been used in humans and animals; however, their usefulness has been hampered by brittleness, fracture, and fragmentation and they must be protected (Figure 2). Ceramic matrices are class III devices, which are not yet approved by the U.S. Food and Drug Administration (FDA) for this use.

Because the use of allograft has a small risk of infection and generates a variable immune response, several substitutes have been developed to provide structural support while depending on synthetic grafts and marrow aspirates or rhBMP to stimulate bone formation. These devices are generally fashioned as rectangular cages constructed of metal, plastic, or bioabsorbable polymers (Figure 3). All of these devices, which are also FDA class III devices, have advantages and disadvantages, but definitive data on their usefulness are lacking.

### Plate Fixation

Anterior cervical plates have been widely used for many years and are a well-accepted device for the surgical treatment of cervical herniated disks, especially when multiple levels are treated. Most studies show that the

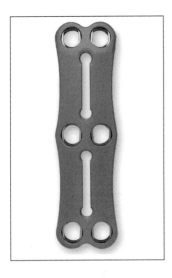

Figure 4 One of many contemporary anterior cervical plate designs includes a bushing to capture the screw and prevent back-out (ACCS, Synthes Spine).

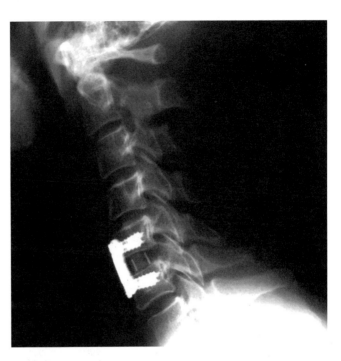

Figure 5 A lateral radiograph of a patient treated with anterior diskectomy. A polyethyletherketone spacer was combined with ceramic that was soaked in bone marrow aspirated from the iliac crest. No iliac bone was harvested.

use of cervical plates improves fusion rates; however, the risk for nonunion is not eliminated. More recently, dynamic plates have been developed that allow for controlled settling of the graft. In theory, these plates should improve the fusion rate while maintaining desired alignment without the need for external bracing. Several designs have been proposed and are currently in clinical use (Figure 4). The impact of dynamic plates is difficult to assess because only small studies have been reported to date. As with total hip arthroplasty, a large number of designs have been marketed, making it difficult to determine the optimal indication and design. Dynamic plates are generally considered equivalent to long bone plates and screws and are FDA class II devices (Figure 5).

## Cervical Disk Arthroplasty

For 50 years, ACDF, using the innovative techniques developed by Smith, Robinson, and Cloward, has been the standard surgical treatment for single- and two-level degenerative disk disease. However, a 1-year study showed that spinal arthrodesis may increase adjacent segment wear at the rate of approximately 2% to 3% per year. Multilevel ACDF leads to a 10% to 15% incidence of dysphagia and increased reports of stiffness. Approximately 175,000 anterior cervical surgeries for disk disease are performed each year in the United States. The patient with degenerative disk disease who is an ideal candidate for cervical disk arthroplasty is the same patient who is a candidate for ACDF. It is estimated that the number of surgeries will grow to 300,000 by 2008, with 70% of patients receiving some form of instrumentation. Of 210,000 patients (70%), at least 30% of surgeries will involve some form of an arthroplasty.

Tribology (the study of friction, lubrication, and wear of interacting surfaces in relative motion) is central to the success of cervical arthroplasty because artificial disk designs that are prone to producing excessive wear debris may cause metal toxicity and foreign-body reac-

tions, which would make their use unacceptable. The subaxial cervical motion segment is a three-joint complex; the disk is a fibrocartilaginous symphysis coupled to the two synovial zygapophyseal joints. Joint movement occurs by deformation of the disk that is constrained by facet geometry. Arthroplasty must replicate these mechanics to prevent prosthetic loosening and preserve facet motion.

Early clinical experience with cervical arthroplasty has shown few instances of periprosthetic osteolysis, probably because of the limited physiologic motion and the lack of synovial tissue in the disk space. Ideally, the cervical arthroplasty should allow simultaneous rotation and translation with shifting of the center of rotation. Mobility is not the only goal. The real benefit of arthroplasty may be the decreased rate of long-term reoperation (surgery at adjacent segments). A critically constrained prosthesis is an ideal treatment option for the cervical motion segment in patients with degenerative disk disease.

The Prestige, Bryan, and Prodisc-C (Figure 6) are current examples of cervical disk replacements. Other designs (all FDA class III) include the PCM cervical artificial disk (Cervitech, Rockaway, NJ), the CerviCore (Stryker, Kalamazoo, MI), and the Pearsall textile design (NuVasive, San Diego, CA). Clinical trials in the United States may begin in 2005. Current cervical disk replacements are discussed in detail in chapter 52.

The putative advantages of cervical disk arthroplasty include preservation of motion, immediate pain relief (potentially cervicalgia in addition to radiculopathy),

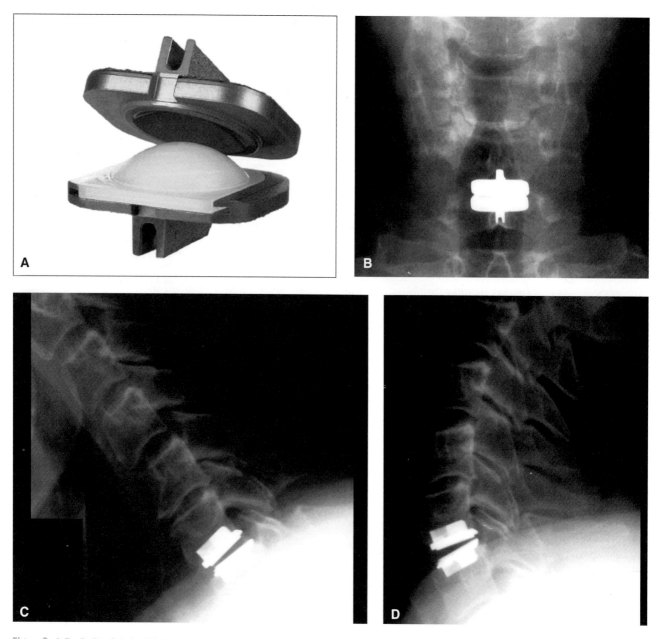

Figure 6 **A,** The ProDisc-C device. This device is limited by United States law to investigational use. **B,** AP radiograph of a patient after C6-7 diskectomy and arthroplasty using the ProDisc-C device. Flexion **(C)** and extension **(D)** lateral radiographs of the same patient showing motion at the treated level.

avoidance of possible fusion failure, reduced or retarded adjacent segment degeneration, and the obviation of autograft bone harvest or substitution.

The long-term effects of motion-preservation technology in the spine must be studied. As has been stated, the disk is not the only spinal structure capable of generating nociception. Degenerative pain also can originate in the facet joints, ligaments, and musculature. ACDF addresses several of these structures, but arthroplasty may not. In the era of evidence-based medicine, well-designed controlled clinical studies are imperative. Although these devices have great potential benefits, they should not be considered panaceas. Proper ran-

domized controlled clinical trials will help preserve the integrity of the development process, producing quantified clinical outcome data rather than unsubstantiated commercial claims. Such trials are needed before spine surgery can be considered a successful joint arthroplasty procedure. Motion-sparing technology is discussed in detail in chapter 52.

## Outcomes

In the past 3 years, there have been changes in the surgical treatment of patients with cervical disk herniation. Many innovations have occurred; however, clinical experience with most of these advancements is limited.

Safety, efficacy, and cost effectiveness must be critically assessed.

Much of the past literature is focused on various objective clinical and radiographic outcomes. Many studies emphasize fusion rates and avoid the assessment of surgical complications and other technical considerations. Although technical factors are important, patients desire relief of disease symptoms and desire improvement in their ability to achieve good daily function. There is a growing appreciation that surgeons and patients differ in their perception of functional outcomes. Surgeons tend to underestimate the prevalence and severity of postoperative morbidity, and to inflate the success rate of treatments.

For example, cervical spine surgeons may underestimate the effect of dysphagia, dysphonia, and bone donor site pain on the patient. The surgical community should gather more accurate data concerning the true incidence and severity of the morbidities associated with medical interventions. This goal is challenging and is further complicated by an ever-increasing array of treatment options. Answers will result from carefully controlled studies.

## Annotated Bibliography

### Diagnosis

Matsumoto M, Chiba K, Ishikawa M, Maruiwa H, Fujimura Y, Toyama Y: Relationships between outcomes of conservative treatment and magnetic resonance imaging findings in patients with mild cervical myelopathy caused by soft disc herniations. *Spine* 2001;26:1592-1598.

Cervical bracing and activity restriction were used to treat 27 patients. Ten patients underwent surgery for deterioration. Mean Japanese Orthopaedic Association scores were similar; however, 77% of nonsurgical and 90% of surgical patients reported satisfactory outcomes. Focal herniation prompted surgery more than the diffuse, median-type of herniation.

### Surgical Treatment

Agrillo U, Mastronardi L, Puzzilli F: Anterior cervical fusion with carbon fiber cage containing coralline hydroxyapatite: Preliminary observations in 45 consecutive cases of soft-disc herniation. *J Neurosurg* 2002;96:273-276.

Results of this study showed that 33 single-level and 12 two-level anterior cervical fusions using a carbon fiber cage containing coralline hydroxyapatite all attained fusion. At a mean follow-up of 22.3 months, all patients reported a decrease or cessation of pain. Patients reported a high rate of satisfaction with the procedure. This is one of many strategies to avoid donor site morbidity.

Bose B: Anterior cervical arthrodesis using DOC dynamic stabilization implant for improvement in sagittal angulation and controlled settling. *J Neurosurg* 2003;98:8-13.

This study presents the results of 37 patients who underwent ACDF using the DOC (DePuy Spine, Raglen, MA) dynamic implant. At 1.3 years mean follow-up, postoperative neck or arm pain was resolved in 52% of the patients and fusion was successful in 80% patients at 88% of the treated levels.

Goffin J, Van Calenbergh F, van Loon J, et al: Intermediate follow-up after treatment of degenerative disc disease with the Bryan Cervical Disc Prosthesis: Single-level and bi-level. *Spine* 2003;28:2673-2678.

This study included 103 patients with one-level and 43 patients with two-level degenerative disk disease. At one-year follow-up, range of motion was maintained and no devices were explanted. Clinical success for single- and bi-level arthroplasty exceeded the study criteria of 85%.

Jho H, Kim W, Kim M: Anterior microforaminotomy for treatment of cervical radiculopathy: Part 1. Disc-preserving "functional cervical disc surgery". *Neurosurgery* 2002;51:S46-S53.

Of 104 patients who underwent anterior cervical microforaminotomies, all except 1 patient with diskitis maintained their motion segment. Results were excellent for 83 patients, good for 20, and fair for 1 patient. Two patients developed transient Horner's syndrome, one patient had transient hemiparesis, and the patient with diskitis developed ankylosis.

McAfee PC, Cunningham B, Dmitriev A, et al: Cervical disk replacement: Porous coated motion prosthesis: A comparative biomechanical analysis showing the key role of the posterior longitudinal ligament. *Spine* 2003; 28(suppl 20):S176-S185.

In an analysis of seven fresh frozen human cadaveric subaxial cervical spines the posterior longitudinal ligament was found to be pivotal to postsurgical stability following anterior cervical diskectomy. The authors concluded that it may be helpful to differentiate between ligament-preserving and ligament-sacrificing arthroplasty designs.

Miccoli P, Berti P, Raffaelli M, Materazzi G, Conte M, Faldini A: Minimally invasive approach to the cervical spine: A proposal. *J Laparoendosc Adv Surg Tech A* 2001;11:89-92.

A video-assisted endoscopic approach through a single 1.5-cm incision was performed in three patients to test the feasibility of the procedure for anterior cervical spine surgery. Surgical instruments and 5-mm and 3-mm endoscopes were inserted through a surgical tube.

Szpalski M, Gunzburg R, Mayer M: Spine arthroplasty: A historical review. *Eur Spine J* 2002;11(suppl 2):S65-S84.

This article presents a chronologic review of published and patented spinal arthroplasty designs up to 2002. The authors discuss the design challenges and need for proper randomized controlled trials to assess the efficacy and indications for spinal arthroplasty.

### Outcomes

Edwards CC II, Karpitskaya Y, Cha C, et al: Accurate identification of adverse outcomes after cervical spine surgery. *J Bone Joint Surg Am* 2004;86-A:251-256.

This article reports on 166 patients who had 342 postoperative visits after anterior cervical arthrodesis performed by four surgeons. The surgeons' records documented 26 reports of dysphagia, whereas 107 patients independently reported dysphagia. Also, the surgeons' records showed only 10 reports of dysphonia, whereas patients reported dysphonia 72 times.

## Classic Bibliography

Boden SD, McCowin PR, Davis DO, Dina TS, Mark AS, Wiesel S: Abnormal magnetic-resonance scans of the cervical spine in asymptomatic subjects: A prospective investigation. *J Bone Joint Surg Am* 1990;72:1178-1184.

Cloward RB: The anterior approach for removal of ruptured cervical disks. *J Neurosurg* 1958;15:602-617.

Cummins BH, Robertson JT, Gill SS: Surgical experience with an implanted artificial cervical joint. *J Neurosurg* 1998;88:943-948.

Herkowitz HN, Kurz LT, Overhoff DP: Surgical management of cervical soft herniation: A comparison between the anterior and posterior approach. *Spine* 1990;15:1026-1030.

Hilibrand AS, Carlson GD, Palumbo MA, Jones PK, Bohlman HH: Radiculopathy and myelopathy at segments adjacent to the site of a previous anterior cervical arthrodesis. *J Bone Joint Surg Am* 1999;81:519-528.

Roh S, Kim D, Cardoso A, Fessler R: Endoscopic foraminotomy using MED system in cadaveric specimens. *Spine* 2000;25:260-264.

Smith GW, Robinson RA: The treatment of certain cervical-spine disorders by anterior removal of the intervertebral disc and interbody fusion. *J Bone Joint Surg Am* 1958;40:607-624.

# Chapter 26

# Cervical Spondylotic Myelopathy: Including Ossification of the Posterior Longitudinal Ligament

John M. Rhee, MD

K. Daniel Riew, MD

## Cervical Spondylotic Myelopathy

Cervical myelopathy describes a constellation of symptoms and signs arising from cervical cord compression. Because symptoms and signs in a patient with myelopathy can be quite subtle in early manifestations, the diagnosis may easily be missed or wrongly attributed to the "normal" epiphenomenon of aging. However, because the natural history of cervical myelopathy is typically one of stepwise progression, early recognition and treatment is essential for optimal patient outcomes before the onset of irreversible spinal cord damage.

### Clinical Presentation

Patients with myelopathy may present with a variety of symptoms. Upper extremity symptoms include a generalized feeling of clumsiness of the arms and hands (tendency to drop things), inability to manipulate small objects such as coins or buttons, difficulty with handwriting, and diffuse numbness (typically nondermatomal). Lower extremity disorders include gait instability, a sense of imbalance during ambulation, and bumping into walls when walking. Family members may comment that the patient walks as if intoxicated. Patients with severe cord compression also may report Lhermitte's sign: electric shock-like sensations that radiate either down the spine or into the extremities with certain offending positions of the neck.

Subjective weakness is a relatively late symptom, and many myelopathic patients deny any loss of motor strength. Similarly, bowel and bladder symptoms, if present, typically arise in the later stages of disease. Despite advanced degrees of spondylosis, many floridly myelopathic patients also have no neck pain. It is the patient without symptoms of pain who is particularly at risk for going undiagnosed until the myelopathy becomes severe. Reports of radicular symptoms such as radiating arm pain may occur with myelopathy if the patient has coexisting symptomatic nerve root compression. However, even though imaging studies may show root compression, many patients have no radicular symptoms or signs. Because pain and weakness may not be present, a high degree of suspicion is necessary to diagnose myelopathy when the disease is in its most treatable, early stages.

A full neurologic examination should be performed; however, just as pain is not a sensitive predictor of myelopathy, a completely normal neurologic examination does not exclude the diagnosis of myelopathy. The motor examination may be completely normal or may show only subtle degrees of weakness. When upper extremity weakness is present, it often manifests as diminished grip and/or intrinsic strength. The finding of severe weakness of the major muscle groups in the upper or lower extremities on manual motor testing is relatively uncommon. Sensory examinations including a pinprick test should be performed; however, findings may be normal. The neurologic examination should also include an assessment of gait to test for instability. Bowel and bladder or dorsal column (proprioceptive) dysfunction occurs with advanced disease and carries a poor prognosis. Hyperreflexia may be present in the upper and/or lower extremities and is suggestive of spinal cord compression. However, because peripheral nerves must be functioning properly to transmit the hyperreflexia characteristic of myelopathy, patients with concomitant myelopathy and peripheral nerve disease from conditions such as diabetes, peripheral neuropathy, or severe multilevel cervical foraminal stenosis can have diminished or absent reflexes. In addition, patients with cervical myelopathy who have coexisting lumbar stenosis may exhibit brisk upper extremity reflexes consistent with upper motor neuron findings yet may have diminished lower extremity reflexes because of root-level compression in the lumbar spine.

There are several provocative tests suggestive of cord compression that can be elicited in the patient with myelopathy. Lhermitte's sign is positive when certain positions of the neck cause an electric shock-like sensation down the arm, legs, and/or spine. Babinski's reflex, when present, is a poor prognostic indicator. Hoffmann's sign occurs when flicking the volar surface of the flexed middle finger distal phalanx results in pathologic flexion of the thumb and index finger. The finger

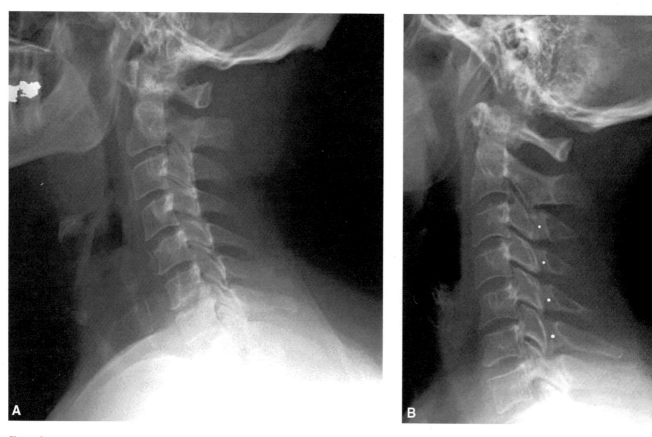

**Figure 1** **A,** Lateral radiograph of a patient with congenital stenosis. Note that the lamina is barely visible. **B,** Lateral radiograph of a normal cervical spine shows a much wider lamina (*white dots*).

escape sign describes the inability to maintain the ulnar digits in an extended and adducted position. An inverted radial reflex is seen when the brachioradialis reflex itself is diminished but causes spastic contraction of the finger flexors instead. Patients with high cervical cord compression may demonstrate the scapulohumeral reflex, in which tapping the tip of the scapula results in brisk scapular elevation and humeral abduction. Sustained clonus of the lower extremities should also be tested in patients with myelopathy. Because some of these upper motor signs can arise from either brain or cervical spinal cord pathology, one method of determining the genesis of the findings is to perform a jaw jerk test. If this test is positive, such that tapping the lower jaw leads to opening of the mouth, the origin of the upper motor neuron findings may be in the brain rather than the spinal cord.

### Differential Diagnosis

The most common cause of cervical myelopathy in patients older than 50 years of age is spondylosis or degenerative changes, producing the condition known as cervical spondylotic myelopathy (CSM). Anterior structures, such as bulging, ossified, or herniated disks, as well as osteophytic anterior spurs, are the usual entities causing cord compression in CSM. Degenerative spondylolisthesis of the cervical spine can also exacerbate or cause compression. Disorders in posterior structures, such as ligamentum flavum hypertrophy or, rarely, ossification of the ligamentum flavum, may also contribute to cord compression, but do so less commonly than their anterior counterparts.

CSM commonly occurs in patients with a congenitally narrowed cervical canal. In these patients, the cord may have had sufficient space and escaped compression when the patient was relatively young; however, with time, an accumulation of space-occupying degenerative changes may reach a threshold level leading to symptomatic stenosis. Although CSM tends to be a disorder found in patients 50 years of age and older, depending on the degree of congenital stenosis and the magnitude of the accumulated spondylotic changes, the disorder can manifest itself in patients who are much younger (even patients in their 30s and 40s).

Ossification of the posterior longitudinal ligament (OPLL) is another major cause of cervical myelopathy. Less common causes of cervical myelopathy include numerous etiologies for cervical cord compression, such as epidural abscess, tumor, and trauma. These entities usually present somewhat differently, with pain, constitutional symptoms, or a history of injury in addition to

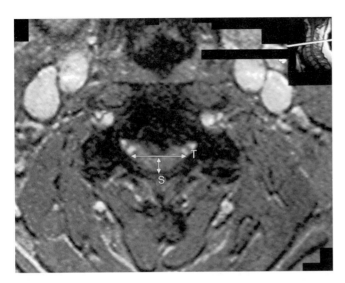

**Figure 2** The compression ratio of the smallest sagittal cord diameter to the largest transverse cord diameter at the same level is measured. A ratio of less than 0.4 carries a poor prognosis. T = transverse cord diameter, S = sagittal cord diameter.

myelopathic symptoms. Kyphosis, whether primary or postlaminectomy, also can cause cord compression and myelopathy. When evaluating the patient who reports myelopathic symptoms, it is important to keep in mind a broad differential diagnosis, including nonspinal disorders such as stroke, movement disorders, and multiple sclerosis.

## Imaging

Plain radiographs can provide useful information but are not diagnostic of cervical stenosis and myelopathy. Routine evaluation may include upright AP and lateral as well as flexion-extension views. A lateral radiograph can be particularly instructive and can be used to determine the degree of congenital cervical stenosis (Figure 1). A Pavlov ratio (AP diameter of canal/AP diameter of vertebral body) of less than 0.8 suggests congenital stenosis. A space available for the cord of 13 mm or less also suggests a narrow sagittal diameter of the spinal canal and has been shown to correlate with neurologic injury after trauma. In many patients, the disk space(s) showing the greatest amount of degeneration will be those associated with the greatest cord compression.

To confirm spinal cord compression, advanced imaging using MRI or CT-myelography is necessary. MRI is noninvasive and provides adequate imaging characteristics for most patients. A closed MRI is preferred over an open study whenever possible because of its superior image quality. Signal changes within the cord may be seen on MRI and are suggestive of severe compression. Another radiographic finding that indicates a poor prognosis is a compression ratio of less than 0.4 (measured as the ratio of the smallest sagittal cord diameter to the largest transverse cord diameter at the same

level) (Figure 2). Conversely, expansion of the compression ratio to greater than 0.4 postoperatively correlates with clinical recovery.

If a patient cannot undergo MRI for medical reasons (for example, the presence of a cardiac pacemakers, aneurysm clips, or because of severe claustrophobia), or if metal or scar tissue from a prior cervical surgery precludes adequate visualization on MRI because of artifact, CT combined with myelography may be considered. Although CT myelography is invasive and is not the best screening test, CT-myelograms provide outstanding resolution of both bony and neural anatomy for surgical planning. Alternatively, if a high quality MRI is obtained but questions remain regarding bony anatomy for the purposes of surgical planning, a noncontrast CT scan can be obtained to provide complementary information. CT may be helpful in diagnosing the presence of OPLL that may not be obvious on MRI or plain radiographs but can have a profound effect on the surgical approach (Figure 3).

## Treatment

Symptomatic myelopathy is typically progressive and is thus considered a surgical disorder. Cord compression may cause myelopathy either by an ischemic effect secondary to compression of the anterior spinal artery, or by a direct mechanical effect on cord function. In a recent prospective study of patients with CSM, surgical treatment has been shown to improve functional outcomes, the amount of pain, and neurologic status. It has also been demonstrated that early intervention improves the prognosis by helping to prevent permanent destructive changes in the spinal cord. Surgery is the treatment of choice unless the patient is unwilling or unable to undergo surgery because of prohibitive medical comorbidities.

The optimal treatment for patients with evidence of cord compression on imaging studies but with mild to no clinical symptoms or signs is unclear. Asymptomatic cord compression may never become symptomatic. Alternatively, acute trauma in a patient with a previously asymptomatic stenosis may present as spinal cord injury. In the end, the decision to provide surgical treatment or to observe a patient with mild or no symptoms is determined by the informed consent of the patient. Depending on the severity of the cord compression seen on MRI scans, however, it can be entirely reasonable to recommend surgery even in the absence of symptoms. If nonsurgical treatment is elected, close and careful follow-up is recommended. The patient should be instructed to immediately report the development of symptoms.

## Surgical Treatment Options

Although there is consensus regarding the need for surgical treatment of cervical myelopathy, considerable debate exists regarding the optimal surgical approach.

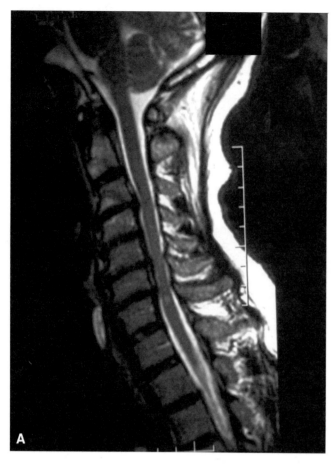

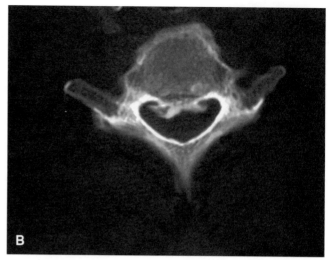

Figure 3　**A,** Sagittal view of a patient with OPLL. On the T2-weighted image, the ossified posterior longitudinal ligament appears dark. It is difficult to differentiate between an ossified posterior longitudinal ligament and a herniated disk on an MRI scan. **B,** CT scan of the same patient. This plain CT scan shows ossification of the posterior longitudinal ligament.

There are several options, including anterior decompression and fusion, laminectomy, laminectomy and fusion, and laminoplasty. Each approach has advantages and disadvantages, and there is no one procedure that is clearly favorable in all circumstances. Considerations that may favor one approach versus another include: the number of stenotic levels present; patient factors, such as comorbidities; the desire to either limit or preserve motion; and alignment of the cervical spine.

### Laminectomy With or Without Fusion

Laminectomy without fusion for the treatment of cervical myelopathy currently has a minor role in the management of this disorder because of its numerous disadvantages. Postlaminectomy kyphosis can occur after laminectomy; however, the true incidence in the adult population is unknown with estimates ranging from 11% to 47%. Although postlaminectomy kyphosis can lead to potential recurrent myelopathy if the cord becomes draped and compressed over the kyphos, the incidence of clinically apparent neurologic symptoms resulting from this complication is unknown. In addition to potential neurologic sequelae, the kyphosis itself can be a source of neck pain or deformity (Figure 4). If an aggressive facetectomy is performed along with laminectomy, spondylolisthesis also can develop and contribute

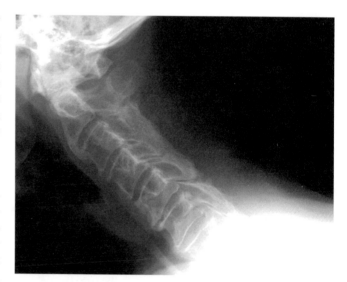

Figure 4　A laminectomy or a laminectomy and fusion without instrumentation can result in the loss of normal lordosis or even kyphosis. This outcome is especially probable if the splenius cervicis, the critical extensor muscle, is detached from C2.

to cord compression. If a patient requires subsequent posterior surgery, the exposed dura over the length of the laminectomy can make the revision more tedious, difficult, and risky to perform.

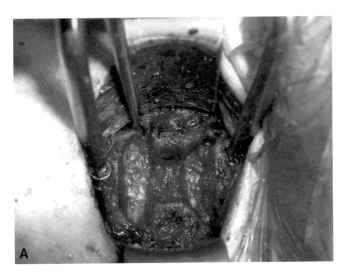
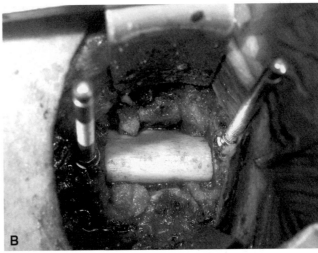

Figure 5 **A,** An anterior single-level cervical corpectomy has been performed. The Penfield 4 is lateral to the uncovertebral joint. A thorough decompression can be achieved anteriorly and direct decompression of uncovertebral spurs, ossified posterior longitudinal ligament, or herniated disks behind the posterior longitudinal ligament can be decompressed. In addition, local autograft can be obtained. **B,** After placing a structural allograft, the locally obtained autograft can be placed into the uncovertebral areas. This local autograft will typically fuse faster than the structural allograft.

A posterior fusion can be added to avoid the disadvantage of performing a laminectomy alone. Laminectomy and fusion is typically performed along with lateral mass screw instrumentation. Fusion has several potential benefits, including improvement of spondylotic neck pain and prevention of postlaminectomy kyphosis. Preexisting kyphosis can be improved after laminectomy by positioning the neck in extension before securing the instrumentation, although for higher degrees of kyphosis an anterior-posterior approach is generally recommended. Despite advantages over laminectomy alone, the literature has shown that laminectomy and fusion may be outperformed by alternative procedures. In a nonrandomized comparison study of laminoplasty versus laminectomy and fusion, laminectomy and fusion showed a trend toward an inferior rate of neurologic improvement based on objective evaluation of the Nurick score as well as patient-reported outcomes. In addition, an analysis of the complication rate strongly favored using laminoplasty, with 14 complications occurring in 13 patients in the laminectomy and fusion group compared with no complications in the laminoplasty group. Most complications were related to fusion and included nonunion, implant failure, adjacent segment degeneration, and significant donor site pain. Based on these findings, laminectomy and fusion with lateral mass instrumentation may be considered an alternative to anterior surgery in certain myelopathic patients with multilevel myelopathy and severe coexisting mechanical neck pain. However, for patients in whom fusion is not necessary, laminoplasty may be a better choice.

Skip laminectomy is a modified procedure that was designed to limit posterior muscle trauma and neck pain. With this approach, two consecutive stenotic disk levels are decompressed via a standard laminectomy of the lamina between the stenotic levels and are combined with a partial laminectomy of the lower adjacent vertebra. For example, a C3-7 decompression can be achieved by performing a laminectomy of C4 and C6, with partial laminectomies and flavum resection at other levels. At the "skipped" lamina (C3, C5, and C7 in this example), the muscular attachments to the spinous processes are left intact, thereby helping to preserve sagittal alignment and preventing postlaminectomy kyphosis. At 2-year follow-up, patients had similar neurologic outcomes with less postoperative neck pain and better range of motion than patients who underwent open-door laminoplasty. However, this procedure may be better suited to patients with moderate stenosis or ossification of the yellow ligament, and may not offer ideal decompression for patients with severe stenosis, congenital stenosis, or extensive OPLL.

### Anterior Decompression and Fusion
The major advantage of the anterior approach for treating cervical myelopathy is the ability to directly decompress structures most commonly responsible for cord compression, such as herniated disks, spondylotic bars, and ossification of the posterior longitudinal ligament (Figure 5, *A*). Anterior decompression, in contrast to posterior approaches, also can directly relieve neural compression resulting from kyphosis by removing the vertebral bodies over which the cord may be draped. In addition, the fusion procedure associated with anterior decompression helps to relieve spondylotic neck pain, can correct and improve kyphosis, immobilizes and therefore protects the segment of decompressed cord,

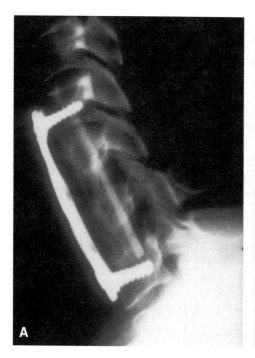
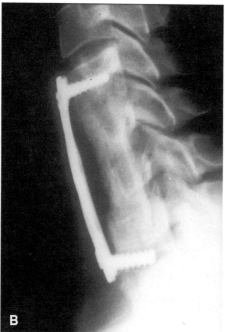

**Figure 6 A,** Radiograph of a patient who had a two-level cervical corpectomy and anterior cervical plating. **B,** Radiograph of the same patient taken at 1-year postoperatively. Although the graft eventually healed, it also subsided and the screws cut into the next disk space, necessitating an arthrodesis of the adjacent level.

and prevents recurrent disease over the fused segments (Figure 5, *B*). Excellent neurologic recovery rates have been reported with anterior surgery for myelopathy.

Several alternative anterior procedures can be performed in the patient with myelopathy, depending on the nature of the stenosis. For myelopathy arising from one or two disk spaces, a single-level or two-level anterior cervical diskectomy and fusion (ACDF) (or a single-level corpectomy for two motion-segment disease) will be the treatment of choice for most patients. For patients with stenosis at three or more disk segments, however, the superiority of an anterior approach is not so clearly established. The traditional anterior approach to multilevel stenosis has been multilevel corpectomy and reconstruction with a long strut graft (Figure 6, *A*). Although effective in treating neural compression, this technique has been plagued by a high rate of graft-related complications (Figure 6, *B*). Pseudarthrosis rates after multilevel anterior corpectomy and fusion range from 11% to 40%. Perhaps less frequent but more troublesome is the rate of graft dislodgement, which has been reported to range from 7% to 20% and can be associated with neurologic compromise, esophageal injury, and airway obstruction leading to death.

### Complications With Multilevel Corpectomy and Long Strut Graft Reconstruction

Although it may seem logical to assume that the addition of an anterior cervical plate would reduce the incidence of graft-related complications in multilevel strut graft reconstructions, clinical studies of plated multilevel corpectomies have shown an association with higher graft complication rates than those without plates. In

one study, graft displacement rates were 9% for a two-level corpectomy and 50% in a three-level corpectomy despite anterior plating. Biomechanical studies which provide insight into these clinical failures suggest that long-plated, strut graft constructs may be mechanically unfavorable because they rapidly lose stability under fatigue loading and reverse load transfer through the strut graft. As a result, buttress plating has been attempted by some authors as an alternative means of stabilizing long anterior strut grafts. A spanning plate fixed to the vertebral body above and below the graft can prevent graft settling as the graft heals and thus acts as a "distraction device." The rationale for the use of a buttress plate is that a buttress plate is fixed only at one end of the construct and thus can allow for settling to occur while preventing graft extrusion. Although theoretically appealing, buttress plates as stand-alone anterior fixation devices are subject to the usual litany of strut graft complications, such as dislodgment and pseudarthroses (Figure 7). Dynamic plates are another alternative to rigid plate fixation of long strut grafts. They also allow for settling and are again theoretically appealing; however, clinical evidence regarding their efficacy in stabilizing long strut grafts is currently unavailable. Excessive settling of dynamic plates can potentially lead to plates overlapping and injuring adjacent disk spaces, as well as kyphosis, foraminal stenosis, and construct failure. Nonplated corpectomies with long strut grafts have shown good clinical results but require cumbersome rigid external immobilization and have been associated with the morbidity of autologous fibular harvest. Supplemental posterior fixation and fusion may be prudent if an anteriorly placed long strut graft is necessary to provide bet-

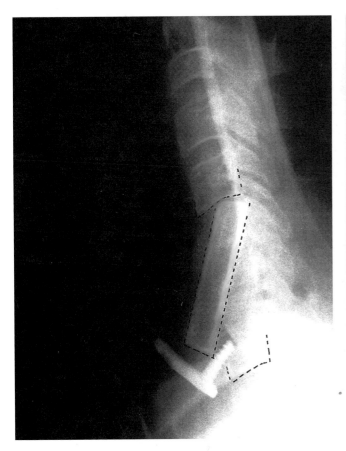

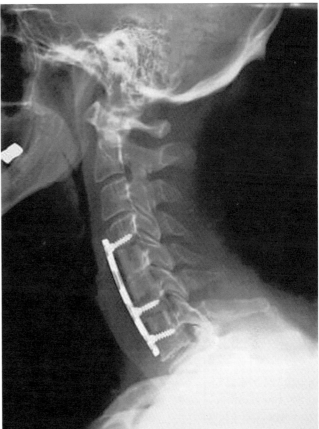

**Figure 7** Radiograph of a patient who had a two-level corpectomy secured with a buttress plate. When the graft extruded, it kicked this plate out at 45° to the pharynx, causing asphyxiation and eventual death. Because of the potential for such catastrophic complications, buttress plates should not routinely be used for an anterior-only construct.

**Figure 8** A corpectomy/diskectomy construct.

ter stability and reduce the incidence of graft kick out and pseudarthrosis.

In addition to the graft complications associated with multilevel corpectomy, it is important to keep in mind that all anterior fusion surgeries carry relatively small but real risks intrinsic to the anterior approach, such as permanent speech and swallowing disturbance, airway obstruction, esophageal injury, and vertebral artery injury. These risks are probably higher for multilevel reconstructions than for a one- or two-level ACDF because of longer surgical times and the number of levels exposed. Another potential disadvantage is that anterior fusion has been associated with accelerated adjacent segment degeneration, although it has never been conclusively proven that fusion actually causes accelerated adjacent segment disease.

### Alternative Corpectomy Constructs
To avoid some of the pitfalls associated with using long strut grafts, several alternative corpectomy constructs can be used if an anterior approach is chosen to treat the myelopathic patient with multilevel (≥ three disk

space involvement) stenosis. Multilevel ACDF is one alternative that can be performed if the stenosis is disk-based and resection of the posterior vertebral body or posterior longitudinal ligament is not necessary. Advantages over a single, long strut graft include the ability to achieve better fixation with segmental screw placement into every vertebral body within the construct, and better preservation or even recreation of lordosis. ACDF grafts, in comparison with long strut grafts, are also much less likely to dislodge. The major disadvantage of multilevel ACDF grafts may be a higher pseudarthrosis rate caused by the increased number of bony surfaces requiring healing (for example, six bony surfaces for a three-level ADCF from C4-7 compared with two surfaces for a two-level corpectomy with a single strut graft from C4-7); however, the literature is not in uniform agreement on this point.

Another alternative treatment option for compression arising from three disk levels is to perform a single-level corpectomy at two disk levels, then an ACDF at the remaining level (corpectomy-diskectomy) (Figure 8). The corpectomy–diskectomy construct is a compromise solution that avoids the biomechanical issues of a single, long strut and decreases the number of healing surfaces (by two) compared with a multilevel ACDF. Segmental plate

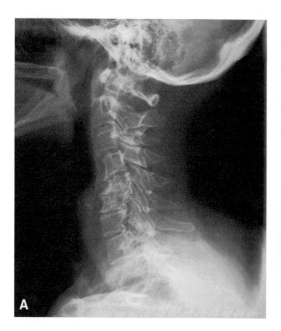 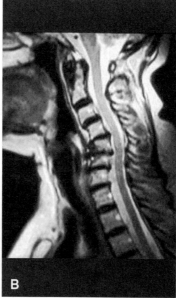 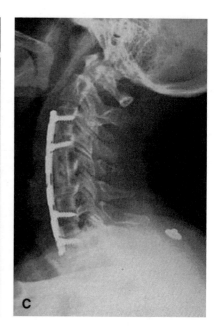

Figure 9　**A,** Preoperative lateral radiograph of a patient with multiple-level spondylosis and stenosis, showing disease from C3-T1. **B,** The MRI scan shows anterolisthesis at C3-4, spondylosis at C4-5 and C5-6 with kyphosis and mild cord compromise; spondylosis is present at C6-7 and C7-T1 with decreased disk height. **C,** Lateral postoperative radiograph. This patient was treated with a combination of corpectomies and diskectomies. This treatment allowed for the restoration of cervical lordosis and a relatively rigid construct that was resistant to graft extrusion. The patient was immobilized in a soft cervical collar and all of the segments eventually healed.

and screw fixation is achievable at every level except for the corpectomy level. If the patient's compressive pathology does not dictate otherwise, the corpectomy is performed at the upper two levels to avoid the mechanical disadvantage of a corpectomy at the bottom end of the construct, where it would be more likely to dislodge.

A final alternative for pathology involving four disk levels is a double corpectomy; for example, two single-level corpectomies separated by an intact intervening vertebra. This construct achieves fewer healing surfaces versus multilevel ACDF and at the same time avoids using a single long strut. Fixation is obtained in three vertebrae: at the top, bottom, and middle of the construct. Before using of one of these alternative corpectomy constructs, however, the surgeon must ensure that the pattern and location of the patient's stenosis are appropriate to the procedure (Figure 9).

### Laminoplasty

Laminoplasty was designed to achieve multilevel posterior cord decompression while avoiding the major complications associated with laminectomy (such as post-laminectomy kyphosis). In most patients, a C3-7 procedure is performed. Many techniques are available for performing a laminoplasty, but the open-door and French-door laminoplasty are the most common. The common element in all variations of laminoplasty is the creation of a hinge at the junction of the lateral mass and lamina by thinning the dorsal cortex but not cutting completely through the ventral cortex, thereby allowing the creation of greenstick fractures. In the open-door

technique, the hinge is created unilaterally; in the French-door technique, the hinge is created bilaterally. The opening is performed on the opposite lateral mass-laminar junction in an open-door procedure, or in the midline with the French-door variation. Opening the laminoplasty increases the space available for the spinal cord, which drifts away from compressive lesions into the space created. The opening can then be held patent with bone (such as autologous spinous process or rib allograft), sutures, suture-anchors, or specially designed plates. Laminoplasty was initially developed in Japan where it has a long record of success, but it is gaining wider acceptance in North America because of proven benefits in properly chosen patients (Figure 10).

In addition to its benefits over laminectomy, laminoplasty has several distinct advantages over anterior surgery. First, because an indirect decompression is performed, laminoplasty is generally a safer and technically easier operation to perform than multilevel anterior corpectomy, particularly in patients with severe stenosis or in OPLLs that require resection. Second, laminoplasty is a motion preserving procedure. No fusion is required; however, a fusion and instrumentation can be done in association with laminoplasty if needed. Thus, all fusion-related complications may be eliminated. Fusions can be avoided in patients at high risk for pseudarthrosis, such as diabetic and elderly patients, and those who are chronic steroid users. Third, a laminoplasty allows the surgeon to decompress segments at future risk for stenosis in one operation without substantially increasing patient morbidity. With a laminoplasty, a C3 to C7

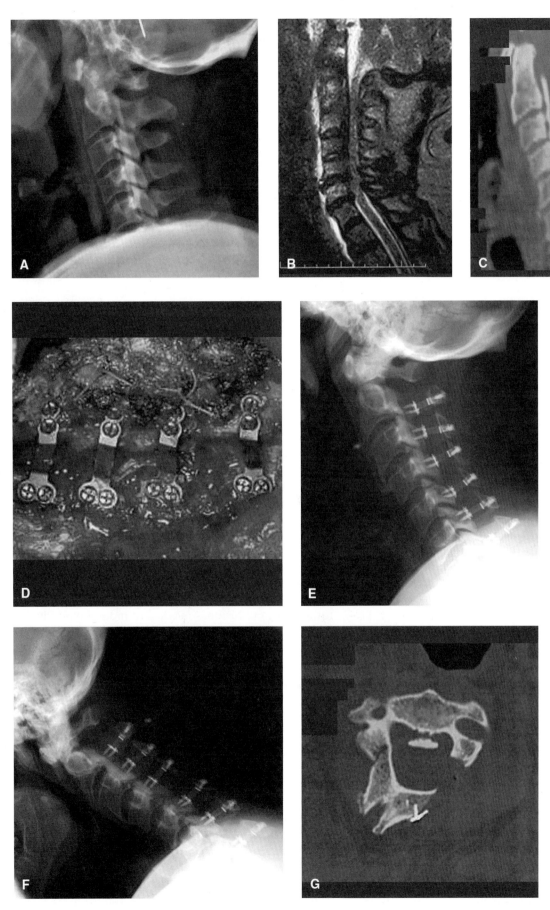

Figure 10 Laminoplasty. A, Preoperative lateral plain radiograph of a patient with OPLL. Notice the shadow of the OPLL as visible from behind C2 down to C5. B, Sagittal MRI scan showing severe stenosis down to C6-7. C, Sagittally reconstructed CT scan showing OPLL. If approached from an anterior approach, the resection would be significantly more difficult and would have to include a resection of the C2 body. D, Intraoperative photograph of the laminoplasty plates. Postoperative neutral lateral (E) and flexion (F) views showing preservation of motion. G, Postoperative CT scan showing adequate decompression of C2. Note that on the hinged side, as well as on the open-door side, the cuts are made just medial to the pedicle to ensure the widest possible canal size.

decompression is performed in one operation. In contrast, if a patient had significant stenosis from C4-C6, a surgeon may hesitate to include mildly stenotic levels at C3-4 and C6-7 anteriorly because of the possibility of increasing complications and morbidity; however, this decision would then leave the patient vulnerable to subsequent disease at those adjacent levels over time. The fourth major advantage of a laminoplasty is that it does not preclude a later anterior procedure. If a patient has persistent stenosis after laminoplasty, focal anterior decompressions can be subsequently performed at needed levels. In addition, laminoplasty can be performed as part of a staged decompression in patients requiring anterior and posterior surgery. The extra space for the cord provided by the laminoplasty (which is performed with the neck in a neutral to slightly flexed, canal-enlarging position) can make the subsequent anterior decompression (which is performed with the neck in an extended, canal-narrowing position) safer to accomplish.

**Clinical Evidence for Laminoplasty** The theoretic advantages of laminoplasty have been proved in clinical trials comparing it with multilevel anterior corpectomy. Laminoplasty and anterior surgery have similar rates of neurologic improvement, but laminoplasty has a much lower complication rate. One study compared 42 patients who underwent laminoplasty with 41 patients who had multilevel anterior corpectomy for CSM. Neurologic outcomes were similar between the two groups, with both groups showing good improvement in the Japanese Orthopaedic Association myelopathy scores. However, the laminoplasty group had a significantly lower complication rate than the corpectomy group (7% versus 29%). As expected, most complications in the corpectomy group were graft-related. In the laminoplasty group, three patients had C5 root paresis, all of which resolved with observation. In North America, another study also found similar neurologic outcomes between the two procedures, but again found a much lower complication rate in the laminoplasty group.

**Potential Issues With Laminoplasty** Laminoplasty has disadvantages and is not appropriate for all patients. Segmental root level palsy remains a concern, with a postoperative incidence ranging from 5% to 12%. It most commonly affects the C5 root, resulting in deltoid and biceps weakness; however, other roots also can be affected. The palsies tend to be motor-dominant, although sensory dysfunction and radicular pain are also possible. Complications that prevent a successful spinal cord decompression may arise at any point postoperatively, from immediately after surgery to 20 days later. The cause of segmental root palsy after laminoplasty is unknown but may be related to nerve root traction because the decompressed cord floats posteriorly. C5 may be preferentially involved because it is usually at the apex of cervical

lordosis, thus the extent of postoperative spinal cord and root drift back will be greatest at that level. Strategies to prevent root palsies include prophylactic foraminotomy and limited opening of the laminoplasty (with an angle of the opened lamina between 45° to 60°) to prevent excessive cord drift back. However, the usefulness of the strategies remains unproved. Recovery usually occurs over weeks to months in most patients, but has been reported to take up to 6 years.

Neck pain can be problematic in patients who have undergone laminoplasty. Because no arthrodesis is performed, laminoplasty is not a procedure that should be used to treat painful spondylosis. Understanding that fact, controversy remains as to whether the neck pain associated with laminoplasty reflects new-onset postoperative symptoms or is simply the persistence of preoperative spondylotic pain. The results of one study on open-door laminoplasty found postoperative axial symptoms in 60% of patients who underwent laminoplasty compared with 19% of patients who had anterior fusion, a statistically significant difference. In addition, 75% of those reporting postoperative neck and shoulder pain in the laminoplasty group had new-onset pain. In contrast, a 2002 study found that spinous process splitting laminoplasty had no effect on either the development or resolution of axial neck and shoulder symptoms. The exact etiology for postoperative neck pain after laminoplasty is unclear, but may be related to stiffening of the facet joints or denervation and injury to the nuchal musculature. However, because pain is not often a major preoperative issue for the myelopathic patient, it usually remains a minor issue or nonissue postoperatively, particularly if the patient has received appropriate preoperative counseling regarding anticipated postoperative neck pain outcomes.

Another limitation of laminoplasty is the potential for loss of motion. Even when laminoplasty is performed without fusion, some loss of motion typically occurs. The cause of this motion loss is probably multifactorial but may be related to facet joint injury with spontaneous stiffening or fusion, or alterations in tissue and muscle elasticity after posterior surgical exposure. Prolonged postoperative immobilization may contribute to this complication. In addition, placing bone graft along the hinge side to assist in healing of the hinge may lead to undesired intersegmental fusion or stiffening. Loss of motion may be controlled with short-term postoperative immobilization and the avoidance of bone grafting on the hinge side.

Preoperative kyphosis is a relative contraindication to laminoplasty. Most of the compressive structures that lead to cervical myelopathy, such as disk herniations, spondylotic bars, and OPLL, arise anteriorly. Thus, laminoplasty and other posteriorly-based procedures for spinal cord decompression rely on the ability of the cord to drift away from the anterior lesions as a result of releas-

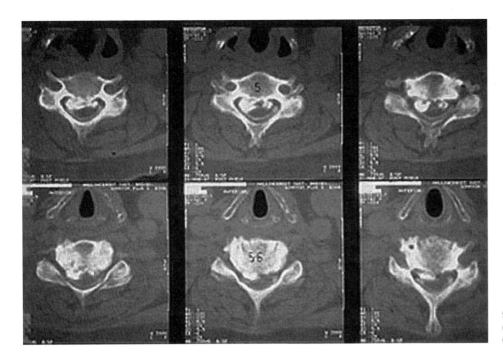

**Figure 11** CT scan of a patient with OPLL taken after myelography. With this degree of canal compromise, it is very likely that the dura also is ossified.

ing the posterior tethers (laminae, ligamentum flavum). Although such posterior drift-back reliably occurs in a lordotic or neutral cervical spine, it may not occur in patients with significant kyphosis. However, the absence of lordosis is not an absolute contraindication to laminoplasty. A 2003 study showed that laminoplasty could be performed with acceptable neurologic recovery when the local kyphosis measured 13° or less. In patients with kyphosis who have compressive lesions arising posteriorly, laminoplasty also may achieve a direct decompressive effect despite the kyphosis. Also, in kyphotic patients with extremely tight cervical stenosis, laminoplasty can be considered as a first stage operation, with subsequent anterior surgery performed if necessary.

### Combined Anterior and Posterior Surgery
Combined approaches are strongly recommended in patients with postlaminectomy kyphosis. If a multilevel corpectomy is performed for these patients to decompress the cord, an extremely unstable biomechanical environment results because of the preexisting laminectomy. In essence, the right and left sides of the spine become disconnected from each other. Supplemental posterior fixation is recommended to improve the stability of the construct. Additionally, in patients with significant kyphosis requiring multilevel anterior decompression, supplemental posterior fixation and fusion should be considered.

## Ossification of the Posterior Longitudinal Ligament
OPLL is a potential cause of cervical myelopathy. Although OPLL-related myelopathy has mainly been described in Japan and its prevalence in the North Amer-

ica population is not known, the disorder is not limited to the Asian population. The cause of OPLL remains unclear, but is most likely multifactorial and related to genetic, hormonal, and environmental influences. Various factors have been implicated, including diabetes, obesity, a diet high in salt intake and low in meat consumption, poor calcium absorption, mechanical stress on the posterior longitudinal ligament, and even sleep habits. OPLL has been noted in approximately 50% of patients with diffuse idiopathic skeletal hyperostosis and may therefore be related to a predisposition for ossification. There also appears to be a familial basis to the disorder, but the mechanism of inheritance is unclear. In Japan, epidemiologic studies have shown a 44% prevalence of OPLL in siblings of patients with known OPLL. More specifically, biochemical studies have linked OPLL to a variety of molecular factors, including collagen XI, transforming growth factor β-1, bone morphogenetic protein-4, and nucleotide pyrophosphatase.

Depending on the severity of OPLL and the amount of associated cord compression, patients may be completely asymptomatic or have severe myelopathy. The pattern of ossification may be segmental, continuous, localized to the disk space, or mixed. As with CSM, the treatment of myelopathy caused by OPLL is typically surgical. However, the surgical treatment of the myelopathic patient with OPLL must take into account two unique variables not usually encountered in the patient with CSM. Depending on the amount and extent of OPLL, direct resection via an anterior approach may be more difficult than in the patient with CSM. OPLL can sometimes erode through the dura, leaving a dural deficiency with attempts at removal (Figure 11). In this circumstance, one way to avoid dural tears is to allow the adherent posterior longitudinal ligament to float anteriorly after corpectomy without necessarily removing it. Another approach is to perform interbody fusion without decompression. This procedure has been suggested for the patient with dynamic myelopathic symptoms and has been reported to have good results. The rationale for this approach is that by immobilizing and fusing the stenotic areas, repeated trauma to the cord by the ossified mass can be avoided. A final means of achieving cord decompression without resection of the posterior longitudinal ligament is to use a posterior approach and perform a laminoplasty.

However, posterior approaches such as laminoplasty and laminectomy that do not resect the ossified posterior longitudinal ligament, introduce the second variable in the surgical treatment of OPLL—namely, the potential for postoperative growth of OPLL. Anterior approaches in which the ossified posterior longitudinal ligament is floated or completely excised have been touted to avoid postoperative growth of OPLL, in contrast to studies of posterior procedures which report a tendency toward radiographic enlargement of OPLL postoperatively. Regardless, postoperative growth of OPLL may be more of a theoretic than a practical concern because the occurrence of recurrent myelopathy as a result of an OPLL has been rare. It may be that extensive enlargement of the spinal canal via laminoplasty is sufficient to keep the cord decompressed as long as growth of OPLL is modest in most patients.

As is the case for CSM, the optimal surgical procedure for treating OPLL remains debatable. The same general guidelines which apply to the choice of approaches in patients with CSM apply to those with OPLL. However, if the OPLL is severe, a posterior approach may be preferable and safer, regardless of the number of stenotic levels involved.

## Summary

Cervical myelopathy is a disorder that is typically treated surgically. Early treatment before the onset of permanent cord injury is recommended. For patients with myelopathy arising from one or two disk segments, the anterior approach is generally preferred. For patients with multilevel involvement (three or more disk spaces), laminoplasty may be a better choice. In patients with multilevel stenosis and kyphosis, or those with postlaminectomy kyphosis, a combined anterior-posterior approach may be best. The surgical procedure chosen must be tailored to the patient's specific pattern of stenosis, comorbidities, and symptoms. Strict adherence to a blind algorithmic treatment protocol should be avoided.

## Annotated Bibliography
### Cervical Spondylotic Myelopathy

Edwards CC, Heller JG, Murakami H: Corpectomy versus laminoplasty for multilevel cervical myelopathy: An independent matched-cohort analysis. *Spine* 2002;27: 1168-1175.

A comparison of the clinical and radiographic outcomes of multilevel corpectomy and laminoplasty using an independent matched-cohort analysis concluded that both multilevel corpectomy and laminoplasty reliably arrest myelopathic progression in multilevel cervical myelopathy and can lead to significant neurologic recovery and pain reduction in most patients.

Hasegawa K, Homma T, Chiba Y, et al: Effects of surgical treatment for cervical spondylotic myelopathy in patients > or = 70 years of age: A retrospective comparative study. *J Spinal Disord Tech* 2002;15:458-460.

A study was performed to compare efficacy of cervical surgery for myelopathy in patients 70 years of age or older and patients 60 years of age or younger. Forty patients age 70 years or older and 50 patients age 60 years or younger with myelopathy (confirmed by MRI and CT) were neurologically assessed using the Japanese Orthopaedic Association score. Three surgical procedures were performed: anterior spinal fusion, laminoplasty, and laminectomy. Postoperatively, patients exhibited comparable outcomes irrespective of age or the surgical procedure performed. The only exception was the increase in postoperative neurologic complications noted for older patients with more comorbidities.

Heller JG, Edwards CC, Murakami H, et al: Laminoplasty versus laminectomy and fusion for multilevel cervical myelopathy: An independent matched cohort analysis. *Spine* 2001;26:1330-1336.

A comparison of the clinical and radiographic outcomes of two procedures that are increasingly used to treat multilevel cervical myelopathy showed a marked difference in the complication rate and functional improvement between matched cohorts. Results of the study suggested that laminoplasty may be preferable to laminectomy with fusion as a posterior procedure for patients with multilevel cervical myelopathy.

Hilibrand AS, Fye MA, Emery SE, et al: Increased rate of arthrodesis with strut grafting after multilevel anterior cervical decompression. *Spine* 2002;27:146-151.

In this study, the reconstruction techniques after multilevel anterior cervical decompression were retrospectively compared. It was determined that because pseudarthrosis resulted in poorer clinical outcomes, strut grafting should be considered after multilevel anterior cervical decompression to increase the rate of successful fusion.

Park AE, Heller JG: Cervical laminoplasty: Use of a novel titanium plate to maintain canal expansion: Surgical technique. *J Spinal Disord Tech* 2004;17:265-271.

A description of the use of a novel plate designed to maintain canal expansion and the technical issues relevant to performing the laminoplasty and securing the laminae showed that the plate was biomechanically equal or superior to the currently used techniques. The use of this plate will allow the patient to engage in an early active rehabilitation protocol while minimizing the risk of restenosis of the canal, which may ultimately lead to better preservation of motion and decreased axial neck pain following laminoplasty.

Samartzis D, Shen FH, Matthews DK, Yoon ST, Goldberg EJ, An HS: Comparison of allograft to autograft in multilevel anterior cervical discectomy and fusion with rigid plate fixation. *Spine J* 2003;3:451-459.

This article presents a retrospective radiographic and clinical review of 80 consecutive patients who underwent ACDF with rigid anterior plate fixation involving two and three levels. The efficacy on fusion rates and clinical outcomes of using allografts or autografts was determined. Fusion was obtained in 97.8% of patients with segmental screw fixation and 97.1% with nonsegmental screw fixation. Proper patient selection and meticulous surgical technique is essential to obtain high fusion rates and optimal clinical outcome, which are more important factors than the type of graft used.

Shiraishi T, Fukuda K, Yato Y, et al: Results of skip laminectomy: Minimum 2-year follow-up study compared with open-door laminoplasty. *Spine* 2003;28:2667-2672.

The results of using skip laminectomy and open-door laminoplasty to treat patients with CSM were compared to verify that skip laminectomy is less invasive to the posterior extensor mechanism of the cervical spine, including the deep extensor muscles, than conventional laminoplasty. Skip laminectomy also was effective in preventing postoperative complications often seen after conventional laminoplasty of the cervical spine, such as persistent axial pain, restriction of neck motion, and loss of cervical lordosis.

Suda K, Abumi K, Ito M, et al: Local kyphosis reduces surgical outcomes of expansive open-door laminoplasty for cervical spondylotic myelopathy. *Spine* 2003;28:1258-1262.

This retrospective study was performed to analyze the effects of cervical alignment on surgical results of expansive laminoplasty (ELAP) for patients with CSM and to determine the limitation of posterior decompression by ELAP for CSM in the presence of local kyphosis. The influence of cervical malalignment on neurologic recovery after ELAP for CSM was shown. In patients with local kyphosis exceeding 13°, anterior decompression or posterior correction of kyphosis as well as ELAP should be considered. ELAP for CSM is best indicated for patients with local kyphosis less than 13°.

Wada E, Suzuki S, Kanazawa A, et al: Subtotal corpectomy versus laminoplasty for multilevel cervical spondylotic myelopathy: A long-term follow-up study over 10 years. *Spine* 2001;26:1443-1447.

A retrospective study was conducted to compare the long-term outcomes of subtotal corpectomy with laminoplasty for patients with multilevel CSM. Subtotal corpectomy and laminoplasty had an identical effect for the surgical treatment of multilevel CSM. Neurologic recoveries usually last for more than 10 years. In the subtotal corpectomy group, the disadvantages were longer surgical time, more blood loss, and pseudarthrosis. In the laminoplasty group, axial pain frequently occurred, and the range of motion was severely reduced.

Yoshida M, Tamaki T, Kawakami M, et al: Does reconstruction of posterior ligamentous complex with extensor musculature decrease axial symptoms after cervical laminoplasty? *Spine* 2002;27:1414-1418.

Postoperative axial symptoms were investigated in 173 of 214 patients (80.1%) who underwent ELAP between January 1989 and December 1998 to determine the prevalence of both preoperative and postoperative axial symptoms of this treatment. The authors concluded that laminoplasty is an appropriate surgery for CSM and did not, in this study, seem to have any significant influence on the development or resolution of axial symptoms.

## Ossification of the Posterior Longitudinal Ligament

Furushima K, Shimo-Onoda K, Maeda S, et al: Large-scale screening for candidate genes of ossification of the posterior longitudinal ligament of the spine. *J Bone Miner Res* 2002;17:128-137.

An extensive nonparametric linkage study with 126 affected pairs of siblings using markers for various candidate genes was performed to detect genetic determinants associated with OPLL. Eighty-eight candidate genes were selected by comparing the genes identified by complementary DNA microarray analysis of systematic gene expression profiles during osteoblastic differentiation of human mesenchymal stem cells with the genes known to be involved in bone metabolism.

Iwasaki M, Kawaguchi Y, Kimura T, Yonenobu K: Long-term results of expansive laminoplasty for ossification of the posterior longitudinal ligament of the cervical spine: More than 10 years follow up. *J Neurosurg* 2002;96:180-189.

Long-term (> 10-year) results of cervical laminoplasty for OPLL of the cervical spine, as well as the factors affecting the long-term postoperative course, showed that when the incidence of surgery-related complications and the strong possibility of postoperative growth of OPLL are taken into consideration, expansive and extensive laminoplasty for OPLL is recommended.

Kamiya M, Harada A, Mizuno M, Iwata H, Yamada Y: Association between a polymorphism of the transforming growth factor-beta1 gene and genetic susceptibility to ossification of the posterior longitudinal ligament in Japanese patients. *Spine* 2001;26:1264-1266.

This study was conducted to determine the association between polymorphism of the transforming growth factor-β1 gene and the prevalence of OPLL. Results showed that transforming growth factor-β1 genotyping may be useful in the prevention of OPLL.

Koshizuka Y, Kawaguchi H, Ogata N, et al: Nucleotide pyrophosphatase gene polymorphism associated with ossification of the posterior longitudinal ligament of the spine. *J Bone Miner Res* 2002;17:138-144.

A case-control association study of 180 patients with OPLL and 265 control patients without OPLL showed that one of these single-nucleotide polymorphisms (IVS15-14T → C substitution), was more frequently observed in OPLL patients ($P = 0.022$), especially in those patients with severe ossification ($P < 0.0001$) and young age of onset ($P = 0.002$), than in controls. A stratified study with the number of ossified vertebrae in patients with OPLL showed that IVS15-14T → C substitution ($P = 0.013$), young age at onset ($P = 0.046$), and female gender ($P = 0.006$) were associated with severe ossification. The authors concluded that the IVS15-14T → C substitution in the human *NPPS* gene is associated not only with susceptibility to, but also with severity of OPLL.

Maeda S, Ishidou Y, Koga H, et al: Functional impact of human collagen alpha2(XI) gene polymorphism in pathogenesis of ossification of the posterior longitudinal ligament of the spine. *J Bone Miner Res* 2001;16:948-957.

A follow-up of earlier studies (providing genetic linkage and allelic association evidence of distinct differences in the human collagen α2[XI] gene [*COL11A2*] that may indicate inherited predisposition to OPLL) was performed to observe a strong allelic association with non-OPLL ($P = 0.0003$) with an intron 6 polymorphism (intron 6 [-4A]), in which the intron 6 (-4A) allele is more frequently observed in patients without OPLL than in patients with OPLL. These results showed that retaining exon 7 together with removal of exon 6 observed in intron 6 (-4A) could play a protective role in the ectopic ossification process because the same pattern was observed in undifferentiated Ob cells and non-OPLL cells.

Matsuoka T, Yamaura I, Kurosa Y, et al: Long-term results of the anterior floating method for cervical myelopathy caused by ossification of the posterior longitudinal ligament. *Spine* 2001;26:241-248.

An investigation of the long-term results of the anterior floating method used to manage OPLL showed that this method appears to yield adequate long-term outcomes.

Onari K, Akiyama N, Kondo S, et al: Long-term follow-up results of anterior interbody fusion applied for cervical myelopathy due to ossification of the posterior longitudinal ligament. *Spine* 2001;26:488-493.

A long-term follow-up study was performed in 30 patients who underwent anterior interbody fusion for cervical myelopathy associated with OPLL. Results showed that anterior interbody fusion without decompression is an effective treatment for cervical OPLL myelopathy that has stable long-lasting outcomes.

Washio M, Kobashi G, Okamoto K, et al: Sleeping habit and other life styles in the prime of life and risk for ossification of the posterior longitudinal ligament of the spine (OPLL): A case-control study in Japan. *J Epidemiol* 2004;14:168-173.

This article presents the results of a study conducted to facilitate early prediction and prevention of OPLL by analysis of life styles such as sleeping habit, physical exercise, smoking, alcohol usage, and the occurrence of hangover in individuals in the prime of life. It was concluded that good sleeping habits in the prime of life may decrease the risk of OPLL.

## Classic Bibliography

Bohlman HH, Emery SE, Goodfellow DB, et al: Robinson anterior cervical discectomy and arthrodesis for cervical radiculopathy: Long-term follow-up of one hundred and twenty-two patients. *J Bone Joint Surg Am* 1993;75:1298-1307.

DiAngelo DJ, Foley KT, Vossel KA, et al: Anterior cervical plating reverses load transfer through multilevel strut-grafts. *Spine* 2000;25:783-795.

Emery SE, Bohlman HH, Bolesta MJ, et al: Anterior cervical decompression and arthrodesis for the treatment of cervical spondylotic myelopathy: Two to seventeen-year follow-up. *J Bone Joint Surg Am* 1998; 80:941-951.

Fernyhough JC, White JI, LaRocca H: Fusion rates in multilevel cervical spondylosis comparing allograft fibula with autograft fibula in 126 patients. *Spine* 1991;16: S561-S564.

Guigui P, Benoist M, Deburge A: Spinal deformity and instability after multilevel cervical laminectomy for spondylotic myelopathy. *Spine* 1998;23:440-447.

Hilibrand AS, Carlson GD, Palumbo MA, et al: Radiculopathy and myelopathy at segments adjacent to the site of a previous anterior cervical arthrodesis. *J Bone Joint Surg Am* 1999;81:519-528.

Hosono N, Yonenobu K, Ono K: Neck and shoulder pain after laminoplasty: A noticeable complication. *Spine* 1996;21:1969-1973.

Isomi T, Panjabi MM, Wang JL, et al: Stabilizing potential of anterior cervical plates in multilevel corpectomies. *Spine* 1999;24:2219-2223.

Kato Y, Iwasaki M, Fuji T, et al: Long-term follow-up results of laminectomy for cervical myelopathy caused by ossification of the posterior longitudinal ligament. *J Neurosurg* 1998;89:217-223.

Macdonald RL, Fehlings MG, Tator CH, et al: Multilevel anterior cervical corpectomy and fibular allograft fusion for cervical myelopathy. *J Neurosurg* 1997;86:990-997.

Mikawa Y, Shikata J, Yamamuro T: Spinal deformity and instability after multilevel cervical laminectomy. *Spine* 1987;12:6-11.

Nurick S: The natural history and the results of surgical treatment of the spinal cord disorder associated with cervical spondylosis. *Brain* 1972;95:101-108.

Resnick D, Niwayama G: Radiographic and pathologic features of spinal involvement in diffuse idiopathic skeletal hyperostosis (DISH). *Radiology* 1976;119:559-568.

Riew KD, Hilibrand AS, Palumbo MA, et al: Anterior cervical corpectomy in patients previously managed with a laminectomy: Short-term complications. *J Bone Joint Surg Am* 1999;81:950-957.

Riew KD, Sethi NS, Devney J, et al: Complications of buttress plate stabilization of cervical corpectomy. *Spine* 1999;24:2404-2410.

Sakou T, Matsunaga S, Koga H, et al: Recent progress in the study of pathogenesis of ossification of the posterior longitudinal ligament. *J Orthop Sci* 2000;5:310-315.

Saunders RL, Pikus HJ, Ball P: Four-level cervical corpectomy. *Spine* 1998;23:2455-2461.

Satomi K, Nishu Y, Kohno T, et al: Long-term follow-up studies of open-door expansive laminoplasty for cervical stenotic myelopathy. *Spine* 1994;19:507-510.

Swank ML, Lowery GL, Bhat AL, et al: Anterior cervical allograft arthrodesis and instrumentation: Multilevel interbody grafting or strut graft reconstruction. *Eur Spine J* 1997;6:138-143.

Tsuyama N: Ossification of the posterior longitudinal ligament of the spine. *Clin Orthop Relat Res* 1984;184: 71-84.

Uematsu Y, Tokuhashi Y, Matsuzaki H: Radiculopathy after laminoplasty of the cervical spine. *Spine* 1998;23: 2057-2062.

Vaccaro AR, Falatyn SP, Scuderi GJ, et al: Early failure of long segment anterior cervical plate fixation. *J Spinal Disord* 1998;11:410-415.

Wang PN, Chen SS, Liu HC, et al: Ossification of the posterior longitudinal ligament of the spine: A case-control risk factor study. *Spine* 1999;24:142-144.

Yonenobu K, Hosono N, Iwasaki M, Asano M, Ono K: Laminoplasty versus subtotal corpectomy: A comparative study of results in multisegmental cervical spondylotic myelopathy. *Spine* 1992;17:1281-1284.

Zdeblick TA, Bohlman HH: Cervical kyphosis and myelopathy: Treatment by anterior corpectomy and strutgrafting. *J Bone Joint Surg Am* 1989;71:170-182.

# Chapter 27

# Disorders of the Spinal Cord

John B. Pracyk, MD, PhD

Vincent C. Traynelis, MD

## Chiari Malformation and Syringomyelia
### History

Chiari malformations are a congenital or acquired group of deformities that result in caudal displacement of the posterior fossa structures below the foramen magnum. The differential extent of hindbrain descent is one of the parameters that constitute the respective Chiari type I, II, III, and IV nomenclature. Other conditions include a spectrum of associated anomalies such as hydrocephalus, myelomeningocele, and syringomyelia. Hindbrain herniation of the cerebellum was first described in 1883 by Cleland in the *Journal of Anatomy and Physiology*. Eight years later, Hans Chiari, a professor of anatomy in Prague, further characterized the malformation but rightfully acknowledged Cleland's earlier work. Today, four respective Chiari malformation types exist, although only three types were originally described.

In the Chiari I malformation (the mildest form), only the cerebellar tonsils descend at least 5 mm below the foramen magnum. The Chiari II malformation represents a more complex herniation involving the cerebellar vermis, medulla, and a portion of the fourth ventricle. In some instances, the pons can even descend below the foramen magnum. The Chiari II malformation is found in most patients with myelomeningocele. If the posterior fossa structures descend beyond the foramen magnum to reside within the cervical canal itself and there is a high cervical or suboccipital encephalomeningocele, a Chiari III malformation exists. These malformations are frequently fatal. The very rare Chiari IV malformation is defined by cerebellar hypoplasia without any herniation.

Syringomyelia is a clinical entity defined as the accumulation of fluid within the spinal cord. The fluid accumulation is usually in the areas immediately adjacent to, but not within, the central canal. Hydromyelia, a specific type of syringomyelia, represents simple dilatation of the central canal itself and is often associated with Chiari malformations (Figure 1).

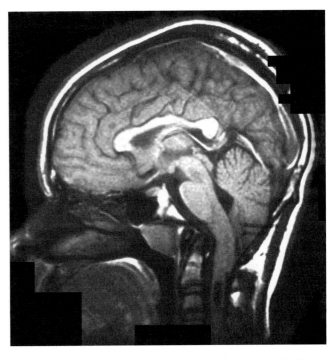

**Figure 1** MRI scan of the brain showing a Chiari II malformation in which the contents of the posterior fossa have descended through the foramen magnum. Note the kinking of the brain stem at the pontomedullary junction and the identifiable syrinx within the cervical cord at the C2 level.

### Pathophysiology

The fundamental abnormality in patients with Chiari malformations is the descent of the posterior fossa contents into the foramen magnum, which may disturb normal cerebrospinal fluid (CSF) flow through the craniovertebral junction. Many theories have been proposed to explain the development of syringomyelia. One theory was that obstruction of the foramen of Magendie (fourth ventricle outlet) was believed to allow the transmission of arterial CSF pulsations, thereby creating a "water hammer" effect through a patent obex, resulting in successive dilatation of the central canal. Alternatively, it was believed that the herniated cerebellar tonsils create an obstruction at the craniocervical junction. A pressure differential between the cranial and cervical compartments creates a syrinx formation along the central canal. Using dynamic (cine) MRI, one author postulated that the descent of the tonsils creates a piston-like effect on the CSF residing within the central canal, which over time creates a syrinx.

### Clinical Signs and Symptoms

The herniation of hindbrain contents through the foramen magnum may produce many of the clinical signs and symptoms of Chiari malformations. Lower brain stem dysfunction produces upper and lower motor neuron signs in the bulbar muscles and nystagmus. Involvement of the descending corticospinal tract produces upper motor neuron and gait disturbances. Truncal ataxia results from compromise of midline cerebellar structures. Few patients have vocal cord paralysis and the resultant respiratory stridor.

Syrinx formation within the adjacent cervical cord explains why many of these symptoms initially begin in the upper extremities. The loss of pain and temperature sensation results from the disruption of pain fibers crossing ventral to the central canal. As the syrinx expands ventrally and approaches the anterior horn, motor neuron destruction produces muscle atrophy and a clinical loss of strength. Similarly, extension of the syrinx dorsally may compromise joint position and vibratory sense carried by the posterior columns. Finally, ascending sensory tracts and descending motor tracts produce upper motor neuron signs, including spasticity, clonus, bowel and bladder dysfunction, and gait disturbances.

### Radiographic Imaging

MRI is the preferred modality for demonstrating the many important anatomic relationships found in patients with Chiari malformations, including (1) the extent of caudal displacement of the cerebellar tonsils, vermis, brain stem, and fourth ventricle through the foramen magnum; (2) the size of the lateral ventricles for the diagnosis of hydrocephalus; (3) the rostral-caudal dimensions and transverse diameter of an associated syrinx cavity; and (4) the presence of a cervical or suboccipital encephalomeningocele. Cine MRI incorporates heart rate information and is useful to visualize CSF flow. With each heartbeat, CSF is forced toward the spine to compensate for the blood entering the brain. Supplemental software fuses disparate images to show the amount of CSF flowing around the hindbrain and spinal cord, particularly at the foramen magnum. This technology is useful in "borderline" cases in which the caudal descent is less than 5 mm and the usefulness of surgical decompression is not indicated by traditional MRI. CT myelography is an alternative imaging modality for patients with contraindications to the use of MRI.

### Surgical Indications and Patient Selection

Surgical decompression is usually recommended for patients who have symptoms clearly referable to a Chiari malformation. Neurologic, sensory, and motor deficits, syringomyelia, cerebellar signs, bulbar dysfunction, hydrocephalus, scoliosis, and respiratory compromise unquestionably warrant surgical intervention. Reasonable expectations of surgical treatment should be communicated to the patient preoperatively. In general, patients with only mild symptoms can expect some degree of resolution. In patients with more moderate deficits, the surgical objective is to prevent the progression of disease rather than to achieve symptom resolution. Headaches alone usually do not warrant surgical intervention. Cine MRI has proved useful in documenting abnormalities in CSF flow in those patients with borderline or uncertain surgical indications.

### Surgical Objectives

The surgical objectives for patients with craniovertebral decompression are focused on increasing the posterior fossa volume and assuring unobstructed CSF flow at the craniocervical junction. Syringomyelia and hydromyelia are intimately associated with abnormal CSF flow dynamics. In most patients, correcting CSF flow abnormalities will lead to resolution of the syrinx. Only in rare, refractory instances should direct drainage of the syrinx be considered.

### Surgical Technique

The patient is usually positioned prone for surgery. Exposure entails a midline muscle-splitting incision from the inion to the C3 spinous process, depending on the caudal extent of the syrinx, if present. Attention to hemostasis is important because blood degradation products induce arachnoid scarring. Leaving a muscle flap attached to the superior nuchal line can be helpful in closure. The craniectomy should be conservative, extending a maximum of 3 cm above the foramen magnum, and should be at least 3 cm in width. The decompression width is far more important than the height. The decompression should extend completely to the lateral aspects of the foramen magnum. In almost all patients a C1 laminectomy is also necessary.

Careful attention must be paid to the opening of the foramen magnum. Occipitalization of the C1 ring, a thickened vascular ligament on the underside of the bone, and ectatic vertebral arteries can easily complicate the bony decompression. An epidural venous plexus is located between the dura and the C1 lamina periosteum. Bipolar cautery and an assortment of thrombolytic agents are important adjuncts for hemostasis.

The dura is opened in a Y-shaped fashion beginning over each cerebellar hemisphere and carried to the midline. Significant dural sinuses and venous lakes can be problematic, and it is advisable to have hemoclips or fine suture available to affix the two layers of the dura together. Bipolar cauterization is usually ineffective and will lead to dural shrinkage. The arachnoid is opened sharply in the transverse plane just below the foramen magnum.

Identification of the posterior inferior cerebellar artery and its relationship to the cerebellar tonsils is fundamentally important. Mobilization of the tonsils through lysis of the arachnoid scar that affixes them together in the midline allows opening to the fourth ventricle. Bipolar electrocautery can then be used to shrink the tonsils away from the midline as well as the foramen magnum. The midline foramen of Magendie should always be inspected. A veil of arachnoid may obstruct the flow from the fourth ventricle. If an arachnoidal obstruction is present, it should be lysed and a fourth ventricular subarachnoid shunt considered. Such shunts consist of small Silastic tubes with one end placed into the fourth ventricle itself and the other end placed in the subarachnoid space caudal to the transverse opening made in the arachnoid. The tube is secured to the arachnoid with a fine suture. Such shunts will prevent reclosure of the foramen of Magendie by an arachnoid membrane.

Closure traditionally incorporates an expansile duraplasty. Many material choices exist to accomplish this, including pericranium, autologous fascia lata, lyophilized cadaveric fascia, bovine pericardium, and synthetic materials. Natural materials decrease the incidence of leakage and inflammation. The dural closure must be careful, meticulous, and watertight. Reinforcing the suture line with fibrin glue is frequently described but has not been scientifically proven to be beneficial. The integrity of the suture line should be tested with a Valsalva pressure maneuver. Increased intracranial pressure and hydrocephalus can compromise a suture line and should be excluded radiographically. Diversion of CSF for children with Chiari II malformation or any patient with hydrocephalus should be performed prior to undertaking the primary posterior fossa decompression. The muscles, fascia, and skin should be reapproximated in a layered fashion.

### Postoperative Management and Complications
If the dural repair is tenuous, it can be managed with a postoperative lumbar drain. Hematoma formation, heralded by new onset neurologic deficits, requires immediate reexploration and evacuation. Respiratory complications can result from the prone position and surgical manipulation near the obex and the respiratory center. Patients with cranial nerve dysfunction may have an impaired gag reflex and are at risk for aspiration and subsequent pneumonia. If a cervical syrinx produced sleep apnea as one of the presenting symptoms, continuous pulse oximetry is warranted until the apnea and/or the syrinx resolves. The presence of a significant syrinx on

follow-up MRI scans may require placement of a syringosubarachnoid, peritoneal, or pleural shunt. If a pseudomeningocele develops, it may be first treated nonsurgically with needle aspiration and a head wrap. A lumbar subarachnoid catheter also may be useful. If it does not resolve promptly and permanently, the wound should be reexplored. Routine MRI follow-up occurs at 3 months postoperatively. Syrinx resolution can usually be documented by this interval. If patients have persistent symptoms, cine MRI is useful to document abnormal CSF flow.

### Results
Approximately 90% of patients will improve or at least stabilize in terms of the progression of symptoms. The remaining 10% of patients will clinically deteriorate despite successful surgical therapy. Persistent muscle weakness, atrophy, pain, ataxia, or any symptoms that persist for longer than 2 years probably reflect permanent disability and are unlikely to improve.

### Conclusion and Perspective
The primary surgical treatment of Chiari malformations and associated syringomyelia consists of posterior fossa decompression, cervical laminectomy, and expansile duraplasty. This surgical strategy will reverse abnormal CSF flow between the cranial and cervical compartments. Surgically addressing an associated syrinx remains a less attractive secondary option.

## Tethered Cord Syndrome
Tethered cord syndrome represents an occult spinal dysraphism. These primary embryonic myelodysplasias also include meningomyelocele, dermal sinus, lipoma, split cord malformations, and tight filum terminale. The basic pathologic entity centers on failure of the spinal cord to ascend within the spinal canal as the patient grows. Tension, abnormal stretching, and distortion produce ischemia and changes in oxidative metabolism within the spinal cord.

### Clinical Signs and Symptoms
Symptoms and clinical signs often occur during the adolescent growth period. Cutaneous stigmata in the dorsal midline include skin tags, dimples, hypertrichosis, hemangiomas, lipomas, and dermal sinus openings. Symptoms can be grouped into orthopaedic, neurologic, and urologic categories. Scoliosis, pedal deformities, and gait disturbances characterize the orthopaedic symptoms. Neurologic symptoms include distal motor weakness in the lower extremities, dermatomal pain, sensory disturbances, and meningitis. Urologic manifestations involve sphincter dysfunction with partial bladder emptying, hydronephrosis, and a history of urinary tract infections. Fecal incontinence is also found.

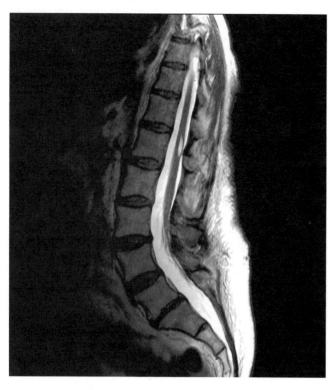

**Figure 2** MRI scan of the lumbar spine showing a tethered cord in which the conus medullaris extends down to the L3-4 disk space. This scan also shows a syrinx within the spinal cord rostral to the tethered cord at the level of the first lumbar vertebra.

### Diagnosis and Patient Selection

External cutaneous stigmata or tethering symptoms should trigger a detailed neurologic evaluation with radiographic assessment to fully delineate the anatomic anomaly. MRI evaluation of the entire axial spine, including the craniocervical junction, should be obtained. The pathologic hallmarks of tethered cord syndrome are a conus lying below the L2 level or a filum terminale greater than 2 mm in thickness (Figure 2). The cord may be displaced dorsally, resulting in a "bowstring" appearance. CT is useful particularly if bony abnormalities exist. After the diagnosis is made, surgical intervention is recommended. Although surgery was a debated treatment in the past, it is now an accepted practice because once symptoms appear they are frequently irreversible.

### Treatment

Surgical detethering of the cord is the treatment objective and must be accomplished without the patient incurring further neurologic loss. Intraoperative electromyogram recordings with electrodes monitoring muscles and sphincters are used in conjunction with intradural nerve root stimulation. Prior to any structure being divided, electrical stimulation is first applied to rule out neurologic function. The approach is a dorsal midline laminectomy with meticulous attention to hemostasis before opening of the dura, as blood degrada-

tion products have been shown to increase the development of arachnoiditis which may lead to complications including retethering. The thickened filum terminale is identified. Frequently there is a lipoma associated with the filum. The filum is coagulated or secured with hemoclips before dividing the structure. This technique will prevent hemorrhage from the associated vessels. The dura is closed primarily. The high incidence of sphincter dysfunction in this patient population mandates the use of a Foley catheter for the perioperative period. If a postoperative cutaneous CSF leak develops, initial reinforcement of the suture line with simple interrupted sutures may be performed; however, surgical exploration is frequently required.

## Intramedullary Spinal Cord Lesions

In 1916, the first of three authoritative works dealing with intramedullary spinal cord lesions were published in which the fundamental principles of successful surgical resection were described. A generous exposure over both poles of the tumor is obtained to allow for adequate resection; careful attention is paid to the vascularity of the cord and tumor. For many years, biopsy and radiation were the mainstays of treatment for these lesions. New technology has transformed the principles of intradural spinal cord surgery. Improved surgical outcomes are a direct and proximate result of the development of better diagnostic radiographic techniques such as MRI, the advent of the surgical microscope, improved surgical instrumentation, intraoperative ultrasound, the use an ultrasonic aspirator, and, possibly intraoperative electrophysiologic monitoring. These advancements have allowed for a philosophic change in clinical treatment. Surgeons can now be aggressive and pursue total resection without simultaneously incurring any neurologic deficits. Surgical treatment of these lesions is now the mainstay of treatment.

### Epidemiology

Intramedullary spinal cord lesions are rare neoplasms, representing about 20% of all spinal cord tumors in adults and 35% to 40% of all pediatric spinal tumors. Compared with their intracranial counterparts, intramedullary spinal cord lesions occur at the ratio of approximately 1:20. Males and females are equally affected. Genetic predispositions are reflected in the association of ependymoma with neurofibromatosis type II, and hemangioblastoma with von Hippel-Lindau disease. Both represent autosomal dominant patterns of inheritance. Pediatric intramedullary tumors have a propensity (46%) for the cervical and thoracic spine and rarely occur in the lumbar spine. In adult patients, the tumors are more evenly distributed.

## Clinical Symptomatology

The onset of clinical symptoms from intramedullary spinal cord lesions is usually slow and insidious, with an average duration from symptom onset to surgery of 3.5 years. Exacerbations and remissions represent changes in peritumoral edema. The most common symptom is pain, with weakness usually manifesting as ataxia. Paresthesias tend to occur late and are not usually painful. Alterations in temperature sensation also may occur. Spinal deformity can occur in up to 30% of pediatric patients. Involvement of the conus medullaris produces sphincter disturbances. Cervicomedullary tumors can manifest with either one of two groups of symptoms. If the tumor predominantly causes brain stem dysfunction, then nausea, emesis, swallowing difficulties, and failure to thrive dominate the clinical picture. Alternatively, chronic neck pain, torticollis, limb motor deficits, and hyperreflexia characterize a cervical lesion. Cranial nerve dysfunction is rare.

## Imaging

Triplanar (axial, sagittal, coronal) MRI with T1-weighted, T1-weighted with contrast, and T2-weighted images constitutes a complete study. Intramedullary lesions typically have both solid and cystic components (Figure 3). The resolution obtained with MRI permits definition of both the rostral and caudal extents of the lesion. Typically, tumor enhancement and a widened spinal cord are seen. Astrocytomas seamlessly integrate into the surrounding spinal cord and frequently present with polar cysts and nonuniform contrast enhancement. Ependymomas typically have a well-defined plane between the spinal cord and the tumor and uniformly display contrast enhancement. Evidence of previous hemorrhage can frequently be seen; cysts also may occur. Hemangioblastomas show intense and eccentric enhancement. If a large hemangioblastoma is suspected, spinal angiography may be useful. Intramedullary metastases represent a rare group of tumors.

## Tumor Types

Of the tumor types discussed, astrocytomas have the widest range of presentations. The pilocytic astrocytoma characteristically presents with an associated cyst. The fibrillary astrocytoma is infiltrative in nature and causes diffuse spinal cord enlargement. Occasionally a syrinx may be associated with this neoplasm. Higher grade tumors include the anaplastic astrocytomas and the glioblastoma multiforme. These tumors are more heterogeneous in their uptake of contrast enhancement and typically display central necrosis. Ependymomas may be classically well-circumscribed intramedullary tumors. Myxopapillary ependymomas present in the caudal spinal canal and are usually intradural extramedullary lesions. Unlike their intracranial counterparts, spinal

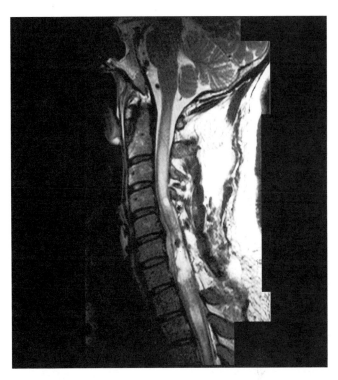

**Figure 3**   MRI scan of the cervical spine showing an intramedullary spinal cord tumor. Note the heterogeneous appearance of the lesion with a diffusely infiltrative component located rostrally and a well-demarcated component caudally at the C6-T1 levels.

ependymomas have a decidedly more encouraging prognosis. Hemangioblastomas account for approximately 2% to 6% of all spinal cord lesions. Patients with von Hippel-Lindau disease may have intracranial and intraspinal hemangioblastomas, retinal hemangioblastomas, cystic lesions of the kidney, liver, pancreas, epididymis, and renal cell carcinoma.

## Patient Evaluation and Selection

The increased availability of MRI has made the diagnosis of these lesions before the onset of major neurologic symptoms a common occurrence. This advancement has produced a philosophical shift in the manner in which these lesions are treated; simply put, early diagnosis drives early treatment. In the past, surgery had been used as a salvage procedure that attempted to restore function that had already been lost; however, it was often too late to realistically recover any function. Surgical intervention should focus on protecting neural elements from future deterioration. In general, patients tolerate surgery better when their baseline preoperative level of functioning is already high.

## Surgical Objectives and Strategies

The goals of surgical treatment of intramedullary spinal cord lesions are tissue diagnosis, neural decompression, and gross total tumor resection. Unfortunately, success is often predicated on the identification of a well-visualized tumor/spinal cord interface. Intuitively, the better defined the dissection plane, the easier the surgical resection. For well-circumscribed tumors such as ependymomas and hemangioblastomas, surgical resection is more straightforward. For more infiltrative lesions such as astrocytomas, the objective of total resection remains more elusive. It is reasonable to resect only what is visibly identifiable as tumor and leave the surrounding transition region of the spinal cord intact. Treatment options can range from a simple biopsy for the diffusely infiltrative lesion that will eventually receive radiation, to a more aggressive resection which would be reserved for a well-circumscribed lesion. Intramedullary lipomas, like astrocytomas, can seamlessly infiltrate into the cord, completely obscuring the tumor margins; therefore, gross total resection is not possible. Internal decompression alone is usually sufficient for effective control.

### Surgical Technique

After appropriate localization, a laminectomy is performed through a dorsal midline incision and subsequent subperiosteal dissection is performed. Alternatively, laminoplasty is a reasonable consideration for preservation of the dorsal tension band that can help reduce postoperative instability, particularly in pediatric patients. Special attention should be paid to maintaining the integrity of the facet joints. After the laminectomy but before the durotomy, intraoperative ultrasound is useful to help delineate the extent of the lesion. Optimal hemostasis is of paramount importance in maintaining a clean field in preparation for the dural opening; lining the surgical field with soaked cottonoids can be helpful. A midline myelotomy is performed to expose both the rostral and caudal extents of the tumor. Enhanced visualization can be accomplished with the aid of pial traction sutures. Bipolar cautery, variable suction, and microsurgical technique are critical. Additionally, the ultrasonic aspirator and $CO_2$ laser aid in debulking lesions that have significant mass. Devices with lower heat transmission are inherently safer alternatives for the preservation of adjacent neural tissues. If gross total resection cannot be achieved, the objective is volumetric reduction of the tumor burden. Hemangioblastomas deserve special mention, as their vascularity precludes traditional internal decompression. Instead, cauterizing the tumor capsule with bipolar cautery may shrink the tumor, which facilitates development of the dissection plane.

Monitoring continuous real-time intraoperative somatosensory and motor-evoked potentials may be helpful. If previously strong signals suddenly deteriorate, the patient's blood pressure should be elevated, the pial traction sutures released, and the dissection halted. If the signals return to normal, the dissection may proceed. If they do not return to baseline, the surgeon must decide whether further tumor resection is warranted. Rotational distortions in the cord may be difficult to appreciate, and neurophysiologic monitoring can aid in identifying the true midline for placement of the myelotomy. Attention to dural closure is of paramount importance. Previous surgery and radiation predispose the patient to the development of an incisional CSF leak. In such circumstances, flat bed rest and the use of a lumbar drain for the first 72 hours is a reasonable consideration.

### Postoperative Management

Adjunctive chemotherapy for intramedullary spinal cord tumors has not been proved to be of universal benefit. For subtotal resections, radiation may prove beneficial but should be used with caution in pediatric patients. As with any surgery, mobilization should be an early goal, although it may be hampered in paretic and plegic patients. Prophylaxis for deep venous thrombosis should be considered for these patients. Postoperative MRI serves to establish the extent of tumor resection as well as provide a basis for future surveillance scans at regular intervals. For the few patients in whom the primary resection was not curative, recurrence will appear on imaging before clinical symptoms occur. Because of the low-grade nature of most spinal cord tumors, most patients with subtotal resections will have a considerable disease-free interval.

### Postoperative Complications

The approach to these lesions through the midline myelotomy corridor can produce dorsal column dysfunction. Dural adhesions along with spinal cord and rootlet tethering may complicate the procedure, particularly when operating on recurrent tumors. Acute transient postoperative deterioration typically represents a neurapraxia that can be treated with aggressive physical therapy. Preoperative deficits often worsen in the immediate postoperative period, but late onset deterioration is uncharacteristic and warrants repeating imaging studies. As in many surgeries, wound healing complications can be a common occurrence, particularly for patients treated with radiation, chemotherapy, and steroids.

### Outcomes

Multiple technological advances have made gross total resection of most intramedullary spinal cord tumors a reality. Mean survival times of 173 months following radical resection compared with 67 months for biopsy alone have established surgery as the fundamental treatment modality. The favorable prognosis and long-term survival rates are directly related to the low-grade status of many of these tumors. Conversely, in those few patients who already have significant neurologic dysfunc-

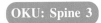

tion, surgical therapy offers effective lesion control but holds less hope for recovery or improvement. Early diagnosis and early surgery offer the best possible promise for preserving neurologic function.

## Summary

Patients with suspected spinal cord pathology should be carefully and completely evaluated with a comprehensive examination and appropriate diagnostic studies. Properly planned and executed surgical procedures will benefit these patients.

## Annotated Bibliography

### Chiari Malformation and Syringomyelia

Mazzola CA, Fried AH: Revision surgery of Chiari malformation decompression. *Neurosurg Focus* 2003;15:E3.

Surgical revision following Chiari decompression is common. The reasons for revision surgery are discussed including initial presentations and surgical indications. Several types of revision strategies are currently available.

Stevenson KL: Chiari type II malformation: Past, present, and future. *Neurosurg Focus* 2004;16:E5.

The author reviews the literature of the Chiari II malformation, typically found in children with myelomeningocele. Embryology, anatomy, symptomatology, pitfalls of diagnosis, and new treatment theories are discussed. The author advocates a proactive and aggressive treatment approach.

Tubbs RS, Smyth MD, Wellons JC, Oakes JW: Arachnoid veils and the Chiari I malformation. *J Neurosurg* 2004;100:465-467.

The authors relate their experience with 140 Chiari I patients and the incidence of foramen of Magendie obstruction by an arachnoid veil. A review of preoperative imaging studies failed to disclose these structural anomalies. The authors present arguments for duraplasty and arachnoid veil fenestration.

Tubbs RS, Webb DB, Oakes WJ: Persistent syringomyelia following pediatric Chiari I decompression: Radiological and surgical findings. *J Neurosurg* 2004;100:460-464.

The authors analyzed a small series of patients to distinguish possible radiographic and surgical findings that may aid in the identification of patients likely to respond to decompression alone. The authors also report their findings in patients requiring reoperative intervention.

### Tethered Cord Syndrome

Kothbauer KF, Novak K: Intraoperative monitoring for tethered cord surgery: An update. *Neurosurg Focus* 2004;16:E8.

The authors review the latest advances in neurophysiologic recording techniques possible for a patient who has had general anesthesia. Technologic advances in digital recording, documentation, and video technology allow for intraoperative identification of neural structures and continuous monitoring of their functional integrity.

Van Leeuwen R, Notermans NC, Vandertop PW: Surgery in adults with tethered cord syndrome: Outcome study with independent clinical review. *J Neurosurg* 2001;94:205-209.

This article presents a retrospective analysis of 57 adults with surgically treated tethered cord syndrome and examines the utility of prophylactic surgery. Postsurgical deterioration was associated with acute preoperative paresis, lipomyelomeningocele, and split cord malformations.

### Intramedullary Spinal Cord Lesions

Cohen-Gadol AA, Zikel OM, Miller GM, Aksamit AJ, Scheithauer BW, Krauss WE: Spinal cord biopsy: A review of 38 cases. *Neurosurgery* 2003;52:806-816.

The authors report on a retrospective study of 38 consecutive patients who underwent spinal cord biopsy. In 26.3% of the patients, the treatment strategy was modified by the biopsy results.

Fassett DR, Schmidt MH: Lumbosacral ependymomas: A review of the management of intradural and extradural tumors. *Neurosurg Focus* 2003;15:E13.

Lumbosacral ependymomas consist of two distinct entities that are treated differently. A literature review showed that the prognosis for the more common intradural lesions is measurably better than the rarer extradural ependymoma. The use of adjunctive radiation therapy is also discussed.

Jallo GI, Kothbauer KF, Epstein FJ: Intrinsic spinal cord tumor resection. *Neurosurgery* 2001;49:1124-1128.

Advances in microsurgical technique and intraoperative monitoring have established surgery as the fundamental treatment for spinal cord lesions. An online digital video can be accessed through the journal's website which demonstrates the authors' surgical techniques and nuances.

Quinones-Hinojosa A, Gulati M, Lyon R, Gupta N, Yingling C: Spinal cord mapping as an adjunct for resection of intramedullary tumors: Surgical technique with case illustrations. *Neurosurgery* 2002;51:1199-1207.

Antidromically elicited somatosensory-evoked potentials and motor-evoked potentials were used to plan a surgical myelotomy. These techniques were also used for direct mapping of spinal cord tracts during tumor resection in an attempt to reduce the risk of neurologic deficits and increase the extent of tumor resection.

Roonprapunt C, Silver VM, Setton A, Freed D, Epstein FJ, Jallo GI: Surgical management of isolated hemangioblastomas of the spinal cord. *Neurosurgery* 2001;49:321-328.

A retrospective study of 19 consecutive patients with isolated intramedullary hemangioblastoma is reported. The role of this study focused on defining the occurrence of these lesions.

## Classic Bibliography

Chiari H: Uber Veranderungen des Kleinhirns in Folge von Hydrocephalie des Grosshirns. *Dtsch Med Wochenschr* 1991;17:1172-1175.

Cleland J: Contribution to the study of spina bifida, encephalocele and anencephalus. *J Anat Physiol* 1983;17: 257-291.

Dyste GN, Menezes AH, VanGilder JC: Symptomatic Chiari malformations: An analysis of presentation, management, and long-term outcome. *J Neurosurg* 1989;71: 159-168.

Gardner W, Angel J: The mechanism of syringomyelia and its surgical correction. *Clin Neurosurg* 1959;6:131-140.

Menezes AH: Chiari I malformations and hydromyelia: Complications. *Pediatr Neurosurg* 1991-92;17:146-154.

Oldfield EH, Muraszko K, Shawker TH, Patronas NJ: Pathophysiology of syringomyelia associated with Chiari I malformation of the cerebellar tonsils: Implications for diagnosis and treatment. *J Neurosurg* 1994;80:3-15.

Reimer R, Onofrio BM: Astrocytomas of the spinal cord in children and adolescents. *J Neurosurg* 1985;63:669-675.

Williams B: A demonstration analogue for ventricular and intraspinal dynamics (DAVID). *J Neurol Sci* 1974; 23:445-461.

Yamada S, Zinke DE, Sanders D: Pathophysiology of "tethered cord syndrome." *J Neurosurg* 1981;54:494-503.

# Chapter *28*

# Head and Neck Injuries in Athletes

Paul A. Anderson, MD

Michael P. Steinmetz, MD

Jason C. Eck, DO, MS

## Introduction

Sports are an important activity played by most people in North America. Because the head and neck are relatively exposed and are subjected to large acceleration and deceleration forces, they are vulnerable to injuries that can be severe. Unlike most appendicular skeletal trauma, injuries to the brain or spinal cord may be irreversible and are commonly associated with long-term disability.

The first role of physicians and trainers is to prevent such injuries through vigilance in physically preparing athletes for competition, ensuring adequate and safe protective equipment, and monitoring the rules of a sport to ensure that they are designed and followed to minimize injuries. Physicians and trainers have an obligation to develop injury prevention programs. This chapter reviews the epidemiology and pathophysiology of athletic head and neck injuries. Although orthopaedic surgeons generally do not treat brain trauma, this subject is discussed because orthopaedic surgeons are often the responsible physician on the field. Cervical spine trauma resulting from participation in sport activities and return to play guidelines after a head and/or neck injury are reviewed.

## Epidemiology

Injuries to the head and neck are common occurrences resulting from sports-related trauma. The annual incidence of traumatic brain injuries in the United States is between 150 to 430 cases per 100,000 people, and 150 to 500 injuries to the cervical spine per 100,000 people. About 14% of these injuries are related to participation in sports activities. The sports with the highest risk for such injuries are football, gymnastics, wrestling, and ice hockey. Football has the greatest number of head and neck injuries because more than 18 times the number of athletes play football compared with other sports. In terms of mortality, 85% of football-related deaths occur as a result of head and neck injury; subdural hematoma is the most common etiology.

An increasing number of injuries are occurring in nonorganized sports such as diving, skiing, trampolining, and surfing. All of these sports have the risk for head impact, usually from a head-first fall to the ground. Injuries to the cervical spine caused by trampolining were considered an epidemic. Work by the American Academy of Pediatrics to ban trampolines in schools except for use by the most skilled athletes virtually eliminated this mechanism of spinal cord injury.

There appears to be an increased risk of injuries with the increasing age of the athlete. For example, no deaths or spinal cord injuries have been reported for those participating in Pop Warner youth football, but the incidence of injury increases proportionally from high school to college to professional football. The size and speed of the athlete are believed to account for this effect. Once a neurologic injury has occurred, recurrent injuries are much more likely.

Efforts by physician groups and researchers have led to prevention strategies that have resulted in a significant reduction in injuries. Rule changes adopted in 1976 to prevent spearing (a common mechanism of spinal cord injury in football) decreased the annual incidence of spinal cord injury resulting from spearing from more than 30 to fewer than 5. When using the spearing technique, the normal lordotic curvature of the cervical spine becomes flattened and is less able to disperse the applied forces of an axial impact. Similarly, traumatic brain injury deaths have also diminished.

## Stingers and Burners

A stinger or burner is a transient neurologic condition characterized by pain and paresthesias in a unilateral upper extremity following an impact to the head, neck, or shoulder. This is a very common injury affecting up to 65% of college football players over the course of a 4-year career. However, the true incidence is unknown because these injuries often go unreported to coaches and trainers. Athletes report sudden unilateral shoulder or arm pain and muscle weakness involving the deltoid, biceps, and spinati. Symptoms are typically transient, but can last from minutes to weeks. Motor symptoms are more likely to persist than sensory symptoms. Electrodiagnostic studies can be performed for patients with persistent symptoms.

Stingers are peripheral nerve injuries and should not be confused with spinal cord injuries. Bilateral symptoms suggest a more serious injury to the spinal cord. Both tensile and compressive etiologies have been suggested. It is believed that in younger athletes a tensile mechanism is most commonly responsible for the stinger. A stretch or traction injury of the brachial plexus occurs when the head is forced away from the symptomatic side. There are no preexisting degenerative changes. Spurling's test is typically negative in these patients. The C5-C6 level is most commonly affected because of greater mobility in the midcervical spine. It was shown that young athletes with a history of stingers are more likely to have low Pavlov ratios indicating that they may have foraminal and central stenosis. Chronic recurrent symptoms in older athletes are more likely to be caused by foraminal stenosis than brachial plexus stretch.

Another mechanism causing a stinger is extension and compression of the nerve root. This condition is more common in adult athletes and is often associated with preexisting degenerative changes. Spurling's test is often positive in these athletes. Direct impact at Erb's point may also cause a stinger. The incidence of these injuries can be reduced through the use of properly fitting shoulder pads that absorb the force of impact and by using proper techniques for blocking and tackling.

## Pathophysiology of Head Injuries

During participation in sports activities, head injuries can occur in many ways. If the head is at rest, but movable, a direct blow may injure the brain below the point of impact. This is termed a coup injury (for example, if the head is struck with a baseball or hockey stick). A moving head that collides with an unyielding object produces brain injury on the side opposite from the site of impact. This is termed a contrecoup injury. The most common location for these types of injuries are at the temporal and frontal poles. Contrecoup injuries may occur when an athlete falls backward and strikes the back of the head, or when two players collide. If the blow is severe, the skull may absorb most of the injury and dissipate it as a fracture. In this circumstance, the fractured skull may be the direct cause of brain injury.

Compression, tensile, and shear forces may result in neuronal injury, neuronal dysfunction (concussion), tearing of arteries or veins, skull fracture, and/or contusion of the brain against the base of the skull (contrecoup injuries).

Acceleration and sudden deceleration via impact may result in contusion of the temporal tips and frontal lobes because shearing forces occur where rotational gliding is hindered, such as the anterior aspects of the anterior and middle cranial fossa. If a bridging vein is torn, a subdural hematoma may ensue. If a meningeal artery is involved, an epidural hematoma may occur. Damage to pial vessels or the vessel at the base of the skull may result in intracranial or subarachnoid hemorrhage. The most common clinical condition that occurs is concussion.

The exact pathophysiology of concussion is unclear. There are no gross or microscopic changes to the cerebral parenchyma. There appears to be a complex cascade of ionic, metabolic, and physiologic events that may adversely affect cerebral function for days or weeks. An early release of large amounts of the excitatory neurotransmitter (glutamate) occurs, there is a major flux of ions, and the brain enters a period of hyerglycolysis. Metabolic instability, mitochondrial dysfunction, decreased cerebral glucose metabolism, reduced cerebral blood flow, and altered neurotransmission also occur. The result is neuronal dysfunction that may present clinically as altered consciousness, cognitive impairment, and/or somatic symptoms.

## Classification of Head Injuries
### Concussion

The definition of concussion remains somewhat vague. It has been defined as a clinical syndrome characterized by immediate and transient posttraumatic impairment of neural function, such as alteration of consciousness, disturbance of vision, or loss of equilibrium resulting from brainstem involvement. In general, there are no gross or microscopic parenchymal abnormalities. Confusion and/or amnesia may occur but loss of consciousness is not a necessary factor.

### Subdural Hematoma

Subdural hematoma is the leading cause of death following a head injury in an athlete. In this condition, a hemorrhage occurs between the brain and the dura and is most often caused by the tearing of a vein that courses from the surface of the brain to the dura. It may also be caused by a skull fracture or venous sinus injury. An underlying brain injury often occurs, which explains the increased morbidity and mortality compared with epidural hematoma. The athlete does not usually recover consciousness (there is no lucid interval) and requires emergent transport for clot evacuation.

Occasionally, the subdural hematoma accumulates over weeks. This condition is most often associated with headache and changes in mental status. The athlete's cognitive or behavioral state does not return to baseline following the injury and requires CT imaging of the brain and evacuation of the clot if appropriate.

## Epidural Hematoma

Epidural hematoma usually results from a tear in the middle meningeal artery, often with an associated temporal bone fracture. The blood rapidly accumulates between the bone and dura, and may reach a fatal size in 30 to 60 minutes. In contrast to an athlete with subdural hematoma, the athlete with an epidural hematoma may regain consciousness following injury and then develop a progressively worsening headache and declining level of consciousness. As intracranial pressure increases, death may occur if the clot is not rapidly evacuated. The underlying brain is not usually injured; therefore, with rapid craniotomy, recovery is expected. Because of the rapidity of decline, an athlete who has a major head injury should be observed in a medical facility with neurosurgical services.

## Intracerebral Hematoma

Intracerebral hematoma is bleeding directly into the brain substance, often from a torn artery. The athlete may not display a lucid interval and the neurologic decline may rapidly progress. Similar to patients with epidural hematoma, these patients should be observed in a medical facility with neurosurgical services.

## Subarachnoid Hemorrhage

A subarachnoid hemorrhage is bleeding into the subarachnoid space, or the space between the arachnoid membrane and pia. It is usually caused by tearing of tiny blood vessels on the surface of the brain. Surgery is usually not required; however, the athlete should be observed for related complications such as edema or seizure.

## Cerebral Contusion

A cerebral contusion is simply a bruise on the brain. This injury occurs with sudden acceleration/deceleration of the brain or direct trauma and may occur with both coup and contrecoup injuries. Contusions often occur in the frontal and temporal poles. The athlete may report headache, and, if severe, there may be neurologic deficit. Surgical evacuation may be required if the contusion is large and life threatening. If not, only medical management of intracranial pressure may be required. As with bruises elsewhere in the body, these bruises may enlarge over the following 24 to 48 hours and require close observation, often in a neurosurgical intensive care unit.

## Second Impact Syndrome

Second impact syndrome has been defined as rapid brain swelling and herniation following a second head injury. It may be more common than previously reported in the medical literature. Typically, the symptoms from the first injury have not resolved when the athlete has a second head injury. The symptoms following the initial injury are postconcussive, and may include headache, difficulty concentrating, difficulty with memory, or visual, motor, or sensory changes.

Interestingly, the second injury may be minor, even a blow to the chest or back. After the second blow, the athlete may remain conscious but appears stunned. Within minutes of the second impact, the stunned athlete may rapidly collapse and display evidence of diffuse brain swelling and herniation, such as pupillary dilation, loss of consciousness, and respiratory collapse. This condition may rapidly progress to death, even before transport to neurosurgical services.

Second impact syndrome is believed to be caused by loss of autoregulation of the brain's circulation following the second injury. This loss leads to vascular engorgement and diffuse edema. The diffuse increase in intracranial pressure leads to eventual herniation with brainstem compromise leading to coma, ocular involvement, and cardiorespiratory failure.

Because this condition can be rapidly fatal, prevention is the only appropriate treatment. It should be emphasized that athletes may only return to play after they are completely asymptomatic from their initial head injury, even if it takes weeks to months. This precaution applies to participation in athletic practices, not just to competitive play.

## Pathophysiology of Spinal Injury

In athletes, spinal injuries usually occur through impact to the cranium. The location and direction of impact and magnitude of acceleration/deceleration determine the patterns of injury. Because most of these injuries result from blows to the cranium, axial compression in either flexion or extension are common. Several biomechanical studies using video fluoroscopy have noted complex patterns of deformations of the cervical spine that occur during impact and within the first 10 milliseconds following impact. The cervical spine is a mobile linkage, which under compressive loads significantly collapses or shortens, with varying amounts of flexion and extension occurring at the same time at different levels. Various patterns of injury occur; however, most patterns can be divided into hyperflexion, axial loading, and extension. In some patients, the deformation of the spine can cause narrowing of the spinal canal with transient cord compression or significant stretching of the cord past the elastic range of the neural tissue.

Hyperflexion injuries can occur in the upper cervical spine with rupture of the transverse ligament and atlantoaxial instability. In the lower cervical spine, hyperflexion causes disruption of the posterior ligamentous complex. Further hyperflexion, especially if the head is initially in a flexed position, can create bilateral facet dislocation.

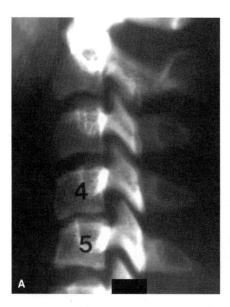 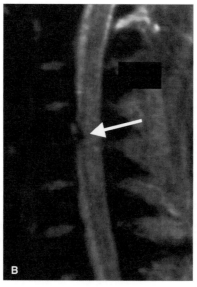 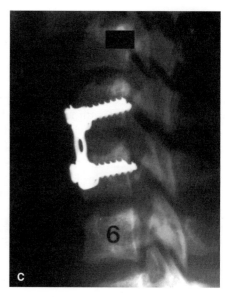

**Figure 1** **A,** A lateral radiograph of 15-year-old wrestler who was dropped on his head and sustained a lateral mass fracture at C4-5 with anterior subluxation. Neurologically the patient had Brown-Séquard syndrome. **B,** MRI shows subluxation of C4-5 with disk space narrowing and disk herniation compressing the spinal cord. **C,** Postoperative lateral radiograph after anterior cervical diskectomy and fusion with a plate. The patient had an excellent recovery but continued to have spasticity and did not return to play.

Hyperextension may be occurring more commonly because of efforts to eliminate axial and flexion-axial loading mechanisms. In these injuries, the athlete is in a heads-up position and, during impact, forces are transmitted to the lateral columns and posterior elements. Additionally, the disk may be disrupted. Compression of the facets can result in lateral mass fractures with or without laminar or spinal process fractures. Occasionally, with a diskoligamentous injury, retrolisthesis of the vertebral body may result. Transient deformation in the neuroforamina may injure nerve roots and be mistaken for a burner. In patients with congenital canal narrowing, transient cord compression may result in neurapraxia.

Axial loading with small amounts of flexion is a head position common to most sports activities. Therefore, associated injury patterns from this position are seen in many athletes. Alignment of the vertebrae in a straight pattern greatly reduces the ability of the spinal column to withstand an axially directed load. In this position, the cervical spine loses its normal lordosis, so that when the head is compressed, axial forces create shearing across the vertebral body and tension on the posterior ligament complex. This creates the classic flexion teardrop fracture or axial loading injury as was described by Schneider.

## Patterns of Spinal Injury

A wide variety of neck injuries can occur from trauma and include muscular strain, transient neurologic deficits, minor fractures, and severe unstable injuries. Any patient or athlete with acute neck pain resulting from impact should be treated as if a fracture is present until proved otherwise.

### Muscular Strains
Muscular strains are the most common sports-related injuries of the neck. These strains, which occur during impact while muscles are contracted, are usually stretch injuries at the musculotendinous junction or in the muscle substance. Other injuries include disruption of the facet capsules from forced flexion, which are more common in children. Patients will report pain, stiffness, and muscle spasm. Paresthesia and neurologic deficits are absent. Radiographs are normal except for perhaps loss of cervical lordosis. The patient's prognosis is good, with expected return to play within 1 to 2 weeks.

### Intervertebral Disk Injuries
Young athletes are at risk for traumatic disk herniation from axial loading. In contrast to adults, this injury usually occurs at C3-4 or C4-5, and in the absence of other signs of disk degeneration (Figure 1). Neurologic consequences can range from only pain to traumatic spinal cord injury. Football players and other athletes who use their heads to strike an object such as a ball or an opponent have a significantly higher incidence of degeneration than the general population. In a radiographic study of high school and collegiate football players in Iowa, degenerative disk disease was seen in only 1% of students in junior high school. By the time these athletes were college football players, more than 24% had degenerative disk disease. Athletes playing certain positions such as defensive back and lineback were more prone to disk degeneration. Other sports activities in which athletes use their head to strike an object or sustain impactions (such as rugby, soccer, and ice hockey) have a similar increase of degenerative disk changes.

## Minor Cervical Fractures

Minor cervical fractures are isolated to a single column or region. Examples are vertebral body compression fractures, lateral mass fractures, facet fractures, or spinous process fractures. Most injuries result from compressive forces that are usually associated with lateral bending or extension. A key component of these injuries is that stability is maintained. Stability is defined as the ability of the spinal column to function under physiologic loads without progressive deformity, neurologic change, or long-term pain and disability. In these injuries, radiographs show no interspinous widening, local kyphosis, or subluxation. Neurologic deficits are usually absent, although a radiculopathy may be present. If a spinal cord injury is present, the spine should be considered unstable.

## Major Cervical Fractures

Major cervical spine injuries represent a full clinical spectrum of all unstable spinal injuries. In athletes, axial loading mechanisms are more common and create injury types such as flexion-axial loading or teardrop fractures. In these types of injury, a flexed spine is axially loaded usually by striking another athlete or the ground. The vertebral body is coronally split and the posterior aspect rotates into the spinal cord. Tension in the posterior ligamentous complex will result in a variable amount of disruption and fractures of the lamina and spinous processes. The anterior aspect of the spinal cord is compressed by the rotated vertebral body, often resulting in anterior spinal cord syndrome or complete cord injury.

Other injury types include unilateral and bilateral facet dislocations with anterior subluxation between 25% and 50%, respectively. Fracture separation of the lateral mass, a fracture frequently seen in athletes, is easily confused with a unilateral facet dislocation. This injury is caused by compression and lateral bending, resulting in an ipsilateral pedicle fracture and lamina fracture at its junction with the lateral mass. The lateral mass is thus separated and free to rotate forward. The spine becomes unstable because of the loss of the facet buttress that normally prevents anterior subluxation. Another potentially dangerous lesion, because it is underappreciated, occurs in a patient with a vertebral body compression fracture and posterior ligamentous disruption. Progressive kyphosis and subluxation will invariably develop.

## Congenital and Developmental Anomalies

Because of the large number of people who participate in sport activities, it is not surprising that preexisting congenital or developmental anomalies are detected in some patients. Common conditions that may predispose an athlete to neurologic injury and deserve the attention of physicians are Klippel-Feil syndrome, os odontoideum, and congenital stenosis. Controversy regarding upper cervical instabilities in disabled athletes, such as in those with Down syndrome, will not be discussed in this chapter.

Klippel-Feil syndrome is the failure of segmentation of the cervical spine. The classic pathognomonic triad is congenital fusion, low hairline, and web neck. The most common lesion is a congenital fusion at C2-3 that has little significance. Multiple fusions with only one or two remaining motion segments or those associated with cranial cervical anomalies are believed to place athletes at significance risk for neurologic injury.

Os odontoideum or other odontoid aplasias are believed to be a developmental or posttraumatic condition in which the dens is no longer fused to the C2 body. This condition results in C1-2 instability. The degree of instability can be impressive, ranging up to 20 mm. This condition should be considered as a contraindication to participation in any contact sport activities and a relative indication for prophylactic fusion even in the asymptomatic patient.

## Congenital Stenosis

The most controversial condition in athletes with head and neck diseases is congenital stenosis. In a classic study, the midsagittal diameter was measured from C1 to C7 in 200 asymptomatic volunteers using standard radiographic techniques and an AP diameter of 21 mm at C1, 20 mm at C2, and 17 mm from C3 to C7 was found. Other researchers have reported that the spinal canal diameter is normally greater than 15 mm and that cervical stenosis is present when the canal diameter is less than 13 mm. Magnification of 15% should be assumed when using plain radiographic measurements; however, radiographs of larger sized athletes or those wearing padding increases magnification. The sagittal diameter of the spinal cord is nearly constant in adults averaging approximately 8 mm from C3 to C7.

To eliminate the effects of magnification, Pavlov and Torg recommended using the ratio of midsagittal diameter to vertebral body diameter to assess stenosis. Significant stenosis is believed to be present when this ratio is less than 0.8. Because the ratio is based on vertebral body diameter, which may be variable among individuals, the positive predictive value of the Pavlov ratio is poor. In one study, the predictive value was reported to be 12%. Using this ratio, another author found that 33% of professional athletes had values less than 0.8. These finding are likely related to the relatively larger vertebral body size found in many large athletes. Therefore, the Torg ratio should be considered unreliable and the literature that is based on its assessment should also be considered unreliable. When in question, the best method to identify stenosis is cross-sectional imaging with CT or MRI. A more important parameter is the functional reserve, which is the adequacy of a protective cushion of cerebrospinal fluid around the spinal cord seen with CT myelography or T2-weighted MRI.

### Transient Quadriplegia

Transient spinal cord injury or neurapraxia is the temporary cessation of spinal cord function after trauma, which usually resolves within 15 to 20 minutes and always resolves by 1 to 2 days (Figure 2). Two mechanisms of spinal cord injury are hypothesized: axial loading and hyperextension. In axial loading, the spinal cord is compressed over a bulging disk or stretched from kyphosis, resulting in direct contusion or indirect tension injury. The hyperextension mechanism of injury is characterized by the ligamentum flavum folding into the spinal canal and compressing the spinal cord. Both of these mechanisms are more severe in the presence of preexisting stenosis.

In a 2002 study, 110 athletes with transient quadriplegia or neurapraxia were reviewed. It was found that 65% of those who continued to participate in the sport activity had a recurrent episode. There was a strong correlation between degree of stenosis and the incidence of another episode. The authors noted that in their experience, no one had gone on to permanent neurologic deficit, although follow-up was incomplete. Others authors have reported instances of spinal cord injuries with long-term deficits in patients with a prior history of neurapraxia. Patients with smaller canals are more likely to have more severe spinal cord injuries when the spine is fractured.

## On-the-Field Management

Because orthopaedic surgeons are commonly the team or event physician they should be prepared to assess injured athletes, provide immediate care for life-threatening injuries, stabilize and transport injured athletes, and make on-the-field decisions regarding return to play. These tasks can be very challenging because they are visible to the public and are performed in an unfamiliar and uncomfortable environment. Although most instances involve minor musculoskeletal system injury and quickly resolve, other life-threatening medical conditions such as traumatic brain injury, heat stroke, or cardiac events can occur. Any physician assuming this function should be certified in basic advanced cardiac life support and advanced trauma and life support skills.

In a 2003 study, five facets of on-the-field management were described: (1) preparation, (2) suspicion and diagnosis, (3) stabilization and safety, (4) immediate treatment, and (5) evaluation of return to play.

### Preparation

Preparation involves proper training and practice in potential life-saving and spinal stabilization techniques in simulated conditions. An emergency plan should be on record and include an ambulance on site for all high-

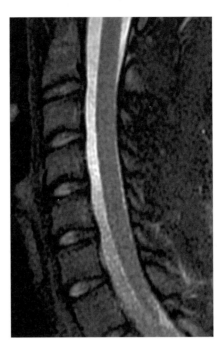

**Figure 2** MRI scan of a 15-year-old quarterback who was tackled and had immediate onset of paralysis and sensory loss in the arms and legs without loss of consciousness. Thirty minutes later he regained all function. The MRI scan is normal with no signs of injury and normal canal dimension. The spinal cord is located posteriorly, which may have been responsible for the transient quadriplegia.

energy or contact sport activities. The National Football League requires all teams to have an on-field trial before the playing season, which includes players with full equipment, team physicians and trainers, and emergency medical personnel. The necessary tools to quickly remove protective equipment should be readily available and in working order. Transport equipment such as a spinal board, extraction collars, and cardiopulmonary resuscitation devices should be available on site and tested before each game.

### Suspicion and Diagnosis

A well-accepted, on-the-field grading scale has been devised that may be easily applied by team physicians and trainers. The scale helps to determine when and which athletes may return to play and which athletes must be transported to a medical facility for further observation and treatment.

On this scale, head injury is divided by level of severity: mild, moderate, and severe (Table 1). Mild head injury is characterized by no loss of consciousness with posttraumatic amnesia lasting less than 30 minutes. If loss of consciousness is less than 5 minutes or the posttraumatic amnesia lasts for more than 30 minutes, the condition is classified as moderate head injury. Those with severe head injury have loss of consciousness for more than 5 minutes or posttraumatic amnesia lasting more than 24 hours.

### Stabilization

Patients with prolonged loss of consciousness, severe head injuries, or neurologic deficits should be stabilized

## Table 1 | Classification of Head Injury in Athletes and Return to Play Criteria

| Grade | Definition | On-the-Field Action | Return to Play |
|---|---|---|---|
| Mild | No LOC, PTA < 30 minutes | Remove from contest<br>Frequent neurologic examinations should be performed | Return to contest if symptoms clear within 30 minutes* |
| Moderate | LOC < 5 minutes or PTA > 30 minutes | Remove from contest<br>Stabilize head and cervical spine on backboard and transport to medical facility for neurologic examination<br>If LOC is brief and patient is fully conscious, may transport off the field with fewer precautions, but professional neurologic examination should be performed | 1 full week without symptoms* if CT/MRI findings are negative[†] |
| Severe | LOC > 5 minutes or PTA > 24 hours | Stabilize head and cervical spine and transport off field on backboard<br>Emergent transport to medical facility with neurosurgical services | 2 weeks without symptoms* and negative CT/MRI findings[†]<br>May be 1 week if LOC was brief and return to asymptomatic state was rapid |

LOC = loss of consciousness; PTA = posttraumatic amnesia
*Evaluations must be made at rest and exertion
[†]If there are positive CT or MRI findings, the athlete should not return to play for the entire season; future return to play should be discouraged

on the field and transported to a hospital. If not supine, patients should be carefully log-rolled supine onto a backboard with the head stabilized by a physician or trainer. For transport, the head or helmet can be taped and sandbags or a collar can be used to immobilize the head and neck. If a face mask is present, it should be quickly removed; however, the helmet or shoulder pads should remain in place. Helmet and shoulder pads can be removed under the following conditions: the helmet and chin pad fit poorly and the head is not stable; there is inadequate access to the airway after the face mask is removed; the face mask cannot be removed; or the helmet interferes with transport. Removal of the helmet and shoulder pads can be done safely but requires a team effort. The National Athletic Trainers Association has described an effective technique involving four people. First, all padding is removed from the helmet and shoulder pads, then one person maneuvers the helmet while another stabilizes the neck posteriorly and the other two stabilize the arms and behind the scapula. In a 2002 study, it was reported that this technique limited cervical motion during helmet and shoulder pad removal.

### Immediate Treatment

Because patients who are unconscious or who have spinal injuries can have respiratory arrest, basic cardiopulmonary resuscitation may be required. This resuscitation requires immediate removal of the face mask or helmet and opening of the shoulder pads. Patients with severe closed head injuries or obvious spinal cord injury should immediately be stabilized on a backboard and transported to a treatment facility. Continuous monitoring of

respiration and blood pressure is required. No attempts at cervical fracture reduction should be performed.

Athletes who have a mild head injury must be removed from the game and allowed to rest on the bench. Although there is no loss of consciousness, the athlete may have difficulty remembering recent events and assimilating and interpreting new information (called having your bell rung). This deficit may escape notice and diligence is required to look for this condition following a collision.

With moderate head injury, the initial management should be similar to that given to athletes with a severe head injury. They should be transported off the field with their head and neck immobilized on a backboard and should be taken to a medical facility with neurosurgical services. If the period of loss of consciousness is brief, and there is no suspicion of neck injury after the athlete regains consciousness, the athlete may be removed from the field without a backboard and should be transported to a medical facility for neurologic observation. CT or MRI may be indicated.

Athletes with a severe head injury should undergo cranial and cervical immobilization on a backboard and should be rapidly transported to a medical facility that has neurosurgical services. The athlete should undergo imaging to evaluate for possible intracranial hemorrhage.

### Return to Play During the Game

Return to play after a head and neck injury may be considered in athletes with minor muscle strains or burners who have recovered full range of motion, have no residual pain or tenderness, and who have no neurologic deficits. Athletes are typically stoic with high pain thresh-

| Table 2 | Contraindications of Return to Play Following Head Injury |
|---|

Persistent postconcussion symptoms

Permanent central nervous system sequelae from head injury (for example, hemiplegia)

Hydrocephalus

Spontaneous subarachnoid hemorrhage

Symptomatic foramen magnum abnormalities (for example, Chiari malformation)

olds and may not initially report significant symptoms because they have an inherent desire to return to play. Therefore, a high index of suspicion is required to prevent more seriously injured athletes from returning to play.

The athlete with a mild head injury should be allowed to rest on the bench for a period of time and should only be allowed to return to play after all symptoms have resolved. Amnesia must resolve within 30 minutes or the player should be classified as having a moderate concussion; that is, there is no headache, dizziness, or impaired concentration or memory. The athlete should be oriented to person, place, time, and recall all of the events occurring immediately before the injury. Additionally, the athlete should demonstrate movement with the usual level of dexterity and speed during exertion. If the symptoms continue while at rest, the athlete requires further observation.

## Return to Play
### After a Head Injury

Many scales have been developed to aid in the determination of when an athlete may return to play. Most scales are based on the grade of concussion. It must be stressed that these scales are only guidelines and athletes should not be allowed to return to play until they are completely asymptomatic. The athlete must be examined at rest and with exertion (such as after running 40 yards, or performing sit-ups or push-ups). Those with a mild concussion may return to play if the symptoms clear within 30 minutes. Athletes with a moderate concussion may be allowed to return to play after 1 full week without symptoms (after symptoms have cleared) both at rest and with exertion, and with normal results on CT scans of the head, if such scans were indicated. These athletes must undergo imaging (CT/MRI) if symptoms persist after 1 week. If positive imaging findings occur, the athlete should not be allowed to return to play for the entire season and should be discouraged from future athletic participation.

Athletes with a severe concussion may be allowed to return to play after 1 to 2 weeks in the absence of symptoms and a normal result on a CT head scan. If the loss

| Table 3 | Return to Play Criteria After Neck Injury Modified From Torg |
|---|

**No Contraindications**

Congenital conditions such as type II Klippel-Feil syndrome (one or two level cervical fusion)

Spina bifida occulta

Healed stable fracture

Asymptomatic disk herniation

Asymptomatic patient status-post one level successful fusion

**Relative Contraindications**

Asymptomatic patients with healed upper cervical fracture such as dens fracture, odontoid fracture, or Jefferson fracture

Healed stable without the vertebral body with normal alignment

Healed stable posterior element fracture

Healed two- to three-level fusion

**Contraindications**

Odontoid abnormalities

Atlantoaxial fusion

Atlantoaxial instability

Complex Klippel-Feil abnormalities

Spear tackler's spine

Cervical instability using White criteria (greater than 3.5 mm translation or 11° angulation compared with adjacent segments

Healed fracture with kyphosis of subluxation

Residual stenosis from bone retropulsion

Symptomatic disk herniation

Fusion with congenital stenosis

| Table 4 | Criteria From Cantu for Return to Play After the First Episode of Transient Quadriplegia |
|---|

Only a single episode

Complete resolution of symptoms

Full range of neck motion

Normal alignment

No instability

Functional reserve space around cord on MRI scan or CT-myelography

of consciousness was brief, consideration should be given to a 1-week respite from play, but if prolonged, the 2-week waiting period should be used. Athletes with positive CT/MRI findings including contusion or edema, should not be allowed to return to play for the entire season; any future return to play should be discouraged. Contraindications for return to play are shown in Table 2. These recommendations are based on a modification of the Cantu and American Academy of Neurology system of concussion grading and management.

It must be emphasized that regardless of the injury level, athletes should never be allowed to return to play unless they are completely asymptomatic. These guide-

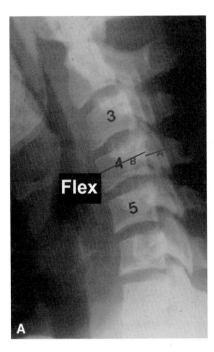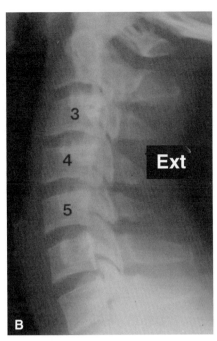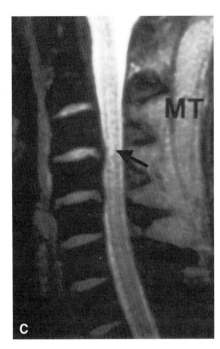

**Figure 3** **A,** Flexion radiograph of 21-year-old collegiate linebacker who speared a quarterback and had transient quadriplegia for 2 hours. His past history was positive for a similar injury 2 years earlier. The radiograph shows a narrow canal at C3-4 and no instability. The Torg ratio is length of A divided by B. **B,** An extension radiograph shows no evidence of instability or fracture. Large posterior osteophytes are present that narrow the spinal canal. **C,** T2-weighted sagittal MRI scan shows cervical kyphosis and anterior cord compression at C3 and C4. A later study showed high-intensity signal in the spinal cord. Although the patient regained neurologic function, he did not return to football.

lines are old concepts and may be replaced by neuropsychologic testing, which may be more sensitive and individualized to the athlete.

### After a Stinger

Return to play for athletes with a stinger can be allowed after full resolution of symptoms. Testing of the deltoid, biceps, brachioradialis, triceps, wrist flexors and extensors, and intrinsic muscles should be performed and compared with the contralateral asymptomatic side. If symptoms resolve, the athlete may be allowed to return to the game. However, athletes with persistent motor or sensory symptoms should not be allowed to return to play until they have complete resolution of symptoms.

### After a Neck Injury

Allowing an athlete to return to play after a neck injury is a difficult decision. Consideration should be given to the short-term and especially the long-term prognosis of the athlete. There are often many interested parties such as the athlete, parents, spouses, school or team officials, agents, the media, and league or sanctioning bodies. For the professional athlete, the discussion becomes a highly complex workers' compensation case. Unfortunately, there is little medical evidence on which to base any decision; all recommendations are currently derived from expert opinion, which varies widely among practitioners.

General concepts apply to athletes with muscle strains, minor fractures that have healed, and patients with resolved disk herniation. Return to play can occur after cessation of pain, restoration of full range of motion, absence of neurologic symptoms, and resolution of loss of any kyphosis. Rehabilitation may speed resolution of symptoms. The goals of rehabilitation should include diminished pain, control of inflammation, restoration of range of motion, and primary tissue healing.

Torg and associates proposed guidelines for return to contact sports for patients with transient neurapraxia, congenital anomalies, and other traumatic conditions (Table 3). Three categories of contraindication were established: no contraindication to return to play, relative contraindication, and absolute contraindication. These contraindications have not been validated and should be considered only expert opinion.

Cantu proposed criteria for return to contact sports after transient quadriplegia (Table 4). He recommended return to contact sports after a single episode of transient quadriplegia, if there was complete recovery, full range of motion, and normal cervical alignment. Also there should be no evidence of stenosis and an adequate reserve of functional cerebral spinal fluid should be present. Contraindications to return to play are a second episode of transient quadriplegia, instability, deformity, or loss of cerebral spinal fluid functional reserve (Figure 3). No validation of these guidelines exists.

## Summary

Head and neck injuries are common in athletes and range from minor muscular strains to potentially life-threatening closed head injuries. Medical staff should be well trained and prepared to deal with on-the-field emergencies and make immediate assessments to determine the severity of injury. Recent protocols have presented criteria for return to play both on the field and after recovery. In general, athletes may only return to play after resolution of symptoms and reversal of any physical findings. The criteria discussed in this chapter have not been validated and are considered only expert opinion.

## Annotated Bibliography

### Epidemiology

Cantu RC, Mueller FO: Catastrophic spine injuries in American football, 1977-2001. *Neurosurgery* 2003;53:358-362.

Over a 25-year period, 223 athletes sustained spinal cord injuries playing football. Since the 1976 rule change that eliminated spearing, a 270% decrease in incidence has been reported.

Ghiselli G, Schaadt G, McAllister DR: On-the-field evaluation of an athlete with a head or neck injury. *Clin Sports Med* 2003;22:445-465.

This article presents a review of the mechanisms of head and spinal cord injury and proper on-field management, including a discussion of transport of injured athletes and helmet removal.

### Stingers and Burners

Shannon B, Klimkiewicz JJ: Cervical burners in the athlete. *Clin Sports Med* 2002;21:29-35.

The syndrome of burners is caused by brachial plexus stretch, intraforaminal compression or compression at Erb's point from poorly positioned protective equipment. Treatment is rest until symptoms resolve and corrective therapy to diminish the effect of the pathologic processes.

### Pathophysiology of Head Injuries

Giza CC, Hovda DA: The neurometabolic cascade of concussion. *J Athl Train* 2001;36:228-235.

The authors reviewed more than 100 articles from the basic science and clinical literature with relevance to concussive brain injury, postinjury pathophysiology, and recovery of function. The authors found that following concussion there is a neuronal depolarization, release of excitatory amino acids, ionic shifts, changes in glucose metabolism, altered cerebral blood flow, and impaired axonal function. These alterations correlate with periods of postconcussive vulnerability and behavioral abnormalities. As the significance and duration of postconcussion physiologic alteration is better delineated, improved guidelines for clinical management of concussion may be formulated.

### Patterns of Spinal Injury

Torg JS, Guille JT, Jaffe S: Injuries to the cervical spine in American football players. *J Bone Joint Surg Am* 2002;84-A:112-122.

This study examined 110 athletes with transient quadriplegia. Those returning to the same contact sport had a 65% incidence of another episode of transient quadriplegia; the presence of cervical stenosis was a strong predictor of recurrence. None of these athletes had a permanent neurologic deficit as a result of additional episodes of the disorder.

Zmurko MG, Tannoury TY, Tannoury CA, Anderson DG: Cervical sprains, disc herniations, minor fractures, and other cervical injuries in the athlete. *Clin Sports Med* 2003;22:513-521.

This article discusses management of mild athletic cervical spine injuries, including overuse syndromes, sprains (the most common injury), disk herniations, and minor fractures.

### On-the-Field Management

Echemendia RJ, Cantu RC: Return to play following sports-related mild traumatic brain injury: The role for neuropsychology. *Appl Neuropsychol* 2003;10:48-55.

Neurophysiologic evaluation identifies neurocognitive changes following traumatic brain injury in atheletes. Using comparison to baseline evaluations, improved decision making regarding return to play can be rendered.

Guskiewicz KM, McCrea M, Marshall SW, et al: Cumulative effects associated with recurrent concussion in collegiate football players: The NCAA Concussion Study. *JAMA* 2003;290:2549-2555.

A prospective study of 1,631 football players was performed. Closed head injury occurred in 95 athletes who recovered by 7 days after injury and had significantly poorer scores on cognitive and balance testing. Neuropsychologic testing appears to identify athletes with brain dysfunction even after resolution of symptoms such as headache.

McCrea M, Guskiewicz KM, Marshall SW, et al: Acute effects and recovery time following concussion in collegiate football players: The NCAA Concussion Study. *JAMA* 2003;290:2556-2563.

In this study, 1,631 football players underwent preseason neuropsychologic testing. During the season, 79 sustained a concussion and had serial repeat neurophysiologic testing. Results showed that significant impairments were present with symptoms, cognitive function, and in balance. These abnormalities resolved usually by 3 to 5 days and no difference was noted at 90 days.

Peris MD, Donaldson WW III, Towers J, Blanc R, Muzzonigro TS: Helmet and shoulder pad removal in sus-

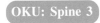
pected cervical spine injury: Human control model. *Spine* 2002;27:995-998.

A technique to remove a helmet from an athlete with a suspected neck injury is validated in this study.

### Return to Play

Morganti C, Sweeney CA, Albanese SA, Burak C, Hosea T, Connolly PJ: Return to play after cervical spine injury. *Spine* 2001;26:1131-1136.

This study examined the decision-making process of return to play and analysis was done using questionnaires to 133 physicians. No consensus of postinjury management was observed. The authors believe that additional research and education are required.

## Classic Bibliography

Alexander MP: Mild traumatic brain injury: pathophysiology, natural history, and clinical management. *Neurology* 1995;45:1253-1260.

Cantu RC: Functional cervical spinal stenosis: A contraindication to participation in contact sports. *Med Sci Sports Exerc* 1993;25:316-317.

Cantu RC: Second-impact syndrome. *Clin Sports Med* 1998;17:37-44.

Cantu RC, Bailes JE, Wilberger JE Jr: Guidelines for return to contact or collision sport after a cervical spine injury. *Clin Sports Med* 1998;17:137-146.

Cantu RC, Mueller FO: Brain injury-related fatalities in American football, 1945-1999. *Neurosurgery* 2003;52:846-852.

Herzog RJ, Wiens JJ, Dillingham MF, Sontag MJ: Normal cervical spine morphometry and cervical spinal stenosis in asymptomatic professional football players: Plain film radiography, multiplanar computed tomography, and magnetic resonance imaging. *Spine* 1991;16:S178-S186.

Kelly JD, Aliquo D, Sitler MR, Odgers C, Moyer RA: Association of burners with cervical canal and foraminal stenosis. *Am J Sports Med* 2000;28:214-217.

Kelly JP, Nichols JS, Filley CM, Lillehei KO, Rubinstein D, Kleinschmidt-DeMasters BK: Concussion in sports: Guidelines for the prevention of catastrophic outcome. *JAMA* 1991;266:2867-2869.

Levitz CL, Reilly PJ, Torg JS: The pathomechanics of chronic, recurrent cervical nerve root neurapraxia: The chronic burner syndrome. *Am J Sports Med* 1997;25:73-76.

Odor JM, Watkins RG, Dillin WH, Dennis S, Saberi M: Incidence of cervical spinal stenosis in professional and rookie football players. *Am J Sports Med* 1990;18:507-509.

Pavlov H, Torg JS, Robie B, Jahre C: Cervical spinal stenosis: Determination with vertebral body ratio method. *Radiology* 1987;164:771-775.

Practice parameter: The management of concussion in sports (summary statement): Report of the Quality Standards Subcommittee. *Neurology* 1997;48:581-585.

Schneider RC: Football head and neck injury. *Surg Neurol* 1987;27:507-508.

Torg JS, Corcoran TA, Thibault LE, et al: Cervical cord neurapraxia: Classification, pathomechanics, morbidity, and management guidelines. *J Neurosurg* 1997;87:843-850.

Torg JS, Sennett B, Vegso JJ: Spinal injury at the level of the third and fourth cervical vertebrae resulting from the axial loading mechanism: An analysis and classification. *Clin Sports Med* 1987;6:159-183.

# Chapter 29

# Degenerative Disorders of the Thoracic Spine

Mark Palumbo, MD

Robert J. Campbell, MD

## Introduction

The age-related process of spinal degeneration produces anatomic and physiologic alterations throughout the vertebral column. As in the cervical and lumbar spine, pathologic structural changes in the thoracic region occur along a continuum with progression through phases of internal disk derangement, disk herniation, and spondylosis. Neurologic consequences can result from compression of the neural elements in the spinal canal or neural foramina.

Symptomatology caused by thoracic diskopathy and spondylosis is relatively rare. The associated clinical syndromes of axial pain, radiculopathy, and myelopathy can occur in isolation or in combination. Diagnosis often proves difficult given the infrequency and variable presentation of thoracic degenerative disorders. Accordingly, the clinician must maintain a high index of suspicion when evaluating the patient with symptoms and signs referable to the thoracic spine.

Decisions regarding treatment can be complicated. Advanced imaging studies must be interpreted carefully given the high prevalence of spinal abnormalities in asymptomatic individuals and the frequent lack of correlation between symptom severity and the magnitude of spinal pathology. Surgical measures are reasonable to consider in patients with intractable pain and/or neurologic dysfunction caused by compression of the thoracic spinal cord or nerve roots.

## Thoracic Disk Herniation

Discogenic pain syndromes caused by a thoracic disk herniation (TDH) are not commonly encountered in clinical practice. It is estimated that only 0.15% to 4% of all symptomatic intervertebral disk protrusions occur in the thoracic region. In recent years, asymptomatic TDHs have been identified with increasing frequency on neuroradiologic imaging studies. Investigational studies using MRI and postmyelographic CT scans have reported incidental detection of a TDH in up to 20% of patients.

## Etiology

Trauma may be a predisposing factor in some patients with TDH. Disk degeneration, however, appears to be the primary causative factor in most patients. Most disk herniations develop in the caudal third of the thoracic spine. This predilection of the degenerative process for the lower thoracic vertebrae may be related to local anatomic features and the unique biomechanical environment of this region. Flexion and torsional forces tend to concentrate between T10 and L1 because the intervening motion segments derive less intrinsic stability from the rib cage. Specifically, the 11th and 12th ribs are not joined to the rib cage anteriorly and do not form a true articulation with the transverse processes of their own vertebra. Additionally, the orientation of the lower thoracic facet joints lies predominantly in the frontal plane and does not effectively resist rotation.

Certain anatomic features of the thoracic spinal column and spinal cord predispose the patient to the development of neurologic dysfunction in association with TDH. Relative to the cervical and lumbar region, the sagittal diameter and cross-sectional area of the thoracic vertebral canal is small. Congenital and/or developmental narrowing of the canal can further reduce the reserve space available to the neural elements. The kyphotic alignment of the thoracic spine also can contribute to the onset of neurologic compromise. Because of kyphosis, the spinal cord tends to translate forward such that it is draped over and closely applied to the posterior surface of the vertebral bodies and disk spaces. The capacity of the cord to migrate posteriorly away from ventral compressive pathology can be limited further by the tethering effect of the dentate ligaments. There is a relatively tenuous blood supply to the cord in the "watershed" zone between T4 and T9 because of the limited intramedullary and radicular circulation.

With respect to the clinical syndromes produced by a TDH, local (such as axial) symptoms and signs are most likely caused by activation of the nerve fibers applied to the anulus fibrosus and posterior longitudinal ligament. Radiculopathy generally results from mechan-

## Table 1 | Differential Diagnosis of Thoracic Pain

**Musculoskeletal**
  Infectious
  Neoplastic
  Degenerative
    Spondylosis
    Spinal stenosis
    Degenerative disk disease
    Facet syndrome
    Costochondritis
  Metabolic
    Osteoporosis
    Osteomalacia
  Traumatic
  Inflammatory
    Ankylosing spondylitis
  Deformity
    Scoliosis
    Kyphosis
  Muscular
    Strain
    Fibromyalgia
    Polymyalgia rheumatica
**Neurogenic**
  Thoracic disk herniation
  Neoplasms
    Extradural
    Intradural
    Extramedullary
    Intramedullary
  Arteriovenous malformation
  Inflammatory
    Herpes zoster
  Postthoracotomy syndrome
  Intercostal neuralgia
**Referred pain**
  Intrathoracic
    Cardiovascular
    Pulmonary
    Mediastinal
  Intra-abdominal
    Gastrointestinal
    Hepatobiliary
  Retroperitoneal
    Renal
    Tumor
    Aneurysm
**Sociopsychogenic**

*(Reproduced from Garfin SR, Vaccaro AR (eds): Orthopaedic Knowledge Update: Spine. Rosemont, IL, American Academy of Orthopaedic Surgeons, 1997, pp 87-96.)*

## Table 2 | Clinical Grades of Symptomatic TDH

Grade 1:  Predominant thoracic central (axial) pain
Grade 2:  Predominant thoracic radicular pain
Grade 3A: Significant axial and thoracic radicular pain
Grade 3B: Significant axial and lower leg pain (with or without thoracic radicular pain)
Grade 4:  Myelopathy but not significant motor weakness
Grade 5:  Paretic-paralytic (significant motor weakness)

*(Adapted with permission from Anand N, Regan J: Video-assisted thoracoscopic surgery for thoracic disc disease. Spine 2002;27(8):871-879)*

to be caused by a combination of mechanical factors (compression and axial tension) and vascular compromise (ischemia and venous congestion).

### Clinical Presentation

Symptomatic TDH affects males and females in a relatively equal distribution. Patients are usually from 30 to 60 years of age. Clinical manifestations are highly variable. The lack of a characteristic symptom profile often leads to delayed or incorrect diagnosis and can contribute to the development of chronic pain. TDH mimics many diseases and the list of differential diagnoses is extensive (Table 1).

Most patients with a TDH have an insidious onset of symptoms. The duration of time between symptom onset and the patient's presentation for treatment typically ranges from months to years, suggesting that degenerative processes are the primary etiologic factor. In a much smaller percentage of patients, there is an acute onset of symptomatology. These patients may seek early medical care and often associate the condition with some form of traumatic event.

The symptoms and physical signs of TDH depend, at least in part, on the level and size of the lesion and whether the herniation is central, centrolateral, or lateral. Pain is the most commonly reported symptom and is usually axial in distribution. Radicular pain, when present, may involve the chest wall (unilaterally or bilaterally), the groin, or the lower extremity. Discomfort typically improves with rest and is aggravated by Valsalva maneuvers. Sensory deficits are generally caused by nerve root compromise and may include numbness, paresthesias, or dysesthesias. Upper motor neuron signs can develop in the presence of spinal cord compression. A clinical classification system has been developed to differentiate the varied presentations of TDH (Table 2).

### Natural History

Research data pertaining to the clinical consequences of abnormal thoracic disks are not conclusive. Despite this fact, patients with asymptomatic TDH are generally considered to have a benign clinical course. Most protrusions

ical distortion and inflammation of the nerve root. Direct compression of the root is typical of a lateral or paracentral herniation. A midline protrusion can produce radicular symptoms by traction on the nerve fibers as the dural sac is displaced in a dorsal direction. Thoracic myelopathy is usually the result of a large central herniation. The associated cord dysfunction is believed incidentally noted on radiologic imaging studies will not progress to produce pain or neurologic dysfunction even though certain imaging characteristics, including cord compression and deformation, are shared between patients with asymptomatic and symptomatic TDH.

The natural history of a patient with symptomatic TDH is influenced by the characteristics of the compressive lesion and the severity of the presenting symptoms. When pain occurs with no major neurologic deficit, nonsurgical treatment leads to clinical improvement in more than 80% of patients and a return to normal functional activities can be expected. In certain patients, radiculopathy may precede the development of spinal cord dysfunction. Factors that may be predictive of progressive symptomatology include lower extremity, bilateral chest wall, or limb symptoms. Younger patients with traumatic disk herniations also may have a less benign clinical course.

## Imaging Studies

The radiologic modalities typically used to diagnose and characterize a TDH include plain radiographs, MRI, and CT myelography. Although advanced imaging studies can effectively identify intervertebral disk abnormalities, the structural changes may not be clinically relevant. Correlation of the radiologic findings with the history and physical examination is critical to distinguish between a symptomatic and an asymptomatic TDH.

### Plain Radiographs

Although not diagnostic, plain radiographs can prove useful in the workup of a patient with TDH. AP and lateral projections allow assessment of coronal and sagittal plane alignment of the thoracic spine. Degenerative changes are identifiable and typically consist of disk space narrowing, end-plate osteophytes, and facet arthrosis. Calcification of the herniated disk is visible on plain radiographs in 4% to 6% of patients.

### Magnetic Resonance Imaging

MRI is the screening study of choice for patients with a suspected TDH. The technique is noninvasive and does not expose the patient to ionizing radiation. Sagittal and axial images can be acquired directly with no need for intrathecal contrast. Degenerative changes, herniated disk material, and neural element compression are delineated with excellent anatomic detail (Figure 1).

The MRI criteria for an intervertebral disk herniation are met when nuclear material extends beyond the posterior margin of the adjacent vertebral body end plates and compromises the space available for the neural elements. The level of the TDH is determined by counting spinal segments down from the second cervical vertebra (or up from the sacrum) on the midsagittal scout view. The herniation can be classified according to

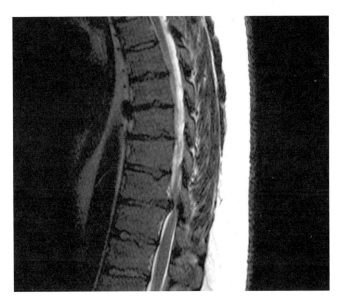

Figure 1   MRI scan showing parasagittal view of a T10-T11 thoracic soft-disk herniation. This soft herniation is characterized as paracentral in location.

its location in the axial plane as: central, if a plane transecting the protruded disk material is coincident with the midsagittal plane; paracentral, if the middle portion of the protrusion is situated to the side of midline but medial to the lateral limit of the dural sac; or lateral, if the major portion of the herniation projects to the side of the lateral edge of the thecal sac.

A relative lack of specificity is the major drawback of using MRI for a TDH. Along with the high prevalence of abnormal findings in asymptomatic individuals, there is no apparent correlation between the size of the herniation and the severity of clinical symptoms. MRI studies are also limited in the capacity to identify calcification within a disk protrusion. When surgical treatment is indicated, MRI alone is generally insufficient for technical planning of the procedure.

### CT Myelography

The sensitivity and specificity of CT myelography is equivalent to that of MRI. However, the myelogram is an invasive procedure that requires injection of an intrathecal contrast agent. Acquisition of CT data necessitates axial cuts at multiple levels, exposing the patient to a relatively high dose of radiation; therefore, CT myelography is not routinely used as an initial screening examination.

When MRI is contraindicated, CT myelography is the procedure of choice to diagnose a TDH. This diagnostic test should also be considered in advance of any surgical procedure. It provides for a more comprehensive analysis of the pathologic anatomy, allowing the surgeon to select the optimal surgical approach.

Dystrophic calcification, reported to occur in 30% to 70% of TDHs, is best delineated on CT scans (Figure 2).

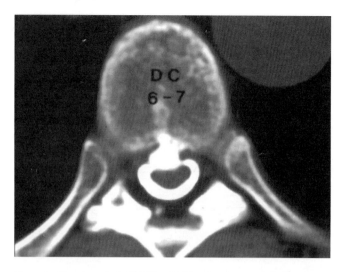

**Figure 2** CT myelograph of a TDH. This axial CT section shows a calcified central disk herniation causing anterior cord compression.

It is important to identify this abnormality before surgery. Calcified disks are often associated with neurologic dysfunction and are more likely to be adherent to the dura.

## Treatment

In treating the patient with a symptomatic TDH, the primary objectives are to arrest the progression of and reverse any neurologic deficits, and to relieve or eliminate pain.

### Nonsurgical Treatment

For the patient who does not have significant neurologic dysfunction or signs of myelopathy, nonsurgical therapy is appropriate. Nonsurgical treatment generally begins with a short period of bed rest followed by gradual mobilization and activity modification. Symptom control can be accomplished with pharmacologic measures, which may include short-term oral corticosteroids, nonsteroidal anti-inflammatory drugs, and, when necessary, opiates. Physical therapy in the form of postural training, core strengthening, and cardiovascular conditioning also may be efficacious. A spinal orthosis can be considered as a means of facilitating early mobilization and pain control.

### Surgical Treatment

**Indications** Surgical treatment of a patient with TDH is reasonable to consider when a clinically significant neurologic deficit caused by compression of the spinal cord or nerve roots is present. Spinal cord dysfunction, especially when accompanied by lower extremity weakness, is a primary indication for surgery. The patient with severe thoracic radicular pain that does not improve after a comprehensive course of nonsurgical management should also be considered a candidate for surgical treat-

ment. Before finalizing any decision to perform surgery, it is imperative that a clear correlation exists between the clinical symptoms/signs and the radiologic findings.

Surgical intervention may not be suitable for the patient with axial pain and a TDH. It has not yet been established that diskography can reliably identify a thoracic disk as the specific pain generator. In addition, no conclusive data are available to confirm that excision and fusion of a symptomatic thoracic disk will alleviate axial symptoms. Additional research is needed to analyze the efficacy of surgical treatment for patients with central thoracic pain.

**Selection of the Surgical Approach** The major technical objective of surgery is to achieve adequate decompression of the neural elements without compromising neurologic function or spinal stability. Avoidance of iatrogenic neurologic injury is an especially important consideration because the thoracic vertebral canal is difficult to access and the spinal cord is easily damaged by surgical manipulation.

It is critical to select a procedure that is both effective and safe. Clinical variables that must be taken into consideration include the age, general health, and neurologic status of the patient. Specific aspects of the pathologic anatomy that should be factored into the decision are the spinal level of the lesion, the location of the herniation relative to the neural structures, and the consistency of the compressive material. The training and experience of the surgeon will also influence the choice of surgical approach.

Several surgical techniques have been developed to treat patients with symptomatic TDH. The relative superiority of one method over another, however, has been difficult to establish because of the low incidence and unclear natural history of the disease process, lack of uniform outcome measures, and limited number of patients analyzed in published reports. Traditional surgical approaches can be characterized as posterior (laminectomy), posterolateral (transpedicular, costotransversectomy), lateral (costotransversectomy), and transthoracic (transpleural, extrapleural, and transsternal). Less invasive procedures also are available and include nonendoscopic laser diskectomy, thoracic microendoscopic diskectomy, and video-assisted thoracoscopic surgery.

**Traditional Surgical Techniques** In early reports, the standard surgical technique to treat patients with symptomatic TDH involved decompressive laminectomy with intradural/extradural excision of the lesion (Figure 3, *A*). With experience, it became evident that this procedure was associated with poor results and an unacceptably high rate of paraplegia. The neurologic complications were most likely related to the need for retraction of the spinal cord to access the disk material. Use of the posterior approach has now been largely abandoned.

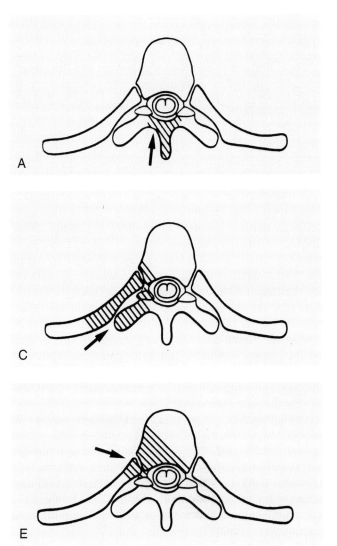

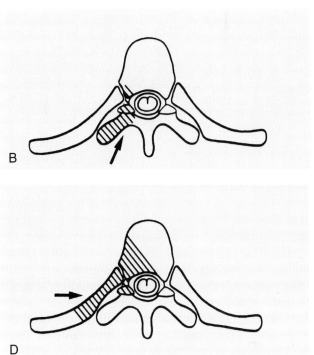

**Figure 3** Traditional surgical approaches for thoracic diskectomy. The angle of approach to the disk space is indicated by the arrow. The cross-hatch area demarcates the extent of osseous resection. **A,** Posterior (laminectomy). **B,** Posterolateral (transpedicular). **C,** Posterolateral (costotransversectomy). **D,** Lateral (extracavitary). **E,** Anterior (transthoracic). *(Reproduced with permission from Cybulski G: Thoracic disc herniation: Surgical technique.* Contemp Neurosurg *1992;14: 1-6.)*

The complications experienced with laminectomy stimulated the development of alternative surgical techniques that do not require manipulation of the spinal cord. The implementation of posterolateral, lateral, and transthoracic approaches for TDH resulted in a significant improvement in surgical outcomes.

**Posterolateral Approach: Transpedicular** The transpedicular approach is relatively popular because the technique and surgical anatomy are familiar to most spinal surgeons (Figure 3, *B*). The procedure is performed through a midline or paramedian incision with the patient prone. On the side of the lesion, the facet joint posterior to the disk space and the pedicle caudal to the herniation are resected. The disk space is entered lateral to the thecal sac and distal to the exiting nerve root. Nucleus pulposus tissue within the intervertebral space is removed after which herniated material can be pushed anteriorly into the central cavity with curets. In general, single level diskectomy cranial to the T10 level does not

require fusion. The thoracic cage prevents destabilization and resultant deformity. At the lower extreme of the thoracic spine at T10-T12 it is reasonable to consider addition of fusion to the decompression.

This surgical option is particularly useful for disk herniations that are soft and situated laterally in the vertebral canal. Compared with other open procedures, the advantages of the transpedicular technique include its simplicity, limited soft-tissue dissection, and lower risk of morbidity. The primary disadvantage is limited visibility of the anterior spinal canal and ventral surface of the dura. This limitation is related to the angle of approach, which is only slightly oblique to the sagittal plane. Given the suboptimal access to the midline, this posterolateral procedure is poorly suited for central TDH, especially when the disk herniation is large, calcified, or associated with spinal cord deformation or intradural penetration.

**Posterolateral Approach: Costotransversectomy** Compared with the transpedicular approach, the costotransversectomy technique allows for a more anterior angle of approach (Figure 3, *C*). The improved exposure is accomplished by removal of the medial portion of the rib and the transverse process immediately caudal to the involved disk space. The disk space is entered lateral to the dural sac and emptied centrally. Using reverse curets, the herniated nucleus pulposus is pushed into the empty interspace and removed.

The major advantage of the costotransversectomy technique compared with the transpedicular procedure relates to improved access and visibility of the lateral and ventral surface of the dura. Costotransversectomy is well suited for resection of lateral and paracentral TDHs. It can be applied to central herniations (especially when thoracotomy is contraindicated) but should be avoided in the presence of disk calcification, large end-plate osteophytes, or intradural penetration.

The major drawback of the approach is that it provides suboptimal exposure of the ventral spinal canal. Other disadvantages relate to more extensive dissection of the paraspinal musculature, extensive removal of osseous structures, and proximity to the pleura.

**Lateral Approach: Extracavitary** The lateral extracavitary procedure involves resection of the facet joint, pedicle, costotransverse articulation, and the medial aspect of the associated rib (Figure 3, *D*). The approach is extrapleural, can be performed at any level of the thoracic spine, and is particularly useful for lateral and paracentral TDHs. It can be considered for midline pathology when thoracotomy would be poorly tolerated.

Relative to the transpedicular and costotransversectomy techniques, the lateral extracavitary approach provides a larger area of access to the posterior and lateral surface of the vertebra and disk. By enhancing access to the midline, it provides some of the advantages of a transthoracic procedure without the morbidity associated with violation of the chest cavity. However, exposure of the ventral spinal canal is still relatively limited. This approach also has an increased potential for morbidity because of the extensive soft-tissue disruption and bone removal, violation of the intercostal neurovascular bundle, and pleural retraction.

**Anterior Approach: Transthoracic** The transthoracic procedure can be used for TDHs situated between the 3rd and 12th thoracic vertebrae (Figure 3, *E*). This technique provides excellent access to the anterior and lateral dural surface. It is favored for central TDHs that are large, calcified, associated with end-plate osteophytes, intradural, or sequestered behind a vertebral body.

In general, the approach is transpleural; an extrapleural exposure is possible at the thoracolumbar junction. The thoracotomy is performed through the rib bed corresponding to the level of the herniation. The base of the rib is excised and the intercostal nerve is followed to identify the appropriate foramen. The caudal pedicle is resected, exposing the underlying dural sac. The midlateral portion of the disk and the posterior aspect of each vertebral body are then removed leaving the dorsal cortex and herniated nucleus in place. The remaining cortical shell and the herniation are then carefully pulled forward away from the dura and into the previously created cavity. The decompression extends across the entire width of the spinal canal to the contralateral pedicle. For a routine thoracic diskectomy, the spine is not destabilized and arthrodesis is not required.

A more extensive decompression may be required in patients with disk fragment migration behind the vertebral body and for calcified herniations which are either adherent to the dura or associated with dural erosion. In these situations, hemivertebrectomy followed by interbody arthrodesis (with or without instrumentation) offers multiple advantages over a more limited anterior approach. The decompressive technique provides better exposure of the pathologic anatomy, improved ability to develop the tissue plane between compressive material and the dura/spinal cord, and enhanced capacity to address a dural defect. Reconstruction of the anterior column maintains sagittal plane alignment and imparts stability to the operated spinal levels.

The advantage of the transthoracic approach is the unrestricted access to the ventral surface of the dural sac and spinal cord. This access allows for optimal decompression of midline pathology without retraction of the spinal cord. Compared with the posterolateral and extracavitary techniques, there is a lower risk of neurologic complications and a higher rate of successful disk excision.

Disadvantages of the transthoracic approach are primarily related to violation of the thoracic cavity. The exposure requires a relatively large incision and extensive muscle dissection along with retraction of the ribs and lung. Significant morbidity can result from pulmonary complications, limb-girdle dysfunction, and prolonged postthoracotomy pain. In patients with marked preoperative respiratory compromise, the anterior approach may be contraindicated because of the potential for hypoxemia with unilateral ventilation.

### *Less Invasive Surgical Techniques*
The surgical treatment of TDH continues to evolve. Less invasive techniques are increasingly being used to access the thoracic disk space and spinal canal. The main objective is to minimize approach-related morbidity without compromising outcome. Compared with traditional approaches, these procedures cause less disruption of normal tissues and can reduce surgical blood loss and operating time. For the patient, the potential advantages of less invasive surgery are reduced postoperative pain, a shortened period of hospitalization, and a more rapid recovery.

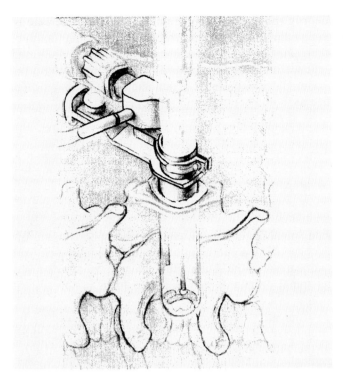

Figure 4  Surgical setup for a thoracic microendoscopic diskectomy. With the tubular retractor in place, the lateral facet complex is resected in preparation for the transforaminal disk excision. *(Reproduced with permission from Perez-Cruet MJ, Kim BS, Sandhu F, Samartzis D, Fessler RG: Thoracic microendoscopic discectomy. J Neurosurg Spine 2004; 1:58-63.)*

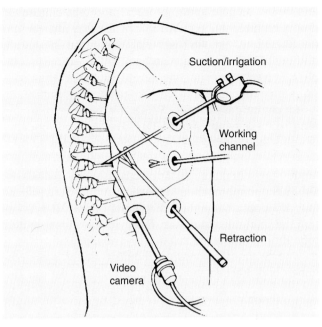

Figure 5  Illustration of VATS for TDH. The approach to the midthoracic disk spaces is accomplished using a three or four trocar strategy to position instruments. *(Reproduced with permission from Regan JJ, Ben-Yishay A, Mack MJ: Video-assisted thoracoscopic excision of herniated thoracic disc: Description of technique and preliminary experience in the first 29 cases. J Spinal Disorders 1998;3:183-191.)*

**Nonendoscopic Percutaneous Laser Diskectomy** Intradiskal percutaneous laser disk decompression and nucleotomy is a nonendoscopic procedure indicated for select patients with symptomatic degenerative disk disease. The technique has gained some acceptance for cervical and lumbar conditions. It has potential applicability to thoracic radicular and/or axial pain syndromes in the absence of significant neurologic dysfunction.

Surgery is performed using regional anesthesia with the patient in a lateral position. Using continuous motor neurologic monitoring and fluoroscopic control, the neodymium-yttrium aluminum garnet (Nd-YAG) 1,064 nm laser is introduced percutaneously into the appropriate disk space. A maximal dose of 1,000 J per disk can be applied. Reports on this technique have documented a high success rate with a very low incidence of complications.

The major advantage of percutaneous laser disk decompression and nucleotomy relates to the minimally invasive nature of the procedure. It is probably best considered as an intermediate treatment option between nonsurgical and surgical care. If the percutaneous disk decompression is not successful, the clinician can proceed with alternative surgical treatment at a later stage.

**Thoracic Microendoscopic Diskectomy** Thoracic microendoscopic diskectomy is a posterolateral approach that accesses the compressive pathology via the neural

foramen (Figure 4). The technique has been applied successfully to the treatment of thoracic radiculopathy and myelopathy caused by lateral, paracentral, and central soft-disk herniations.

This procedure is performed with the patient prone. An incision is made 3 to 4 cm lateral to the midline at the appropriate level. After positioning tubular muscle dilators using fluoroscopic control, the endoscope is passed down the center of a tubular retractor. Exposure requires resection of the lateral portion of the facet joint and the cranial edge of the lower transverse process. After accessing the foramen and identifying the nerve root, the pedicle of the caudal vertebra is followed to the involved disk space. Specialized instruments are used to perform the annulotomy and diskectomy. Use of the 30°-angled endoscope provides enhanced medial visualization, reduces manipulation of the neural elements, and facilitates the decompression.

Compared with traditional posterolateral approaches, thoracic microendoscopic diskectomy is associated with less approach-related morbidity. It requires limited muscle dissection and less bone resection to access the disk herniation. Although medial visualization is enhanced by the endoscope, the technique still provides suboptimal access to the ventral spinal canal.

**Video-Assisted Thoracoscopic Surgery** Video-assisted thoracoscopic surgery (VATS) is a modified anterior approach to the thoracic vertebral column (Figure 5). This less invasive technique allows the surgeon to visualize and manipulate the spinal structures using an endoscope and specialized instruments which are introduced into the thoracic cavity via small incisions in the chest wall. Although technically demanding, VATS permits complete decompression of the neural elements while substantially reducing approach-related surgical trauma.

Over the past decade, VATS has been increasingly used to treat symptomatic TDH. This surgical modality is well-suited for the excision of soft, lateral disk herniations. The experienced surgeon also can use the technique for complex midline compressive pathology. VATS is not appropriate for patients with severe pulmonary disease, an inability to tolerate unilateral ventilation, or pleural symphysis. Prior thoracotomy and/or tube thoracostomy are relative contraindications.

The technical procedure requires use of a double-lumen endotracheal tube for unilateral ventilation. The patient is positioned lateral with a partial forward tilt to allow the collapsed lung to shift anteriorly away from the vertebral column. Neurophysiologic monitoring of somatosensory- and motor-evoked potentials should be considered. A three- or four-portal approach is used to access the thoracic cavity. Trocars are inserted through small incisions made in the intercostal spaces. The 30° endoscope and surgical instruments are introduced, and the ribs are counted internally to identify the appropriate disk space. The surgical level is then confirmed using a marker and fluoroscopy. The procedural steps for diskectomy and decompression are essentially the same as for the open anterior transthoracic approach.

Recent reports indicate that VATS is a safe and effective treatment option for the patient with a symptomatic TDH. A long-term follow-up study documented an overall patient satisfaction rate of 84% and objective clinical success in 70% of patients. The more common complications consist of intercostal neuralgia, atelectasis, and epidural bleeding. Other potential complications include pneumothorax, pleural effusion, dural tear, and neurologic compromise.

The major advantage of VATS is the ability to achieve complete decompression while reducing approach-related trauma. Use of the high-resolution endoscope provides excellent visualization, illumination, and magnification of the spinal structures without the need to significantly retract the ribs or disrupt the soft tissues of the chest wall. Compared with thoracotomy, the endoscopic technique is associated with a decreased incidence of pulmonary morbidity, intercostal neuralgia, and shoulder girdle dysfunction. Other potential advantages include reduced intraoperative blood loss, less incisional pain, and a shortened period of hospitalization. In comparison with the open posterolateral and lateral procedures, thoracoscopy provides more complete access to the ventral spinal canal enabling resection of midline disk herniations.

The main disadvantage of VATS is the technically demanding nature of the procedure. The steep learning curve for the surgeon necessitates a period of dedicated practice on animals. Safe and effective surgery also requires the assistance of a thoracic surgeon with expertise in thoracoscopy.

## Thoracic Stenosis

Narrowing of the spinal canal in the thoracic region is much less common than in the cervical and lumbar spine. Although isolated instances of thoracic stenosis occur in patients with generalized skeletal disorders, canal compromise more frequently results from the localized spinal conditions of hypertrophic spondylosis, ossification of the posterior longitudinal ligament, and ossification of the ligamentum flavum. Stenosis caused by spinal degeneration will be the focus of this discussion.

Clinically significant stenosis is typically caused by circumferential epidural constriction in the lower third of the thoracic spinal column. In most patients, the results of acquired degenerative changes are superimposed on preexisting developmental narrowing of the thoracic canal. Because of the unique anatomy and biomechanical behavior of the T10-T12 vertebral segments, mechanical forces tend to concentrate at the thoracolumbar junction. As a result, the process of spinal degeneration more frequently affects the caudal thoracic levels compared with the more proximal vertebrae of the thoracic spine.

Prompt recognition of thoracic stenosis as a cause of neurologic compromise is important but often difficult to achieve. The clinical presentation, similar to that of TDH, is highly variable. Symptoms and signs frequently suggest the more common diagnoses of cervical and lumbar stenosis. The spectrum of neurologic dysfunction observed in this patient population can be explained, in part, by the neural anatomy of the lower end of the thoracic spinal canal. Because this zone contains both the lumbosacral cord enlargement and portions of the lower thoracic through first sacral nerve roots, compressive pathology can produce mixed upper and lower motor neuron lesions. Spondylotic changes also can cause intermittent claudication by dynamic canal compromise with resultant neural element compression and/or transient circulatory impairment.

Appropriate radiologic investigation is critical to confirm the diagnosis and to define the pathologic anatomy of thoracic stenosis. Plain radiographs are useful for evaluating overall spinal alignment in the sagittal and coronal plane. MRI is the most effective method of screening for neural element compression. In patients with advanced spondylosis, CT scanning after myelography provides the most accurate definition of the compressive pathology. Given the substantial number of pa-

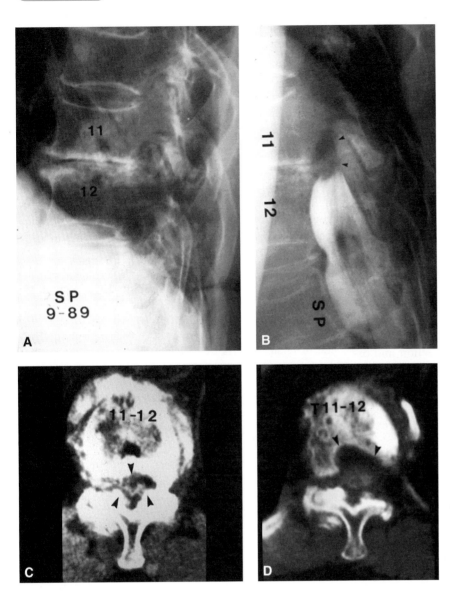

Figure 6  Degenerative stenosis of the thoracic spinal canal. **A,** Lateral plain radiograph showing advanced spondylotic changes at the T11-12 spinal segment. **B,** The lateral myelogram shows a complete block to the flow of intrathecal contrast at the level of the T11-12 disk space. **C,** The postmyelographic axial CT scan shows circumferential canal stenosis secondary to disk protrusion, end-plate osteophyte formation anteriorly, and bilateral facet arthrosis posteriorly. Left and right arrows point to bilateral posterior facet arthrosis. Top arrow points to disk protrusion. **D,** A CT scan (axial section) obtained subsequent to transthoracic diskectomy showed adequate decompression of the neural elements. *(Reproduced with permission from Palumbo MA, Hilibrand A, Hart R, Bohlman HH: Surgical treatment of thoracic spinal stenosis: Two to nine year follow-up.* Spine *2001;26:558-566.)*

tients with concurrent lumbar stenosis, advanced imaging of the lumbosacral spinal canal also should be performed. When the physical examination cannot rule out a neurologic lesion at the cervical level, the entire spinal axis should be imaged.

In part, the limited data available regarding the natural history of thoracic spinal stenosis, make treatment decisions difficult. Nonsurgical treatment is reasonable in the absence of myelopathy or a major neurologic deficit. Nonsurgical treatment options include short-term bed rest, activity modification, thoracolumbar bracing, pharmacologic measures, and physical therapy. Surgical intervention for the patient with documented neural element compression is indicated in the presence of debilitating neurologic dysfunction and/or myelopathy. When major neurologic compromise is not present, the decision to perform surgery should be based on a significant alteration in the patient's quality of life. Typically, such patients have profound restriction in performing the ac-

tivities of daily living caused by pain, sensory abnormalities, or weakness in one or both lower limbs.

All levels that are determined to be stenotic on the preoperative imaging studies should be decompressed. Selection of the surgical approach should be based predominantly on the location of the primary compressive pathology within the spinal canal. Additional factors to consider include the total number of stenotic levels, the need for simultaneous lumbar decompression, and the medical status of the patient. An anterior approach should be strongly considered for patients with one- or two-level disease caused primarily by spondylotic changes involving the end plates and/or disk (Figure 6). Decompressive laminectomy is the standard procedure for patients with canal narrowing caused primarily by facet arthrosis. Posterior decompression is also the preferred initial intervention for the patient with multiple levels of thoracic stenosis and/or concurrent lumbar canal narrowing.

Although satisfactory early results can be expected in most patients, the long-term prognosis after decompression is guarded. Late deterioration after initial improvement is especially problematic after surgery on the lower thoracic segments. Symptoms can recur because of the development of recurrent stenosis, mechanical instability, or progressive deformity at the operated levels. To lower the risk of late complications, a more aggressive surgical approach may be warranted in select patients at the time of the index procedure. Arthrodesis (with or without instrumentation) spanning the thoracolumbar junction should be strongly considered in the presence of local deformity or instability and whenever extensive resection of the stabilizing spinal structures is performed.

## Summary

The successful treatment of degenerative disorders of the thoracic spine represents a great challenge to the spine surgeon. Successful outcomes are intimately linked to proper diagnosis and careful selection and execution of the surgical technique. The incorporation of new technologies will become increasingly important as each is critically evaluated and finds its proper place in the arsenal used to treat these conditions.

## Annotated Bibliography
### Thoracic Disk Herniation

Anand N, Regan JJ: Video-assisted thoracoscopic surgery for thoracic disc disease: Classification and outcome study of 100 consecutive cases with a two year minimum follow-up period. *Spine* 2002;27:871-879.

One hundred consecutive patients undergoing VATS for disk disease were followed prospectively for an average of 4 years. Successful outcomes were defined as improvement of 20% or greater in the Oswestry score from preoperative to 2-year and final follow-up. Clinical success was noted in 73% of patients at 2 years and 70% at final follow-up. Patient satisfaction was quoted at 84% overall. The authors concluded that VATS is safe and efficacious in the treatment of symptomatic thoracic disk herniations.

Debnath UK, McConnell JR, Sengupta DK, Mehdian SM, Webb JK: Results of hemivertebrectomy and fusion for symptomatic thoracic disc herniation. *Eur Spine J* 2003;12:292-299.

A retrospective review of 10 consecutive patients treated surgically for symptomatic TDH between T6 and T12 is presented. Hemivertebrectomy followed by diskectomy and fusion was used in all patients. Results were excellent or good in six patients, fair in three, and poor in one. The authors advocate this approach because it increases access to the thoracic disk, which is likely to reduce the risk of iatrogenic injury to the spinal cord.

Hellinger J, Stern S, Hellinger S: Nonendoscopic Nd-YAG 1064 nm PLDN in the treatment of thoracic discogenic pain syndromes. *J Clin Laser Med Surg* 2003;21:61-66.

In this prospective controlled clinical study, 42 patients with symptomatic thoracic disk protrusions and extrusions were treated with Nd-YAG 1064 nm percutaneous laser disk decompression and nucleotomy. Disk puncture was accomplished with a dorsolateral approach and a maximal laser dose of 1,000 J was applied to each affected disk. Results were successful in 41 patients based on subjective patient pain scale, McNab score, neurologic findings, and peripheral electromyography. The authors concluded that laser treatment of symptomatic TDH is safe and effective and recommend it prior to any open surgery.

Perez-Cruet MJ, Kim BS, Sandhu F, D Samartzis RG Fessler: Thoracic microendoscopic discectomy. *J Neurosurg Spine* 2004;1:58-63.

A case series of seven patients with symptomatic soft lateral or midline TDHs treated with thoracic microendoscopic diskectomy is presented. Clinical success assessments were based on a modified Prolo scale and resulted in five excellent, one good, and one fair outcome. The authors concluded that thoracic microendoscopic diskectomy is a safe, effective, and less invasive alternative for the treatment of TDHs.

### Thoracic Stenosis

Palumbo MA, Hilibrand A, Hart R, Bohlman HH: Surgical treatment of thoracic spinal stenosis: Two to nine year follow-up. *Spine* 2001;26:558-566.

A retrospective investigation of the results of surgical treatment of patients with symptomatic thoracic spinal stenosis is presented. The study documents 12 patients who had undergone decompression for symptomatic stenosis and had an average follow-up time of 62.4 months. Study conclusions include the expectation of short-term success following decompression, but warn of common deterioration of results over a longer term secondary to recurrent stenosis and deformity/instability at the thoracolumbar junction.

## Classic Bibliography

Bohlman HH, Zdeblick TA: Anterior excision of herniated thoracic discs. *J Bone Joint Surg Am* 1988;70:1038-1047.

Wood KB, Blair J, Aepple D, et al: The natural history of asymptomatic thoracic disc herniations. *Spine* 1997;22:525-529.

Wood KB, Garvey TA, Gundry C, Heithoff KB: Magnetic resonance imaging of the thoracic spine: Evaluation of asymptomatic individuals. *J Bone Joint Surg Am* 1995;77:1631-1668.

# Chapter 30

# Acute Low Back Pain

James J. Yue, MD

Ajit V. Patwardhan, MD

Andrew P. White, MD

## Introduction

Acute low back pain (LBP) is most commonly defined as back pain that is present for 6 weeks or less. It can alternatively be defined as functionally limiting pain that lasts for less than 3 months. Acute LBP is the fifth most common reason for all visits to orthopaedic physicians and is the second most common reason that patients seek medical attention. Some of the common causes of LBP include injury, poor muscle conditioning and/or obesity, and episodic degenerative processes. However, most acute LBP occurs without an obvious or diagnosable cause. Socioeconomic, psychologic, biochemical, and biomechanical factors also may play a role in the etiology of acute LBP. The prevalence of LBP has been estimated to be 60% to 80% in industrialized countries. Acute LBP is a major determinant of physical disability and can have devastating socioeconomic effects.

Patients with acute LBP typically present with nonspecific back symptoms, without radiculopathy or underlying systemic disease. Despite a large volume of evolving literature on the subject, and despite an expanding differential diagnosis, a distinct etiology is rarely identified. A musculoligamentous process, herniated nucleus pulposus, degenerative changes in the spine, or a combination of these factors is often suspected. Patients with social and psychologic stressors, depression, substance abuse, pending or past litigation for disability or disability compensation, low socioeconomic status, dissatisfaction with work, and a history of previous back pain are more likely to have persistent LBP.

Most episodes of acute LBP are self-limiting. The chief causes of LBP include: spondylogenic factors (degenerative, infectious, neoplastic, and inflammatory), arising from the paraspinal musculature, ligaments and tendons, facet joints, disks, and vertebrae; neurogenic factors, arising from the cauda equina and lumbosacral plexus; viscerogenic factors, arising from the abdominal viscera (vascular, from abdominal aortic aneurysms; or peripheral, from vascular disease); and psychogenic/inorganic causes.

## Federal Agency Clinical Categories

In the first half of the 1990s, the Agency for Health Care Policy and Research (AHCPR) of the United States Department of Health and Human Services, the predecessor of the present day Agency for Healthcare Research and Quality (AHRQ), developed and published practice guidelines for use by physicians and patients in formulating appropriate health care plans. In 1994, the AHRQ published clinical practice guidelines on the management of acute LBP. Instead of defining practice guidelines for patients and professionals, the current focus of the AHRQ is in preparing evidence-based practice reports. This agency critically reviews medical evidence to formulate sound clinical practice guidelines in cooperation with professional societies and other organizations.

The original AHCPR guidelines grouped back pain into three categories: potentially serious spinal conditions, sciatica, and nonspecific back symptoms. Potentially serious spinal conditions include fractures, infections, spinal tumors, and cauda equina syndrome. Urgent evaluation and treatment is required for patients with these conditions. Sciatica involves lower extremity symptoms caused by nerve root compression. In most patients, sciatic pain regresses with nonsurgical therapy. Nonspecific back symptoms, however, suggest neither neurologic compromise nor any serious underlying condition. Mechanical back pain is included in this category. Symptoms are usually self-limiting and improve with nonsurgical therapy.

## Screening for Red Flag Conditions

A detailed medical history is critical in the initial evaluation of a patient with acute LBP. The timing, character, location, intensity, and effect of the pain on daily activities should be elicited. Activities or positions that affect the pain and any previous trauma should be noted. Acute onset of pain may indicate a disk herniation, whereas slowly progressing pain may be caused by degenerative changes or a tumor. Localized pain in the paraspinal muscles typically has a musculoskeletal cause, such as a muscle strain.

Radiculopathy is a symptom of nerve root irritation and can be associated with pain radiating to one or both lower extremities. Although mechanical back pain may last days to several weeks, the usual natural history of radicular pain will commonly last for 6 to 8 weeks or longer. Nonradiating musculoskeletal pain may be mild to severe. Radicular pain caused by a herniated nucleus pulposus is typically severe. Lumbar radiculopathy often occurs on awakening in the morning. Radicular pain often is reduced when the patient is supine and accentuated in the standing or sitting positions. The presence of pain in recumbency may be the result of an infection or a metastatic cause.

An employment and psychosocial history may reveal significant information related to the cause of the pain. Work-related LBP syndromes are the most common disorder reported to primary care physicians and occupational health providers.

The suspicion of an underlying serious condition warrants immediate intervention. Clinical conditions that are considered potentially serious are referred to as red flag conditions in the AHCPR clinical practice guidelines. These red flag conditions are described in Table 1 with typical symptoms, risks, and physical findings. The initial history should include questions that are appropriately focused and relevant based on the mechanism of injury; past medical, social, and family history; as well as a review of organ systems. A history of weakness, loss of bowel or bladder control, fever, malignancy, night pain or pain in the back and legs when at rest, and the occurrence of nausea or vomiting should be sought.

An evaluation of the pain's character, location, and aggravating or relieving factors will help in determining the underlying pathology. This appraisal of the chief complaint should be accompanied by a complete medical history, then augmented by a systematic physical examination if the physician suspects any serious underlying condition. The rationale for the initial evaluation is to identify potentially serious symptoms or findings and screen for serious conditions. These patients are at increased risk for persistent LBP symptoms and also may have more serious pathology requiring surgical treatment.

## Physical Examination

The physical examination should narrow the differential diagnoses that may cause episodes of acute LBP. A focused physical examination will follow a comprehensive and complete patient history. A complete objective physical evaluation should be later integrated with subjective reports of the complaints to confirm clinical suspicions. Patients should be dressed in a gown and should be examined standing, supine, and prone. In the standing position, the back should be palpated to assess alignment, location of tenderness, and the presence or absence of masses and/or signs of trauma. Range of motion including flexion-extension, lateral bending, and rotation should be documented. In the supine position, the abdomen should be palpated for pulsatile masses and lower extremity pulses should be assessed. In the prone position, compression of the spinous processes and facet joints also can provide information to assist in diagnosing the etiology of LBP. The body mass index should be documented.

General examination of the lumbar spine and paraspinal tissues should be followed by a comprehensive neurologic examination including motor, sensory, reflex, and long-tract evaluation. The presence or absence of nerve tension signs should be confirmed. Signs of muscle atrophy should be noted. The rectal and perineal examination should be documented when clinically indicated. An effort to discern physiologic and nonphysiologic etiologies should be attempted. The so-called Waddell's signs can often be elicited and include an exaggerated tenderness to light touch; the presence of back pain with vertical compression of the skull, pain with rotation of the shoulders and pelvis in the same plane, discrepancy of the straight-leg raising test in the supine and sitting positions, exaggerated facial or verbal expression, tremor, and nondermatomal and myotomal symptoms.

## Diagnostic Evaluation

The performance of a diagnostic test in a patient with acute LBP should be guided by the anticipation of how the test will direct the patient's treatment. Approximately 90% of acute back pain episodes have no identifiable cause and are designated as nonspecific. Diagnostic studies can be divided into those that may identify physiologic causes and those that may identify structural causes.

Physiologic assessment of extremity pain may include electromyography (EMG) with nerve conduction velocity (NCV) studies. EMG/NCV testing can identify nerve root involvement and may indicate if the nerve injury is old, active, or improving. Physical examination findings (for example, the straight-leg raising test) with supporting evidence from EMG and NCV studies can confirm the specific nerve root involved. The diagnosis of nonneurologic medical diseases may be aided by general laboratory screening tests such as erythrocyte sedimentation rate, a complete blood count, urine analysis, prostate specific antigen analysis, and serum protein electrophoresis. There is a strong correlation between the high intensity C-reactive protein and acute sciatic pain, but not with chronic pain.

There is no clear consensus as to the best imaging studies to evaluate the patient with acute LBP. Plain radiographs may not be helpful in the first month after symptoms occur, primarily because the correlation of

## Table 1 | Types, Signs, Symptoms, and Physical Findings of Red Flags

| Category | Symptoms/Risk Factors | Physical Findings |
|---|---|---|
| Cancer | History of cancer | Tenderness over the spinous process |
| | Unexplained weight loss > 10 kg within 6 months | Range of motion is decreased because of protective muscle spasm |
| | Age older than 50 years or younger than 17 years | |
| | Failure to improve with therapy | |
| | Pain persists for more than 4 to 6 weeks | |
| | Night pain or pain at rest | |
| Infection | Persistent fever (temperature > 100.4°F) | Tenderness over spinous process |
| | History of intervenous drug abuse | Decreased range of motion |
| | Recent bacterial infection, urinary tract infection, or pyelonephritis | Vital signs consistent with systemic infection |
| | Cellulitis | Tachycardia |
| | Pneumonia | Tachypnea |
| | Immunocompromised states | Hypotension |
| | Systemic corticosteroids | |
| | Organ transplant | Elevated temperature |
| | Diabetes mellitus | Pelvis or abdominal mass or tenderness |
| | Human immunodeficiency virus | |
| | Rest pain | |
| Vertebral fracture | Corticosteroids | Findings related to the site of fracture |
| | Mild trauma in patients older than 50 years | |
| | Age older than 70 years | |
| | Osteoporosis | |
| | Recent significant trauma at any age | |
| | Ejection from a motor vehicle | |
| | Fall from a substantial height | |
| Cauda equina syndrome | Urinary incontinence or retention | Unexpected laxity of bladder or anal sphincter |
| | Saddle anesthesia | Major motor weakness: quadriceps (knee extension weakness) |
| | Anal sphincter tone decreased or fecal incontinence | Anal plantar flexors, everters, and dorsiflexors |
| | Bilateral lower extremity weakness or numbness | Spastic (thoracic) or flaccid (lumbar) paraparesis |
| | Progressive neurologic deficit | Increased (thoracic) or decreased lumbar reflexes |
| Acute abdominal aneurysm | Abdominal pulsating mass | |
| | Atherosclerotic vascular disease | |
| | Pain at rest or nocturnal pain | |
| | Age older than 60 years | |
| Renal colic | Excruciating pain at costovertebral angle radiating to testis | Possible tenderness at costovertebral angle |
| | History of urolithiasis | |
| Pelvic inflammatory disease | Vaginal discharge | Uterine tenderness |
| | Pelvis pain | Pelvic mass |
| | Prior episode | Cervical discharge |
| Urinary tract infection | Dysuria | Suprapubic tenderness |
| | History of urinary tract infection | |
| Retrocecal appendix | Subacute onset without inciting event | Low grade fever |
| | Constipation | |

*(Data from Bratton RL: Assessment and management of acute low back pain. Am Fam Physician 1999;60:2299-2308).*

symptoms with radiographic findings is poor. Plain radiographs of the lumbosacral spine are recommended if there are red flag conditions of fracture, malignancy, or infection. Routine plain radiographs of the lumbosacral spine may be indicated if pertinent red flag conditions are present or if the patient has had pain for more than 4 to 6 weeks. Initial radiographs should include AP and lateral projections.

Advanced studies such as radionuclide scintigraphy, CT, MRI, myelography, or CT myelography are recommended if the patient's history is suggestive of a serious underlying pathology such as spinal stenosis, osteomyelitis, cauda equina syndrome, disk herniation, epidural abscess, or recent fracture. These advanced studies also are warranted in patients with persistent or progressive neurologic deficits. MRI is the most commonly used advanced study and allows visualization of the disks and neural elements; no radiation is involved. Patients with a history of prior surgery also may benefit from MRI evaluation with or without contrast. Specific indications for a CT scan include an obese patient, the presence of suspected fracture, facet joint abnormality, or severe degenerative changes, as well as patients with nontitanium hardware, cochlear implants, pacemakers, and other medical devices that preclude the use of MRI. Clinical correlation between imaging studies, the patient's symptoms, and neurologic findings is imperative.

## Management

Following a well-organized and thorough patient history and physical examination, the physician can usually differentiate acute LBP syndromes that are likely to resolve with limited nonsurgical care from those that are associated with red flag conditions and require further evaluation and may require more aggressive treatment. There are currently more than 600 randomized controlled trials evaluating nonsurgical treatments for LBP. The North American Spine Society and the American Academy of Orthopaedic Surgeons have jointly developed clinical guidelines and algorithms that are updated periodically and can be reviewed in the National Guidelines Clearinghouse (NGC) website (http://www.ngc.gov). The NGC is a free Internet database of evidence-based clinical guidelines and is produced jointly by the AHRQ and the American Medical Association.

### Nonsurgical Treatment

The mainstay of treatment for patients with LBP is nonsurgical. There is strong evidence that acetaminophen, nonsteroidal anti-inflammatory drugs (NSAIDs), and muscle relaxants relieve pain better than placebos. The serious side effects of both NSAIDs and muscle relaxants must be taken into consideration. A moderate amount of evidence exists that indicates that analgesics and spinal manipulations are also effective for pain relief. Bed rest has been shown to have no beneficial effect, and in some patients has a negative overall impact on recovery. Physical therapy has a slightly greater benefit than medical treatment alone. Interestingly, continuous low-level heat wrap therapy has been shown to be superior to the use of acetaminophen and NSAIDs. At the present time, no firm conclusions can be made regarding the use of other alternative treatments such as acupuncture, dry needle therapy, or botanical medicine. Clinically, spinal manipulation has been shown to be equally effective when compared with other conservative therapies and more effective than sham manipulation. An active lifestyle accelerates symptomatic recovery and reduces chronic disability. The routine use of passive treatment modalities is not recommended because they promote chronic pain behavior.

### Surgical Treatment

Surgery is used for acute LBP only when serious underlying spinal pathology is diagnosed. Cauda equina syndrome is a spinal emergency and requires immediate evaluation and decompressive surgery. Fracture, infection, and tumor also require urgent surgical consultation for possible stabilization, culture, biopsy or removal, and decompression. Surgery for patients with sciatica caused by a herniated lumbar disk or spinal stenosis is usually elective. It is appropriate to consider surgery for a patient if a static or progressive neurologic deficit exists and/or there has been no response to nonsurgical therapy for 6 to 8 weeks for patients with a herniated lumbar disk, or 8 to 12 weeks for those with spinal stenosis when imaging shows a lesion corresponding to symptoms.

## Annotated Bibliography
### Federal Agency Clinical Categories

The National Guideline Clearinghouse website. Available at http://www.ngc.gov. Accessed January, 2006.

The NGC is a free internet database of evidence-based clinical guidelines and their related publications. Produced by the AHRQ in partnership with the American Medical Association and the American Association of Health Plans, the NGC is updated weekly. The NGC offers guideline abstracts, links to full-text articles, ordering information, a comparison utility for comparing guidelines side-by-side, guideline syntheses, and annotated bibliographies. Search utilities, update services, and discussion lists are also available.

### Screening for Red Flag Conditions

Grotle M, Brox JI, Veierød MB, Glomsrød B, Lønn LH, Vøllestad NK: Clinical course and prognostic factors in acute low back pain patients consulting primary care for the first time. *Spine* 2005;30:976-982.

This study included 123 patients with acute LBP of less than 3 weeks duration who consulted a primary care physician for the first time. One hundred twenty of the patients completed the 3-month follow-up. Baseline assessments included sociodemographic characteristics, back pain history, current status, psychological questionnaires, and clinical examination. During a period of 3 months, 24% of the patients had not recovered. Psychological factors and neurologic signs were strongly associated with nonrecovery. The authors concluded that in addition to the traditional examination of neurologic symptoms and signs, psychological factors should be considered at the initial visit of a patient with an episode of LBP.

## Physical Examination

Atlas SJ, Deyo RA: Evaluating and managing acute low back pain in the primary care setting. *J Gen Intern Med* 2001;16:120-131.

This review article describes a recommended approach to examining the patient with acute LBP in the primary care setting. A patient history and physical examination usually provide clues to the rare but potentially serious causes of LBP and identify patients at risk for prolonged recovery. Diagnostic testing, including plain radiographs are often unnecessary during the initial evaluation. For patients with acute, nonspecific LBP, the primary emphasis of treatment should be nonsurgical care, time for symptom resolution, reassurance, and education.

## Diagnostic Examination

Bartleson JD: Low back pain. *Curr Treat Options Neurol* 2001;3:159-168.

This opinion statement directed toward the clinical neurologist describes LBP as a symptom rather than a specific disease. Most patients (90%) with acute LBP recover within 1 month with very limited treatment. Because of the multiple possible musculoskeletal causes and because of the self-limiting nature of most LBP, only about 15% of patients can be given a specific diagnosis. Recurrent episodes of pain are common; approximately 10% of patients develop chronic LBP. When red flag conditions are not present, patients with LBP should be treated with comfort control measures only.

Sturmer T, Raum E, Buchner M, et al: Pain and high sensitivity C reactive protein in patients with chronic low back pain and acute sciatic pain. *Ann Rheum Dis* 2005;64:921-925.

This study reviewed the association between pain as assessed by a visual analog scale and high-intensity C-reactive protein in patients with chronic LBP and acute sciatic pain. The mean intensity of pain during the previous 24 hours, as assessed by the visual analog scale, was independently associated with high levels of high-intensity C-reactive protein in patients with acute sciatic pain but not in those with chronic LBP.

van Tulder M, Koes B, Bombardier C: Low back pain. *Best Pract Res Clin Rheumatol* 2002;16:761-775.

LBP is not simply either acute or chronic but fluctuates over time with frequent recurrences or exacerbations. Although epidemiologic studies have identified many individual, psychosocial, and occupational risk factors for the onset of LBP, their independent prognostic value is usually low. Several factors have now been identified that may increase the risk of chronic disability, but no single factor seems to have a strong impact. Consequently, the most efficient strategy for primary and secondary prevention is unclear. In general, multimodal preventative approaches seem better able to reflect the clinical reality than single-modal interventions.

## Management

Bernstein E, Carey TS, Garrett JM: The use of muscle relaxant medications in acute low back pain. *Spine* 2004; 29:1346-1351.

A cohort of 1,633 patients was followed for up to 24 weeks after the onset of acute LBP. Muscle relaxants were used by 49% of patients. In patients who had a greater functional status impairment at baseline, those using muscle relaxants had slower recovery. This finding persisted after controlling for baseline functional status, age, workers' compensation status, and the use of NSAIDs.

Clarke J, van Tulder M, Blomberg S, et al: Traction for low-back pain with or without sciatica. *Cochrane Database Syst Rev* 2005;4:CD003010.

The evidence suggests that traction is probably not an effective treatment for LBP. Neither continuous nor intermittent traction by itself was more effective in improving pain, disability, or work absence than placebo, sham, or other treatments for patients with a mixed duration of LBP, with or without sciatica. Although studies of patients with sciatica had methodological limitations and inconsistent results, moderate evidence indicated that autotraction was more effective than mechanical traction for global improvement in this population of patients.

Furlan AD, van Tulder M, Cherkin D, et al: Acupuncture and dry-needling for low back pain: An updated systematic review within the framework of the Cochrane collaboration. *Spine* 2005;30:944-963.

This study assessed the effects of acupuncture and dry-needling for the treatment of nonspecific LBP. Randomized controlled trials of acupuncture or dry-needling for adults with nonspecific acute/subacute or chronic LBP were considered. Thirty-five randomized clinical trials were included with only three trials of acupuncture for acute LBP. Firm conclusions could not be made because of the small sample sizes and low methodologic quality of the studies. No clear recommendations could be made concerning the most effective acupuncture technique.

Hagen KB, Hilde G, Jamtvedt G, Winnem MF: The Cochrane review of advice to stay active as a single treatment for low back pain and sciatica. *Spine* 2002;27:1736-1741.

This study was done to assess the effects of the recommendation to stay active as a single treatment for patients with acute LBP or sciatica. Four trials, with a total of 491 patients were included. In all the trials, advice to stay active was compared with advice for bed rest. The results from one high-quality trial of patients with acute, simple LBP found small differences in functional status and length of sick leave in favor of staying active compared with staying in bed for 2 days. The other high-quality trial compared advice to stay active with advice to rest in bed 14 days for patients with sciatic syndrome, and found no differences between the groups. Evidence suggests that advice to stay active alone has little beneficial effect for patients with acute, simple LBP and little or no effect for patients with sciatica. There is no evidence that advice to stay active is harmful.

Hayden JA, van Tulder MW, Tomlinson G: Systematic review: Strategies for using exercise therapy to improve outcomes in chronic low back pain. *Ann Intern Med* 2005;142:776-785.

The purpose of this analysis was to identify particular exercise intervention characteristics that decrease pain and improve function in adults with nonspecific chronic LBP. The study included 43 trials of 72 exercise treatments (31 comparison groups were included). Bayesian multivariable random effects meta-regression found improved pain scores for patients in individually designed programs and supervised home exercise, group, and individual programs compared with those in home exercise programs alone. High-dose exercise programs fared better than low-dose exercise programs. Patients in stretching and strengthening exercise programs showed the largest improvement over comparison groups.

Jellema P, van Tulder MW, van Poppel MN, Nachemson AL, Bouter LM: Lumbar supports for prevention and treatment of low back pain: A systematic review within the framework of the Cochrane Back Review Group. *Spine* 2001;26:377-386.

The systematic review of therapeutic trials showed that there is limited evidence that lumbar supports are more effective than no treatment for patients with LBP; however, it is still unclear whether lumbar supports are more effective than other interventions for the treatment of LBP.

Nadler SF, Steiner DJ, Erasala GN, et al: Continuous low-level heat wrap therapy provides more efficacy than ibuprofen and acetaminophen for acute low back pain. *Spine* 2002;27:1012-1017.

This prospective, randomized, single investigator, blinded, comparative trial was conducted to compare the efficacy of continuous low-level heat wrap therapy with that of ibuprofen and acetaminophen in patients with acute nonspecific LBP. Continuous low-level heat wrap therapy was superior to both acetaminophen and ibuprofen for treating LBP.

Rozenberg S, Delval C, Rezvani Y, et al: Bed rest or normal activity for patients with acute low back pain: A randomized controlled trial. *Spine* 2002;27:1487-1493.

This study compared 4 days of bed rest with continued normal daily activity in patients with acute LBP, taking into account the type of work performed by the patients (physical or sedentary labor). This open, comparative multicenter study included 281 ambulatory patients, age 18 to 65 years, with LBP (onset < 72 hours). The patients were randomized into two treatment groups: one instructed to continue normal activity (insofar as the pain allowed), and the other prescribed 4 days of bed rest. It was found that normal activity is at least equivalent in efficacy to bed rest for patients with LBP. The findings of this study indicate that prescriptions for bed rest should be limited when the physical demands of a patient's job are similar to those for daily life activities.

van der Roer N, Goossens ME, Evers SM, van Tulder MW: What is the most cost-effective treatment for patients with low back pain: A systematic review. *Best Pract Res Clin Rheumatol* 2005;19:671-684.

Seventeen studies from 1966 to July 2004 were used to assess the most cost-effective treatment for patients with LBP. The consensus health economic criteria list was used to assess the quality of the studies. Six of the studies concluded that the intervention of interest was superior to the control intervention. Definite conclusions about the most cost-effective intervention could not be drawn because of the heterogeneity of interventions, controls, and study populations. More high-quality economic evaluations are needed before a conclusion can be made.

van Tulder MW, Furlan AD, Gagnier JJ: Complementary and alternative therapies for low back pain. *Best Pract Res Clin Rheumatol* 2005;19:639-654.

The effectiveness of complementary and alternative medicine therapies compared with placebo, no intervention, or other interventions for acute/subacute and chronic nonspecific LBP was evaluated. Results from Cochrane reviews on acupuncture, botanical medicine, massage, neuroreflexotherapy, and spinal manipulation were used. Spinal manipulation was more effective than sham manipulation or ineffective therapies, and equally effective as other conventional therapies.

van Tulder MW, Touray T, Furlan AD, Solway S, Bouter LM: Muscle relaxants for nonspecific low back pain: A systematic review within the framework of the Cochrane collaboration. *Spine* 2003;28:1978-1992.

Studies involving patients diagnosed with nonspecific LBP who were treated with muscle relaxants as monotherapy or in combination with other therapeutic methods were included in this review. Results showed that there is strong evidence that muscle relaxants are more effective than placebos for patients with acute LBP for short-term pain relief. Adverse events were significantly more prevalent in patients receiving muscle relaxants.

## Classic Bibliography

Atlas SJ, Volinn E: Classics from the spine literature revisited: A randomized trial of 2 versus 7 days of recommended bed rest for acute low back pain. *Spine* 1997;22: 2331-2337.

Bigos SJ (ed): *Acute Low Back Problems in Adults.* Rockville, MD, United States Department of Health and Human Services, AHCPR Publication 95-0642, Clinical Practive Guideline Number 14, 1994.

Boden SD, Davis DO, Dina TS, Patronas NJ, Wiesel SW: Abnormal magnetic resonance scans of the lumbar spine in asymptomatic subjects: A prospective investigation. *J Bone Joint Surg Am* 1990;72:403-408.

Boos N, Lander PH: Clinical efficacy of imaging modalities in the diagnosis of low back pain disorders. *Eur Spine J* 1996;5:2-22.

Borenstein DG, Wiesel SW, Boden SD (eds): *Low Back Pain: Medical Diagnosis and Comprehensive Management.* Philadelphia, PA, WB Saunders, 1995.

Bratton RL: Assessment and management of acute low back pain. *Am Fam Physician* 1999;60:2299-2308.

Cherkin DC, Deyo RA, Battie M, Street J, Barlow W: A comparison of physical therapy, chiropractic manipulation, and provision of an educational booklet for the treatment of patients with low back pain. *N Engl J Med* 1998;339:1021-1029.

Deyo RA, Andersson G, Bombadier C, et al: Outcome measures for studying patients with low back pain. *Spine* 1994;19:2032S-2036S.

Deyo RA, Phillips WR: Low back pain: A primary care challenge. *Spine* 1996;21:2826-2832.

Gehweiler JA, Daffner RH: Low back pain: The controversy of radiologic evaluation. *Am J Roentgenol* 1983; 140:109-112.

Hagen KB, Hilde G, Jamtvedt G, Winnem MF: The Cochrane review of bed rest for acute low back pain and sciatica. *Spine* 2000;25:2932-2939.

Hall H, Hadler NM: Controversy: Low back school, education or exercise? *Spine* 1995;20:1097-1098.

Malmivaara A, Hakkinen U, Aro T, et al: The treatment of acute low back pain: Bed rest, exercises or ordinary activity? *N Engl J Med* 1995;332:351-355.

McKenzie RA: *The Lumbar Spine: Mechanical Diagnosis and Therapy.* Waikanae, New Zealand, Spinal Publications, 1989.

Rush AJ, Polatin P, Gatchell R: Depression and chronic low back pain: Establishing priorities in treatment. *Spine* 2000;25:2566-2571.

van Tulder MW, Scholten RJ, Koes BW, Deyo RA: Nonsteroidal anti-inflammatory drugs for low back pain: A systematic review within the framework of the Cochrane Collaboration Back Review Group. *Spine* 2000; 25:2501-2513.

Vroomen PC, de Krom MC, Knottnerus JA: Consistency of history taking and physical examination in patients with lumbar nerve root involvement. *Spine* 2000;25:91-97.

Waddell G, McCulloch JA, Kummell E, Venner RM: Nonorganic physical signs in low back pain. *Spine* 1980; 5:117-125.

# Chapter 31

# Lumbar Disk Herniation

John A. Bendo, MD

John N. Awad, MD

## Introduction

Evidence-based medicine is becoming the standard of care throughout the medical field. The treatment of low back pain has changed little since the establishment of evidence-based guidelines by the Agency for Health Care Policy and Research in the early 1990s. The treatment of lumbar disk herniations (LDHs) also has evolved slowly over the past two decades. The principles of treatment are still based on a classic study performed in the early 1980s. Multiple investigations and trials have both supported and criticized these findings. This chapter presents the current trends in both nonsurgical and surgical treatment for patients with LDHs.

## Anatomy and Pathophysiology

The intervertebral disk is one of the primary motion segments in the spine. It consists of three components: (1) the outer anulus fibrosus, a ring of highly oriented, densely packed type I collagen fibers that insert onto the vertebral bodies; (2) the fibrocartilaginous inner anulus fibrosus, which consists of a less dense random array of type II collagen fibers; and (3) the central nucleus pulposus, which has a high concentration of proteoglycans creating a highly viscoelastic core. Vascular supply and innervation to the disk are quite limited. The blood supply is located on the periphery of the outer anulus fibrosus where the vertebral body's blood vessels penetrate the end plates, but do not enter the disk itself. Nutrition is therefore supplied by diffusion of nutrients and wastes through the nucleus pulposus. Terminal nerve endings exist on the surface of the outer anulus fibrosus; however, no innervation has been identified within the central disks. The cause of annular fissures is largely unknown but is presumed to be the result of degeneration of the anulus fibrosus, intradiskal dehydration and fragmentation, and/or altered biomechanics that results in excessive loading. Other proposed risk factors include lifting heavy loads, torsional stress, physical activity, and prolonged sitting. Interestingly, most disk herniations occur in the morning soon after the patient arises from a supine position. It is hypothesized that the disk rehydrates and expands during recumbency, thereby making it more prone to herniation when pressure is applied. Herniations most commonly occur at the insertion of the outer anulus fibrosus onto the vertebral body.

From a biochemical standpoint, disk changes are evident before disk herniation. As the aging process proceeds, the nucleus pulposus slowly degrades from a resilient well-hydrated proteoglycan gel to a more desiccated fibrocartilaginous substance that more closely resembles the inner anulus fibrosus. This process leads to a degradation of the viscoelastic properties resulting in a greater load being placed on the collagen matrix itself and further degradation.

The mechanistic cause for the resulting pain is still under investigation. The fragmentation and fissuring of the nucleus pulposus and inner anulus fibrosus is largely asymptomatic secondary to the lack of innervation. This fact is clinically supported by the observation of degenerated, dehydrated intervertebral disk seen on MRI scans in 20% to 30% of asymptomatic individuals. When the outer anulus fibrosus is torn, pain ensues. The mechanism is most likely multifactorial often involving mechanical stimulation of the nerve ending in the outer anulus fibrosus, direct compression on the nerve root, and/or the chemical inflammatory cascade induced by the exposed nucleus pulposus.

## Clinical Presentation and History

Most disk herniations are characterized by varying degrees of back and leg pain. The leg pain commonly follows the dermatomal path of the compressed nerve roots. The sudden onset of back pain often coincides with the tearing of the highly innervated outer annular fibers. The back pain will often abate shortly after herniation occurs, secondary to the depressurization of the intervertebral space and relief of annular tension, concomitant with the onset of radicular pain. The typical radicular pain may be accompanied by paresthesias along with varying degrees of motor, sensory, and reflex loss. The presence of sciatica is both the most sensitive and specific finding for LDH, and can be critical in determining the level of herniation, especially in patients younger than 30 years of age. Symptoms may present insidiously or may be preceded by a minor traumatic event (such as a sneeze), or may occur after a notable load-bearing event (such as lifting a heavy object). It is important to differentiate this type of radicular pain from a less well-defined deep aching sclerotomal pain that is commonly known as referred pain. Typically, lateral herniations will often present with a predominance of leg pain, whereas central herniations often present with isolated back pain secondary to irritation of the posterior longitudinal ligament. Activities that increase intraspinal and intradiskal pressure such as sitting, coughing, sneezing, and the Valsalva maneuver often accentuate pain.

During the initial consultation, the clinician should inquire about the presence of specific aspects of the patient's history, which strongly suggest the possibility of serious underlying pathology (known as red flags), specifically tumor, infection, or fracture. These red flags include a history of trauma, cancer, constitutional symptoms, immunosuppression, recent infection, bladder/bowel dysfunction, bilateral neurologic deficits, saddle anesthesia, progressive neurologic deficit, and night or unremitting pain. If any of these symptoms or signs exist, further workup is warranted on an urgent basis; this is especially true for large central herniations that cause cauda equina syndrome. Cauda equina syndrome, one of the few surgical emergencies, consists of a triad of symptoms: acute onset of bowel and bladder incontinence or retention, bilateral lower extremity motor weakness, and perianal saddle anesthesia.

A family history also can be informative. Several reports exist of a familial as well as genetic predisposition to developing LDH. Patients with LDH who are younger than 30 years of age tend to have a strong hereditary predisposition to the condition.

Although rare, children and adolescents have LDHs. This group accounts for 0.5% to 3.8% of all patients undergoing diskectomy. Trauma is an important inciting factor for children and adolescents with LDH; in adults, disk degeneration is the predominate causative factor. Apophyseal ring fractures or avulsions are a common finding in this population. LDHs are usually encountered in children older than 10 years of age. Any child younger than 10 years with LDH should undergo an extensive workup to rule out any red flag conditions. Sciatica and/or back pain are the main clinical symptoms. As in adults, L4-5 and L5-S1 are the levels most commonly affected. Surgical indications are the same as in the adult population, although a longer course of nonsurgical treatment should be undertaken. Short-term surgical results in children are comparable with those of adults. Long-term results in children are less promising. In one study with long-term follow-up, only 42% of patients were completely without pain, 50% reported occasional pain and disability, and 8% had disabling pain. Also, a significant incidence (67%) of disk degeneration was found at the index and adjacent levels.

## Physical Examination

The first step in the physical examination is observation of the patient's gait and standing positions. Patients with an LDH will frequently have guarded range of motion of the spine as well as a slow antalgic gait. The classic posture or "list" acts to relieve tension on the nerve root as illustrated by the patient leaning away from the side of neural compression. With herniations into the axilla of the nerve root, patients commonly lean toward the side of the leg pain. Recently these findings have been questioned, as multiple studies have shown that the direction of the list may not be related to the anatomy or location of the affected disk. Palpation and percussion of the lumbar spine often reveals paraspinal muscular spasms. Palpation should continue along the axis of the sciatic nerve including the sciatic notch, which may be painful. This sign is nonspecific although it correlates with nerve irritation.

A full neurologic examination including an evaluation of muscle strength, tactile sensation, proprioception, vibration, and deep tendon reflexes should be performed. A variety of tests/maneuvers have been developed to delineate the level of herniation. These maneuvers are based on the premise that normal nerve roots have an average excursion of 1.5, 3, and 6 mm for L4, L5, and S1, respectively. The more proximal lumbar roots reveal little motion with lower extremity motion. When a nerve root is compressed, the lack of mobility and subsequent tension creates pain during provocative maneuvers.

The supine straight-leg raise (SLR), which produces Lasègue's sign, is performed by the examiner slowly elevating the affected lower extremity by the heel with the knee fully extended. A positive test corresponds to reproducible concordant leg symptoms at 30° to 75° of elevation and corresponds to L4, L5, or S1 compression. Pain is often relieved by knee flexion, which then relaxes the sciatic nerve. Palpation within the popliteal fossa that recreates leg discomfort is known as the bowstring sign. Reproduction of back pain is not considered a positive test. The sensitivity of the SLR is age dependent. Positive results from an SLR are seen in nearly all patients with lumbar disk herniations younger than 30 years of age. In patients older than 30 years, the result of the SLR may be negative even in the presence of a true symptomatic disk herniation. The test also can be performed in the sitting position by extending the flexed knee with the hip already flexed. When the patient leans backward during this maneuver to avoid pain, it is called a positive flip test or tripod sign. The contralateral SLR (ipsilateral radicular pain with elevation of the contralateral asymptomatic lower extremity) is more specific for an axillary herniation. A positive femoral stretch test (anterior leg pain with hip hyperextension and knee flexion in the prone position) is indicative of upper lumbar (L2, L3, L4) nerve root dysfunction.

A drop foot, or ankle dorsiflexion weakness, is commonly associated with an L4 or L5 radiculopathy. It also may be a manifestation of a peripheral neuropathy secondary to diabetes or compression of the peroneal nerve at the level of the fibular head. Etiology differentiation can be performed via careful examination. Trendelenburg's sign is caused by gluteus medius weakness from an L5 radiculopathy and is not present with a more distal neuropathy. Sensory examination will show a stocking/glove distribution of sensory dysfunction in patients with peripheral neuropathy. Also, motor testing of the foot everter (S1) will be normal with an L5 radiculopathy but may be abnormal with common peroneal nerve dysfunction.

## Imaging and Classification
The goal of any imaging study is to confirm a clinical diagnosis. By itself, imaging may lead to overdiagnosis. Significantly high rates of LDHs are found on MRI scans of asymptomatic individuals. Therefore, clinical correlation is of paramount importance when interpreting imaging studies. Upright lumbar radiographs are not particularly helpful for the diagnosis of a herniated disk, but are indicated in patients with more than 6 weeks of back pain and in those with a clinical history suggestive of a red flag condition as previously discussed.

MRI has become the diagnostic test of choice for LDH. MRI is useful to identify different constituents of the disk based on the differing concentration of water, proteoglycan, and collagen. The high water content of the nucleus pulposus and inner anulus fibrosus produces a high signal on T2-weighted images, whereas the low water content of the anterior and posterior longitudinal ligaments and the outer anulus fibrosus generate a low-intensity signal. This difference in signal intensity allows the visualization of the tear. The sensitivity and specificity of MRI in detecting annular tears, disk herniations, and nerve root swelling has been confirmed in several studies. Furthermore, MRI findings have been correlated to clinical findings and are strong predictors of surgical outcomes. Newer technologies such as "stand up," or "dynamic MRI," in which the patient is scanned in several positions have recently gained popularity, but have yet to show clinical correlation or added benefits.

CT scans with multiplanar reconstructions may serve as a tertiary test in certain distinct clinical situations. These scans are particularly helpful in assessing the bone anatomy (especially in patients who had previous surgery) when an occult pars interarticularis fracture is

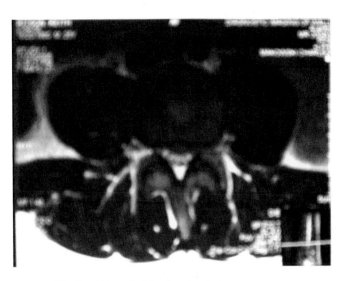
Figure 1  T2-weighted image of axial contained protrusion.

suspected. CT can also be useful in visualizing lateral disk herniations. CT myelograms are rarely used in the diagnosis of LDH. Most experts agree that a good quality MRI scan along with a CT scan obviates the need for a CT myelogram.

When reviewing an MRI scan it is important to correctly classify the state of the disk. Confusion exists concerning terminology. A herniation is defined as a focal displacement of nuclear, annular, or end-plate material beyond the normal peripheral margin of the disk. The most subtle finding is a "disk bulge." A bulge is defined as a generalized outpouching of the peripheral margin of the anulus fibrosus (> 25%) with loss of disk height. There is no focal displacement of inner disk material. It is important to realize that, to date, these descriptive terms have no direct implications with respect to clinical significance. A true disk herniation may be asymptomatic and a bulge may cause symptomatic compression in combination with other degenerative changes. Protrusion refers to a displacement of the inner disk material within a partially torn or thinned anulus fibrosus. The base of the herniation is broader than the apex. Protrusions are synonymous with contained herniations (Figures 1 and 2). In a noncontained disk herniation, the inner disk material is displaced through a complete defect of the anulus fibrosus. Generally, the circumference of the displaced disk material is larger than the actual defect in the anulus fibrosus. Extrusions and sequestrations represent noncontained herniations. Extrusions are considered subligamentous or transligamentous relative to the posterior longitudinal ligament (Figures 3 and 4). Once the disk material becomes separated from its origin and remains as a completely free fragment (within the spinal cord) it is defined as sequestered. There are several documented cases of intradural herniations as well.

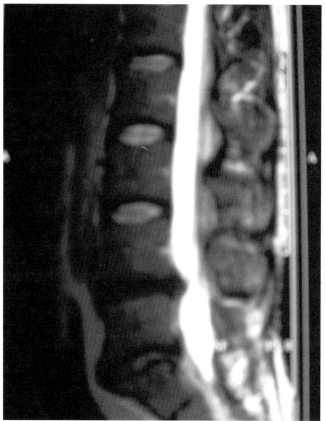

Figure 2   T2-weighted MRI scan of L4-5 contained protrusion.

Figure 3   Sagittal T2-weighted MRI scan of L4-5 disk extrusion.

LDHs also can be classified by their anatomic location within zones along the circumference of the anulus fibrosus. When in the midline, the herniation is in the central zone. A large central herniation may affect the traversing nerve roots bilaterally as well as all the nerve roots caudal to the herniation. When the herniation rests between the pedicle and center of the spinal canal, the herniation is in the posterolateral or subarticular zone. This zone is the most common location; the displaced disk material generally impinges on the anterior and lateral aspect of the traversing nerve root. Within the intervertebral foramen, a herniation is in the foraminal zone, and lateral to the foramen is the extraforaminal or far lateral zone. LDHs in these locations impinge on the exiting nerve root. An axillary disk herniation implies that disk material has migrated medial to the compressed nerve root, generally either superiorly from the posterolateral position affecting the exiting nerve root cephalad to the disk space (most commonly L4-5 affecting the L4 nerve root), or inferiorly impinging the traversing nerve root (most commonly at L5-S1 affecting the S1 root).

## Differential Diagnosis

Once a clinical diagnosis is established it is imperative to rule out any other causes. These other etiologies include other space occupying lesions (such as abscesses,

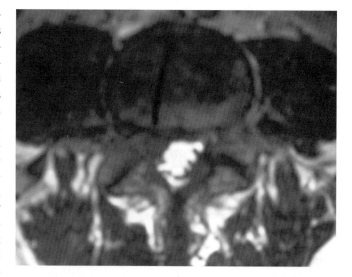

Figure 4   Axial T2-weighted image of L4-5 extrusion (on the right). The patient had preoperative foot drop.

tumors, and epidural hematomas), stenosis, and intradural pathology. Direct compression of the sciatic nerve in the pelvis and upper thigh (extraspinal region) also may present as sciatica. Further workup including CT of the abdomen and pelvis, as well as electrophysiologic monitoring may be warranted in unusual situations.

## Natural History and Nonsurgical Treatment

The natural history of lumbar radiculopathy is quite favorable. The peak incidence of LDHs occurs in the forth and fifth decades of life. LDHs are relatively uncommon during childhood and adolescence. Only 4% to 6% of LDHs become symptomatic throughout an individual's lifetime; males are up to three times more likely than females to have symptomatic LDH. The lifetime prevalence for surgical intervention varies from 1% to 3%. Up to 90% of patients will experience gradual resolution of symptoms without the need for surgical intervention within 3 months from the onset of symptoms. Over time, most LDHs, particularly with large noncontained disk fragments, will resorb and reduce in size. Proposed mechanisms include loss of initial water content, reduction of inflammatory mass, and macrophage removal of disk material by the incited inflammatory response. This improvement in the LDH is the main reason why radiographs and MRI are not always indicated in the first 6 weeks following the onset of radiculopathy.

Most practitioners advise a short period of bed rest and/or activity modification for severe radiculopathy. The supine position places the least amount of pressure on the intervertebral disk. However, there have been no prospective randomized studies to show the efficacy or appropriate duration of bed rest. Some authors suggest a maximum of 1 week of bed rest followed by the gradual resumption of normal activity. A randomized trial compared the consequences of recommending 2 days compared with 7 days of bed rest. The group that was assigned 2 days of bed rest missed 45% fewer days (3.1 versus 5.6 days) of work than those assigned to the 7-day period of bed rest. No differences were observed in other functional, physiologic, or perceived outcomes. Oral analgesics are also a mainstay of treatment. The use of nonsteroidal anti-inflammatory drugs has shown mixed results in achieving long-term reduction of back pain and sciatica. In the acute setting, the literature shows a clear benefit to the use of nonsteroidal anti-inflammatory drugs and muscle relaxants for acute low back pain and radiculopathy. Short-term use of an oral steroid also can prove effective for severe, recalcitrant sciatica.

Physical therapy has been shown to be beneficial for patients with low back pain and LDHs. Multiple studies have shown that physical therapy reduces long-term use of narcotics and limits the number of days off from work. It is suggested that prolonged bed rest deconditions the paraspinal and abdominal musculature. Although still controversial, the current trend of using specific unidirectional exercises for a certain identified pain generator appears to be beneficial. The premise behind a unidirectional exercise program is the avoidance of the painful position while the muscles that maintain that posture are strengthened. In a prospective trial of limiting early morning lumbar flexion (compared with sham exercises), pain was significantly reduced; the effect continued for at least 3 years. The current standard of care includes both abdominal and paraspinal muscle strengthening and overall body conditioning.

Another commonly prescribed modality is spinal manipulation. The literature shows mixed results on its efficacy. In a recent meta-analysis, most studies were found to be of low quality and most had no long-term results beyond 3 months. Over 50% of the studies showed limited positive short-term results. A trend showed a beneficial effect for patients with acute onset (< 4 weeks) of low back pain. Traction appears to offer no added benefit in the treatment of lumbar radiculopathy.

With the growing evidence that inflammatory agents released by the herniation are a significant contributor to the pain and nerve root irritation, the use of epidural steroids to decrease this inflammation has increased. Epidural steroids can be administered via an interlaminar or a transforaminal route; both methods should be performed under fluoroscopic guidance to ensure application of the steroid to the proper level and prevent intravascular penetration. A recent prospective, randomized study of the use of up to four selective nerve root injections in patients with lumbar radiculopathy showed significant improvement in symptoms and an almost 50% decrease in the need for surgery. Complications are extremely uncommon, but transient paresis and paralysis, epidural hematoma, infection, chemical meningitis, and arachnoiditis have been reported. The incidence of these complications appears higher in patients with significant medical comorbidities and a history of previous lumbar surgery.

## Surgical Treatment

Since the first documented surgical decompression for LDH, countless debates and clinical investigations comparing the results of surgical with nonsurgical treatment have been published.

Most patients can be treated successfully by nonsurgical methods if the patient complies with participation in a physical therapy regimen, maintains proper medication and epidural steroid usage, and, most importantly, is willing to allow ample time for symptom resolution. Treatment options should be explained and discussed with the patient. Society has placed too great an emphasis on short-term outcomes. Patients who undergo early decompression will have a faster resolution of the symptoms, a quicker recovery period, will return to work in less time, and will place less of a financial and social burden on the health care system when compared with those who have nonsurgical treatment. However, studies also indicate that at 4 years following the onset of radiculopathy the outcomes of patients undergoing surgical decompression appear comparable with those treated nonsurgically. However, the results with either treatment are not as promising for patients who have long-standing low back pain or chronic sciatica.

Emergent surgical indications include a progressive neurologic deficit or the presence of cauda equina syndrome. A static neurologic deficit without profound functional impairment does not require immediate surgical intervention. Relative surgical indications include persistent radiculopathy despite an adequate trial of nonsurgical treatment (minimum 6 weeks), recurrent episodes of incapacitating sciatica, a persistent motor deficit with tension signs and pain, and pseudoclaudication caused by concomitant canal stenosis. The failure of nonsurgical treatment remains the most common indication for surgical intervention.

Limited open lumbar laminotomy and microdiskectomy remain the standard of surgical care. The surgical field is generally magnified using either loupes or an operating microscope. A limited diskectomy with removal of the herniation and nearby loose fragments is advised. Radical diskectomy has not been shown to be effective in lowering the reherniation rate. In some studies, the incidence of recurrent herniation has been reported to be as high as 20%.

Proper patient selection is the key to a successful outcome. Patients who have a predominance of lower extremity symptoms, a paucity of low back pain, strong correlation with preoperative images, preoperative tension signs, and large herniations that have been documented intraoperatively, tend to have the best surgical outcomes. Isolated back pain in the absence of radicular signs and symptoms is a contraindication to diskectomy because the outcome in this situation is quite unpredictable. The exception to this rule is a patient with large central herniations that may benefit from a simpler diskectomy versus arthrodesis or arthroplasty. In the short term, surgery results in nearly 85% to 95% excellent to good outcomes. These results deteriorate with time to approximately 55% to 70% excellent to good outcomes. Several studies show that 18% of patients require recurrent back surgery. Persistent low back pain may limit long-term patient satisfaction. It is unclear whether this persistent pain is a direct result of surgery or just the natural history of lumbar degeneration. Although no clear timeline has been delineated, there is a general trend of poorer surgical outcomes in patients who have undergone a lengthy period of unsuccessful nonsurgical care; some authors have suggested that the critical time period is between 4 months to 1 year. Patients with documented psychosocial issues, involvement in a lawsuit, or patients receiving workers' compensation also tend to have poorer surgical outcomes.

To minimize the dissection and scar tissue, arthroscopic techniques have emerged as an alternative to microdiskectomy. These techniques allow the surgeon to perform the procedure with minimal access; however, the laminotomy and the amount of disk removed are the same as in open microdiskectomy. Patient selection is of paramount importance when using these techniques. Reports have shown that the arthroscopic results are comparable for both primary and revision herniations, especially far lateral herniations. The proposed advantages of arthroscopic techniques are less surgical time, the use of limited anesthetic for conscious sedation and local anesthesia, minimal blood loss, and less epidural scarring. A higher incidence of retained disk material with residual symptoms has been reported. Another less popular technique is chemonucleolysis with chymopapain. This technique uses enzymatic dissolution of the herniated portion of the nucleus pulposus via percutaneous injection. This procedure is no longer used in the United States secondary to drastic complications such as anaphylaxis; however, a recent resurgence of its use has occurred in Europe. The overall short-term rate of satisfaction for chemonucleolysis with chymopapain is approximately 75%, well below that achieved by standard laminectomy. Further investigations, including prospective randomized trials, are warranted to accurately assess the utility of these procedures.

Postoperative care is quite variable. A recent meta-analysis concluded that there was no evidence that postoperative activity restriction was required after a primary diskectomy. Physical therapy initiated 4- to 6-weeks following surgery was beneficial in the short term with regard to a faster return to work and an increase in general functional status. There is no evidence that therapy decreases the rate of recurrence or the need for reoperation.

## Complications

Perioperative complications of LDH surgery include wrong-level and wrong-side surgery, incidental durotomy, retained disk fragments with persistent radiculopathy, and postoperative wound infections. Inexperienced surgeons appear to have the highest rate of wrong-side surgery. This complication can be avoided by adequate intraoperative radiographic localization. Inadvertent durotomy occurred in 0.8% to 7.2% of patients in different studies with the incidence decreasing with the surgeon's level of experience. Recognition and timely intraoperative repair of this complication should not alter the long-term outcome. The average incidence of nerve root injury is 0.2% and the incidence of infection is approximately 1%. These complications generally respond to a short course of intravenous antibiotics and occasionally require surgical débridement. These possible complications should be discussed with the patient.

Late complications of LDH surgery include disk space infection, postoperative instability, and recurrent herniation. Patients with disk space infection will

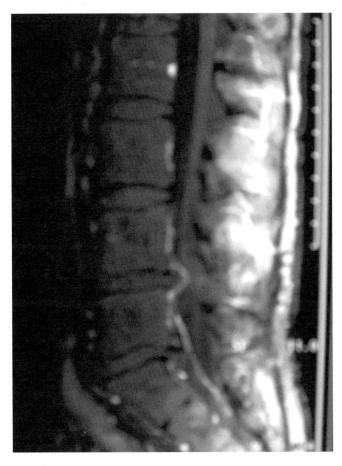

Figure 5 T1-weighted MRI scan with contrast of L4-5 recurrent herniated nucleus pulposus.

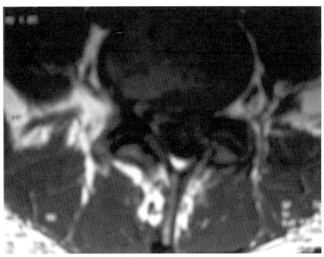

Figure 6 Recurrent L4-5 (left) extrusion. Note that the recurrent disk herniation does not absorb contrast.

present with disabling back pain as early as 3 to 6 weeks postoperatively or at any later period. The erythrocyte sedimentation rate and C-reactive protein are usually elevated; however, the white blood cell count may be normal. Radiographs will show progressive loss of disk space height and erosion. An increased signal within the disk space on T2-weighted MRI is characteristic. Percutaneous biopsy is recommended with identification of the organism before beginning a 6-week regimen of intravenous antibiotic. *Staphylococcus aureus* is the most common infecting organism. Surgical débridement with interbody arthrodesis with autograft may be recommended for patients with recalcitrant infections or significant deformity or instability.

Distinguishing between recurrent disk herniation and epidural fibrosis can be difficult. Gadolinium-enhanced MRI has become the study of choice to differentiate between nonenhancing disk material and vascularized scar tissue (Figures 5 and 6). Although there is no direct correlation between the amount of fibrosis and the degree of the patient's symptoms, those with extensive fibrosis may be more likely to experience radicular symptoms. Symptomatic herniations with predominant leg pain often require revision lumbar diskectomy.

Severe back pain requires erect radiographs as well as lateral flexion/extension radiographs to rule out instability. Oblique radiographs and/or CT with reconstructions may help to reveal an occult pars interarticularis fracture. The presence of instability or a pars fracture would necessitate a concomitant lumbar fusion. Children and adolescents show a high rate of symptomatic recurrence. Nearly 60% may have recurrent symptoms and approximately 30% require a reoperation during their lifetime.

The patient who experiences severe back pain following a diskectomy without evidence of significant degenerative facet disease or spinal instability may be a candidate for total disk arthroplasty. This technology has recently been approved by the U.S. Food and Drug Administration for single level lumbar disk disease in the treatment of axial low back pain.

## Summary
Multiple treatment strategies exist for treating patients with LDHs. Each strategy has proponents and critics. Because of the differing opinions on treatment options, the physician should place importance on the subtleties of the individual patient. A trial of nonsurgical therapy consisting of oral analgesics, activity restrictions, and physical therapy programs for a minimum of 6 weeks is warranted unless a red flag condition is present. If no improvement occurs, radiological workup including plain radiographs and MRI to confirm the clinical diagnosis is essential. Epidural steroids may be considered as well. If a disk herniation is confirmed and there is no improvement with the use of steroids, timely surgical treatment should be discussed with the patient. Providing patient education throughout the process is the most important aspect of treatment. The patient's concerns and expectations will guide the practitioner in both non-

surgical and surgical treatment. As technology advances, it is the responsibility of the caregivers including general practitioners, physical therapists, interventional radiologists, and spine surgeons to stay abreast of the current evidence-based modalities available. A cohesive effort will ensure that the patient receives proper treatment, timely consultations, and a faster recovery of functional status.

## Annotated Bibliography
### Clinical Presentation and History

Ala-Kokko L: Genetic risk factors for lumbar disc disease. *Ann Med* 2002;34:42-47.

This review article highlights the recent advances made in identifying genetic markers for disk degeneration including two collagen IX alleles, aggrecan gene polymorphisms, a vitamin D receptor, and matrix metalloproteinase-3 gene alleles associated with sciatica and LDH.

### Natural History and Nonsurgical Treatment

Buttermann GR: Treatment of lumbar disc herniation: Epidural steroid injection compared with discectomy: A prospective, randomized study. *J Bone Joint Surg Am* 2004;86-A:670-679.

A prospective randomized study was done to determine the efficacy of epidural steroid injection for the treatment of patients with symptomatic LDHs who had an initial 6-week course of failed nonsurgical treatment. The patients were randomized to surgical versus epidural injection groups. The patients who had undergone diskectomy had the most rapid response, with more than 90% of the patients reporting that the treatment had been successful. Approximately 50% of the patients in the epidural group reported that the treatment had been effective. Those who did not obtain pain relief had a subsequent diskectomy; their outcomes did not appear to have been adversely affected by the delay in surgery resulting from the trial of epidural steroid injection.

Kool J, de Bie R, Oesch P, et al: Exercise reduces sick leave in patients with non-acute non-specific low back pain: A meta-analysis. *J Rehabil Med* 2004;36:49-62.

A meta-analysis of 14 studies identified and demonstrated that exercise reduces the number of sick days taken by patients in the year following treatment for nonacute, nonspecific low back pain.

Long A, Donelson R, Fung T: Does it matter which exercise?: A randomized control trial of exercise for low back pain. *Spine* 2004;29:2593-2602.

This article presents the findings of a multicenter, randomized controlled trial to determine if patient-specific, directional preference physical therapy programs are beneficial for treating low back pain. The patients' directional preference (an immediate and lasting improvement in pain using either repeated lumbar flexion, extension, or side-glide/rotation tests) was identified if any existed. The patients were randomized to

a group using directional exercises that matched the patient's directional preference; a group using exercises directionally opposite to the patient's directional preference; or a group performing nondirectional exercises. Outcome measures included pain intensity, location, the presence of disability, use of medication, and degree of recovery, depression, and work interference. A directional preference was elicited in 74% of patients. One third of patients in both the opposite and nondirectional exercise groups withdrew from the trial within 2 weeks because of no improvement or worsening symptoms. Significantly greater improvements occurred in the group using directional exercises that matched the patient's directional preference when compared with the other treatments. A threefold decrease in medication use was found in this group.

van Tulder MW, Touray T, Furlan AD, Solway S, Bouter LM: Cochrane Back Review Group: Muscle relaxants for nonspecific low back pain: A systematic review within the framework of the cochrane collaboration. *Spine* 2003;28:1978-1992.

This article presents a meta-analysis reviewing the efficacy of muscle relaxants in the treatment of low back pain. The relaxants appear to produce a beneficial effect when compared with a placebo. There were no differences in efficacy between the pharmacologic classes of muscle relaxants used.

### Surgical Treatment

Ahn Y, Lee SH, Park WM, Lee HY, Shin SW, Kang HY: Percutaneous endoscopic lumbar discectomy for recurrent disc herniation: Surgical technique, outcome, and prognostic factors of 43 consecutive cases. *Spine* 2004;29:E326-E332.

This article presents a retrospective study of 43 consecutive patients who underwent percutaneous endoscopic lumbar diskectomy for recurrent disk herniation. With an average follow-up of 31 months, approximately 82% of patients showed excellent or good outcomes based on the MacNab criteria. The mean visual analog scale decreased from an average of 9 to 3. The authors noted that patients younger than 40 years of age, patients who had symptoms for less than 3 months, and patients without concurrent lateral recess stenosis had better outcomes. The authors concluded that percutaneous endoscopic lumbar diskectomy is an effective treatment for recurrent disk herniation in selected patients and that the posterolateral approach through unscarred virgin tissue can prevent nerve injury and can preserve spinal stability.

Ng LC, Sell P: Predictive value of the duration of sciatica for lumbar discectomy: A prospective cohort study. *J Bone Joint Surg Br* 2004;86:546-549.

The authors attempted to identify whether timing of surgery affected the surgical outcome. A significant association was found between the duration of radiculopathy, Oswestry Disability Index scores, and low back outcome scores. Patients with an uncontained LDH had a shorter duration of symptoms and a better functional outcome than those with a contained LDH. Patients with sciatica for more than 12 months have a less favorable outcome. The authors found no difference in outcome for those patients who underwent surgery within 12 months of symptom onset.

Ostelo RW, de Vet HC, Waddell G, Kerckhoffs MR, Leffers P, van Tulder M: Rehabilitation following first-time lumbar disc surgery: A systematic review within the framework of the cochrane collaboration. *Spine* 2003;28: 209-218.

This article presents a meta-analysis of randomized controlled trials of postoperative rehabilitation. Thirteen studies met the criteria for inclusion in this review. The authors concluded that there is no strong evidence for the effectiveness of any therapy that is started immediately in the postoperative period. However, there is strong evidence (level 1) that intensive exercise programs are more effective on functional status and faster return to work compared with mild exercise programs when started 4 to 6 weeks after a diskectomy. In long-term follow-up, the difference between the two groups became insignificant. There was no difference in the rate of reoperation. No difference could be identified between patients undergoing supervised training compared with those doing home exercises. Limited evidence was found that work hardening treatments are more effective than usual care in improving return-to-work rates.

Yorimitsu E, Chiba K, Toyama Y, Hirabayashi K: Long-term outcome of standard discectomy for lumbar disc herniation: Over 10 years follow-up. *Spine* 2001;26:652-657.

This retrospective study presented an analysis of the long-term (minimum of 10 years) outcomes of diskectomy for lumbar disk herniation. The Japanese Orthopaedic Association scoring system was used to evaluate the outcomes. The average recovery rate was 73.5 ± 21.7%. Residual low back pain was found in approximately 75% of patients, but only 13% of those classified the pain as severe. Most patients with severe low back pain were under 35 years of age at the time of surgical intervention. The final Japanese Orthopaedic Association scores in the patients with radiographic evidence of disk degeneration were significantly lower than those in patients with no degeneration.

## Complications

Kara B, Tulum Z, Acar U: Functional results and the risk factors of reoperations after lumbar disc surgery. *Eur Spine J* 2005;14:43-48.

Risk factors for LDH include driving a motor vehicle, sedentary occupations, exposure to vibration, smoking, previous full-term pregnancies, physical inactivity, an increased body mass index, and a tall stature. Protective factors include regular physical activity. This prospective study found that patients who have a disk reherniation requiring a second diskectomy have poorer outcomes from both a functional and economic standpoint. The author showed that lack of regular physical exercise was a significant predictor for reoperation, whereas gender, age, body mass index, occupation, and smoking were not significant predictors, although a trend did exist for these factors.

Toyone T, Tanaka T, Daisuke K, Kato D, Kaneyama R: Low-back pain following surgery for lumbar disc herniation: A prospective study. *J Bone Joint Surg Am* 2004;86-A:893-896.

This prospective study investigated the effect of standard open versus microendoscopic diskectomy on low back pain associated with LDH. The mean duration of follow-up was 40 months. All patients in either group were satisfied with the outcome. There was no significant difference in leg pain or low back pain in either group.

## Classic Bibliography

Ahn UM, Ahn NU, Buchowski JM, et al: Cauda equina syndrome secondary to lumbar disc herniation. *Spine* 2000;25:1515-1522.

Boden SD, Davis DO, Dina TS, Patronas NJ, Wiesel SW: Abnormal magnetic resonance scans of the lumbar spine in asymptomatic subjects: A prospective investigation. *J Bone Joint Surg Am* 1990;72:403-408.

Buckwalter JA, Mow VC, Boden SD, Eyre DR, Weidenbaum M: Intervertebral disk structure, composition, and mechanical function, in Buckwalter JA, Einhorn TA, Simon SR (eds): *Orthopaedic Basic Science: Biology and Biomechanics of the Musculoskeletal System*, ed 2. Rosemont, IL, American Academy of Orthopaedic Surgeons, 2000, pp 547-556.

Deyo RA, Deihl AK, Rosenthal M: How many days of bed rest for acute low back pain?: A randomized clinical trial. *N Engl J Med* 1986;315:1064-1070.

Weber H: Lumbar disc herniation: A controlled, prospective study with ten years of observation. *Spine* 1983; 8:131-140.

# Chapter 32

# Lumbar Spinal Stenosis and Degenerative Spondylolisthesis

Elliot Carlisle, MD

Jeffrey S. Fischgrund, MD

## Introduction

Lumbar spinal stenosis is defined as reduction in the diameter of the spinal canal, lateral nerve canals, or neural foramina. The stenosis may involve multiple levels of the spinal canal or may be localized or segmental. Degenerative spondylolisthesis is forward displacement of a proximal vertebra in relation to its adjacent vertebra in association with an intact neural arch, and in the presence of degenerative changes.

The natural history of spinal stenosis and degenerative spondylolisthesis is unclear because of a lack of prospective studies following the course of patients who have been untreated. A review of the literature shows progression of symptoms in approximately 20% of untreated patients with spinal stenosis. Because most studies are not randomized or prospective, it is difficult to predict the natural history of the disease and to compare the available treatment options. A slow progression may be expected to occur in most affected patients. Even with significant canal narrowing, patients are unlikely to develop acute cauda equine syndrome in the absence of a significant disk herniation. One study that concentrated on the natural course of lumbar spinal stenosis reported on 32 patients who were followed for an average of 49 months (range, 10 to 103 months). The condition of 15% of these patients improved, 70% remained the same, and 15% were worse. On clinical examination, 41% were improved, 18% were worse, and 41% were unchanged. The authors concluded that severe progression was unlikely.

The natural history of degenerative spondylolisthesis also is poorly understood. A meta-analysis was performed using studies in the literature from 1970 to 1993. Only three studies were believed to adequately address the natural history of degenerative spondylolisthesis. Results showed that 32% of the patients in these studies had satisfactory outcomes without treatment. One study of 40 patients untreated for at least 5 years showed progression of spondylolisthesis in 12 patients. There was no correlation between progression of the slip and worsening of symptoms in the 12 patients. Only 4 patients had clinical deterioration, and none had slip progression.

Overall, the natural history of spinal stenosis and degenerative spondylolisthesis is not well understood, but appears to be favorable, with approximately 15% of patients showing clear clinical deterioration. Clinical improvement appears to occur in approximately one third to one half of patients with these conditions.

## Lumbar Spinal Stenosis

The decreased diameter of the canal or neural elements may be caused by bone or ligamentous hypertrophy, disk protrusion, spondylolisthesis, or any combination of these conditions. Pain in the back and leg (or legs) and claudication are the main symptoms. Patients often present with few objective physical findings; up to 95% of patients treated surgically have only subjective symptoms, usually pain. Vascular claudication must be considered in the differential diagnosis, as well as peripheral neuropathy.

Spinal stenosis usually affects patients older than 50 years and is uncommon in younger patients unless they are predisposed to the disease by a congenitally narrowed canal, previous trauma, or deformity. Patients typically report pain, paresthesias, weakness, or heaviness in the buttocks radiating into the lower extremities as a result of prolonged standing or walking. Importantly, there is a relationship of symptoms to posture. Symptoms occur with extension and are relieved with flexion. Patients can walk farther with less pain when leaning forward (such as when using a grocery cart while shopping).

In a review of 68 patients with spinal stenosis proved by myelography and surgically confirmed, the most prevalent symptoms were pseudoclaudication and standing discomfort (94%), followed by numbness (63%), and weakness (43%). Discomfort was noted both above and below the knee in 78% of patients, in the buttocks or thigh in 15%, and below the knee in 7%.

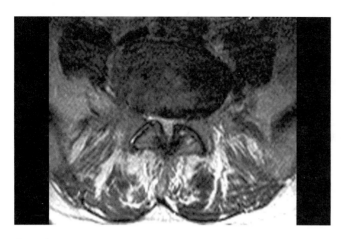

Figure 1   MRI scan showing central and lateral recess stenosis.

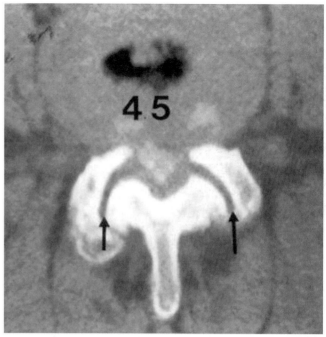

Figure 2   CT scan showing sagittal orientation of the L4-5 facets.

The physical examination of patients with lumbar stenosis is often normal or shows only nonspecific findings. Many older patients have reduced spinal mobility, with or without spinal stenosis. Extension is usually more limited than flexion, and may reproduce lumbar or lower extremity symptoms of pain and/or paresthesias. Some patients assume a characteristic "simian stance," with their hips and knees flexed and the trunk forward. This posture may allow patients to stand or walk longer distances. Hamstring tightness is common and may produce a false-positive straight-leg raising test. The neurologic examination typically is normal or may show subtle weakness, sensory changes, and reflex abnormalities. Weakness of the muscles innervated by the L5 nerve root may occur. A positive lumbar extension test is strongly predictive of spinal stenosis. The patient is asked to stand with the spine hyperextended for 30 to 60 seconds; a positive test is defined by reproduction of buttock or leg pain.

Symptoms of pseudoclaudication are associated primarily with central lumbar stenosis. In contrast, patients with purely lateral recess stenosis usually do not develop symptoms of neurogenic claudication, and typically have radicular symptoms in a specific dermatomal pattern. Patients with lateral recess stenosis often have pain at rest and with the Valsalva maneuver, and tend to be younger (mean age, 41 years) than patients with central canal stenosis (mean age, 65 years) (Figure 1).

The differential diagnosis of spinal stenosis is broad, and many conditions must be ruled out. Peripheral neuropathy, vascular disease, and disorders of the hip are common disorders with similar symptoms. Significant weight loss and intractable night pain should raise the suspicion of possible malignancy. Fever with localized back tenderness, recent infection, or after an invasive procedure should raise the suspicion of a spinal infection. Patients with vascular claudication may have diminished pulses and are not expected to have both pain with standing and relief of pain with flexion as would be

the case for those with spinal stenosis. Patients with peripheral neuropathy usually have a stocking-glove distribution of pain or paresthesias. Vibratory sensation is often diminished, and numbness is typically constant in patients with peripheral neuropathy. A careful examination of the hips and surrounding soft tissues should be done to exclude significant hip arthritis and gluteal or trochanteric bursitis from the diagnosis.

Overall, no objective criteria for using the patient history and results of the physical examination have been reported as a means of diagnosing lumbar spinal stenosis. The only quantitative evidence correlating diagnostic information with outcomes is imaging findings. Radiographic studies usually begin with routine AP and lateral radiographs. Degenerative changes include disk space narrowing, end-plate irregularities, osteophytes, traction spurs, and facet hypertrophy. Lateral radiographs should be obtained in the standing position because the slip may be reduced on the supine radiographs. Flexion and extension views should also be obtained because frequently the listhesis may not be visible on the static views. Electromyography is useful for distinguishing peripheral neuropathy from spinal stenosis. Noninvasive vascular studies are required if the patient has diminished peripheral pulses or symptoms consistent with vascular claudication.

Further imaging studies are indicated for patients with persistent back pain that is unresponsive to nonsurgical treatment, significant radicular pain, or neurologic decompensation. Imaging studies include CT, myelography, contrast enhanced CT, and MRI (Figures 2 and 3).

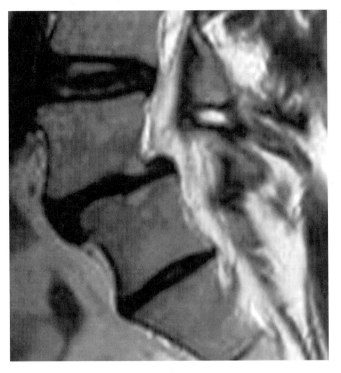

Figure 3  MRI scan showing degenerative spondylolisthesis and spinal stenosis

The degree of spinal stenosis is best evaluated by MRI. If an MRI scan cannot be obtained (because of pacemaker or cardiac stent implantation), a lumbar myelogram followed by CT is required to visualize the degree of neural compression. A decreased cross-sectional area at the level of the spondylolisthesis is often noted on imaging studies. There may be hypertrophy of the superior facet with entrapment of the L5 nerve root. Parasagittal images on MRI may show encroachment of the nerve root in the foramina by disk or hypertrophic bone.

Radiographic abnormalities are often present in asymptomatic individuals. Clinical decisions must be made on an individual basis by carefully evaluating a collection of data, including the patient history, physical findings, and relevant imaging and other adjunctive studies.

## Nonsurgical Treatment

Nonsurgical treatment for patients with spinal stenosis and degenerative spondylolisthesis is similar to conservative treatment for low back pain. Careful use of nonsteroidal anti-inflammatory drugs may give partial relief of symptoms. Narcotic prescriptions should be used only on a short-term basis. Physical therapy is often prescribed as the initial form of nonsurgical intervention. Although improvement in lumbar range of motion and axial muscle strength can be achieved, these passive and active modalities have little effect on the natural history of symptom progression. A series of epidural steroid in-

jections may give temporary relief of radicular symptoms and are frequently used for those patients who may not be candidates for surgery.

## Surgical Treatment

There are a variety of procedures that are commonly used for the surgical treatment of lumbar spinal stenosis and these are often divided into decompressive procedures with or without concomitant fusion. The decompressive procedures may be limited to single-level unilateral laminotomy for isolated neurologic compression to much larger global procedures including multilevel bilateral laminectomy with bilateral facetectomies and foraminotomies. Multilevel laminotomies may be most appropriate for patients with degenerative lumbar spinal stenosis with predominantly radicular pain. In these patients, the narrowing is usually maximal at the level of the facet joints and disks, whereas the canal is otherwise patent. In contrast, laminotomies are generally not appropriate in patients with congenital stenosis and global spinal canal narrowing.

The fusion procedures are equally varied and include posterolateral or intertransverse fusion, posterior fusion, posterior lumbar interbody fusion, transforaminal lumbar interbody fusion, and anterior lumbar interbody fusion, or some combination of these procedures. Neural decompression can be accomplished indirectly via anterior lumbar interbody fusion or posterior lumbar interbody fusion/transforaminal lumbar interbody fusion if disk space distraction and/or spondylolisthesis reduction occurs, which would enlarge the central canal as well as the involved foramina. Importantly, fusion may be either instrumented or noninstrumented. The instrumented fusions may include historically nonsegmental hook-wire techniques, or more commonly used segmental instrumentation with pedicle screws.

### Laminectomy

The most common surgical procedure for patients with lumbar spinal stenosis is decompressive lumbar laminectomy. Because spinal stenosis is often a global degenerative process that involves multiple levels and nerve roots bilaterally, a multilevel bilateral laminectomy is often required. For bilateral laminectomy, the spinous processes and the lamina and ligamentum flavum are removed on either side of the stenotic levels, laterally to the lateral recesses. Typically, decompression begins at the distal extent of the neurologic compression and proceeds in a caudal-to-cranial manner. Entry to the spinal canal is often obtained by the use of dissection with a small curet between the ligamentum flavum and the lamina at the inferior aspect of the involved lamina. Decompression is extended laterally from the midline until the lateral edge of the nerve root is observed and determined to be free of compression. Care is taken to preserve the pars interarticularis to prevent iatrogenic fracture to minimize the risk of iatrogenic instability. Instability also may be caused by inadvertent removal of the superior articular facet.

The presence of a concomitant disk herniation should be determined and removed because it can contribute to neural compression. However, diskectomy in the presence of laminectomy should generally be avoided unless the disk herniation contributes to significant neurologic compression because subsequent instability is more likely to occur when both anterior and posterior supporting structures are violated. This factor may be more important when significant amounts of the disk and anulus material are removed. When laminectomy is accompanied by a significant amount of diskectomy, arthrodesis at the time of surgery should be considered.

After decompression centrally and at the lateral recesses, the lateral decompression of the foramina is performed. Decompression is believed to be complete when a bent probe can be easily passed out of the neural foramen, both dorsal and ventral to the nerve root; the nerve root can be gently retracted approximately 1 cm medially; and there is no significant tension on the nerve root.

Controversy exists on whether to decompress levels that appear to be stenotic and do not seem to correlate with the patient's symptoms. When there is doubt regarding the symptomatic level, further diagnostic studies (such as a diagnostic nerve root block), which may help to identify symptomatic levels, should be considered. The risk of decompressing an apparently asymptomatic level and causing symptoms or complications must be weighed against the possible risk of further degeneration. Because spinal stenosis is a degenerative process that is believed to progress over time, it is possible that asymptomatic stenotic levels may eventually become symptomatic. Several studies have indicated that inadequate decompression results in long-term deterioration in clinical outcome following initially successful surgery, and may be a cause of failed back surgery and/or may necessitate additional spinal procedures.

### Hemilaminectomy
Hemilaminectomy includes unilateral removal of bone and ligamentum flavum, compared with bilateral removal in a complete laminectomy. It is an appropriate treatment for patients with unilateral spinal stenosis and with unilateral symptoms. The spinous processes and interspinous and supraspinous ligaments are preserved in the midline. For this reason, normal stabilizing structures are retained that reduce the risk of postoperative instability. Hemilaminectomy also avoids exposure and potential injury to the contralateral facet joint. The surgeon must preserve the pars interarticularis to avoid iatrogenic instability. One disadvantage of hemilaminectomy

is the increased technical difficulty of performing contralateral decompression and obtaining enough medial exposure to perform an adequate ipsilateral decompression in patients with foraminal stenosis. The intact medial structures of the spinous process and interspinous/supraspinous ligament complex may make it difficult to obtain the correct angle on the Kerrison rongeur laterally, which will enable the jaw of the rongeur to adequately decompress the neural foramen. In this situation, removal of the midline structures for the spinous process and interspinous/supraspinous ligament complex may be necessary to allow the correct angulation of the rongeur to perform an adequate decompression.

Nerve roots on the contralateral side of the hemilaminectomy can often be decompressed by tilting the operating table away from the surgeon and angling the operating microscope. The contralateral neural foramen can usually be seen and decompressed, and the more distal portion can be palpated with a long, bent probe. This technique may preserve normal, noncompressing midline structures and may minimize scar tissue on the opposite side. However, the technique is more demanding than bilateral laminectomy because the decompression is performed with limited exposure; the determination of adequate foraminal decompression depends on palpation rather than observation. An increased potential for dural laceration from the rongeur may exist while working through a more distant, smaller opening. When the surgeon cannot be sure of adequate neural decompression, bilateral laminectomy with adequate exposure may be necessary. If a dural laceration occurs from the rongeur while working through a small opening, complete bilateral laminectomies should be performed for adequate exposure and repair of the dura.

### Laminectomy Alternatives
Alternatives to laminectomy and hemilaminectomy have been described to avoid removal of normal, noncompressing structures. These alternative procedures, which include hemilaminotomy and laminoplasty, are believed to minimize the risk of postoperative instability and scarring. Hemilaminotomy involves a more limited decompression than hemilaminectomy. The procedure involves removing only ligamentum flavum and smaller adjacent caudal and cranial portions of the two hemilaminae, as opposed to removing the entire hemilaminae. This procedure is commonly performed in younger patients with unilateral focal neural compression. It may, however, also be considered in older patients with localized stenosis. Resection of the distal half of the superior hemilaminae is generally required to visualize and remove the proximal extent of the insertion site of the ligamentum flavum on the inferior aspect of the lamina. Lateral decompression also may require partial facetectomy. Similar to a hemilaminectomy, contralateral decompression with preservation of the spinous

processes and midline supraspinous/interspinous ligaments can be done by tilting the operating table away from the surgeon and by removing the midline and contralateral ligamentum flavum with a 45°-angled rongeur.

Lumbar laminoplasty is similar to cervical laminoplasty and involves hinging open the lamina on one side and inserting the excised spinous processes into the open hinge to keep it patent. This procedure was initially proposed as an alternative to laminectomy for active manual workers. In a 3-year follow-up study of 10 patients who underwent lumbar laminoplasty, the mean evaluation score improved an average of 73%, and the size of the spinal canal increased an average of 119% following surgery.

*Results of Surgical Treatment*
Although a large number of studies have been performed to assess the results of surgical treatment for patients with spinal stenosis, a recent review of the literature did not identify a randomized controlled trial comparing surgical versus nonsurgical treatment. An attempted meta-analysis of the literature on surgical outcomes for patients with lumbar spinal stenosis concluded that the poor scientific quality of the literature precluded conducting the intended meta-analysis. Of 625 articles that were identified as potentially relevant, only 74 (12%) met inclusion criteria for the study. Only 3 of the 74 studies were prospectively designed, 7 had an independent rating of outcome, and none were randomized. The average proportion of good to excellent outcomes was 72%. There was no statistically significant relationship between outcome and patient age, gender, presence of previous lumbar spinal surgery, or number of levels operated on. An important finding of this attempted meta-analysis was that there was no statistically significant difference in the outcome of decompression, with or without concomitant fusion, for patients with lumbar spinal stenosis. This finding has been corroborated in other surveys of the literature for outcomes following lumbar spinal fusion for a variety of diagnoses. This information is particularly important because of the obvious increased morbidity associated with lumbar fusion, with or without instrumentation.

In a recent prospective, nonrandomized study, a cohort group of patients with spinal stenosis who were treated surgically or nonsurgically were followed for 1 year. Seventy-one of 81 patients (88%) who had surgery had a decompressive lumbar laminectomy. At 1-year follow-up, 28% of the nonsurgical group reported definite improvement in predominant symptoms compared with 55% of the patients treated with surgery. After adjustment for covariates, surgery was believed to increase the relative odds of definite improvement by 2.6-fold when compared with nonsurgical treatment. Unfortunately, this study included only a 1-year

follow-up period, was nonrandom in nature, and examined only 22% of those eligible to be enrolled. Also, no standardization of nonsurgical methods was used. Although the results of the study should be interpreted with caution, some indication is provided of the expected short-term outcomes for patients receiving decompressive lumbar laminectomy for lumbar spinal stenosis.

A study compared 44 patients with lumbar spinal stenosis treated surgically with 19 patients who were treated nonsurgically. The results showed that 26 patients (59%) who underwent surgery improved, whereas 7 (16%) were unchanged, and 11 (25%) deteriorated or worsened. Six patients who did not undergo surgery (32%) improved, and 13 (68%) had the same or worse symptoms of neurogenic claudication at an average follow-up of 31 months. This study showed that the percentage of patients in the surgical group who improved were nearly twice that of the number in the nonsurgical group who improved. A larger percentage of the surgical group was worse at follow-up (25% versus 10%). This study was neither prospective nor random and it is not clear whether the nonsurgical group was untreated or had some type of conservative treatment.

Another retrospective study of 88 patients treated with decompressive lumbar laminectomy and followed for 2.8 to 6.8 years showed that 11% of the patients reported poor outcome at 1-year follow-up and 43% at final follow-up. Six percent of the patients had repeat lumbar surgery within the first year and 17% had additional surgery by the time of the final follow-up. Risk factors for poor outcome included preoperative comorbidities and limited single-level decompression. The authors concluded that long-term outcome for patients undergoing decompressive lumbar laminectomy for spinal stenosis was not as good as commonly believed because of the progressive deterioration of the results over time. The authors recommended more extensive decompression at the time of initial surgery. Another prospective, consecutive surgical study of 105 patients undergoing decompressive lumbar laminectomy for lumbar spinal stenosis also reported the deterioration of surgical results over time. Excellent results were reported by two thirds of the patients at 2-year follow-up; however, outcomes deteriorated to only 52% excellent results by 5-year follow-up. In the 5-year period of the study, 16% of the patients had resurgery for severe back pain or recurrent stenosis. Importantly, a significant correlation was noted between excellent outcome and preoperative duration of symptoms of less than 4 years with no preoperative low back pain and no significant comorbidities.

Although decompressive lumbar laminectomy in the treatment of spinal stenosis is a well-recognized form of treatment, the role of fusion in the treatment of spinal stenosis remains controversial. In patients with stenosis and no associated degenerative spondylolisthesis or other deformity in the sagittal or coronal plane, most studies indicate that decompression alone is the preferred method of surgical treatment. In a prospective, randomized study of 45 patients who underwent either decompression alone or decompression with fusion for lumbar spinal stenosis without associated instability, there were no significant differences in the outcome between the groups. The authors concluded that surgical decompression altered the natural history of spinal stenosis and resulted in a generally favorable outcome with improved quality of life in most patients. They also reported that arthrodesis in patients with lumbar spinal stenosis was not justified in the absence of radiographically proven segmental instability. Similarly, for patients with associated degenerative spondylolisthesis or degenerative scoliosis, concomitant fusion is recommended. The use of supplementary spinal instrumentation remains unresolved.

Predictors of outcome after spinal surgery for lumbar spinal stenosis have been studied. A retrospective review of 88 patients who underwent decompressive lumbar laminectomy for lumbar spinal stenosis found that 6% of patients required a second operation by 1 year after surgery and 17% required a second operation by the time of the last follow-up (between 2.8 and 6.8 years). Several predictors of poor outcome were identified, such as increasing length of time since surgery, single-level decompression, and increased number of comorbidities; only the latter was significant after adjusting for multiple comparisons. In patients with the highest comorbidity scores, only 40% had a good outcome at final follow-up compared with 75% of patients with the lowest comorbidity scores. The most common comorbidities included osteoarthritis (32%), cardiac disease (22%), rheumatoid arthritis (10%), and chronic pulmonary disease (7%). No single comorbidity was significantly associated with worse outcome; this fact was interpreted to indicate that comorbidities may be additive. In a subsequent study by the same authors, comorbidity was found to be second only to preoperative reports of predominant low back pain as a determinate of disability in lumbar spinal stenosis.

The effects of comorbidities on other outcome measures have also been studied. In patients with an increased number of comorbidities, both the cost of lumbar spinal surgery and the length of the hospital stay after surgery were increased. Patients with three or more comorbidities were found to have 25% longer hospital stays, 35% higher hospital costs, and a 73% higher rate of transfer to nursing facility after surgery than those without comorbidities.

A recent retrospective study of 118 consecutive patients (age 70 to 101 years) who were surgically treated for lumbar spinal stenosis produced different conclusions. Overall morbidity occurred in 24 patients (20%). Of 118 patients, 109 expressed satisfaction with the sur-

gery and resumed daily activities, whereas 9 had fair or poor results. The authors concluded that advanced age did not increase the morbidity associated with spinal stenosis surgery.

## Degenerative Spondylolisthesis

Anterior displacement of one vertebral body on another in the presence of an intact neural arch is termed degenerative spondylolisthesis. This condition may be a source of low back pain, as well as radicular or referred leg pain, and often produces symptoms of neurogenic claudication. Degenerative spondylolisthesis occurs five to six times more frequently in women and usually occurs after the age of 40 years. The L4-5 interspace is 6 to 10 times more frequently involved than adjacent levels. Also, a transitional vertebra with sacralization of L5 is four times more frequent in patients with degenerative spondylolisthesis.

The degenerative lesion is believed to be the result of long-standing intersegmental instability. Degeneration of the disk accompanied by degeneration of the facet joints allows vertebral translation. The articular processes may be sagittally or horizontally oriented and therefore parallel to each other, or they may be anomalous in their orientation and asymmetric. In both of these instances the articular processes are free to glide forward one on the other, causing slippage as the joints degenerate. Forward displacement results from a failure of the apophyseal joints to restrain shear. The slip seldom exceeds 30% unless there has been prior surgical intervention.

A thorough patient history and physical examination are always the first steps in the diagnosis. Back pain is the most commonly reported symptom, often follows a variable course, and is usually unrelated to trauma. The back pain is mechanical and is usually relieved by rest. Radiation of pain into the posterolateral thighs is common. The second most common symptom is neurogenic claudication. The pain is usually diffuse in the lower limbs, involving dermatomes and muscles innervated by the L4, L5, and S1 nerve roots. The leg pain is classically accentuated by walking and relieved by rest. Patients may have "drop episodes" characterized by unexpected falls during ambulation.

The results of a physical examination in patients with degenerative spondylolisthesis may be nonspecific. Hamstring tightness is a common finding and patients may have a type of waddling gait. When stenotic symptoms are severe, a fixed forward-flexed posture may be observed. Except in very thin patients, the deformity is not usually appreciated on examination or palpation. Although a neurologic examination is critical, results are often normal and/or nonspecific. Findings may include bilaterally absent reflexes, spotty sensory loss, and possible muscle weakness or atrophy.

## *Surgical Treatment*

### *Decompression Without Fusion*

The surgical treatment of lumbar spinal stenosis with associated degenerative lumbar spondylolisthesis involves either decompression alone or decompression with arthrodesis. A meta-analysis of the literature from 1970 to 1993 included 11 articles that met inclusion criteria on decompression without fusion. Overall, only 69% of patients were found to have satisfactory results following surgical decompression without concomitant fusion. Thirty-one percent of the patients in nine studies in which slip progression was recorded showed an increase in the degree of slip. However, in most studies, there was no correlation between clinical outcome and the amount of slip progression.

A retrospective review of 290 patients who had limited lumbar decompression for spinal stenosis with degenerative spondylolisthesis, with 10-year follow-up, reported excellent results in 69% of patients, good results in 13%, fair results in 12%, and poor results in 6% of patients. Because only 2.7% of patients required secondary fusion, the authors concluded that routine concomitant fusion for spinal stenosis with degenerative spondylolisthesis was not warranted. In a prospective, randomized study comparing decompression alone and combined decompression with noninstrumented fusion for degenerative spondylolisthesis, only 11 of 25 patients (44%) having decompression without fusion had satisfactory results. This group also had significantly more postoperative low back and leg pain than the fusion group, and had an average increase of 50% in slip from preoperative levels.

### *Decompression With Fusion*

A meta-analysis of the literature on degenerative spondylolisthesis found only six studies that met the inclusion criteria for treatment using decompression with noninstrumented fusion. In these studies, 79% of patients reported satisfactory outcome following decompression without arthrodesis. Only three of the studies were prospective and randomized; the most widely quoted study compared decompression alone to decompression with noninstrumented spinal fusion in the treatment of L3-4 and L4-5 degenerative spondylolisthesis with spinal stenosis. The authors reported improved results when concomitant intertransverse process arthrodesis was performed in addition to decompression when compared with decompression alone. Ninety-six percent good to excellent results were noted in the arthrodesis group and only 44% good to excellent results in the nonarthrodesis group. Thirty-six percent of those undergoing arthrodesis had a pseudarthrosis; however, all had either an excellent or good result. The authors concluded that the results of surgical decompression with in situ arthrodesis was superior to those of decompression alone in the treatment of spinal stenosis associated with L3-4 and L4-5 degenerative spondylolisthesis. The authors also concluded that the decision to perform arthrodesis should be based on the presence or absence of preoperative spondylolisthesis rather than other factors such as patient age or gender, disk height, or the amount of bone resected during decompression.

The relationships between bone regrowth following surgical decompression for lumbar spinal stenosis and long-term outcome have also been evaluated. In general, satisfactory outcome has been found to be inversely related to the amount of bone regrowth. Although patients with degenerative spondylolisthesis do show some bone growth following lumbar decompression and fusion, the degree of regrowth is less than in those patients who undergo decompression alone without arthrodesis. These results are also reflected in the outcome following surgery; outcome was shown to be significantly improved in patients undergoing decompression with spinal fusion. Although this study was retrospective, results suggest that arthrodesis stabilizes the spine, resulting in less bone regrowth and subsequent recurrent stenosis.

The benefit of the use of additional instrumentation for fusion in patients with degenerative spondylolisthesis remains controversial. A prospective, randomized study of 124 patients who underwent either instrumented or noninstrumented fusion for degenerative spondylolisthesis using two types of spinal instrumentation (rigid and a nonrigid systems) found that 65% of the patients in the noninstrumented group achieved fusion, compared with 50% of patients in the group treated with semirigid fixation, and 86% of the rigid fixation group. The authors concluded that the fusion rate and outcome were improved in patients undergoing fusion with more rigid fixation systems. A retrospective, multicenter study of 2,684 patients with degenerative spondylolisthesis treated with pedicle screw fixation was performed. Solid fusion was noted radiographically in 89% of the patients who underwent pedicle screw fixation compared with 70% of those without instrumentation. Clinical outcome also improved in the group of patients undergoing instrumented fusion.

A prospective, randomized study of 76 patients with symptomatic lumbar spinal stenosis and associated degenerative spondylolisthesis who underwent decompression and either noninstrumented in situ posterolateral fusion or instrumented fusion with segmental fixation was performed. Sixty-seven patients were available for a 2-year follow-up. The clinical outcome was good to excellent in 76% of patients in whom instrumentation was used, and in 85% of those with no instrumentation. Successful fusion occurred in 82% of the patients with instrumentation compared with 45% of those with no instrumentation. Overall, successful fusion did not influence patient outcome. The authors concluded that in patients who undergoing single-level posterolateral fusion for degenerative spondylolisthesis with spinal stenosis, the use of pedicle screws may lead to a higher fusion rate, but clinical outcome 2 years after surgery shows no improvement in pain levels in the back and lower limbs.

A recent prospective, randomized study on patients who underwent posterior lumbar decompression with posterolateral arthrodesis without instrumentation was performed to determine the influence of pseudarthrosis on clinical outcome. The study included 47 patients with an average follow-up of 7 to 8 months. Clinical outcome was excellent to good in 86% of patients with a solid arthrodesis and 56% of patients with a pseudarthrosis. The authors concluded that in patients undergoing single-level decompression and posterolateral arthrodesis for stenosis and concurrent spondylolisthesis, solid fusion improves long-term clinical results. Because earlier studies have shown a higher fusion rate, it may be inferred that instrumented fusion may be indicated for patients with degenerative spondylolisthesis (Figure 4).

Decompressive lumbar laminectomy with fusion is generally recommended for patients with spinal stenosis associated with degenerative spondylolisthesis. In elderly, low-demand patients with more pain resulting from radiculopathy than from pseudoclaudication, laminotomies without fusion may be performed. This procedure may have less risk of subsequent slip progression if there is significant collapse of disk spaces and vertebral osteophyte formation.

Multiple studies have shown a higher fusion rate with the addition of rigid spinal instrumentation. To date, no study has determined what radiographic criteria can be identified preoperatively to predict the probability of a successful noninstrumented fusion. If a clinician believes that a noninstrumented fusion will lead to a successful arthrodesis, pedicle screw instrumentation can be avoided. However, because a solid arthrodesis is beneficial for successful long-term outcome, instrumentation should be used in those patients who are determined to be at risk for pseudarthrosis following a noninstrumented fusion.

## Summary
The natural history of untreated spinal stenosis either with or without degenerative spondylolisthesis is relatively benign but progressive. However, because few long-term studies are available it is difficult to evaluate the results of treatments of these conditions. Although the role of decompression in the treatment of spinal stenosis is fairly well defined, the role of arthrodesis in the treatment of spinal stenosis with or without degenerative spondylolisthesis is less well characterized because of the paucity of controlled, prospective, and randomized studies comparing different treatment options.

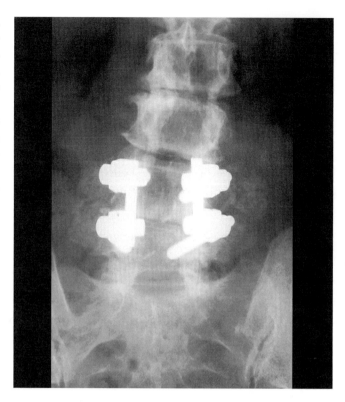

Figure 4 Solid posterolateral fusion following instrumentation and autograft is shown.

The literature to date suggests that the natural history of spinal stenosis, with or without degenerative spondylolisthesis, is characterized by improvement in approximately one third of patients and deterioration in approximately 10% of patients. The remaining patients have a generally static clinical course over time, with little if any improvement.

There are few data to support the routine use of fusion with or without instrumentation in the surgical treatment of patients with lumbar spinal stenosis that is not associated with degenerative spondylolisthesis. However, in patients who undergo extensive decompression either by excessive bone removal, extensive number of levels decompressed, removal of the pars interarticularis, or removal of more than one facet joint at one level, arthrodesis is often recommended. Support exists for the use of decompression and arthrodesis in the treatment of lumbar spinal stenosis associated with degenerative spondylolisthesis. Many studies indicate that the fusion rate is improved in patients undergoing instrumented fusion, although the relationship between outcome improvement and fusion rate is less clear. The future role of bone graft substitutes and/or bone morphogenetic proteins in spinal fusion continues to be studied. These biologic agents will likely have an increased role in the future of the surgical treatment of patients with these complicated spinal ailments.

## Annotated Bibliography
### General

Sengupta D, Herkowitz H: Lumbar spinal stenosis treatment strategies and indications for surgery. *Orthop Clin North Am* 2003;34:281-295.

This review article describes the natural history and treatment options, both nonsurgical and surgical, for patients with lumbar spinal stenosis. Important discussions on degenerative spondylolisthesis, iatrogenic instability, recurrent or junctional stenosis, and treatment algorithms are also included.

### Lumbar Spinal Stenosis

Arinzon Z, Adunsky A, Fidelman Z, Gepstein R: Outcomes of decompression surgery for lumbar spinal stenosis in elderly diabetic patients. *Eur Spine J* 2004;13: 32-37.

This retrospective study on decompressive surgery for spinal stenosis compared elderly diabetic patients with gender and age-matched controls. The authors found poorer results for diabetic patients with regard to basic activities and pain improvement after surgery. The outcome for patients with diabetes depends on the presence of other comorbidities, concurrent diabetic neuropathy, duration of diabetes, and insulin treatment.

Bridwell KH, Lenke LG, Lewis SJ: Treatment of spinal stenosis and fixed sagittal imbalance. *Clin Orthop Relat Res* 2001;384:35-44.

This review article discusses the treatment options for patients with sagittal imbalance associated with spinal stenosis. The authors recommend that fixed deformities are most suitably treated with a pedicle subtraction procedure with decompression and extension of the fusion.

Epstein NE: Lumbar laminectomy for the resection of synovial cysts and coexisting lumbar spinal stenosis or degenerative spondylolisthesis: An outcome study. *Spine* 2004;29:1049-1055.

This article reviews the outcomes of surgical treatment for patients with synovial cysts and stenosis, with or without concomitant spondylolisthesis. The author noted the high percentage of patients who had postoperative development or progression of spondylolisthesis after laminectomy. Because synovial cysts reflect disruption of the facet joint and some degree of instability, the author recommended consideration of primary fusion to improve surgical results for patients in both categories.

Gunzburg R, Keller TS, Szpalski M, Vandeputte K, Spratt KF: A prospective study on CT scan outcomes after conservative decompression surgery for lumbar spinal stenosis. *J Spinal Disord Tech* 2003;16:261-267.

The postoperative CT scans of patients who underwent conservative lumbar laminarthrectomy were analyzed in this prospective study. This procedure involved decompressing the central and nerve root canals while respecting the integrity of the neural arches, facet joints, and most muscle attachments. The authors noted a statistically significant increase in interfacet bony canal diameter of the operated levels.

Gunzburg R, Keller TS, Szpalski M, Vandeputte K, Spratt KF: Clinical and psychofunctional measures of conservative decompression surgery for lumbar spinal stenosis: A prospective cohort study. *Eur Spine J* 2003; 12:197-204.

The authors prospectively evaluated psychometric and functional outcomes for patients who had conservative lumbar laminectomy. With short-term follow-up, the authors reported outcomes to be as successful as standard more aggressive decompressive procedures presented in the literature. The authors noted that even in a highly organic disorder such as spinal stenosis, illness behavior plays an important role in predicting surgical outcomes.

Khoo LT, Fessler RG: Microendoscopic decompressive laminotomy for the treatment of lumbar stenosis. *Neurosurgery* 2002;51(suppl 5):S146-S154.

This study compared the outcomes of patients undergoing microendoscopic percutaneous midline-sparing lumbar decompression with standard open decompression. The authors reported similar short-term clinical outcomes for the patients treated with the microendoscopic technique and the standard technique. Those treated with the microendoscopic technique had a reduction in blood loss, shorter postoperative hospital stay, and needed fewer narcotics than the other group. Lower surgical stress, decreased tissue trauma, and quicker recovery rate are believed to be important factors for the patients treated.

Ragab AA, Fye MA, Bohlmann HH: Surgery of the lumbar spine for spinal stenosis in 118 patients 70 years of age or older. *Spine* 2003;28:348-353.

A consecutive case retrospective review evaluating the outcome of lumbar spine surgery for spinal stenosis in elderly patients is presented. The authors report on a 2-year follow-up of 118 patients from 70 to 101 years of age who were surgically treated for lumbar spinal stenosis. Advanced age did not increase the morbidity associated with this surgery when compared with other studies of a younger population, nor did advanced age decrease patient satisfaction or return to activities.

Stoll TM, Dubois G, Schwarzenbach O: The dynamic neutralization system for the spine: A multicenter study of a novel non-fusion system. *Eur Spine J* 2002;11(suppl 2):S170-S178.

This article presents the results of a prospective, multicenter study that evaluated the safety and efficacy of a dynamic nonfusion neutralization system for various degenerative lumbar spine conditions in 83 consecutive patients. Nine complications were reported that were unrelated to the implant, and one complication was caused by screw misplacement. The authors reported that the results compared well with those obtained by conventional procedures, and that mobile stabilization is less invasive than fusion. Dynamic neutralization is believed to be a safe and effective alternative in the treatment of unstable lumbar conditions.

Zucherman JF, Hsu KY, Hartjen CA, et al: A prospective, randomized multicenter study for the treatment of lumbar spinal stenosis with the X STOP interspinous implant: 1-year results. *Eur Spine J* 2004;13:22-31.

This article reviews a prospective, randomized multicenter trial of a new interspinous implant (X STOP, St. Francis Medical Technologies, Concord, CA) for patients with lumbar spinal stenosis. One hundred patients received the X STOP implant and a control group of 91 patients received nonsurgical therapy. At 1-year follow-up, 59% of the patients who received the X STOP implant and 12% of the control group had successful results. The authors report these success rates to be comparable with published reports for decompressive laminectomy, but with considerably less morbidity.

### Degenerative Spondylolisthesis

Kornblum MB, Fischgrund JS, Herkowitz HN, Abraham DA, Berkower DL, Ditkoff JS: Degenerative lumbar spondylolisthesis with spinal stenosis: A prospective long-term study comparing fusion and pseudoarthrosis. *Spine* 2004;29:726-733.

This article presents the result of a prospective, randomized study on patients who underwent posterior lumbar decompression with bilateral posterior arthrodesis for degenerative spondylolisthesis and spinal stenosis to determine the long-term influence of pseudarthrosis. The authors showed that a solid fusion improves long-term clinical results for back and lower limb symptomatology compared with prior shorter-term studies, which indicated no significant difference in clinical outcome between solid fusion and pseudarthrosis.

Vaccaro AR, Patel T, Fischgrund J, et al: A pilot safety and efficacy study of OP-1 putty (rh-BMP-7) as an adjunct to iliac crest autograft in posterolateral lumbar fusions. *Eur Spine J* 2003;12:495-500.

This article presents the results of a multicenter pilot study to evaluate the safety of a bone morphogenetic osteogenic protein-1 (OP-1), in the form of OP-1 putty combined with autograft, for intertransverse process fusion of the lumbar spine in 12 patients with symptomatic spinal stenosis and degenerative spondylolisthesis following decompression. No instrumentation was used. Radiologists used blinded methods to assess fusion status with stringent criteria for fusion. A successful fusion was achieved in slightly over half the patients. No adverse events were reported; findings were in agreement with other studies supporting the safety of bone morphogenetic proteins.

Zheng F, Cammisa FP Jr, Sandhu HS, Girardi FP, Khan SN: Factors predicting hospital stay, operative time, blood loss, and transfusion in patients undergoing revision posterior lumbar spine decompression, fusion, and segmental instrumentation. *Spine* 2002;27:818-824.

This article presents the results of a retrospective chart review of 112 patients who underwent revision posterior lumbar spine decompression, fusion, and segmental instrumentation, to determine factors predicting length of hospital stay, surgical time, blood loss, and transfusion requirements. Patient demographics, comorbid conditions, factors related to previous lumbar surgery, diagnosis, number of levels fused, and preoperative hemoglobin and hematocrit were used as independent variables. The authors noted that the number of levels fused and patient age seemed to be the most significant factors predicting length of hospital stay, surgical time, intraoperative blood loss, and transfusion requirements in this patient population.

## Classic Bibliography

Atlas SJ, Deyo RA, Keller RV, et al: The Maine Lumbar Spine Study: Part III: One-year outcomes of surgical and non-surgical management of lumbar spinal stenosis. *Spine* 1996;21:1787-1795.

Deyo RA, Cherkin DC, Loeser JD, Bigos SJ, Ciol MA: Morbidity and mortality in association with operations on the lumbar spine: The influence of age, diagnosis, and procedure. *J Bone Joint Surg Am* 1992;74:536-543.

Deyo RA, Ciol MA, Cherkin DC, Loeser JD, Bigos SJ: Lumbar spinal fusion: A cohort study of complications, reoperations, and resource use in the Medicare population. *Spine* 1993;18:1463-1470.

Fischgrund JS, Mackay M, Herkowitz HN, Brower R, Montgomery DM, Kurz LT: Degenerative lumbar spondylolisthesis with spinal stenosis: A prospective, randomized study comparing decompressive laminectomy and arthrodesis with and without spinal instrumentation. *Spine* 1997;22:2807-2812.

France JC, Yaszemski MJ, Lauerman WC, et al: A randomized, prospective study of posterolateral lumbar fusion: Outcomes with and without pedicle screw instrumentation. *Spine* 1999;24:553-560.

Frymoyer JW: Degenerative spondylolisthesis: Diagnosis and treatment. *J Am Acad Orthop Surg* 1994;2:9-15.

Hall S, Bartleson JD, Onofrio BM, Baker HL Jr, Okazaki H, O'Duffy JD: Lumbar spinal stenosis: Clinical features, diagnostic procedures, and result of surgical treatment in 68 patients. *Ann Intern Med* 1985;103:271-275.

Herkowitz HN: Spine update: Degenerative lumbar spondylolisthesis. *Spine* 1995;20:1084-1090.

Herkowitz HN, Kurz LT: Degenerative lumbar spondylolisthesis with spinal stenosis: A prospective study comparing decompression with decompression and intertransverse process arthrodesis. *J Bone Joint Surg Am* 1991;73:802-808.

Johnsson KE, Rosen I, Uden A: The natural course of lumbar spinal stenosis. *Clin Orthop Relat Res* 1992;279: 82-86.

Johnsson KE, Uden A, Rosen I: The effect of decompression on the natural course of spinal stenosis: A comparison of surgically treated and untreated patients. *Spine* 1991;16:615-619.

Katz JN, Stucki G, Lipson SJ, Fossel AH, Grobler LJ, Weinstein JN: Predictors of surgical outcome in degenerative lumbar spinal stenosis. *Spine* 1999;24:2229-2233

Macnab I: Spondylolisthesis with an intact neural arch: The so-called pseudo-spondylolisthesis. *J Bone Joint Surg Br* 1950;32:325-333.

Mardjetko SM, Connolly PJ, Shott S: Degenerative lumbar spondylolisthesis: A meta-analysis of literature, 1070-1993. *Spine* 1994;19(suppl 20):2256S-2265S.

Postacchini F: Surgical management of lumbar spinal stenosis. *Spine* 1999;24:1043-1047.

Postacchini F, Cinotti G: Bone regrowth after surgical decompression for lumbar spinal stenosis. *J Bone Joint Surg Br* 1992;74:862-869.

Sidhu KS, Herkowitz HN: Spinal instrumentation in the management of degenerative disorders of the lumbar spine. *Clin Orthop Relat Res* 1997;335:39-53.

Tenhula J, Lenke LG, Bridwell KH, Gupta P, Riew D: Prospective functional evaluation of the surgical treatment of neurogenic claudication in patients with lumbar spinal stenosis. *J Spinal Disord* 2000;13:276-282.

Weinstein MA, McCabe JP, Cammisa FP Jr: Postoperative spinal wound infection: A review of 2,391 consecutive index procedures. *J Spinal Disord* 2000;13:422-426.

Yuan HA, Garfin SR, Dickman CA, Mardjetko SM: A historical cohort study of pedicle screw fixation in thoracic, lumbar, and sacral spinal fusions. *Spine* 1994; 19(suppl 20):2279S-2296S.

Zdeblick TA: A prospective, randomized study of lumbar fusion: Preliminary results. *Spine* 1993;18:983-991.

# Chapter 33

# Adult Isthmic Spondylolisthesis

Elisha Ofiram, MD

Timothy A. Garvey, MD

## Introduction

The term "spondylolisthesis" (SPL), from the Greek words spondylos (vertebra) and olisthesis (slip), is defined as a forward slippage of one vertebra on the caudal level. Wiltse and associates established the classic classification system for SPL that included five types of slippage. Type II slippage is isthmic or spondylolytic SPL, in which the slip is secondary to a defect in the pars interarticularis. Type II SPL has been divided into three subtypes: IIA, characterized by a lytic lesion with fatigue fracture of the pars and complete bony separation; IIB, elongation of the pars without separation; and IIC, an acute pars fracture. Marchetti and Bartolozzi proposed a new classification system for SPL that primarily relied on developmental components rather than observed anatomic pathology. This was the first classification system that suggested a possible etiology for SPL and provided a predictive quality. In patients with isthmic lytic SPL, a developmental condition, the bilateral defects in the pars enable the body of the superior vertebra to slip on the vertebra below, reaching a state of canal expansion, which explains the low incidence of neurologic symptoms. The most accepted theory on the etiology of isthmic SPL is that the condition is caused by a stress fracture, which results from either an acute event or secondary to fatigue during repetitive stress. The pars interarticularis is more prone to lysis because it offers less resistance compared with other cortical parts of the vertebra when subjected to comparable forces. A weakened posterior arch, under the influence of upright posture with flexion and extension of the spine and repetitive microtrauma, finally yields to those repetitive forces leading to a stress fracture of the pars.

Isthmic SPL is a common pathology of the lumbar spine, particularly at the L5-S1 level. The incidence of isthmic SPL has been reported to be 4% by the age of 6 years and 6% in adulthood. In a biomechanical analysis and a retrospective clinical review, it was reported that an L4-5 isthmic SPL lesion often progresses more than an L5-S1 lesion in adult patients because it is more

unstable; the iliolumbar ligament does not provide stability as it does at L5-S1.

## Slip Progression

Although the progression of isthmic SPL in children and adolescents has been well documented, its occurrence in adults has been questioned. One study reported on the progression of isthmic SPL in 21 adult patients. Documented slip progression ranged from 8% to 30% during a period of 3 to 20 years, beginning after the fourth decade of life. The increased slippage was always associated with degeneration of the disk below the pars defect. It may be hypothesized that the slip progression results from the inability of the degenerated disk to resist translation as effectively as a normal disk. The anterior shear forces cause the increased olisthesis; this process may result in an asymptomatic developmental lesion becoming symptomatic.

## Clinical Presentation

Most adults with isthmic SPL are asymptomatic. If symptoms develop, they usually consist of back pain, leg pain, or both. Back pain appears to be more prevalent in adults with isthmic SPL than in the general population. The possible sources of pain are the disk, nerve entrapment caused by foraminal stenosis, facet joint arthrosis, and segmental instability. Disk degeneration with associated discogenic pain is a possible source of back pain. Although isthmic SPL causes central canal expansion, the forward slippage applies traction to the free neural arch, causing it to rotate on the pivot formed by its articulation with the sacrum. The free neural arch can encroach on the foramen and compress the emerging nerve root of L5 (in patients with L5-S1 SPL). This process, as well as degenerative uncal osteophyte formation, can bring about foraminal stenosis and radiculopathy. Extraforaminal sources of nerve root compression include the corporotransverse ligament and the ileotransverse ligament.

Segmental instability is an important and common cause of back pain because of the stabilizing affects of

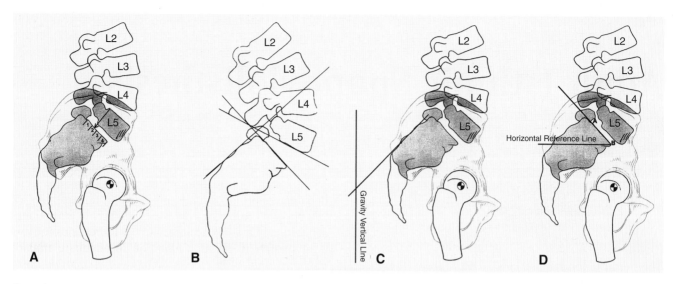

Figure 1 **A,** The Meyerding classification provides a simple and common quantification of the slip of L5 on S1. Grade I defines a slip from 0 to 25%, grade II from 26% to 50%, grade III from 51% to 75%, and grade IV from 76% to 100%. **B,** To determine the slip angle, a line is drawn parallel to the posterior aspect of the sacrum with a perpendicular line at the level of the cephalad border of the sacrum (because of remodeling), and then a line is drawn at the undersurface of the body of L5. This angle represents the relationship of L5 to the sacrum. **C,** In higher-grade slips, the sacrum becomes more vertical and the kyphotic deformity increases, as measured by the sacral inclination. **D,** Sacral slope is defined as the angle between the horizontal reference line and the end-plate line of S1. *(Courtesy of Medtronic Sofamor Danek USA, Inc.)*

the ileotransverse ligament and the position of L5, which typically is set deep in the pelvis. Radicular pain is frequently reported by adult patients, in contrast to tight hamstring muscles that more commonly occur in children. It is important to differentiate whether the pain is acute, chronic, or an acute exacerbation of a chronic condition. Determining how much of the reported pain is low back pain versus leg pain is important for an understanding of the source and mechanism of the pain. This determination allows the physician to individualize the best treatment for each patient.

## Imaging Evaluation

Plain weight-bearing PA and lateral radiographs of the thoracolumbar and the lumbosacral spine including the pelvis are the primary imaging studies for the diagnosis and treatment of SPL. It is of paramount importance that the radiographs are obtained with the patient in an upright position using standard techniques. Variations in technique can lead to misinterpretation of the progress of the slip. The lateral thoracolumbosacral view allows basic measurements to be obtained that help in quantifying and following the course of slip.

The Meyerding four-grade classification system for slip, slip angle, sacral inclination, and sacral slope identifies common parameters that can be measured using the weight-bearing lateral radiograph (Figure 1). It is important to consistently choose a set of measurements that document the magnitude of the slip, the effective sagittal deformity, and the shear force of L5 in relationship to the sacrum.

When considering sagittal alignment of the spine, it has been recognized that the orientation of the lum-

bosacral pelvic junction plays a critical role in the overall alignment of the spine. Since Legaye and associates introduced the concept of pelvic incidence, more studies have been done to try to determine the association between isthmic SPL and pelvic parameters (Figure 2). A significant correlation between pelvic incidence and the degree of isthmic SPL in adolescence as well as in adults was found in a 2002 study.

Flexion and extension lateral radiographs may be helpful in the evaluation of instability or potential instability following decompression. The evaluation of the disk adjacent to the isthmic slip level can provide important preoperative planning information for the surgeon because this disk has a predisposition for degeneration. MRI is the most common modality to assess disk degeneration at the slip and at adjacent levels, as well as to evaluate nerve or thecal sac compression. Preoperative diskography is another diagnostic tool that is widely used because of its capability of relating pathoanatomy to disk symptomatology. It is particularly important to assess the adjacent level to the slip, especially if there are degenerative changes seen on MRI scans. This information can impact the surgeon's decision as to where the fusion should be stopped.

## Treatment

### Nonsurgical Treatment

In symptomatic adults, the mere presence of low-grade isthmic SPL on radiographs does not necessarily indicate the source of the pain. There are many possible causes for low back or leg pain that must be distinguished from pain secondary to the slip. The nonsurgical treatment of adults with symptoms caused by the slip is

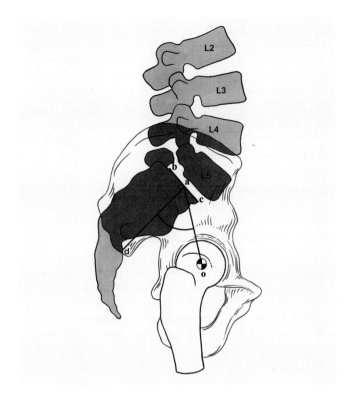

Figure 2 Pelvic incidence is defined as an angle subtended by a line which is drawn from the center of the femoral head to the midpoint of the sacral end plate (oa) and a line perpendicular to the center of the sacral end plate (ad).

similar in concept to the treatment for any type of mechanical low back pain. In patients with predominant radiculopathy, nonsurgical management may not be as effective as in patients with mechanical low back pain. The nonsurgical treatment regimens for adults with isthmic SPL are controversial and ill-defined; randomized controlled trials are lacking. The efficacy of the treatment often is based on subjective data. Because pain is the most common presenting symptom and often can spontaneously improve, it is difficult to assess the efficacy of treatments. Many patients respond to nonsurgical treatment; however, advanced age and the presence of neurologic symptoms and chronic pain are indicators of a poor prognosis. Several studies have investigated the benefit of exercise for patients with adult isthmic SPL. One study showed a significant reduction in pain intensity and disability level for an exercise group compared with a control group without an exercise program. Another short-term study compared exercise with posterolateral fusion, and showed better functional outcome, less pain, and an improvement in the disability rating index for patients in the surgical group. Recently, a randomized long-term study that compared fusion with a 1-year exercise program showed that in contrast to the short-term study of the same patients, in which fusion produced significantly better results than conservative treatment for all variables studied, a significant

long-term difference remained only for the global outcome variable. Although no data exist regarding the efficacy of using nonsteroidal anti-inflammatory drugs, narcotics, muscle relaxants, and selective injections to the epidural space, facet joints, or pars, these modalities are frequently used by the clinician as part of a nonsurgical treatment program.

### Surgical Treatment

The goals of surgical treatment for the patient with adult isthmic SPL include stabilization of the slip level, decompression of neural elements, reconstruction of disk height, and restoration of the three-dimensional alignment of the lower lumbar spine. Indications for surgical treatment include failure of an adequate trial of nonsurgical therapy for disabling back and/or leg pain, radiographic evidence of symptomatic instability, progressive neurologic deficit, bowel or bladder dysfunction related to the isthmic SPL, and documented symptomatic slip progression.

When surgery is chosen for a patient with symptoms caused by isthmic SPL, a key decision is whether to perform specific nerve root decompression. During the process of surgical decision making, it is critical to elucidate the dominant symptom complex (for example, it should be determined whether the patient's back pain is greater than or equal to leg pain or vice versa). If a patient has little or no leg pain and no neurologic dysfunction, then consideration of a fusion alone is reasonable. If buttocks and/or leg pain predominate, if there is documentable impairment of neurologic function, and/or if significant hamstring tightness exists, surgical decompression must be considered.

### Surgical Options

There are many surgical treatment options for the adult patient with symptomatic isthmic SPL. Decompression, fusion, instrumentation, reduction, and the use of autogenous bone graft are all possible options. No choice should be made in a void. Each subselection of a procedure can impact on the others. Each surgical intervention must be customized to the needs of the individual patient.

### Decompression

The decision whether to perform a component of a procedure often is based on a continuum, determined by the surgeon's assessment of the risk-benefit ratio for that patient. The treating surgeon must assess what symptoms brought the patient to the need for surgical intervention. Reports of greater radicular leg pain favor the choice for decompression. The greater the presence and magnitude of objective findings from the physical examination (such as paresthesias, weakness, hamstring tightness, or bowel and bladder dysfunction), the greater is the support for the decision to formally decompress. The so-called Gill laminectomy, without a fusion, is currently not commonly performed as a stand-alone procedure. The traditional approach was direct surgical decompression followed with posterolateral arthrodesis and, more recently, with instrumentation. Indirect decompression by anterior structural interbody fusions with titanium cages had some recent popularity that has now waned.

### Fusion Alone

On the opposite end of the decompression and/or fusion continuum is the decision to perform only fusion. The younger the patient, the more likely that fusion alone is a treatment choice. One study reported on eight adults with grade III or IV isthmic SPL who had severe sciatica. An in situ arthrodesis without decompression was performed on these patients. At 5.5-year follow-up, all had excellent relief of both back pain and sciatica. Another report on 45 patients with adult isthmic SPL who were treated with fusion alone correlated fusion rate and clinical outcome. Results showed that clinical success correlated with fusion success.

### Decompression and Fusion

Decompression and fusion is the standard surgical treatment for adults with symptomatic low-grade isthmic SPL. An instrumented in situ posterolateral fusion is the most commonly used technique because of the favorable risk-benefit ratio to the patient; high successful clinical and radiographic results are achieved. Fusion is necessary when instability and low back pain exist and when performing primarily decompressive surgery in a patient whose main symptom is radiculopathy and who has SPL and degenerative disk disease. Decompression is particularly important whenever a focal neurologic deficit is present. One study reported on single-level posterolateral arthrodesis, with or without posterior decompression, for the treatment of isthmic SPL in adults. It was found that adding decompression to arthrodesis, with or without instrumentation, in those patients who did not have a serious neurologic deficit, did not appear to improve the results and could significantly increase the rate of pseudarthrosis with potential for unsatisfactory results. Another study reported on a similar group of patients who had lumbar decompression and fusion related to a principal diagnosis at 5-year follow-up. In a subset, 58 of the patients had grade I or grade II SPL (38 lytic and 20 degenerative). Most patients were treated with both decompression and an instrumented fusion. Of these patients, 46 of 58 (84%) reported a successful outcome and 47 of 58 (86%) reported that they would have the procedure again and would recommend it to others (Figure 3).

### The Fusion Technique

Anterior and posterior procedures, either in combination or alone and with or without instrumentation, are used to establish stability and obtain fusion. Posterior procedures may involve posterior lumbar interbody fusion (PLIF), transforaminal lumbar interbody fusion (TLIF), or posterolateral fusion.

In most patients, posterolateral fusion has fewer risks for complications and leads to reported pain relief and fusion rates of 70% to 100%. However, in patients with a significant collapse of the disk space, high-grade slip, or in those requiring extensive decompression, it may not be sufficient treatment. PLIF and TLIF both provide circumferential stabilization through a single posterior approach. In the TLIF technique, the access to the disk space is more lateral, thus requiring less retraction of the thecal sac and neural elements than the traditional PLIF technique. Recently, a radiographic analysis of TLIF for the treatment of 30 adults with isthmic SPL showed that translational slippage and disk height can be restored; however, the ability to induce lordosis at the slip level was found to be marginal. Because this study lacked data regarding radiographic fusion rates and clinical outcome and did not have a control group, it is impossible to evaluate the efficacy of the technique. The anterior lumbar interbody fusion (ALIF) procedure provides the most direct access to the disk space through which a more complete diskectomy and a greater restoration of disk space height can be achieved. ALIF provides increased surface area for the structural interbody device compared with the posterior approach, but it allows only indirect nerve root decompression compared with the nerve root release afforded by a posterior approach.

ALIF has potential complications of graft dislodgment, injury to great vessels, and injury to the sympathetic plexus that may result in retrograde ejaculation in males. Most spine surgeons will not perform stand-alone ALIF for patients undergoing first time surgery. If an ALIF procedure is desired, a posterior instrumented stabilization is advisable.

A combined approach has the advantages of achieving rigid fixation, direct posterior decompression if needed, restoration of height at the affected level, and high fusion rates. Circumferential fusion is the preferable choice for patients undergoing revision surgery following failed posterolateral fusion or for those with high-grade SPL.

## High-Grade SPL

The pathology of high-grade SPL typically involves lumbosacral kyphosis of L5 on S1 and hyperlordosis above L5 leading to pain, facet joint arthrosis, central and lateral recess stenosis, and nerve root stretching. Patients typically have a vertical pelvis, loss of trunk height, a flattened buttock, and a crouched stance with flexion of

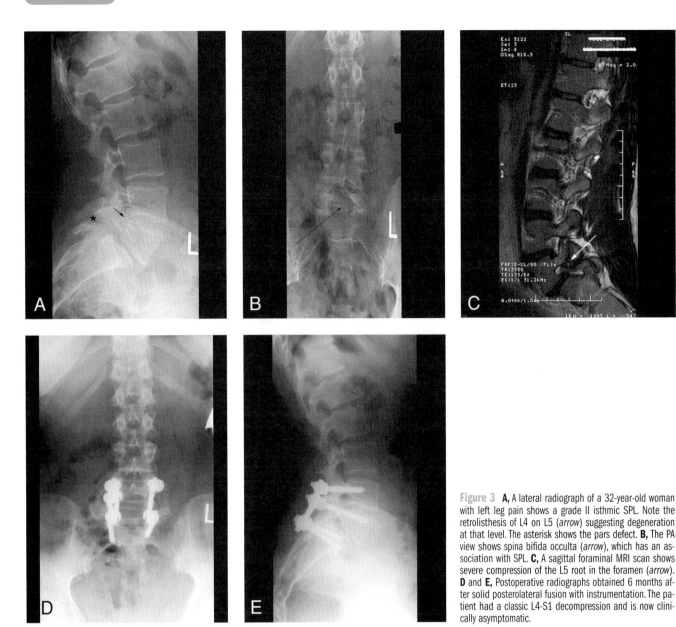

Figure 3  **A,** A lateral radiograph of a 32-year-old woman with left leg pain shows a grade II isthmic SPL. Note the retrolisthesis of L4 on L5 (*arrow*) suggesting degeneration at that level. The asterisk shows the pars defect. **B,** The PA view shows spina bifida occulta (*arrow*), which has an association with SPL. **C,** A sagittal foraminal MRI scan shows severe compression of the L5 root in the foramen (*arrow*). **D** and **E,** Postoperative radiographs obtained 6 months after solid posterolateral fusion with instrumentation. The patient had a classic L4-S1 decompression and is now clinically asymptomatic.

the hip and knees to maintain an upright posture. Hip and knee flexion contractures may help maintain sagittal balance. Reversing lumbosacral kyphosis is a more important goal of treatment than reducing translation because lumbosacral kyphosis has the most deleterious effect on the balance of the lumbar spine.

Reduction can be performed through a combined anterior and posterior approach or as a stand-alone posterior procedure. Although most authors agree that the symptomatic adult with a high-grade slip requires surgical stabilization and would benefit from partial lumbosacral kyphosis reduction, there is still debate regarding the surgical technique for obtaining these goals.

The literature concerning a high-grade slip is based on a small number of studies of adolescents and young adults; therefore, there are no clearly established indica-tions for treatment choices in adults. Partial reduction of a high-grade slip allows direct neural decompression, improves sagittal lumbosacral alignment, places the fusion mass in more compression, and achieves a better cosmetic appearance by spontaneous correction of the thoracic hypokyphosis and lumbar hyperlordosis. The main disadvantages of complete reduction are the high risk for neurologic injury and the need for an additional anterior procedure.

The fibula dowel procedure has been used for the surgical treatment of high-grade slips. Using a posterior stand-alone approach, a fibula dowel has been placed through the sacrum into the body of L5. Drilling techniques are used through the sacrum to then place the fibula dowel into the body of L5 both for fusion and sta-bilization.

## Outcomes Following Surgery

There are several documented predictors of outcomes following surgical treatment of patients with SPL. In one study, patients with workers' compensation or disability claims resulting from new onset low back pain in the setting of low-grade SPL were found to be less likely to have pain relief or improvement of function after fusion with or without decompression. Patients should typically anticipate an 80% to 85% incidence of self-rated good to excellent outcome with surgical decompression and fusion for SPL. The rate of fusion was significantly affected by the use of the combined anterior and posterior fusion approach and by rigid postoperative immobilization in a cast. A solid fusion was found to be the main parameter that improved patient outcomes and was more significant than the use of a specific fusion technique (various surgical fusion techniques were included in the studies).

## Annotated Bibliography

### Imaging Evaluation

Hanson DS, Bridwell KH, Rhee JM, et al: Correlation of pelvic incidence with low-and high-grade isthmic spondylolisthesis. *Spine* 2002;27:2026-2029.

This study used a radiographic analysis of 20 pediatric and 20 adult patients with isthmic SPL in an attempt to identify correlations between pelvic incidence and low-grade or high-grade slips. Pelvic incidence was significantly higher in the group with higher-grade slips than in the group with lower-grade slips ($P = 0.007$). Pelvic incidence may be a predictive factor for both high- and low-grade SPL and should be considered a factor in treatment as well as in the assessment of the risk of progression.

### Treatment

Ekman P, Moller H, Hedlund R: The long-term effect of posterolateral fusion in adult isthmic spondylolisthesis: A randomized controlled study. *Spine J* 2005;5:36-44.

This article presents the results of a long-term prospective randomized study to determine whether posterolateral fusion in 77 patients (37 noninstrumented and 40 with pedicle screws) with adult isthmic SPL resulted in an improved outcome compared with an exercise program for 34 patients. The average long-term follow-up was 9 years (range, 5 to 13 years). At long-term follow-up, pain and functional disability were significantly better than before treatment in both surgical groups regardless of whether instrumentation was used. In the exercise group, pain was significantly reduced, but functional disability did not decrease.

### High-Grade SPL

Bartolozzi P, Sandri A, Cassini M, et al: One-stage posterior decompression-stabilization and trans-sacral interbody fusion after partial reduction for severe L5-S1 spondylolisthesis. *Spine* 2003;28:1135-1141.

The authors present the results of a study of 15 adults with high-grade SPL who were treated with posterior decompression and partial reduction followed by circumferential stabilization performed in one stage combining pedicle fixation with transsacral titanium cage interbody fusion. Good radiologic and clinical outcomes were achieved using the technique.

Boachie-Adjei O, Do T, Rawlins BA: Partial lumbosacral kyphosis reduction, decompression, and posterior lumbosacral transfixation in high-grade isthmic spondylolisthesis: Clinical and radiographic results in six patients. *Spine* 2002;27:E161-E168.

This article presents the results of a study of six patients with grade IV and V isthmic SPL. In patients with high-grade SPL, the posterior approach is safe and effective in obtaining a solid arthrodesis, restoring sagittal balance, and improving function. The partial reduction of the slip angle rather than the percentage of slip is important in obtaining optimal results in patients with high-grade SPL.

Lauerman WC Jr: Adult isthmic spondylolisthesis, in Frymoyer JW (ed): *The Adult and Pediatric Spine*, ed 3. New York, NY, Lippincott Williams & Wilkins, 2004.

This chapter provides in-depth coverage of adult isthmic SPL and an extensive bibliography.

### Outcomes Following Surgery

L'Heureux EA Jr, Perra JH, Pinto MR, et al: Functional outcome analysis including preoperative and postoperative SF-36 for surgically treated adult isthmic spondylolisthesis. *Spine* 2003;28:1269-1274.

A prospective and retrospective outcome analysis of 31 adult patients with isthmic SPL who had arthrodesis is presented. Significant functional improvement was seen following surgical arthrodesis of the painful segment ($P = 0.001$). The improved patient outcomes in this study were dependent on the achievement of solid fusion in the adult isthmic patient rather than on the specific fusion technique used. Various surgical fusion techniques were included in the study.

## Classic Bibliography

Buttermann GR, Garvey TA, Hunt AF, et al: Lumbar fusion results related to diagnosis. *Spine* 1998;23:116-127.

Carragee EJ: Single-level posterolateral arthrodesis, with or without posterior decompression, for the treatment of isthmic spondylolisthesis in adults: A prospective, randomized study. *J Bone Joint Surg Am* 1997;79:1175-1180.

Farfan HF, Osteria V, Lamy C: The mechanical etiology of spondylolysis and spondylolisthesis. *Clin Orthop Relat Res* 1976;117:40-55.

Floman Y: Progression of lumbosacral isthmic spondylolisthesis in adults. *Spine* 2000;25:342-347.

Fredrickson BE, Baker D, McHolick WJ, et al: The natural history of spondylolysis and spondylolisthesis. *J Bone Joint Surg Am* 1984;66:699-707.

Grobler LJ, Novotny JE, Wilder DG, et al: L4-5 isthmic spondylolisthesis: A biomechanical analysis comparing stability in L4-5 and L5-S1 isthmic spondylolisthesis. *Spine* 1994;19:222-227.

Kim SS, Denis F, Lonstein JE, et al: Factors affecting fusion rate in adult spondylolisthesis. *Spine* 1990;15:979-984.

Legaye J, Duval-Beaupere G, Hecquet J, et al: Pelvic incidence: A fundamental pelvic parameter for three-dimensional regulation of spinal sagittal curves. *Eur Spine J* 1998;7:99-103.

Marchetti PC, Bartolozzi P: Classification of spondylolisthesis as a guideline for treatment, in Bridwell K, DeWald R (eds): *The Textbook of Spinal Surgery*, ed 2. Philadelphia, PA, Lippincott-Raven, 1997, pp 1211-1254.

Meyerding HW: Spondylolisthesis. *J Bone Joint Surg* 1931;13:39-48.

Moller H, Hedlund R: Surgery versus conservative management in adult isthmic spondylolisthesis: A prospective randomized study: Part 1. *Spine* 2000;25:1711-1715.

Peek RD, Wiltse LL, Reynolds JB, et al: In situ arthrodesis without decompression for Grade-III or IV isthmic spondylolisthesis in adults who have severe sciatica. *J Bone Joint Surg Am* 1989;71:62-68.

Schoenecker PL, Cole HO, Herring JA, et al: Cauda equina syndrome after in situ arthrodesis for severe spondylolisthesis at the lumbosacral junction. *J Bone Joint Surg Am* 1990;72:369-377.

Transfeldt EE, Dendrinos GK, Bradford DS: Paresis of proximal lumbar roots after reduction of L5-S1 spondylolisthesis. *Spine* 1989;14:884-887.

Vaccaro AR, Ring D, Scuderi G, et al: Predictors of outcome in patients with chronic back pain and low-grade spondylolisthesis. *Spine* 1997;22:2030-2034.

Wiltse LL, Newman PH, Macnab I: Classification of spondylolisis and spondylolisthesis. *Clin Orthop Relat Res* 1976;117:23-29.

# Chapter 34

# Discogenic Back Pain

Rob D. Dickerman, DO, PhD

Jack E. Zigler, MD

## Introduction

Although widely recognized, discogenic back pain remains a disease that at times is difficult to unequivocally diagnose. The multiplicity of etiologies responsible for low back pain and the mixed bag of symptoms associated with it are two of the main reasons why the diagnosis of this disease entity remains controversial. The accurate workup of a patient with discogenic back pain requires a logical stepwise progression through the diagnostic process. This chapter discusses the pathophysiology, diagnostic algorithm, and treatment options for patients with presumed lumbar discogenic pain.

## Incidence

Low back pain is an essentially ubiquitous phenomenon. The annual incidence of back pain is projected to be 5% per year, with an associated prevalence of 60% to 90%. Only medical visits to primary care physicians for upper respiratory infections outnumber those for back pain. Back pain has been reported in more than 50% of people engaged in light physical activity and in more than 60% of those performing heavy labor; it is the most common reason for limited activity in individuals younger than 45 years. Back pain is the third most common cause for disability in patients 45 to 65 years of age. The potential for return to work following disabling back pain correlates directly with the length of time away from work; patients who are away from work more than 6 months have a 50% rate of returning to work, those away more than 1 year have a 25% rate, and those away more than 2 years have less than a 5% chance of returning to work. Despite the aforementioned statistics, only 7% of patients have low back pain that persists more than 2 weeks, and only 1% require long-term treatment. Less than 1% of patients with low back pain ultimately require surgery. Surprisingly, approximately 85% of patients who report back pain cannot be given a pathoanatomic diagnosis. This common medical condition results in an estimated medical cost of $30 to $50 billion annually in the United States.

## Etiologies

Obesity is a known risk factor for numerous diseases, including degenerative disk disease (DDD). The mechanical load on the disk space increases in obese patients and may lead to premature degeneration through several progressive pathophysiologic processes. Smoking also has been associated with an increased incidence of both DDD and disk herniation. Nicotine has been shown to limit oxygenation to tissues leading to accelerated degeneration by inhibiting the daily restorative properties at the cellular level within the intervertebral disk. This process may cause hyalinization and necrosis of the nucleus pulposus. Nicotine inhibits osteoblastic function, bone metabolism, and cellular exchange within the disk space, leading to disk degeneration. One study showed a 32% increased rate of pseudarthrosis in smokers who underwent a two-level lumbar spinal fusion. The overall success rate for surgical and nonsurgical treatments of low back pain has been shown to be significantly lower in patients who smoke.

Genetics has always been considered an important factor in DDD. MRI investigations have found a 74% heritability of DDD in twins. Molecular biology studies have attempted to identify some of the genetic loci for DDD and have found that genes encoding polypeptide chains for collagen IX, which is produced in the disk space, may play an important role in the development of DDD.

Other studies have attempted to determine the role of heavy labor or weight-bearing exercise (such as bodybuilding or weight lifting) as possible risk factors for DDD. One study addressed the question of whether long-term compressive loading on the intervertebral disk predisposes an individual to disk degeneration; no increased incidence of DDD was found. However, alterations in the intradiscal distribution of proteoglycan and collagen were identified. A recent 5-year prospective study for the assessment of DDD in 41 asymptomatic patients that examined physical job characteristics, participation in sports activities, and various morphologic changes from baseline MRI found that nonparticipation

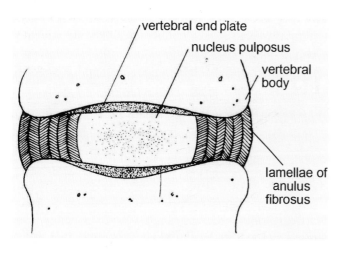

Figure 1  A coronal illustration of the anulus fibrosus, disk, and vertebral end plates.

in sports activities, night-shift work, and a previously injured disk on initial MRI were significant risk factors. Despite the logical conclusion that athletes who use their lumbar spines to perform weight-bearing exercises over a long period will increase their risk for DDD, studies have determined that exercise alone is not a factor in DDD and may be protective in preventing DDD.

The incidence of DDD in athletes is likely to be increased not from the mechanical loading associated with weight lifting (which in most instances is a static exercise in which the joints are loaded in a fixed physiologic manner, limiting the risk for injury), but rather the athlete is at increased risk during sports competitions when the spine is loaded in a nonphysiologic manner and in a mechanically more vulnerable position. A 2004 study analyzed a large cohort of identical twins and determined that multiple social factors and work experience had little influence on the development of DDD. It was concluded that genetics played the most important role, accounting for up to 74% of the variance in the adult population.

## Anatomy and Physiology

Intervertebral disks are amphiarthrodial joints, having no synovial membrane. The disks contribute approximately 30% of the height to the lumbar spine. The disk consists of cartilaginous end plates, the anulus fibrosus, and nucleus pulposus (Figure 1). Hyaline cartilage connects the end plates to the vertebral body. The lamina cribrosa, a calcified layer within the cartilaginous end plate, has a porous surface that permits diffusion of nutrients and plays an important role in the pathophysiologic cascade of DDD.

The anulus fibrosus has collagen fibrils in concentric laminae. Each lamina has parallel fibrils obliquely oriented to the end plates; the direction of the fibrils alternate between laminae, analogous to the belts of a radial

tire. Sharpey's fibers, which are predominately type I collagen, are the outer most layer of fibrils attaching directly to the epiphyses of the vertebral body. The inner layer of fibrils is type II collagen, which are also attached to the cartilaginous end plates.

The nucleus pulposus is an embryonic remnant of the notochord and contains type II collagen. The nucleus makes up approximately 40% of the intervertebral disk volume and is located in the posterior central portion of the disk. The nucleus is more gelatinous than the anulus fibrosus and thus permits the nucleus to perform as a hydrostatic load-bearing structure, contained by the less elastic anulus fibrosus.

The intervertebral disk is made up of collagen, proteoglycans, connective tissue, and water. Type I and type II collagen are the major forms of collagen in the intervertebral disk. The molecular structure of collagen leads to its enormous tensile strength, which provides the secure attachment to the vertebral bodies and assists in the ability to withstand daily shearing forces.

Proteoglycans are macromolecules that are synthesized by the disk and diffuse throughout the disk. These proteoglycans are composed of a hyaluronic acid core with an attached glycosaminoglycan (chondroitin or keratan sulfate), which yields a negatively charged group. For the disk to remain electrically neutral, sodium, potassium and calcium cations are concentrated within the disk space, causing an osmotic gradient for water to enter the disk. This gradient is opposed by the hydrostatic pressure applied to the disk as a result of axial loading in the upright posture, which compresses the disk. The constant reciprocal forces allow water to constantly flow in and out of the disk.

Innervation to the disk is provided by the sinovertebral nerve, which arises from the primary ventral ramus and gray ramus communicans. The sinovertebral nerve supplies innervation to the annular fibers, the posterior portion of the intervertebral disk, the dura, and the posterior longitudinal ligament. The anterior portion of disk and anterior longitudinal ligament are innervated by branches from the gray ramus. The primary dorsal ramus supplies innervation to the facet joints, interspinous ligaments, and paraspinal musculature (Figure 2).

## Pathophysiology

Disk degeneration begins in early childhood as vessels within the disk space slowly regress. The etiology of this vascular regression is thought to be secondary to the change from quadripedal to bipedal locomotion in childhood, thus loading the disk in the upright posture, increasing intradiskal pressure, and causing involution of the blood supply. By 4 years of age, chondrocytes are dependent on diffusion alone for metabolic supply. The porous surface in the lamina cribrosa decreases with age. With increasing age the metabolic strain to the in-

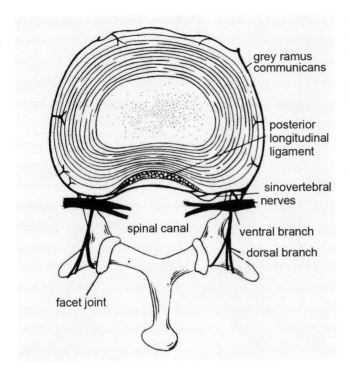

Figure 2  An axial illustration of the spinal canal, posterior longitudinal ligament, and neural innervation.

tervertebral disk increases because of decreasing blood supply and decreasing diffusion. These metabolic changes lead to alterations in the overall charge in the disk space, decreasing the net inward flow of fluid and decreasing water content from 90% to 70%; this change ultimately leads to loss of disk height and expandability. Once the degenerative cascade begins, spinal mechanics are altered, and abnormal loading on adjacent levels may result in ligamentous strain causing pain in linked structures (facet joints, sacroiliac joints, and adjacent disk levels).

An MRI study examined 50 patients with chronic low back pain under axial loading and found that 20% of patients showed no changes, whereas 80% had accentuation of their lumbar disease (stenosis, disk protrusion, or listhesis). The authors concluded that axial loading may not cause the initial disease, but a prior injury may lead to a degenerative cascade allowing axial loading that negatively affects the intervertebral disk.

The DDD process also has an inflammatory component that can often be seen on the anterior disk space on MRI scans or intraoperatively during anterior lumbar spine surgical exposures. This inflammatory component may explain why intradiskal corticosteroid injections and/or oral anti-inflammatory medications have occasionally been reported as beneficial in some patients. A comparative study on inflammatory mediators in disk tissue that were removed from patients undergoing routine diskectomy for a herniated disk compared with disk tissue from patients undergoing total diskectomy and fusion for discogenic pain, found significantly higher levels of proinflammatory mediators (interleukin-6 and interleukin-8) in the group with discogenic pain. These findings suggest an inflammatory role within the nucleus pulposus as one of the possible components of the degenerative cascade.

## Neural Innervation

Studies of the anulus fibrosus and end plate have shown that end-plate innervation is concentrated centrally and a similar innervation pattern exists in the anulus fibrosus. Immunohistochemistry studies have defined neuron populations within the dorsal root ganglion that affect the lumbar disks and alter their activity during physiologic and pathologic states. It is well known that the dorsal root ganglion plays an essential role in innervation at the disk level. This fact is further supported by recent studies that have attempted to clarify the possible invasive, nonsurgical treatment options for patients with discogenic pain. A recent study of patients with diagnosed discogenic concordant pain during diskography were given an intradiskal injection of corticosteroid compared with normal saline to demonstrate the possible beneficial anti-inflammatory effects of the corticosteroid. No significant difference was found. In another study, a significant benefit was found with the use of spinal steroid injections in a select pool of patients with definitive inflammatory changes at the end plate and positive diskography. A retrospective study on outcomes of intradiskal electrothermal therapy for patients with discogenic pain found that 50% were dissatisfied with their outcome. These results were likely secondary to the inability of intradiskal electrothermal therapy to remove the pain generator. A recent study implementing percutaneous radiofrequency thermocoagulation of the dorsal ramus communicans demonstrated significant benefit in patients with discogenic pain; these results are probably related to denervation of the end plates and anulus fibrosus.

## Clinical Presentation

The patient history and physical examination are extremely important in determining the etiology of the patient's back pain. Several historic and physical examination findings can help direct the physician to the appropriate diagnostic test or treatment option. The patient with DDD typically presents with daily pain that is worse with weight bearing (standing and sitting) for prolonged periods. Patients may occasionally report subjective radicular irritability, but it is not the primary reported condition. Back pain is generally daily and persistent, whereas radicular symptoms are usually transient.

## Physical Examination

Results of the physical examination may be nearly normal; therefore, a diagnosis by exclusion will be required. Patients will typically have a normal neurologic examination with intact motor, reflex, and sensory findings. Patients generally deny radiculopathy, and although the gait may be guarded or antalgic, it is generally normal. A small percentage of patients may have transient radicular symptoms if their DDD has caused a loss of disk height and subsequent foraminal stenosis with weight bearing. A common physical finding is mild transverse low back tenderness that may not be associated with true paraspinous muscle spasm. The most typical subjective symptom is a deep aching pain that is relieved with bed rest and aggravated by weight bearing. The classic question to ask the patient is: "Can you sit through a movie without fidgeting?" It is a consistent finding that patients with true discogenic pain cannot sit with comfort for even short periods. Examination findings regarding straight-leg raising and other radicular tests are normal. The range of motion in the lumbar spine may be limited in flexion and extension because of aggravation caused by loading of the intervertebral disks.

The surgeon should always question the patient about common red flags such as pain at night, unexplained systemic symptoms, fever, and weight loss. The patient should also be examined for tenderness with percussion over the lower ribs (suggestive of renal stones) or palpable masses in the abdomen (suggestive of tumors or abdominal aortic aneurysm), which also may cause back pain. The patient should have a complete history and physical examination because back pain may be associated with other disease processes.

Psychological evaluation is required for patients with any history of mental illness, including depression, or in those who have a long history of narcotic use. Patients should routinely undergo a mental health evaluation by a psychologist before diskography and surgery to ensure that the patient has reasonable expectations regarding postoperative management and rehabilitation. Numerous studies have demonstrated the relationship between preoperative psychological status and outcomes.

## Diagnostic Evaluation

Plain radiography is the best initial study. The normal degenerative processes in the foramen and intervertebral space such as disk space narrowing with osteophyte formation or sclerosis at the end plates should be evaluated (Figure 3). With severe narrowing, there may be the characteristic "vacuum phenomenon" or gas formation within the disk space. Other possible sources for back pain should be excluded by analyzing the plain radiograph for any suspicious areas, absent pedicles, compression fractures, and other possible degenerative, oncologic, or infectious changes.

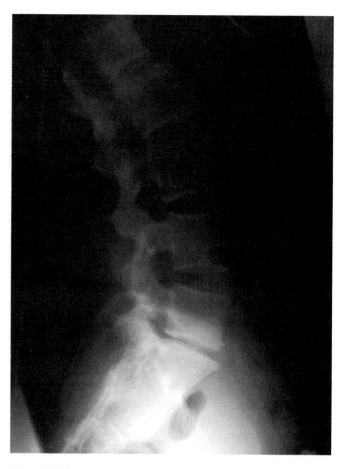

Figure 3 Plain lateral radiograph of the lumbar spine showing loss of disk space height at L5-S1.

MRI has become one of the most commonly used tools in the diagnostic workup of a patient with back pain. Sagittal T2-weighted MRI yields the best initial view of the dessicated disk space. In the typical degenerated disk segment, the T2-weighted MRI scan will show decreased signal intensity (dark) within the affected disk space and increased signal intensity in the normally hydrated disk spaces (Figure 4). The appearance of degeneration of the vertebral bodies adjacent to the affected disk level on MRI scans has been described by Modic as three different signal intensity patterns. A type I pattern is defined as decreased signal intensity on T1-weighted MRI scans and increased signal on T2-weighted MRI scans. Type II changes have increased signal intensity on T1-weighted MRI scans and are isointense on T2-weighted MRI scans. Type II changes have been examined pathologically to reveal end-plate disruption with increased lipid content in the marrow, which are believed to represent an inflammatory response to the painful disk. Type III changes have decreased signal intensity on T1- and T2-weighted MRI scans, which corresponds pathologically to significant loss of marrow and end-plate sclerosis. The clinical significance of these findings of DDD on T2-weighted

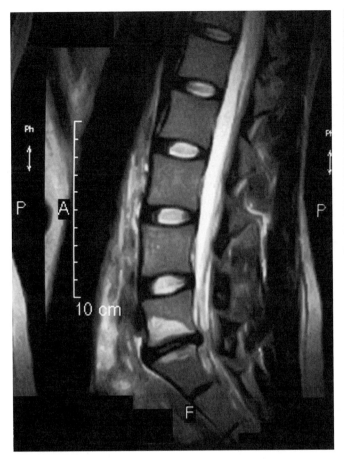

Figure 4 Sagittal T2-weighted MRI scan showing loss of L5-S1 disk space height, decreased disk space signal intensity, and vertebral body Modic changes.

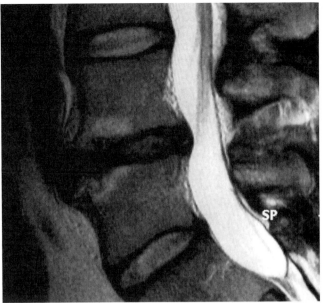

Figure 5 Sagittal T2-weighted MRI scan showing loss of L4-L5 disk space height, decreased disk space signal intensity, and inflammatory changes along the ventral disk space, with small ventral disk protrusion.

MRI scans and Modic changes at the end plate is yet to be elucidated. One study found no significant correlation between an MRI scan that is positive for vertebral end-plate changes and concordant pain with provocative diskography. The results of additional biomechanical studies have led to the conclusion that there is no direct correlation between degenerative changes to the disk and the adjacent vertebral bodies. Thus, Modic changes may demonstrate degenerative changes within the body and/or disk but have failed to clinically correlate with findings on provocative diskography.

Few studies have found definitive correlations between various pathologic findings within the disk space on MRI scans and positive findings on diskography. One study examined over 100 patients and found that radial tears on MRI scans are not reliable predictors of a positive pain response on diskography, whereas high-intensity zones on T2-weighted images are reliable predictors for painful diskography. Severe disk degeneration with loss of height is also a good predictor, and although posterior annular tears are likely pain generators, they are not good predictors of discogenic pain. Loss of disk height and abnormal intensity on T2-weighted MRI have remained consistent in the litera-

ture as good predictors of disk disruption (Figure 4). In a few patients, obvious ventral disk space inflammatory changes can be found intraoperatively as well as on preoperative MRI scans (Figure 5). An interesting study attempted to differentiate disk protrusions, disk bulges, and disks with normal height but with abnormal signal intensity to diskography. In this study, it was found that 100% of disk protrusions and 80% of disk bulges were associated with annular disruption and a high rate of positive diskography. Surprisingly, there was no significant difference between disk protrusions, disk bulges, and disks with normal contour but abnormal signal with respect to the degree of disk degeneration, extent of disk disruptions, or presence of discogenic pain. It was concluded that the loss of disk height or abnormal signal intensity is highly predictive of symptomatic annular tears. However, disk protrusions or bulges seen on MRI scans do not represent disks with significantly different internal architecture based on diskography and are no more suggestive of symptomatic tears than disks showing normal contour but loss of height or abnormal signal intensity.

Diskography is strictly a confirmatory examination and not a stand-alone test. The test itself is a provocative examination requiring a cooperative effort from the radiologist and the patient. The test is beneficial to confirm the definitive DDD level, but should always include at least one (or preferably two) normal levels. The rationale for including the normal levels is to exclude the adjacent levels as a source for pain and to further confirm that the disk with abnormal internal architecture is the concordantly painful disk. Should two levels be suspected as a source of pain, the surgeon can request that the radiologist test the first level with a lidocaine diskogram, which blocks the level from possible hydraulic stimulation from the diskogram at the adjacent level, thus further isolating the level in question. Diskography is an invasive examination. Although the reported risk of diskitis is less than 1%, it is a risk that requires discussion with the patient. The situation is complicated when a patient has postdiskography diskitis in a previously normal disk space. These studies should be conducted by experienced physicians because the rate of complications is inversely proportional to the experience of the physician.

All surgeons do not find clinical significance in diskography results, and reports exist concerning the validity of diskography. The specificity of diskography has been questioned since its introduction as a diagnostic tool. In a study using the diskographic examination of patients without low back pain, including 10 control patients without pain or a psychiatric history, 10 patients with chronic neck pain, and 6 patients with somatization disorder, a positive pain response was found in only 10% of the pain-free group, 40% of the group with chronic cervical pain, and 83% of those with a somatization disorder. More recent studies have concluded that the specificity of diskography when used by an experienced physician is nearly 90% in healthy patients without psychiatric illness, and only 20% in patients with chronic pain and psychiatric risk factors. Experienced diskographers have suggested techniques to improve accuracy that include always having "control levels" (normal disks) on MRI, knowing the patient's psychiatric risk factors, and not providing audible clues as to the onset or conclusion of the injection or the levels being injected. It must be reiterated that diskography is a dynamic provocative test; therefore, the patient's pain response during the injection is the most important component of the examination. It is not a passive imaging study.

An example of a diagnostic radiographic algorithm for a patient who has back pain without radiculopathy and for whom conservative therapy has failed would include the following steps: (1) Obtaining plain radiographs (AP, flexion, and extension); classic findings include loss of disk height and a degenerative disk space. (2) The use of MRI, with findings that include T2-weighted "dark disk" at the suspicious level, loss of height, and possible high-intensity zones within the disk space coinciding with annular tears. (3) The use of facet blocks if there is suspicion of facet arthropathy or facetogenic pain is contributing to the symptom complex. (4) The use of diskography (should include two normal levels). A provocative examination requiring patient-radiologist interaction should be done, with a final report on the subjective findings and pressures generated within the disk spaces. A psychological evaluation should be done before diskography if clinically indicated. (5) Psychological screening should be considered for most patients being considered for surgical treatment of disabling axial pain.

## Nonsurgical Treatment

Most patients with low back pain will recover without surgery. All patients (excluding those with a neurologic emergency) should be managed initially with nonsurgical treatment options that are supported by the literature. Exercise programs are strongly encouraged for a variety of reasons. Strengthening the abdominal wall muscle groups and lumbar musculature (core muscle groups) have demonstrated a definitive benefit in relieving low back pain of discogenic origin. The physiologic basis of strengthening the muscles to unload the joints is well-supported in the literature. Patients who improve their strength through a trial of physical therapy but still require surgery tend to better tolerate surgery and recover faster. Several studies have analyzed the use of bracing for patients with discogenic pain and found limited benefit, with some studies showing aggravation of the pain. Bracing has typically been used for the diagnosis and treatment of mechanical back pain and has limited use in treating discogenic pain. Special orthoses that unweight the lumbar spine by pneumatic pistons may have diagnostic as well as therapeutic use.

Chiropractic manipulation has been shown to be more beneficial in the treatment of acute low back pain than placebo and has been recommended for acute treatment of low back pain in the neurologically intact patient. Data suggest, however, that chiropractic treatment of chronic back pain (pain lasting > 12 weeks) is of no greater benefit than the use of a placebo.

Traction is often used in the cervical spine for temporary relief of DDD and mild cervical disk herniations. It is more difficult to use traction in the lumbar spine, and the literature supporting its use for patients with discogenic pain is limited.

Several pharmacologic studies have demonstrated the benefits of nonsteroidal anti-inflammatory medications in the treatment of discogenic back pain, thus adding support to the hypothesis of an inflammatory factor in the disease process. Each patient undergoing treatment of acute or chronic low back pain should be initially prescribed a trial of nonsteroidal anti-inflammatory medications along with other nonsurgical treatments such as physical therapy or chiropractic manipulation that have evidence-based benefits.

Outcome studies have examined the efficacy of nonsurgical treatment on patients with debilitating discogenic back pain and positive diskography. Over a 3-year follow-up period, 68% of patients improved, 8% remained unchanged, and 24% worsened. Factors influencing positive outcome included a shorter history of back pain, and older age at the onset of the pain. The main predictive factor of a poor outcome was psychiatric disease, which was present in 67% of the patients who worsened.

## Surgical Treatment

In the past decade, the most common surgical treatment for discogenic lower back pain has been disk excision with interbody fusion performed either anteriorly, posteriorly, or circumferentially, depending on the surgeon's experience and the clinical findings. The main goal in the treatment of discogenic pain is removal of the pain source (for example, diskectomy and fusion of the diseased segment, thus prohibiting motion. The success rate of posterolateral fusion surgery for relieving discogenic pain without removal of the disk has been fairly poor. Several studies on posterolateral fusion for DDD have shown high fusion rates (upward of 90%), but with only a 60% clinically beneficial result. Posterolateral fusions have a definite role in the elimination of mechanical back pain because of their ability to reduce motion; however, laboratory investigations have demonstrated that posterolateral fusions can reduce motion within a spinal segment by 40%, whereas anterior lumbar interbody fusions reduce motion in the segment by 80% and eliminate all motion within the disk space. One study reported on five patients who had persistent discogenic pain after posterolateral fusions and subsequently had positive diskography leading to an anterior interbody fusion, which provided pain relief in all patients. An essential factor in the treatment of discogenic pain is the complete removal of the pain generator. Anterior and posterior interbody fusions have reports of fusion rates of more than 90%, but posterolateral interbody fusions show a lower success rate in discogenic pain relief (ranging from 60% to 90%). Anterior interbody fusions have been found to be consistently superior for pain relief.

An additional negative factor associated with the posterior approach to the lumbar spine is violation of the posterior paraspinal musculature. Muscle damage by dissection and retraction can be a significant source for early postoperative pain. If significant muscle ischemia occurs during surgery, muscles may scar postoperatively and lead to postfusion syndrome. In addition to the muscles, the posterior approach exposes the dura and neural elements to possible damage and risks for postoperative perineural fibrosis.

The anterior approach for interbody fusion avoids the risk of posterior paraspinal muscle damage, reduces risks for direct injury or scarring to the neural elements, and permits a total diskectomy with restoration of disk space height. Achieving a total diskectomy and implanting an appropriate interbody device allows restoration of the disk space height and indirectly increases the vol-

ume of neural foramen. When placing interbody devices for fusion, the anterior approach allows for higher fusion rates by obeying the essential rules of successful fusion: allowing a better graft-bone contact area than can be achieved using the posterior approach; easier compression of the graft-bone interfaces, which are more evenly distributed; and obtaining segmental stabilization, which can be achieved by numerous routes, either through posterior percutaneous pedicle screws, an anterior plate, or in certain instances, by stand-alone anterior lumbar interbody fusion with the addition of recombinant human bone morphogenetic protein (rhBMP).

Traditional stand-alone anterior lumbar interbody fusions with autogenous iliac crest grafts have been reported to have a high rate of pseudarthrosis, graft extrusions, and subsidence. Subsidence is governed by the cross-sectional area of contact and the relationship of the strut to the margin of the end plate. Three essential factors for the prevention of subsidence should be addressed intraoperatively. (1) It is necessary to appropriately size the bone graft to the vertebral body. A good fit will permit Wolff's law (bone placed under appropriate stress is remodeled, whereas bone not under stress is resorbed) to operate. (2) The contact surface area between the graft and the vertebral body should be maximized. The extent of subsidence is inversely proportional to the surface area of contact between the graft and the vertebral body. (3) The character and quality of contact surfaces should be optimized. The cartilaginous end plate must be removed to expose the cortical bone surface and allow access to bleeding subchondral bone. Increased fusion rates without increased subsidence have been shown by burring off the end plate to allow the cortical vertebral body to fuse. With the introduction of rhBMP, fusion rates have increased substantially. A comparative study analyzing rhBMP with allograft versus iliac crest autograft found similar clinical outcomes; however, the rhBMP group had significantly higher fusion rates (95% versus 89%). In addition, surgical time and blood loss were both lower in the rhBMP group.

Circumferential surgery has gained acceptance as a means of addressing graft subsidence noted in stand-alone anterior lumbar interbody fusion procedures. Circumferential spinal fusions have resulted in fusion rates of 90% to 100%, with more than 80% of patients having clinical improvement. Patient selection and the need for circumferential fusions should be clearly identified before surgery. In a recent Swedish study that examined three surgical techniques for patients with chronic low back pain and analyzed both fusion rates and long-term outcome scales, patients were grouped into those treated with posterior lateral fusion alone, posterior lateral fusion with pedicle screws, and posterior lateral fusion with pedicle screws and interbody graft. The fusion rates were highest in the circumferential fusion group

(91%), followed by the group with posterior lateral fusion with pedicle screws (87%). The lowest fusion rates were in the group treated with posterior lateral fusion alone (72%). In terms of surgical time, postoperative hospital days, blood loss, and complications, all were highest in the circumferential group and lowest in the onlay fusion group without instrumentation. The patient outcomes did not differ among the three groups, leading the authors to conclude that, in this study population, there was no disadvantage to using the least surgically demanding and lowest cost procedure (uninstrumented onlay posterolateral fusion) despite the low fusion rate.

Circumferential surgery can and should be used in appropriate clinical situations for either an additional posterior tension band or to prevent graft subsidence in a high-risk patient. When circumferential surgery is necessary, the anterior lumbar interbody fusion can be performed first, followed by a posterior Wiltse muscle-splitting approach with placement of percutaneous pedicle screws unilaterally or bilaterally. The tissue-sparing retroperitoneal anterior approach to the lumbar spine and the minimally invasive percutaneous pedicle screw insertion posterolaterally allow mobilization of the patient on the afternoon of surgery, and result in relatively short hospital stays of 1 to 3 days.

Artificial disk replacement is now approved for use in the treatment of discogenic pain. Arthroplasty may become more commonly recommended than fusion for the surgical treatment of discogenic pain for several reasons. Arthroplasty involves less intraoperative blood loss, shorter surgical times, and shorter hospitalization than fusion surgery. Patients who receive disk replacements are rehabilitated faster and return to work sooner than patients treated with fusion. It is believed that motion preservation may decrease the incidence of adjacent level disease (transition syndrome) that occurs with fusion surgery. Large prospectively randomized cohorts of patients have been identified for the US Food and Drug Administration Investigational Device Exemption studies of several lumbar artificial disks. These cohorts will be followed over time to more scientifically evaluate the long-term outcomes of arthroplasty versus fusion.

## Summary

Discogenic back pain has a multifactorial pathogenesis, with substantial published research showing a degenerative cascade occurring after an initial insult, probably beginning at the molecular level. Discogenic back pain, often referred to as internal disk derangement, DDD, mechanical back pain, or segmental instability all require the appropriate diagnostic algorithm and eventual treatment based on that algorithm. The importance of following the diagnostic algorithm to identify the pa-

tients with true discogenic pain as opposed to an internal pain generator cannot be overemphasized. With appropriate patient selection, the treatment of discogenic back pain can be successful.

## Annotated Bibliography

### General

Saal JS: General principles of diagnostic testing as related to painful lumbar spine disorders: A critical appraisal of current diagnostic techniques. *Spine* 2002;27: 2538-2545.

The available information and data on invasive diagnostic tests to evaluate chronic low back pain were reviewed. Inherent limiations in the accuracy of the diagnostic tests were found.

### Incidence

Devereaux MW: Neck and low back pain. *Med Clin North Am* 2003;87:643-662.

This article discusses cases that represent a sample of conditions that affect the spine and paraspinous structures.

Frymoyer JW, Wiesel SW: *The Adult and Pediatric Spine*, ed 3. Philadelphia, PA, Lippincott Williams & Wilkins, 2004, pp 899-905.

A discussion of low back pain and other conditions that affect the spine is presented.

Pauza KJ, Howell S, Dreyfuss P, et al: A randomized, placebo controlled trial of intradiscal electrothermal therapy for the treatment of discogenic low back pain. *Spine J* 2004;4:27-35.

The efficacy of intradiskal electrothermal therapy is compared with that of placebo treatment.

Pawl RP: Pain treatment and spine surgery. *Surg Neurol* 2004;61:320-322.

This article discusses methods of pain treatment during spine surgery.

### Etiologies

Ala-kokko L: Genetic risk factors for lumbar disc disease. *Ann Med* 2002;34:42-47.

The hypothesis that genetic factors play a role in lumbar disk disease is strengthened by the identification of two collagen IX alleles associated with sciatica and lumbar disk herniation.

Battie MC, Videman T, Parent E: Lumbar disc degeneration: Epidemiology and genetic influences. *Spine* 2004; 29:2679-2690.

A review of the scientific literature discussing the prevalence of lumbar disk degeneration and genetic influences is presented.

Chung SA, Khan SN, Diwan AD: The molecular basis of intervertebral disk degeneration. *Orthop Clin North Am* 2003;34:209-219.

Molecular evidence involved in intervertebral disk degeneration is still being investigated. The involvement of cytokines and other inflammatory mediators in this process is controversial.

Elfering A, Semmer N, Birkhofer D, Zanetti M, Hodler J, Boos N: Risk factors for lumbar disc degeneration: A 5-year prospective MRI study in asymptomatic individuals. *Spine* 2002;27:125-134.

Risk factors involved in the development of lumbar disk degeneration are studied.

Hartvigsen J, Christensen K, Frederiksen H, Pedersen HC: Genetic and environmental contributions to back pain in old age: A study 2108 Danish twins aged 70 and older. *Spine* 2004;29:897-901.

A discussion of the relative contribution of genetic and environmental factors to back pain in old age is presented.

Iwashashi M, Matsuzaki H, Tokuhashi Y, et al: Mechanism of intervertebral disc degeneration caused by nicotine in rabbitts to explicate intervertebral disc disorders caused by smoking. *Spine* 2002;27:1396-1401.

The effects of nicotine on the vascular buds of rabbits were studied to determine the mechanism of nicotine-induced vertebral disk degeneration.

Manenti G, Liccardo G, Sergiacomi G, et al: Axial loading MRI of the lumbar spine. *In Vivo* 2003;17:413-420.

According to this study, axial loading MRI provides important information for specific nonsurgical or surgical treatment of low back pain.

Sobajima S, Kim JS, Gilbertson LG, Kang JD: Gene therapy for degenerative disc disease. *Gene Ther* 2004; 11:390-401.

The ability of gene therapy to affect biologic processes in the degenerated intervertebral disk is reviewed.

### Anatomy and Physiology

Aoki Y, Takahashi Y, Ohtori S, Moriya H, Takahashi K: Distribution and immunocytochemical characterization of dorsal root ganglion neurons innervating the lumbar intervertebral disc in rats: A review. *Life Sci* 2004;74: 2627-2642.

This study suggests that nerve growth factor is involved in the generation of discogenic low back pain.

Burke JG, Watson RW, Conhyea D, et al: Human nucleus pulposis can respond to a pro-inflammatory stimulus. *Spine* 2003;28:2685-2693.

This study set out to confirm that human intervertebral disk is responsive to a proinflammaotry stimulus and to identify the specific mediators involved.

Butterman GR: The effect of spinal steroid injections for degenerative disc disease. *Spine J* 2004;4:495-505.

Spinal steroid injections are beneficial to some patients with advanced degenerative disk disease and chronic low back pain.

Norcross JP, Lester GE, Weinhold P, Dahners LE: An in vivo model of degenerative disk disease. *J Orthop Res* 2003;21:183-188.

An animal model of degenerative disk disease using the intervertebral disks in the tails of rats was studied in order to determine possible treatments.

### Neural Innervation

Davis TT, Delamarter RD, Sra P, Goldstein TB: The IDET procedure for chronic discogenic low back pain. *Spine* 2004;29:752-756.

The purpose of this study was to assess the functional status, symptoms, and treatments of patients treated with intradiskal electrothermal therapy.

Fagan A, Moore R, Vernon R, et al: The innnervation of the intervertebral disc: A quantitative analysis. *Spine* 2003;28:2570-2576.

This article presents the first quantitative analysis of the innervation of the lumbar intervertebral disk.

Khot A, Bowditch M, Powell J, et al: The use of intradiscal steroid therapy for lumbar spinal discogenic pain: A randomized controlled trial. *Spine* 2004;29:833-836.

This study determined whether intradiskal steroid injection influenced clinical outcome after 1 year in patients with chronic discogenic low back pain.

Oh WS, Shim JC: A randomized controlled trial of radiofrequency denervation of the ramus communicans nerve for chronic discogenic low back pain. *Clin J Pain* 2004;20(1):55-60.

The efficacy of percutaneous radiofrequency thermocoagulation of the ramus communicans nerve in patients with chronic discogenic low back pain was studied.

### Diagnostic Evaluation

Anderson MW: Lumbar discography: An update. *Semin Roentgenol* 2004;39:52-67.

Diskography remains the only test that can provide physiologic information about the role an intervertebral disk plays in a patient's symptom complex. Assessment of the patient's pain response is the most important component of the procedure.

Carragee EJ, Alamin TF: Discography: A review. *Spine J* 2001;1:364-372.

Current uses of discography, technique involved, and recent studies on its validity are discussed.

Ferguson SJ, Steffen T: Biomechanics of the aging spine. *Eur Spine J* 2003;12(suppl 2):S97-S103.

Advancing age is not the only factor in spine degeneration. Additional study is needed for full understanding of the aging spine's unique biomechanical function.

Willems PC, Jacobs W, Duinkerke ES, De Kleuver M: Lumbar discography: Should we use prophylactic antibiotics?: A study of 435 consecutive discograms and a systematic review of the literature. *J Spinal Disord Tech* 2004;17:243-247.

According to this study, not enough evidence was found that prophylactic antibiotics can prevent diskitis.

### Nonsurgical Treatment

Borman P, Keskin D, Bodur H: The efficacy of lumbar traction in the management of patients with low back pain. *Rheumatol Int* 2003;23:82-86.

The efficacy of lumbar traction in the treatment of patients with low back pain was studied. No specific effect of traction on standard physical therapy was observed.

Jellema P, van Tulder MW, van Poppel MN, Nachemson AL, Bouter LM: Lumbar supports for prevention and treatment of low back pain: A systematic review within the framework of the Cochrane Back Review Group. *Spine* 2001;26:377-386.

The effects of lumbar supports for the prevention and treatment of low back pain were assessed.

### Surgical Treatment

Burkus JK, Gornet MF, Dickman CA, et al: Anterior lumbar interbody fusion using rhBMP-2 with tapered interbody cages. *J Spinal Disord Tech* 2002;15(5):337-349.

Lumbar fusion with rhBMP-2 and tapered interbody fusion cages can lead to solid union and eliminate the need to harvest iliac crest bone graft.

Fritzell P, Hagg O, Wessberg P, et al: Chronic low back pain and fusion: A comparison of three surgical techniques: A prospective multicenter randomized study from the Swedish lumbar spine study group. *Spine* 2002; 27:1131-1141.

Three commonly used surgical techniques to achieve lumbar fusion were compared according to their ability to reduce pain and decrease disability in patients with chronic low back pain.

McAfee PC, Fedder IL, Saiedy S, Shucosky EM, Cunningham BW: SB Charite disc replacement: Report of 60 prospective randomized cases in a US center. *J Spinal Disord Tech* 2003;16:424-433.

This study is the first to show improvement of functional outcome measures in a prospective randomized design, with disk arthroplasty treating mechanical back pain and achieving comparable results to lumbar fusion-interbody fusion cage and bone morphogenetic protein or interbody autograft and pedicle screw instrumentation.

Park P, Garton HJ, Gala VC, et al: Adjacent segment disease after lumbar or lumbosacral fusion: Review of the literature. *Spine* 2004;29:1938-1944.

The etiology, incidence, and risk factors associated with adjacent segment disease are discussed.

Zigler JE: Lumbar spine arthroplasty using the Prodisc II. *Spine J* 2004;4:260S-267S.

Results from this study suggest that total disk arthoplasty may be an option to lumbar fusion for surgical treatment of disabling mechanical low back pain secondary to lumbar disk disease.

## Classic Bibliography

Annunen S, Paassilta P, Lohiniva J, et al: An allele of COL9A2 associated with intervertebral disc disease. *Science* 1999;285:409-412.

Blumenthal SL, Baker J, Dossett A, et al: The role of anterior lumbar fusion for internal disc disruption. *Spine* 1988;13:566-569.

Boden SD, Davis DO, Dina TS, et al: Abnormal magnetic resonance scans of the lumbar spine in asymptomatic subjects: A prospective investigation. *J Bone Joint Surg Am* 1990;72(3):403-408.

Brown WC, Orme TJ, Richardson HD: The rate of pseudoarthrosis in patients who are smokers and patients who are nonsmokers: A comparison study. *Spine* 1986;11:942-943.

Burdorf A: Exposure assessment of risk factors for disorders of the back in occupational epidemiology. *Scand J Work Environ Health* 1992;18(1):1-9.

Carragee EJ, Paragioudakis SJ, Khurana S: Lumbar high-intensity zone and discography in subjects without low back pain. *Spine* 2000;25:2987-2992.

Carragee EJ, Tanner CM, Khurana S, et al: The rates of false-positive lumbar discography in select patients without low back symptoms. *Spine* 2000;25:1373-1380.

Cloward RB: Posterior lumbar interbody fusion updated. *Clin Orthop Relat Res* 1985;193:16-19.

Cloward RB: Lesions of the intervertebral discs and their treatment by interbody fusion methods. *Clin Orthop Relat Res* 1963;27:51-77.

Cypress BK: Characteristics of physician visits for back symptoms: A national perspective. *Am J Public Health* 1983;73:389-395.

de Vernejoul MC, Bielakoff J, Herve M, et al: Evidence for defective osteoblastic function: A role for alcohol and tobacco consumption in osteoporosis in middle-aged men. *Clin Orthop Relat Res* 1983;179:107-115.

Dennis S, Watkins R, Landaker S, et al: Comparison of disc space heights after anterior lumbar interbody fusion. *Spine* 1989;14(8):876-878.

Deyo RA, Bass JE: Lifestyle and low back pain: The influence of smoking and obesity. *Spine* 1989;14:501-506.

Dickerman RD, Pertusi R, Smith GH: The upper range of lumbar spine bone mineral density? *Int J Sports Med* 2000;21:469-470.

Emery SE, Bolesta MJ, Banks MA, et al: Robinson anterior cervical fusion: Comparison of the standard and modified techniques. *Spine* 1994;19:660-664.

Frymoyer JW, Pope MH, Clements JH, Wilder DG, Macpherson B, Ashikaga T: Risk factors in low-back pain: An epidemilogical survey. *J Bone Joint Surg Am* 1983;65:213-218.

Glassman SD, Anagnost SC, Parker A, et al: The effect of cigarette smoking and smoking cessation on spinal fusion. *Spine* 2000;25:2608-2615.

Guiot BH, Fessler RG: Molecular biology of degeneration disc disease. *Neurosurgery* 2000;47:1034-1040.

Hanley EN Jr, Shapiro DE: The development of low back pain after excision of lumbar disc. *J Bone Joint Surg Am* 1989;71(5):719-721.

Hollo I, Gergely I, Boross M: Smoking results in calcitonin resistance. *JAMA* 1977;237(23):2470.

Hopper JL, Seeman E: The bone density of female twins discordant for tobacco use. *N Engl J Med* 1994;330:387-392.

Horton WC, Daftari TK: Which disc as visualized by magnetic resonance imaging is actually a source of pain? *Spine* 1992;17:S164-S171.

Hutton WC, Ganey TM, Elmer WA, et al: Does long-term compressive loading on the intervertebral disc cause degeneration? *Spine* 2000;25:2993-3004.

Ito M, Incorvaia KM, Yu SF, Fredrickson BE, Yuan HA, Rosenbaum AE: Predictive signs of discogenic lumbar pain on magnetic resonance imaging with discography correlation. *Spine* 1998;23(11):1252-1258.

Jackson RK, Boston DA, Edge AJ: Lateral mass fusion: A prospective study of a consecutive series with long-term follow-up. *Spine* 1985;10:828-832.

# Chapter 35

# Adult Scoliosis

D. Greg Anderson, MD

Todd Albert, MD

Chadi Tannoury, MD

## Introduction

Adult scoliosis may be defined as a lateral curvature of the spine of greater than 10° in a skeletally mature patient. Several types of adult curves are commonly seen. Prior idiopathic scoliosis and de novo degenerative scoliosis resulting in asymmetric degeneration of the disks are the most common types of adult curvatures. Less common causes of adult spinal curvatures include congenital deformities that present in adulthood, paralytic curves, posttraumatic deformities, iatrogenic deformities, and curves related to severe osteoporosis. Adults with idiopathic scoliosis are much more likely than children or adolescents to report that pain is the primary reason for seeking medical treatment. Adult deformities have the potential for curve progression and the development of sagittal or coronal imbalance that can lead to substantial disability.

The clinical presentation of adult patients is somewhat different than for adolescents. Older adults often have increasing back pain or progressive trunk imbalance. Some patients also may report neurogenic symptoms resulting from stenosis in the lumbar region of the spine. Another challenge in treating adults with a spinal deformity is the presence of complications from prior surgeries such as iatrogenic flat back deformity, pseudarthrosis, postlaminectomy scoliosis, or adjacent spinal segment disease. The surgical treatment of patients with adult spinal deformity presents a greater challenge than the treatment of adolescent patients with idiopathic scoliosis. One long-term follow-up study estimated the risks related to the surgical treatment of an adult deformity to be as high as a 5% risk of death, 6% risk of a major neurologic deficit, 20% risk of significant correction loss, 10% risk of a deep infection, and a 40% risk of a major medical complication. Although surgical techniques, anesthesia, spinal instrumentation, and medical support have improved in the years since that study, adult patients with a spinal deformity continue to present a great challenge to the reconstructive spinal surgeon.

The surgical treatment of spinal deformities has advanced in recent years because of improvements in spinal instrumentation (beginning with the Harrington rod), and because of the contributions of many researchers who have played a significant role in the development of current understanding of spinal deformities and in the development of newer instrumentation systems. Harrington rods provided a major improvement over body casting and functioned reasonably well in patients with simple thoracic curves; however, the use of these rods often led to sagittal imbalance or pseudarthrosis when applied to the lumbar spine. Early nonsegmental instrumentation systems required long-term postoperative immobilization with a body cast. With the advent of posterior segmental fixation systems and contoured rods, the incidence of complications decreased and earlier mobility for patients was possible.

Equal in importance to the developments in spinal instrumentation are the improvements in techniques of anesthesia, spinal cord monitoring, perioperative medical support, and postoperative rehabilitation. These improvements have increased the safety of surgical procedures and have made surgical treatment possible for patients with more severe deformities and for older patients with disabling spinal deformities. Adults with spinal deformities are currently treated most efficiently by a team of specialists, including the reconstructive spinal surgeon, anesthesiologist, intensive care specialist, internist, physical therapist, nutritionist, rehabilitation physician, and orthotist.

## Prevalence of Adult Deformities

One study suggested that about 2.9% of adults displayed evidence of a structural spinal curve. Curve progression in adults with scoliosis was noted in 69 of 102 patients (68%) with idiopathic scoliosis over an average 40.5-year follow-up period. Curves of less than 30° tended to be stable, whereas curves of 50° to 75° were at high risk for progression. Other risk factors for progression included involvement of the lumbar spine, significant trunk imbalance, and curvature of the lumbosacral junction.

The degree of disability in adults is highly variable. Although some authors have suggested that patients

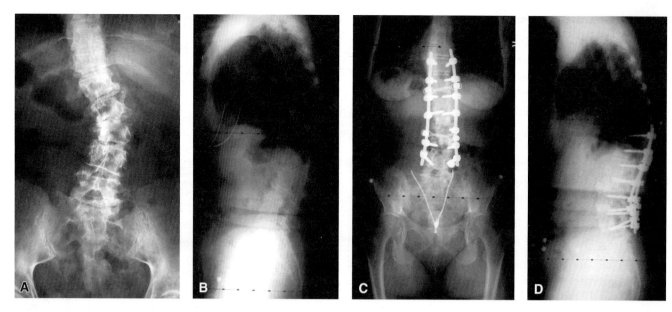

Figure 1  PA (**A** and **C**) and lateral (**B** and **D**) weight-bearing long radiographs of a woman with a major spinal deformity before (**A** and **B**) and after (**C** and **D**) surgical correction.

with idiopathic scoliosis rarely have disabling pain as adults, other authors have concluded that severe adult spinal deformity has a great potential for causing disabling symptoms, which may be seen in approximately 25% of adult scoliosis patients. The prevalence of pain in patients with adult spinal deformity has been reported to be about 60%, a rate similar to that found in age-matched control groups. However, those with lumbar curves and curves greater than 45° have a high incidence and more severe level of pain. Other risk factors for disability from spinal deformity include thoracolumbar kyphosis, rotatory translations (subluxations) of the lumbar spine, and degenerative changes at the lumbosacral joint. Decreased gait velocities were found in patients with lumbar deformities compared with an age-matched control group.

Using data from the Medical Outcomes Study 36-Item Short Form (SF-36), the psychosocial well being of adult scoliosis patients was reported to be lower in seven of eight categories compared with results from the general population of the United States. The most important predictor of poor scores in the social functioning, emotion, well being, and overall general health categories was the presence of a lumbar deformity with poor lordosis. Poor scores on the Scoliosis Research Society questionnaire also have been shown to correlate with poor scores on the SF-36 for adult patients with spinal deformities.

## Patient Evaluation
### Patient History
A patient history should be obtained to ascertain a thorough understanding of the location and severity of any symptoms and the effectiveness of any prior treatments

of the condition. The effects of the spinal condition on the patient's quality of life (such as the performance of the activities of daily living, occupational activities, social functioning, participation in recreational activities, and sexual functioning) should be assessed. In some patients, the cosmetic effects of the deformity may be a major concern and should be discussed. Evidence of progression of the deformity should be sought. Clinical clues of progression include changes in trunk height, fit of clothing, or body shape (such as an altered waistline). When possible, prior radiographs should be reviewed to objectively measure the degree of progression of the deformity.

Pain should be quantified descriptively and can be measured using the visual analog scale. The location of the pain should be determined, which can provide a clue to the underlying cause of the pain. For example, pain at the apex of the curve is often attributed to the deformity, whereas distal leg pain is more likely the result of spinal stenosis. Patients with severe deformities may present with pain from rib impingement on the iliac crest or from intercostal neuralgia caused by rib cage deformity.

### Physical Examination
The physical examination should include details of the spinal deformity, musculoskeletal system, and neurologic status. The three-dimensional aspects of the spine should be defined, including the magnitude and location of the spinal curves, the sagittal plane (for example, the degree of kyphosis or lordosis relative to normal), the magnitude of any rib hump and/or lumbar prominence, the coronal and sagittal balance (such as decompensation), the flexibility of the deformity, and the presence of any pelvic obliquity. The musculoskeletal examination should focus on the large lower extremity joints

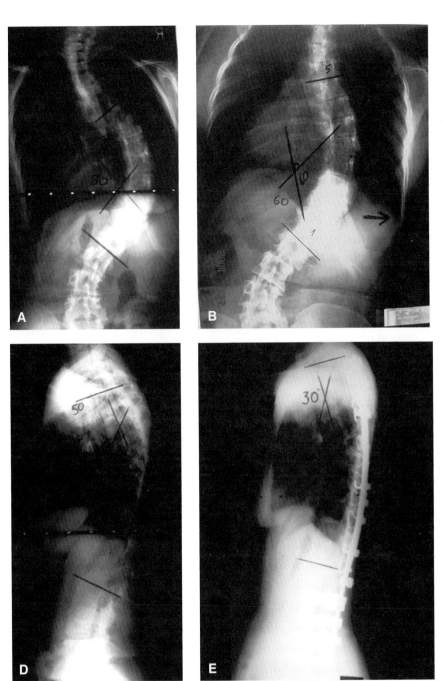

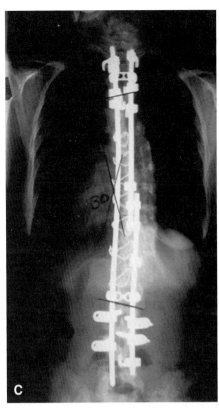

Figure 2  PA (**A**, **B**, and **C**) and lateral (**D** and **E**) long radiographs of a woman with adult scoliosis. Note the curve correction after surgical instrumentation (**C** and **E**).

(hip and knee) and leg lengths to rule out any contractures that may affect the ability of the patient to function following correction of the deformity. In patients with severe deformities, abutment of the rib cage against the iliac wing may be observed.

A thorough neurologic examination should be performed to determine any evidence of spinal cord or nerve root dysfunction. Any evidence of upper motor neuron dysfunction should be further examined to ensure that the progressive curve does not have a neurologic basis. Examples of significant findings may include a left thoracic curve, clawing of the toes, hyperreflexia, asymmetry of the abdominal reflexes, or difficulties in balance and/or gait.

When considering surgery, it is important to take into account the body habitus and nutritional status of the patient because these factors can significantly impact the risks of surgery. Prior to elective surgery, it is imperative to correct any nutritional deficiencies that will increase the risk of perioperative healing problems or may contribute to complications such as infection.

## Imaging Studies

Weight-bearing, 36-inch PA and lateral plain radiographs generally are the first radiographic studies obtained (Figure1, *A* and *B*, and Figure 2, *A*, *B*, and *D*). These studies are imperative for measuring the magnitude of the spinal curves and determining and measuring spinal balance in the sagittal and coronal planes. To accurately measure sagittal balance on the lateral radiograph, the patient's knees must be straight when the radiograph is taken. Additional plain radiographs or coned views should be obtained to focus on specific areas of degenerative changes or congenital abnormalities. Stagnara views (oblique views that image the rotated spine in a true lateral projection) may be helpful in patients with severely rotated deformities to more accurately assess kyphosis or sagittal plane deformity.

Curve flexibility can be estimated using lateral bending views; however, these views may not accurately predict the degree of correction obtained at surgery. Flexion and extension views may be used to assess sagittal plane flexibility and expose subtle degrees of spondylolisthesis. Some surgeons find push-prone or traction views useful in assessing curve flexibility. Lateral views obtained with a bolster under the apex of a kyphosis can be used to estimate the flexibility of a sagittal plane kyphosis.

In patients with neurologic symptoms, an MRI scan or CT/myelogram is obtained to determine the presence of spinal cord or nerve root compression. In patients with severe spinal deformities, CT/myelography is often more useful than MRI, which can be difficult to interpret unless specifically aligned with the vertebral end plates over each region of the deformed spine. MRI scans, however, are advantageous in allowing visualization of the status (such as hydration) of the lumbar disks, which can be useful when choosing distal fusion levels. Diskography has also been used to define pain generators at the lower end of the proposed fusion, which can be included in the fusion construct. In patients at higher risk for spinal dysraphism (such as those with left thoracic curves, congenital abnormalities, or hairy patches), MRI of the entire neuraxis is recommended to rule out spinal cord abnormalities that could place the patient at higher risk for neurologic injury during surgical correction.

## Nonsurgical Treatment

Nonsurgical treatment is appropriate for most adult patients with a spinal deformity. A variety of therapies are useful, and the treatment approach is similar to that used for degenerative spinal pain. Treatment options include exercise, the administration of nonsteroidal anti-inflammatory drugs, and activity modification. Patient education is an important part of any nonsurgical treatment program. The patient should be aware that the goal of nonsurgical treatment is to decrease spinal symptoms and to improve function, stamina, and quality of life. Nonsurgical treatment will not diminish the magnitude of the spinal deformity. Low-impact aerobics, cycling, and swimming are particularly useful in the older

adult with painful spinal deformities. Osteoporosis may worsen a deformity or contribute to pain and thus should be detected and treated. Rigid bracing is generally poorly tolerated by adult patients. However, in selected patients a well-molded brace or a soft brace may be useful to diminish spinal symptoms.

## Surgical Treatment

The primary indications for surgery in adult patients with spinal deformity include (1) a progressive deformity, (2) the development of poor spinal balance causing functional difficulties, (3) a large deformity threatening cardiopulmonary compromise, or (4) the presence of neurologic manifestations. Other factors that may be considered in choosing surgery may include the presence of persistent pain (that fails to respond to nonsurgical measures) or an unsatisfactory cosmetic appearance. Rarely, if ever, should the issue of pain or cosmesis be the sole reason for surgery.

The progression of the deformity is the most common reason for surgery in the young adult patient or in an elderly patient with a curve progression caused by severe degenerative disease. Neurologic deficits secondary to idiopathic scoliosis alone are rare; however, patients may develop degenerative changes in the lumbar region leading to stenosis with neurogenic leg symptoms. When severe compression of the neural elements is present on preoperative imaging studies, a formal decompression is required in addition to the procedure to correct the deformity. Although not the primary reason for surgery, cosmesis is a common concern. Studies have shown that cosmetic improvements can play a major role in the patient's desire for surgical correction and ultimately influence the perceived benefit of the surgery and the patient's postoperative perception of health status. A careful discussion of the patient's goals is needed before surgery. Patients with poor spinal balance will often have a combination of pain, poor functional capacity, and concerns with a poor cosmetic appearance because of the spinal deformity. Successful surgery may be able to address all of these issues. The surgeon should discuss the risks and benefits of the surgery and should provide a realistic assessment of the expected outcome.

Achieving proper sagittal and coronal balance are the most important goals of surgery. After surgery, the patient should be able to stand erect with the trunk positioned directly over the pelvis in both the coronal and sagittal planes (Figure 1, *C* and *D*, and Figure 2, *C* and *E*). This alignment reduces the energy expenditure of upright posture, reduces the pain and fatigue that are often present in the patient with poor sagittal balance, and also may reduce the risks of adjacent segment degeneration following surgery.

## Surgical Techniques

A variety of surgical options have been developed to treat adult spinal deformities. Available approaches include anterior only, posterior only, and combined anterior and posterior surgery. The primary factors to consider when determining the approach for a particular patient include the location, magnitude, and flexibility of the deformity and the medical status of the patient. In adults with spinal deformity, thoracoscopic and minimally invasive techniques, although used at some centers, have not yet been widely validated.

## Thoracic Deformities

In adults, isolated thoracic deformities are less likely to require surgery because these deformities, unless large, are generally stable. Occasionally, a patient will present with an isolated large thoracic curve (> 75°) that may benefit from surgery. Large thoracic curves, especially those with significant rotational deformities, have the potential to cause restrictive lung disease and may eventually lead to right-sided heart failure. Posterior instrumented fusion is used most often to correct an isolated thoracic curve in an adult patient. Rigid deformities may also benefit from anterior release. Patients with severe hypokyphosis (thoracic lordosis) also benefit from anterior release. When kyphoscoliosis is present, multiple Smith-Petersen type osteotomies in conjunction with a posterior column shortening procedure can be used to correct coronal plane deformity.

Although hooks have traditionally been used as anchors in the thoracic spine, pedicle screws have become popular, particularly at the upper end of the deformity where hook dislodgement can cause complications. With proper training, these implants can be safely used and have reduced the rate of anchor dislodgement and lamina fracture compared with hook constructs. In patients with severe kyphoscoliosis, the addition of a sublaminar wire at the ends of the construct appears to further reduce the odds of screw pullout. To prevent the development of a junctional kyphosis adjacent to the upper end of the fusion, the construct should be initiated high in the thoracic spine at the T2 or T3 level, and the ligaments between the upper fused level and the supraadjacent level should be spared.

## Thoracolumbar and Lumbar Curves

In the lumbar spine, symptoms of pain, sagittal plane imbalance, and occasionally neurogenic claudication are common reasons for surgery. The choice of a surgical approach depends on the flexibility of the curve and the location of the spinal segments believed to be causing the pain. For isolated lumbar curves, the fusion begins proximally at the T10 or T11 level, crossing the thoracolumbar junction to avoid junctional kyphosis. The lower end of the fusion is usually stopped at the stable vertebrae or the L5 level unless there is a fractional curve at the L5-S1 level of more than 15°, or there is painful degeneration or a spondylolisthesis at the lumbosacral disk. Thoracolumbar curves generally require fusion from the upper thoracic region to the lower stable vertebrae (often L4 or L5). It is particularly important to avoid stopping a fusion near the apex of a spinal kyphosis, such as in the midthoracic area.

In adults, there is a low threshold for using a combined anterior and posterior approach when treating structural lumbar curves because, in part, poor fusion results have been achieved with multilevel posterolateral fusions, especially those extending to the sacrum. In addition, older adults with spinal deformities tend to have rigid curves, which benefit from circumferential release. Structural interbody grafting at the lower L1-2 levels is helpful to prevent loss of fixation in the postoperative period at the lower end of a long construct. Anterior release with morcellized grafting improves the flexibility of the curve and enhances the degree of correction achieved. Lumbar pedicle screws have largely supplanted hooks and wire constructs for adult lumbar curves. Pedicle screws improve the degree of segmental purchase, allow derotation of the deformity, and provide secure fixation even in the absence of the posterior elements (such as laminectomy).

An anterior-only approach is occasionally useful for the young adult (with good bone quality) with a relatively flexible thoracolumbar curve. Anterior instrumentation can often save one or two fused levels by stopping at the neutral vertebrae (often L3) rather than extending to the L4 or L5 level (stable vertebrae). Single- or dual-rod instrumentation in conjunction with structural interbody support is used to achieve a rigid construct and prevent kyphosis of the lumbar region. An important technical tip is to place a structural graft in the anterior disk spaces of the lumbar region to prevent the kyphosing tendency of anterior rod instrumentation. Anterior stand-alone deformity correction should be avoided in the older patient with osteopenic bone in whom curve rigidity and poor bone quality increase the risk of construct failure.

## Fusion to the Sacrum

Fusion to the sacrum versus stopping fusion at the L5 level remains controversial for curves in many adults. In younger patients, fusion to the L4 or L5 segment results in a high rate of subsequent painful disk degeneration below the fusion during the subsequent decade. However, this complication has not been shown conclusively to affect older patients. Fusion to the sacrum markedly increases the rate of pseudarthrosis and other complications. Long fusions to the sacrum also lead to sacroiliac joint degeneration, although in most patients the symptoms are not severe. Rarely, an older, osteopenic patient will develop an insufficiency fracture of the sacrum and pelvis, which can be debilitating following a long fusion to the sacrum. For these reasons, some surgeons advocate stopping the construct short of the sacrum whenever possible. Certain situations mandate extending the fusion to the sacrum, including symptomatic spondylolisthesis, severe disk disease at the L5-S1 level, or a fractional curve (oblique take-off) of the lumbosacral joint of greater than 15°. Less common deformities requiring fusion to the sacrum include a fixed sagittal imbalance with kyphosis of the lumbosacral junction.

When performing fusion to the sacrum in the patient with adult spinal deformity, anterior column structural grafting and adequate fixation are mandatory. Of the various fixation procedures, the Galveston technique of placing iliac bolts or rods into the iliac regions is the most biomechanically sound. The Galveston technique has been shown to maintain lordosis and enhance the rate of successful fusion in these difficult deformities. In addition to the Galveston technique, other methods of obtaining secure sacropelvic fixation include placing four sacral screws (S1 and S2), Jackson intrasacral rods, or using a transsacral bar.

Anterior column structural grafting may theoretically be achieved using anterior lumbar interbody fusion, posterior lumbar interbody fusion, or transforaminal lumbar interbody fusion; however, in most patients anterior lumbar interbody fusion provides the best structural reconstruction of the disk space and also allows release and grafting of disk spaces above the L5-S1 level. The use of an anterior release and interbody grafting of multiple levels in patients with challenging deformities is generally more efficient and associated with less blood loss than multilevel transforaminal lumbar interbody fusion.

## Intraoperative Management

Adult scoliosis surgery is often associated with significant blood loss and substantial fluid resuscitation. It is critical to work with a team of anesthesiologists that has experience in managing major spinal procedures and is vigilant in replacing and correcting the various coagulation deficits that may arise. A discussion of the surgical plan should be undertaken prior to starting surgery and appropriate blood products should be available. Fluid overload with crystalloids should be avoided because it can increase the risk of postoperative pulmonary complications and intensive care requirements.

Packed red blood cells should be administered early in the surgical procedure, by the time that the estimated blood loss reaches 800 to 1,000 mL, because delay is often associated with hypotension and coagulopathy. The use of cell salvage systems for this type of surgery is routine, but may increase the degree of coagulopathy because of the loss of clotting factors and because of

the anticoagulants used in these systems. It is imperative to replace coagulation factors using fresh-frozen plasma, calcium, and occasionally platelets in patients who lose large quantities of blood (generally in the 1,500 to 2,000 mL range).

Spinal cord monitoring has become routine for most surgeons during the correction of major deformities at the spinal cord level. Although monitoring with somatosensory-evoked potentials has been used successfully by many centers, other modalities such as transcranial electrical motor-evoked potentials appear to be more sensitive for detecting early spinal cord insult and therefore may increase the time in which the surgeon can take corrective action in the situation of an evolving neurologic deficit. Stimulated electromyograms are useful to ensure that transpedicular implants have not breached the confines of the bony pedicle. With modern neurophysiologic monitoring, many surgeons no longer routinely use an interoperative wake-up test unless there has been an aberration in intraoperative spinal cord monitoring.

## Postoperative Care

The neurologic status of the patient should be determined as soon as possible after surgery. Patients generally stay in a monitored setting for the first 24 to 48 hours following major reconstructive spinal surgery. To minimize the risks of prolonged recumbency, early mobilization on the first postoperative day is attempted. Bracing may be used depending on the fixation technique used and preference of the surgeon.

The length of the hospital stay depends on the age and medical status of the patient. After hospitalization, inpatient rehabilitation that focuses on achieving functional gains and improving the ability to perform activities of daily living is often recommended. Return to work varies depending on the individual situation and type of work. Full, unrestricted activities are generally allowed when the fusion appears to be solid and the patient is well rehabilitated.

## Surgical Outcome

One study reviewed the outcome of 110 adult patients with scoliosis at an average follow-up of 12.5 years after surgical reconstruction of a spinal deformity. Although most patients had some back pain, most did not feel disabled. Seventy-five percent of the patients participated in recreational activities and only 11% were receiving disability compensation. Eighty-five patients said that they would undergo the same surgical procedure again for the same degree of benefit.

Another study compared 197 adult patients with scoliosis with 180 control patients who did not have a spinal deformity. Prior to surgery, the patients with scoliosis had significantly more pain, especially when a structural lumbar curve was present. At a mean follow-up of 5 years after surgery, 83% of the patients with scoliosis reported significant pain relief.

In one study, a 36% incidence of adjacent segment degeneration was found in 83 patients treated surgically for a spinal deformity. No differences were observed on the basis of the surgical approach (posterior versus anterior/posterior); however, more severe adjacent segment degeneration was noted in patients with poor postoperative sagittal plane balance.

## Summary

Adult deformities include a diverse spectrum of conditions and present a significant challenge to the spinal reconstructive surgeon. Fortunately, the methods used to treat these patients have improved in recent years. With careful evaluation and meticulous technique, it is possible to obtain rewarding results in most patients. Reconstructive surgery in this patient population requires an experienced team to manage the many issues involved and to provide an optimal outcome for patients. The importance of achieving proper sagittal plane balance cannot be overemphasized. Other techniques that improve the rate of surgical success in adults with spinal deformity include the use of structural interbody support at the lower end of long constructs, and the achievement of stable, segmental spinal instrumentation along with meticulous grafting and fusion techniques. When treating an adult with a spinal deformity, the surgeon should strive for good balance and symptom relief rather than for a high degree of deformity correction.

## Annotated Bibliography

### General

Engsberg JR, Bridwell KH, Reitenbach AK, et al: Preoperative gait comparisons between adults undergoing long spinal deformity fusion surgery (thoracic to L4, L5, or sacrum) and controls. *Spine* 2001;26:2020-2028.

The results of this study supported subjective observations regarding the preoperative gait of patients with spinal deformity and presented results difficult to observe in a clinical setting. The techniques used appear useful in providing objective information regarding the gait abilities of patients with spinal deformity prior to long fusion surgery.

### Prevalence of Adult Deformities

Berven S, Deviren V, Demir-Deviren S, Hu SS, Bradford DS: Studies in the modified scoliosis research society outcomes instrument in adults: Validation, reliability, and discriminatory capacity. *Spine* 2003;28:2164-2169.

This study supports the use of the Scoliosis Research Society Outcomes Instrument as a valid tool for assessing the impact of adult spinal deformity on the general health status of adults. This fact was determined using a correlation analysis with comparable domains of the SF-36. However, poor corre-

lation between radiographic parameters of outcome and patient self-assessment of health status was found.

Schwab FJ, Smith VA, Biserni M, Gamez L, Farcy JP, Pagala M: Adult scoliosis: A quantitative radiographic and clinical analysis. *Spine* 2002;27:387-392.

Assessment techniques for the adult scoliosis population are discussed.

### Patient Evaluation

Deviren V, Berven S, Kleinstueck F, Antinnes J, Smith JA, Hu SS: Predictors of flexibility and pain patterns in thoracolumbar and lumbar idiopathic scoliosis. *Spine* 2002;27:2346-2349.

This retrospective study showed that curve magnitude and patient age are the main predictors of structural flexibility. Every 10° increase in curve magnitude over 40° results in a 10% decrease in flexibility; every 10-year increase in age decreases flexibility of the structural curve by 5% and the lumbosacral fractional curve by 10%. These associations offer useful information for estimating how surgical options for deformity correction may change over time.

### Nonsurgical Treatment

Schwab F, Dubey A, Pagala M, Gamez L, Farcy JP: Adult scoliosis: A health assessment analysis by SF-36. *Spine* 2003;28:602-606.

An analysis comparing the SF-36 scores to benchmark data for patients with comorbid conditions such as back pain and hypertension clearly demonstrates the severe impact of adult scoliosis on patients' perceptions of their health status.

### Surgical Treatment

Bridwell KH: Selection of instrumentation and fusion levels for scoliosis: Where to start and where to stop: Invited submission from the Joint Section Meeting on Disorders of the Spine and Peripheral Nerves, March 2004. *J Neurosurg Spine* 2004;1:1-8.

This article discussed fusion levels for the adult scoliosis patient.

Bridwell KH, Edwards CC II, Lenke LG: The pros and cons to saving the L5-S1 motion segment in a long scoliosis fusion construct. *Spine* 2003;28:S234-S242.

A paucity of data is available on whether to save the L5-S1 motions segment in a long scoliosis fusion construct. Further study on this issue is required. Complications of stopping fusion at L5 include fixation at that segment and subsequent breakdown at L5-S1. The problems with stopping fusion at the sacrum include additional surgical requirements and an increased potential for pseudarthrosis.

Islam NC, Wood KB, Transfeldt EE, et al: Extension of fusions to the pelvis in idiopathic scoliosis. *Spine* 2001; 26:166-173.

The analytical process in fusing to the sacrum is discussed in this article.

### Intraoperative Management
Nahtomi-Shick O, Kostuik JP, Winters BD, Breder CD, Sieber AN, Sieber FE: Does intraoperative fluid management in spine surgery predict intensive care unit length of stay? *J Clin Anesth* 2001;13:208-212.

The perioperative management of the adult scoliosis patient is discussed in this article.

### Surgical Outcome
Kumar MN, Baklanov A, Chopin D: Correlation between sagittal plane changes and adjacent segment degeneration following lumbar spine fusion. *Eur Spine J* 2001;10:314-319.

After lumbar spinal fusion, 36.1% of patients showed radiographic evidence of adjacent segment degeneration, mostly retrolisthesis. Patients with a normal C7 plumb line and normal sacral inclination on the immediate postoperative radiographs had the lowest incidence of adjacent level change compared with patients who had abnormality in one or both of these parameters.

## Classic Bibliography

Allen BL Jr, Ferguson RL: The Galveston technique for L rod instrumentation of the scoliotic spine. *Spine* 1982;7:276-284.

Cochran T, Irstam L, Nachemson A: Long-term anatomic and functional changes in patients with adolescent idiopathic scoliosis treated by Harrington rod fusion. *Spine* 1983;8:576-584.

Dickson JH: An eleven-year clinical investigation of Harrington instrumentation: A preliminary report on 5/8 cases. *Clin Orthop Relat Res* 1973;93:113-130.

Fowles JV, Drummond DS, L'Ecuyer S, Roy L, Kassab MT: Untreated scoliosis in the adult. *Clin Orthop Relat Res* 1978;134:212-217.

Harrington PR: The history and development of Harrington instrumentation. *Clin Orthop Relat Res* 1973;93:110-112.

Hu SS, Fontaine F, Kelly B, Bradford DS: Nutritional depletion in staged spinal reconstructive surgery: The effect of total parenteral nutrition. *Spine* 1998;23:1401-1405.

Jackson RP, Simmons EH, Stripinis D: Incidence and severity of back pain in adult idiopathic scoliosis. *Spine* 1983;8:749-756.

Kostuik JP, Israel J, Hall JE: Scoliosis surgery in adults. *Clin Orthop Relat Res* 1973;93:225-234.

Lonstein JE: The Galveston technique using Luque or Cotrel-Dubousset rods. *Orthop Clin North Am* 1994;25:311-320.

Luque ER: Segmental spinal instrumentation for correction of scoliosis. *Clin Orthop Relat Res* 1982;163:192-198.

Nachemson A: A long term follow-up study of nontreated scoliosis. *Acta Orthop Scand* 1968;39:466-476.

Ponder RC, Dickson JH, Harrington PR, Erwin WD: Results of Harrington instrumentation and fusion in the adult idiopathic scoliosis patient. *J Bone Joint Surg Am* 1975;57:797-801.

Vauzelle C, Stagnara P, Jouvinroux P: Functional monitoring of spinal cord activity during spinal surgery. *Clin Orthop Relat Res* 1973;93:173-178.

Weinstein SL, Ponseti IV: Curve progression in idiopathic scoliosis. *J Bone Joint Surg Am* 1983;65:447-455.

Weinstein SL, Zavala DC, Ponseti IV: Idiopathic scoliosis: long-term follow-up and prognosis in untreated patients. *J Bone Joint Surg Am* 1981;63:702-712.

Zielke K, Stunkat R, Beaujean F: Ventrale derotationsspondylodesis. *Arch Orthop Unfallchir* 1976;85:257-277.

# Chapter 36

# Inflammatory Arthritis of the Spine

Nilesh M. Patel, MD

Louis G. Jenis, MD

## Introduction

Inflammatory arthropathy of the spine is an all-encompassing term that includes rheumatoid arthritis and the seronegative spondyloarthropathies. These conditions result in inflammatory changes of the bone, connective tissue, and/or synovium of the spine. Rheumatoid arthritis presents primarily in the synovial tissues of the upper cervical spine leading to deformity and instability. The spondyloarthropathies include ankylosing spondylitis, reactive arthritis (including Reiter syndrome), psoriatic arthritis, inflammatory bowel disease-associated spondyloarthropathy, and undifferentiated spondyloarthropathy. These diseases are linked by their association with the *HLA-B27* gene and by the presence of enthesitis as the basic pathologic lesion leading to spondylitis. Surgical care for these conditions requires an in-depth understanding of the disease processes and detailed preoperative planning. Recent advances in medical intervention may dramatically decrease the necessity for surgical care in many patients.

## Rheumatoid Arthritis

Rheumatoid arthritis is a chronic systemic autoimmune disorder affecting 1% to 2% of the population. Disease manifestations are primarily seen in synovial-lined joints secondary to an erosive synovitis. The cause of the destructive synovitis is based on the immune complex theory and appears to stem from an autoimmune response against an antigenic expression of synovial cells. This response is detected by the production of rheumatoid factor, an immunoglobulin that is directed against antigens of targeted synovial cells. This antigen-antibody interaction leads to release of proteolytic enzymes that destroy local structures, including ligaments, tendons, cartilage, and bone. The upper cervical spine is primarily affected in patients with rheumatoid arthritis because of the extensive presence of synovial tissue in the occiput-C1 and C1-2 articulations. The eventual soft-tissue and bony destruction leads to instability and subluxation. The most common instability patterns are atlantoaxial sublux-

ation, superior migration of the odontoid, and subaxial subluxation.

Atlantoaxial subluxation occurs after weakening or destruction of the joint capsule and the transverse, alar, and apical ligaments of the C1-C2 joint. The resulting instability in combination with retro-odontoid pannus can lead to significant dynamic or static spinal cord compression. Superior migration of the odontoid (also termed atlantoaxial impaction, pseudobasilar invagination, or cranial settling) occurs from bony erosion between the occipitoatlantal and atlantoaxial joints. Bilateral erosion of the lateral masses can lead to settling of the occiput on the cervical spine and a relative superior migration of the odontoid into the foramen magnum. The resulting anatomic anomaly can cause brainstem compression and vascular compromise to the basivertebral and anterior spinal arterial systems. Appearances of these subluxations differ based on pathogenesis: atlantoaxial subluxation occurs secondary to soft-tissue destruction and is typically an early event in rheumatoid arthritis, whereas superior migration of the odontoid results from bony destruction over time and is seen as a late manifestation in the cervical spine. Subaxial subluxation occurs as a result of facet joint, interspinous ligament, and intervertebral disk disruptions caused by inflammatory and degenerative processes. Multiple level subaxial subluxation may lead to a stepladder spine appearance or a kyphotic deformity.

### Clinical Presentation

The clinical presentation of rheumatoid arthritis is variable and ranges from an asymptomatic patient to those with severe deformity and neurologic compromise. Neck pain is the most common initial complaint and is often localized to the upper cervical spine and associated with occipital headaches. Greater occipital nerve root irritation (C2) can lead to pain patterns in the face, ear, and mastoid region. Vertebrobasilar insufficiency may cause vertigo, nausea, vomiting, dysphagia, and dysarthria. Patients with myelopathy typically present with unsteadiness of gait, loss of dexterity, hyperreflexia below the

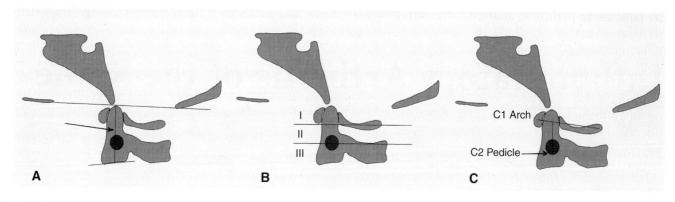

**Figure 1** **A,** Schematic representation of the Redlund-Johnell criterion. The distance between the McGregor line and the midpoint of the caudal margin of the second cervical vertebral body is measured (*arrow*). A measurement of less than 34 mm in males and less than 29 mm in females indicates basilar invagination. **B,** Schematic representation of the Clark station. The station of the first cervical vertebra is determined by dividing the odontoid process into three equal parts in the sagittal plane. If the anterior ring of the atlas is level with the middle third (station II) or caudal third (station III) of the odontoid process, basilar invagination is diagnosed. **C,** Schematic representation of the Ranawat criterion. The distance between the center of the second cervical pedicle and the transverse axis of the atlas is measured along the axis of the odontoid process. A measurement of less than 15 mm in males and less than 13 mm in females is indicative of basilar invagination. *(Reproduced with permission from Riew KD, Hilibrand AS, Palumbo MA, Sethi N, Bohlman HH: Diagnosing basilar invagination in the rheumatoid patient: The reliability of radiographic criteria. J Bone Joint Surg Am 2001;83-A:194-200.)*

level of compression, and weakness. The Ranawat classification is often used for myelopathy classification in patients with rheumatoid arthritis: class I includes patients with no neurologic deficit; class II includes patients with subjective weakness, dysesthesias, and hyperreflexia; and class III includes patients with objective signs of weakness and upper motor signs and is subclassified as IIIA (ambulatory) or IIIB (nonambulatory).

### Radiographic Evaluation

Lateral radiographs are used initially for evaluation of patients with rheumatoid arthritis. The key features to evaluate are the posterior atlanto-dens interval, anterior atlanto-dens interval, subaxial subluxation, and superior migration of the odontoid. Dynamic lateral views are used to evaluate for changes in the posterior and anterior atlanto-dens intervals. An anterior atlanto-dens interval greater than 5 mm is considered abnormal in patients with rheumatoid arthritis, but the posterior atlanto-dens interval has more prognostic value and is the critical determinant for further evaluation or treatment because this is a true measurement of the space available for the spinal cord.

Diagnosing superior migration of the odontoid can be difficult. A screening test with high sensitivity is imperative so as to not miss a potentially life-threatening condition; such a test must also have a high negative predictive value to reliably determine the absence of superior migration of the odontoid. The validity and reliability of the most commonly used radiographic criteria have recently been evaluated. The most reliable measurements are those that do not involve finding the tip of the odontoid, which is often obscured in patients with rheumatoid arthritis. The best combination of the above parameters is the analysis of the station of the atlas referenced to the C2 body as proposed by Clark (a sensi-

tivity of 83% and a negative predictive value of 85%) and the Wackenheim line (a sensitivity of 88%, a negative predictive value of 90%, and a low specificity of 20%). Therefore, it was determined that a combination of three criteria would maximize sensitivity and negative predictive value while maintaining a reasonable specificity. If any of the three test results are positive, then a sensitivity of 94% is reached. If all three test results are negative, then there is a 91% chance that the patient does not have superior migration of the odontoid. The three tests are the atlas stations, the Redlund-Johnell criterion, and the Ranawat criterion (Figure 1).

If any of the test results are positive or the examination is suggestive of brainstem dysfunction with no evidence of injury on plain radiographs, further evaluation with MRI or CT is indicated. CT with sagittal reconstruction is useful for evaluating the altered bony anatomy and for preoperative planning. MRI reveals the space available for the spinal cord by including the posterior odontoid soft-tissue pannus and subluxation. MRI also allows for an accurate evaluation of the cervicomedullary angle, which is measured by the intersection of lines drawn anterior to the spinal cord and along the brainstem. A cervicomedullary angle less than 135° is consistent with superior migration of the odontoid and has been reported to correlate with signs of neural compression in all patients.

### Natural History

Spinal disease eventually occurs in approximately 60% of patients with rheumatoid arthritis. This trend may be on the decline because of new medical treatments. Patients with arthritis mutilans or severe peripheral disease and longer disease duration are at higher risk for cervical spine involvement. Once instability begins, the disease tends to progress toward more complex instability patterns. In particular, atlantoaxial subluxation tends to progress toward superior migration of the odontoid. Although it may often appear that atlantoaxial subluxation has improved, in reality the odontoid may have migrated into the foramen magnum with a secondary stabilizing effect on atlantoaxial subluxation.

Long-term studies on the natural history of spinal disease are difficult to interpret because of variations in disease duration at presentation and diagnostic yield of radiographic interpretations. A study of 546 patients showed that spinal disease of 14-year duration had cervical involvement in 39% of patients; by 24-year duration, 56% of patients had cervical disease. Recent studies have also shown that all patients with mutilating type rheumatoid arthritis will eventually develop cervical disease. With the appearance of myelopathy, the mortality rate increases dramatically. A long-term follow-up study of 40 matched myelopathic patients who were treated with or without surgery revealed the advantage of early surgery. In the surgical cohort (C1 laminectomy with occipitocervical fusion), 13 of 19 patients (68%) improved neurologically, with 5- and 10-year survival rates of 84% and 37%, respectively. The nonsurgical treatment group did not achieve any significant neurologic improvement; all patients were bedridden at 3-year follow-up and none survived at 8-year follow-up. A similar study showed nonsurgical mortality rates of 47% at 6 months and 73% at 5 years versus 27% for patients who underwent surgical treatment. Overall, the literature has shown that progression of instability, neurologic deficit, and mortality rates support the use of surgical intervention.

### Treatment

Current treatment of rheumatoid arthritis is based on medical and surgical care to alleviate intractable pain and prevent neurologic injury or deterioration.

### Pharmacotherapy

During the past decade, improved understanding of the pathophysiology of rheumatoid arthritis has led to changes in therapeutic strategies. Early diagnosis and implementation of disease-modifying antirheumatic drugs (DMARDs) such as methotrexate, hydroxychloroquine sulfate, and sulfasalazine gold within 3 months is critical. During the first few weeks of symptoms, nonsteroidal anti-inflammatory drugs (NSAIDs) can be used until a definitive diagnosis is made. Methotrexate is usually the first-line DMARD, with the addition of oral steroids as a bridge to effective DMARD therapy. If symptoms continue after 2 to 3 months of methotrexate therapy, additional DMARDs may be added to the regimen. The use of agents that target tumor necrosis factor-α and interleukin-1 can be added for patients with inadequately controlled disease. Three types of tumor necrosis factor-α (infliximab, etanercept, and adalimumab) and one type of interleukin-1 (anakinra) inhibitors are currently available. With modern medical therapy and early intervention, patients can achieve the realistic goal of prevention and actual remission of active disease. Recent data from the California hospitalization database suggest that rheumatoid cervical spine surgery declined by 37% from 1998 to 2001 compared with 1983 to 1987; these data, however, were not statistically significant.

### Surgical Decision Making and Management

Patients with intractable pain or neurologic deficits from cervical subluxation are considered candidates for surgery. Surgical intervention should be attempted before the onset of Ranawat class III myelopathy because afterward improvement of neurologic status is limited at best. A dilemma arises from the approach to management of asymptomatic patients or those who are mildly affected with instability. Based on radiographic criteria, three categories of instability have been described for surgical stabilization of the rheumatoid spine in patients with or without neurologic deficits based on a long-term analysis of 73 patients. Category 1 includes patients with atlantoaxial subluxation with a posterior atlanto-dens interval of 14 mm or less, category 2 includes those with atlantoaxial subluxation and 5 mm or more of superior migration of the odontoid as determined by McGregor's line, and category 3 includes those with subaxial subluxation with 14 mm or less of space available for the spinal cord. In this study, patients with neurologic deficits, atlantoaxial subluxation, and a preoperative posterior atlanto-dens interval of less than 10 mm showed no recovery, whereas those with a posterior atlanto-dens interval of at least 10 mm showed some recovery, and those with a posterior atlanto-dens interval of at least 14 mm showed complete neurologic recovery after surgery. Patients with a postoperative posterior atlanto-dens interval between 10 and 14 mm experienced recovery of at least one Ranawat class.

In asymptomatic patients with a subaxial sagittal diameter of 14 mm or less, MRI can be used to evaluate the true space available for the spinal cord. If the true space available for the spinal cord is less than 13 mm or if there is more than 3.5 mm of segmental mobility, stabilization and decompression should be considered.

The goals of surgical management are to prevent further neurologic deterioration and alleviate pain by neural decompression and stabilization of deformity. Over the past decade, advances in modern instrumentation have increased the options for cervical stabilization. The traditional method of C1-C2 fusion involves the use of sublaminar wires and bone grafting. In patients with spinal cord compression and an irreducible atlantoaxial subluxation, the use of posterior C1 arch wires should be avoided and a laminectomy performed. Although

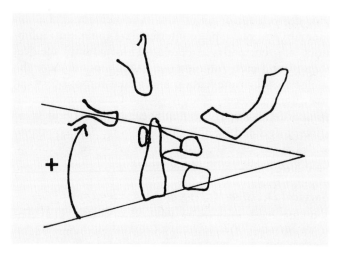

Figure 2 Schematic representation showing how the association between the occipital bone and the axis is determined by the angle (*curved arrow*) made by the McGregor line and the inferior surface of the axis. (*Reproduced with permission from Matsunaga S, Onishi T, Sakou T: Significant of occipitoaxial angle in subaxial lesion after occipitocervical fusion. Spine 2001;26:161-165.*)

transarticular C1-C2 screws provide improved biomechanical strength, they may not be feasible for use in patients with a large or aberrant foramen transversarium in C2. Fusion rates of 97% have been obtained with transarticular screws and iliac crest bone graft. Alternative techniques include the use of C1 lateral mass screws coupled with C2 isthmic, pedicle, or laminar screws. When a solid fusion is obtained, the periodontoid pannus tends to regress and slow the progression of cranial settling.

If cranial settling has occurred, then the fusion may need to be extended to the occiput to prevent further collapse. Many choices are available for posterior occipitocervical fusion stabilization, including loop-wire constructs, plate fixation, and plate-rod combinations. In patients with neural compression, traction may be attempted; if reduction is not successful, then decompression should also be performed. Decompression may be accomplished by posterior C1 arch removal or transoral odontoid resection. Modern screw, plate, and rod systems have shown biomechanical superiority, and the literature has shown they have some clinical superiority to loop-sublaminar wiring. Care should be taken in the alignment of occipitocervical fusions because an occiput-C2 angle greater than 30° has been associated with early onset subaxial subluxation; intraoperative radiographs should confirm an angle between 0° and 30° (Figure 2).

For patients with subaxial subluxation requiring surgery, a posterior arthrodesis with interspinous wiring or lateral mass fixation is often adequate. When multilevel disease is present, often as a stepladder deformity, lateral mass fixation may be the preferable technique.

Severe chin on chest or rotational deformities can occur in patients with long-standing rheumatoid arthri-

tis. A recent report of five patients showed excellent results with full correction to neutral gaze using a halo-dependent or a halo-Ilizarov apparatus. Emphasis was placed on the time in traction rather than an increase in weight (5 to 20 lb); reduction occurred within 4 days to 4 weeks. Traction first was applied parallel with the deformity to distract and unlock the involved joints before attempting correction.

All of the aforementioned conditions can appear alone or in combination. Care must be taken to address all cervical instability and deformity to avoid additional surgery and extension of the arthrodesis. Recent long-term data illustrate the success of surgical intervention in the appropriate patients. Prior reports stated that surgery for patients with Ranawat class IIIB disease had no benefit other than pain relief; however, recent reviews have shown neurologic benefit in up to 55% of these patients. A strong predictor of postoperative neurologic recovery still appears to be preoperative neurologic status, and early surgical intervention before the development of severe myelopathy is preferable.

## Seronegative Spondyloarthropathies
### Ankylosing Spondylitis
Ankylosing spondylitis is a chronic inflammatory disease that affects the axial skeleton. It often begins in the third decade of life, and has a 3:1 male to female incidence. Those afflicted with the disease can have severe functional limitations secondary to stiffness, pain, fatigue, and deformity.

Ankylosing spondylitis is a member of a class of seronegative spondyloarthropathies, a term that is used to describe a group of inflammatory arthropathies that share similar characteristics, including sacroiliitis with or without spondylitis, peripheral inflammatory arthritis, tendency for familial aggregation, and negative rheumatoid factor serology. The other seronegative spondyloarthropathies include spondylitis associated with inflammatory bowel disease, psoriatic arthritis, Reiter syndrome, and reactive arthritis.

Ankylosing spondylitis has a definite genetic predilection, with identical twins having concordance of up to 63%. Ankylosing spondylitis occurs in 0.2% of North Americans and Western Europeans. HLA-B27 is present in 6% to 8% of Caucasians and in 95% of patients with ankylosing spondylitis. Ankylosing spondylitis is rare in Africa, where HLA-B27 is practically absent. A few dominant theories exist for disease susceptibility associated with HLA-B27, including an arthritogenic peptide in tissues affected with disease that binds to the HLA-B27 antigen and stimulates the pathologic cascade. HLA-B27–positive individuals also may be more susceptible to certain microorganisms because the prolonged intracellular presence of these arthritogenic organisms may lead to a disease-producing synovitis. *Klebsiella pneumoniae* has common amino acid sequences with the HLA-B27 antigen, and patients with ankylosing spondylitis have shown increased immune responses to this disease. Autoimmunity against HLA-B27 itself by cytotoxic T cells may also play a role.

There are fundamental differences in the distribution and morphology of osteoarticular lesions in the seronegative spondyloarthropathies compared with rheumatoid arthritis. Seronegative spondyloarthropathy produces abnormalities in the enthesis—bony insertions of ligaments and tendons, whereas a synovial process causes rheumatoid arthritis lesions. The inflammation in patients with seronegative spondyloarthropathy leads to bony erosions followed by new or reactive bone formation and eventual ankylosis. Inflammation of the anulus fibrosus eventually leads to formation of bridging syndesmophytes. The manifestations of seronegative spondyloarthropathy will often involve the entire axial skeleton, whereas manifestations of rheumatoid arthritis are limited primarily to the cervical spine.

The unifying feature of all the spondyloarthropathies is sacroiliitis and distinctive patterns in the appendicular skeleton. In the peripheral skeleton, ankylosing spondylitis involves the enthesis; patients with psoriatic arthritis typically have interphalangeal destruction, whereas Reiter syndrome affects the synovial joints of the lower extremity. Ankylosing spondylitis usually begins with the axial skeleton, but it can involve other organ systems. The nonspinal manifestations of ankylosing spondylitis may include peripheral large joint arthritis (hip and shoulder), acute anterior uveitis, renal amyloidosis, ascending aortic abnormalities (stenosis, aortitis, and regurgitation), and cardiac conduction abnormalities.

### Radiographic Evaluation

The earliest radiographic sign of ankylosing spondylitis is erosion on the iliac side of the sacroiliac joint. Continued erosions appear as joint space widening, new bone formation, and eventual ankylosis. Ankylosing spondylitis has a predilection for bilateral sacroiliitis and marginal thin flowing syndesmophytes leading to a pathognomonic bamboo spine appearance. Plain radiographic changes are often seen late and may delay diagnosis by years. The sacroiliac joint is difficult to evaluate with plain radiography because of the undulating and oblique nature of the joint. Other diagnostic modalities include scintigraphy, CT, and MRI. Scintigraphy is sensitive to the inflammation in sacroiliac joints, but lacks specificity. CT detects early bony changes, but is unable to show active inflammation. MRI can detect active inflammation; thus, it is critical for assessing early changes in spondyloarthropathies.

### Clinical Presentation

The axial spine manifestations of ankylosing spondylitis commonly present as chronic low back pain in early adulthood. Pain is often localized to the gluteal and sacroiliac regions. With further inflammatory changes, back stiffness begins that is typically exacerbated by periods of inactivity (characteristic morning stiffness and/or rest pain). As spine mobility decreases, patients may develop hip flexion contractures as a result of the loss of overall lumbar lordosis and inflammatory changes around the hip articulations.

The natural history of radiographic findings involves a steady linear progression, with 35% radiographic progression every 10 years based on studies using radiographic indices. After disease duration of 25 years, 85% of patients have lumbar spine involvement and 75% have cervical spine involvement.

### Treatment

Until recently, treatment options for patients with ankylosing spondylitis have been limited. Despite the relatively high prevalence of the disease, no disease-modifying agents have been available as they have been for patients with rheumatoid arthritis. NSAIDs have been the mainstay of therapy and provide minimal pain relief. Recent studies have shown excellent clinical and radiographic efficacy of tumor necrosis factor-α blocking agents for both ankylosing spondylitis and psoriatic arthritis. Radiographic studies with serial MRI have shown significant improvements in inflammatory changes at 3 months after initiation of tumor necrosis factor-α blocking agent therapy. Tumor necrosis factor-α blocking agents can be considered the first-line therapy for patients whose axial symptoms are not controlled with NSAIDs. In addition to the medical management of symptoms, physical therapy including a program to improve flexibility and strength should be advised. Bracing may also be considered as an adjunct for pain management.

### Fractures

Any patient with ankylosing spondylitis and sudden onset of neck or back pain regardless of how trivial the inciting factor should be considered to have a fracture until proven otherwise. Most fractures are located in the midcervical to cervicothoracic junction and at the thoracolumbar junction. A fractured ankylosed spine may be extremely unstable because any fracture universally extends across three columns, creating two rigid segments that move independently. Rapid neurologic deterioration can occur from subtle movements or from developing epidural hematomas. Strict spine precautions and careful positioning that equally support all areas of the spine are required. Radiographs and fine-cut CT scans with sagittal reconstructed images should be obtained to rule out a fracture because up to 50% of fractures can be missed using plain radiography. In a recent study of

11 ankylosing spondylitis cervical fractures, 4 were found to have epidural hematomas that required surgical evacuation. MRI should be considered to evaluate patients for epidural hematomas that can occur with minimal fractures in the ankylosed spine. Fibrous tissue associated with chronic fracture pseudarthrosis may be differentiated from acute hematomas with contrast-enhanced T1 images.

Stable fractures without neurologic involvement often heal without complication and may be immobilized in an external brace or a halo device; however, neurologic deterioration can occur quickly even in patients with well immobilized fractures. Unstable fractures or those difficult to brace may require internal fixation and fusion. Because of the risks for neurologic deterioration and difficulties of halo vest immobilization caused by thoracic kyphosis in most patients with ankylosing spondylitis, internal fixation for all cervical fractures has been recommended. Because the ankylosed anterior column provides adequate anterior support, most fractures can be managed by a posterior approach with lateral mass fixation and interspinous wiring. In patients with osteopenia or chronic fracture with pseudarthrosis in whom the anterior support has been compromised by granulation tissue, additional anterior support may be required.

### Deformity

A flexion deformity may develop secondary to multiple microfractures over time, leading to a severe sagittal imbalance. The resulting kyphosis may be centered at the cervicothoracic junction or over the thoracolumbar region. Cervicothoracic kyphotic deformity can result in a chin on chest posture that leads to difficulty of jaw opening and horizontal gaze. The goals for corrective osteotomies are restoration of sagittal balance and leveling of horizontal gaze. The correction in the gaze angle is in direct relation to the angular correction at the osteotomy site. However, the magnitude in sagittal balance correction varies according to the location of the osteotomy. As the osteotomy site progresses caudally, a larger correction in sagittal balance for the same angular correction is obtained. This can lead to an iatrogenically created abnormal gaze angle (Figure 3).

If the primary deformity is at the CT junction in the absence of thoracolumbar kyphosis, sagittal balance may not be a significant issue; in this instance a cervicothoracic osteotomy is required. This procedure is usually performed between C7-T1 where the canal is widest; the exiting eighth root is more resistant to stretch and compression and below the entry of the vertebral artery.

Few modifications of the basic technique of spinal osteotomy have occurred over the past 25 years. The most useful preoperative evaluation comes from the clinical chin-brow to vertical angle by observing the patient from the side with the neck in neutral position and the hips and knees fully extended (Figure 4). The result-

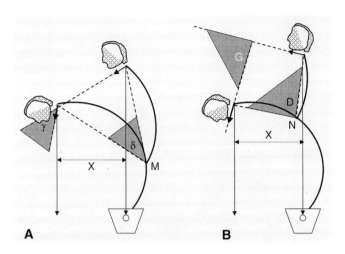

Figure 3  Schematic representation showing the effect that the level of osteotomy has on sagittal balance and gaze angle. Restoration of sagittal balance is achieved by posterior shift of the plumb line (X). The correction of the gaze angle ($\gamma$ and G) is always the same as the corresponding osteotomy angle ($\delta$ and D), respectively; ($\delta = \gamma$ and D = G). **A,** When osteotomy is performed at a lower level (M), an osteotomy angle $\delta$ is needed for restoration of the sagittal balance (X). **B,** When osteotomy is performed at a higher level (N), a larger osteotomy angle (D) is needed (D > $\delta$) for the same degree of sagittal balance restoration (X). Because the osteotomy angle is always the same as the gaze angle correction (D = G), the correction of the gaze angle will be larger (G > $\gamma$) with a higher level of osteotomy. This may lead to overcorrection of the gaze angle upward. *(Reproduced with permission from Sengupta DK, Khazin R, Grevitt MP, Webb JK: Flexion osteotomy of the cervical spine: A new technique for correction of iatrogenic extension deformity in ankylosing spondylitis. Spine 2001;26: 1068-1072.)*

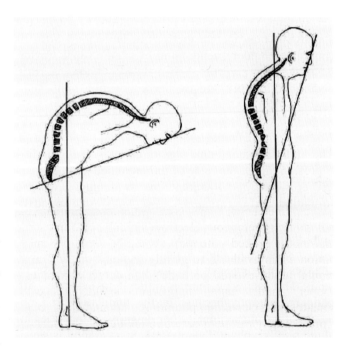

Figure 4  Schematic representation of the chin-brow to vertical angle measurement of flexion deformity of the spine, which is obtained from the intersection of a chin-brow line with the vertical line in a patient with neutral or fixed neck and full hip and knee extension. *(Reproduced with permission from Kostuik JP: Ankylosing spondylitis: Surgical treatment, in Frymoyer JW (ed): The Adult Spine: Principles and Practice. New York, NY, Raven Press, 1991, p 724.)*

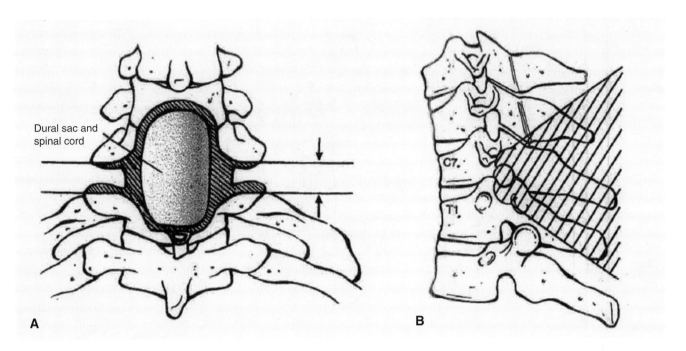

**Figure 5** Posterior **(A)** and lateral **(B)** view schematic representations of the bony resection required for cervicothoracic osteotomy. In the posterior view, the pedicles must be undercut to avoid impingement of the C8 root and the cut surface is beveled on its deep surface to avoid dural impingement. The lines (see arrows) show the upper and lower limit of the osteotomy. (*Adapted with permission from Simmons EH: The cervical spine in ankylosing spondylitis, in Bridwell KH, DeWald RL (eds): The Textbook of Spinal Surgery, ed 3. Philadelphia, PA, Lipincott-Raven, 1997, p 1143.*)

ing angle is useful for surgical planning of the extent of the osteotomy required to obtain a horizontal gaze. The procedure may be performed with the patient under general anesthesia or, as originally described, under local anesthesia with sedation (Figure 5). The 36-year experience with this technique in 131 patients was reported recently. The number of C8 root palsies was decreased with experience as wider decompression was being performed. Spinal cord injury occurred in three patients, and all patients had excellent correction of visual fields. Pseudarthrosis occurred in only 6 of 131 patients. Some authors now recommend use of segmental instrumentation with lateral mass cervical screws and thoracic pedicular fixation. Modern anesthetic technology, such as fiberoptic intubation and hypotensive anesthesia, and intraoperative neuromonitoring allow for general anesthesia to be used. Somatosensory-evoked potentials, spontaneous electromyography, and transcranial motor-evoked potentials should be used in combination when available to greatly increase safety. Transcranial motor-evoked potentials can detect cord injury sooner and have improved sensitivity over somatosensory-evoked potentials. Spontaneous electromyography can help detect eighth nerve root injuries that can otherwise be missed when only somatosensory-evoked potentials are used.

Thoracolumbar osteotomies can be performed to correct global sagittal alignment and gaze alignment. Classically, an anteriorly opening osteotomy that pivots on the posterior edge of the vertebral body had been

used (Figure 6). This procedure has an increased risk of major vascular injuries in elderly patients with reduced arterial compliance. Vascular complications occurred when the osteotomies were done at L2 or above the point at which the renal vessels tether the aorta and above the bifurcation. Another option is to perform polysegmental posterior V-shaped osteotomies. Although there is less risk to anterior structures because of the gradual correction, this procedure can lead to insufficient correction when the anterior column is spontaneously fused. Recent studies advocate the use of a closing wedge procedure in the lumbar and thoracic region (Figure 7). These osteotomies involve removal of the posterior elements of one vertebra (usually below L2) and removal of a posterior wedge of the vertebral body by a transpedicular decancelization procedure. The closing osteoclasis hinges on the anterior cortex, leading to direct bony apposition and rapid consolidation. One report describes 78 patients who underwent 98 closing wedge osteotomies for ankylosing spondylitis. The authors found a high patient satisfaction rate (> 95%), average correction of 34° per osteotomy, and no vascular complications. Corrections of up to 100° were obtained with double osteotomies. Another study reported on 45 patients with similar angular correction and no vascular complications. A structured review of 523 osteotomies that were performed from 1945 to 1998 reported that the average correction ranged from 37° to 40°. Closing wedge osteotomy achieved 3.8° less correction than the other methods, but loss of correction was more common

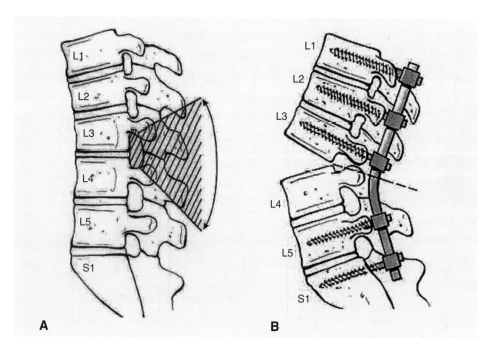

Figure 6 **A** and **B,** Schematic representations of bony resection for an L3-4 open wedge osteotomy and pedicle screw fixation. *(Reproduced with permission from Simmons ED, Zeng Y: Ankylosing spondylitis, in Bono C, Garfin S (eds): Orthopaedic Surgery Essentials: Spine. Philadelphia, PA, Lipincott Williams & Wilkins, 2004, p 201.)*

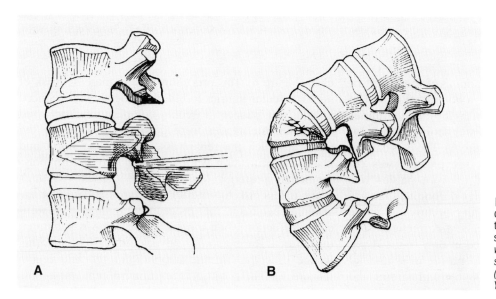

Figure 7 Schematic representation of a closing wedge osteotomy (pedicle subtraction: three-column osteotomy). **A,** Area of bony resection. **B,** Closed osteotomy. *(Reproduced with permission from Bridwell KH: Pedicle subtraction osteotomy, in Vaccaro A, Albert A (eds): Spine Surgery Tricks of the Trade. New York, NY, Thieme Med Pub, 2003, p 147.)*

with opening wedge and polysegmental osteotomies. For the whole group, neurologic complication occurred in 2% to 2.7%. Aortic injury occurred in only the open wedge group at a rate of 0.9% (4 of 451 patients).

## Psoriatic Spondylitis

Approximately 10% of patients with psoriatic arthritis will develop a spondyloarthropathy. Seventy percent of those with axial involvement are HLA-B27 positive compared with 20% without axial involvement. In contrast to ankylosing spondylitis, discovertebral erosions and axial ankylosis occur in a noncontiguous asymmetric pattern with both marginal and nonmarginal syndesmophytes. Patients with psoriatic spondylitis may also

develop a synovial proliferative process in the cervical spine, with clinical presentation similar to that in patients with rheumatoid arthritis. Medical treatment is similar to that for patients with rheumatoid arthritis, with early use of DMARDs and tumor necrosis factor-α blocking agent. Surgical indications are the same as those for patients with rheumatoid arthritis cervical disease or ankylosing spondylitis and deformity.

## Reiter Syndrome

Reiter syndrome is thought to occur as a postinfectious reactive arthritis, and it usually affects patients in the third and fourth decades of life, with a typical presentation occurring within 1 month of an episode of urethritis or enteritis. Lumbar spine involvement occurs in 50% of patients, but cervical spine involvement is rare. In contrast to ankylosing spondylitis, asymmetric sacroiliitis and nonmarginal syndesmophytes are characteristic in patients with Reiter syndrome. Treatment is symptomatic and rarely involves spinal surgery.

### Enteropathic Arthritis
Spondylitis can occur in association with ulcerative colitis or Crohn's disease. The clinical presentation and treatment is identical to that for idiopathic ankylosing spondylitis. Eighty percent of patients who develop axial disease are HLA-B27–positive. Axial involvement is independent of the bowel disease course and may occur before the onset of intestinal symptoms.

### Diffuse Idiopathic Skeletal Hyperostosis
Diffuse idiopathic skeletal hyperostosis is an enthesopathy of the spine, shoulder, elbow, knee, and calcaneus, and it typically occurs in patients who are middle-age or older. The spinal enthesopathy leads to large nonmarginal anterolateral syndesmophytes and does not involve the sacroiliac joints. Four contiguous vertebral bodies need to be involved for diagnosis. Thoracic and lumbar involvement leads to stiffness and pain, and cervical disease with large anterior osteophytes can cause dysphasia and stridor. Ossification of the posterior longitudinal ligament can lead to myelopathy, whereas large segmental ossification makes the spine vulnerable to fracture as with ankylosing spondylitis.

## Summary
Inflammatory conditions of the spine represent a wide category of conditions. Appropriate early medical intervention can result in a decline in the rate of surgical interventions. Early diagnosis, aggressive medical therapy, modern diagnostic imaging, and modern instrumentation have significantly improved the ability to care for this patient population.

## Annotated Bibliography
### Rheumatoid Arthritis

Asano S, Mine K, Kiya T, Imura J, Nohara Y: Long-term follow up study of cervical lesions in rheumatoid arthritis, in *Proceedings of the 32nd Annual Meeting.* Rosemont, IL, Cervical Spine Research Society, 2004. Available at: http://www.csrs.org/searchabstr/2004_papers_44.pdf. Accessed November 28, 2005.

The authors conducted this study to assess the incidence and natural history of cervical lesions in patients with rheumatoid arthritis. They found that the incidence of cervical lesions was 39% in patients with a 14-year duration of rheumatoid arthritis and 56% in those with a 24-year duration.

Falope ZF, Griffiths ID, Platt PN, et al: Cervical myelopathy and rheumatoid arthritis: A retrospective analysis of management. *Clin Rehabil* 2002;16:625-629.

The authors of this retrospective review of 40 patients compared the outcomes of 18 patients who were managed nonsurgically (5-year mortality rate was 73% and no neurologic improvement was noted) and 22 patients who were treated surgically (5-year mortality rate was 27%; 30% of patients improved at least one Ranawat grade, and 55% of nonambulators [those with Ranawat grade IIIB] became ambulators).

Graziano GP, Hensinger R, Patel CK: The use of traction methods to correct severe cervical deformity in rheumatoid arthritis patients: A report of five cases. *Spine* 2001;26:1076-1081.

In this article, the authors describe the successful management of severe flexible cervical deformity from rheumatoid arthritis using a combination of traction techniques and surgical stabilization.

Haid RW Jr, Subach BR, McLaughlin MR, Rodts GE Jr, Wahlig JB Jr: C1-C2 transarticular screw fixation for atlantoaxial instability: A 6-year experience. *Neurosurgery* 2001;49:65-68.

The authors of this study report experience with 75 consecutive patients who underwent C1-C2 transarticular screw fixation to treat atlantoaxial instability. They report a 96% fusion rate at mean follow-up of 2.4 years (range, 1 to 5.5 years).

Matsunaga S, Onishi T, Sakou T: Significance of occipitoaxial angle in subaxial lesion after occipitocervical fusion. *Spine* 2001;26:161-165.

The authors of this study reported a high correlation between abnormal position of occiput-C2 fusion and subsequent subaxial subluxation. They also found that the best results were achieved if the occipitoaxial angle was maintained between 0° and 30°.

Matsunaga S, Sakou T, Onishi T, et al: Prognosis of patients with upper cervical lesions caused by rheumatoid arthritis: Comparison of occipitocervical fusion between c1 laminectomy and nonsurgical management. *Spine* 2003;28:1581-1587.

In this study, 19 surgical patients were compared with a cohort of 21 patients who underwent nonsurgical management. Improvement was found in 68% of the patients who underwent surgery. The survival rate was 84% at 5-year follow-up and 37% at 10-year follow-up. In the patients who did not undergo surgical treatment, no neural improvement was reported; neurologic deterioration was found in 76% during the follow-up period, and none survived at 8-year follow-up.

O'Dell JR: Therapeutic strategies for rheumatoid arthritis. *N Engl J Med* 2004;350:2591-2602.

The author presents a comprehensive review of current recommendations and future directions for the treatment of rheumatoid arthritis, discusses treatment algorithms, adverse effects, and reviews the results of recent clinical trials.

Omura K, Hukuda S, Katsuura A, Saruhashi Y, Imanaka T, Imai S: Evaluation of posterior long fusion versus conservative treatment for the progressive rheumatoid cervical spine. *Spine* 2002;27:1336-1345.

In this study, 17 seropositive patients with rheumatoid arthritis with mutilating-type joint involvements were assessed; 11 patients underwent surgical treatment and 6 patients underwent nonsurgical management. The authors reported that the patients without surgical intervention either went on to experience sudden death from minor trauma or became bedridden, whereas those who underwent surgical stabilization improved or the progressive natural history of the disease was halted.

Riew KD, Hilibrand AS, Palumbo MA, Sethi N, Bohlman HH: Diagnosing basilar invagination in the rheumatoid patient: The reliability of radiographic criteria. *J Bone Joint Surg Am* 2001;83-A:194-200.

In this study, the cervical spine radiographs of 131 patients with rheumatoid arthritis were examined. Data suggest that none of the radiographic screening tests for basilar invagination has a highly sensitive or a high negative predictive value. The authors recommend MRI or tomography whenever there is doubt about the diagnosis of basilar invagination based on plain radiographs.

Shad A, Shariff SS, Teddy PJ, Cadoux-Hudson TA: Craniocervical fusion for rheumatoid arthritis: Comparison of sublaminar wires and the lateral mass screw craniocervical fusion. *Br J Neurosurg* 2002;16:483-486.

The authors compared the outcomes of 21 patients who underwent craniocervical fusion using either sublaminar wires (N = 10) or plate/lateral mass constructs (N = 11). Three of the 10 patients with sublaminar wires had complete relief of pain, whereas 8 of 11 with skull plate and lateral mass cervical fixation had complete relief of pain. Neurologic improvement was similar in both groups.

Sutterlin CE, Bianchi JR, Kunz DN, et al: Biomechanical evaluation of occipitocervical fixation devices. *J Spinal Disord* 2001;14:185-192.

The authors of this biomechanical evaluation of occipitocervical fixation devices reported that plate systems were biomechanically superior to rod-wire constructs.

## Seronegative Spondyloarthropathies

Braun J, Sieper J: Biological therapies in the spondyloarthritides: The current state. *Rheumatology (Oxford)* 2004;43:1072-1084.

The authors reviewed the current literature and indications for the use of tumor necrosis factor-α blocking agents in the treatment of spondyloarthropathies.

Brophy S, Mackay K, Al-Saidi A, Taylor G, Calin A: The natural history of ankylosing spondylitis as defined by radiological progression. *J Rheumatol* 2002;29:1236-1243.

The authors of this study conducted a radiographic analysis of 571 patients with ankylosing spondylitis over a 25-year period. Ankylosing spondylitis is a linearly progressive disease with about 35% change every 10 years. They concluded that spinal involvement is largely an expression of disease duration, whereas the hips become involved in approximately 25% of patients and may predict a more severe outcome for the cervical spine.

Chen IH, Chien JT, Yu TC: Transpedicular wedge osteotomy for correction of thoracolumbar kyphosis in ankylosing spondylitis: Experience with 78 patients. *Spine* 2001;26:E354-E360.

The authors report experience with 78 patients who underwent 98 transpedicular wedge osteotomies; 14 patients had two-level osteotomies. Most osteotomies were at the L2 or L3 level, with an average 34° correction. At an average 46-month follow-up, the authors reported good to excellent results in greater than 90% of patients and no incidence of major vascular or neurologic injuries.

Grigoryan M, Roemer FW, Mohr A, Genant HK: Imaging in spondyloarthropathies. *Curr Rheumatol Rep* 2004; 6:102-109.

The authors review the various modalities available for the imaging of axial skeleton in patients with seronegative spondyloarthropathies.

Grisolia A, Bell RL, Peltier LF: Fractures and dislocations of the spine complicating ankylosing spondylitis: A report of six cases: 1967. *Clin Orthop Relat Res* 2004; 422:129-134.

In this report of six fractures and dislocations of the spine that occurred in patients with ankylosing spondylitis, the authors reported characteristic injury patterns and management options.

Hilibrand AS, Schwartz DM, Sethuraman V, Vaccaro AR, Albert TJ: Comparison of transcranial electric motor and somatosensory evoked potential monitoring during cervical surgery. *J Bone Joint Surg Am* 2004;86-A:1248-1253.

In this study, 427 patients undergoing surgery were reviewed. The authors found that somatosensory-evoked potential monitoring findings may lag transcranial motor-evoked potentials by 30 minutes. They also reported that somatosensory-evoked potential monitoring failed to detect any changes in one patient with new motor deficits.

Kim KT, Suk KS, Cho YJ, Hong GP, Park BJ: Clinical outcome results of pedicle subtraction osteotomy in ankylosing spondylitis with kyphotic deformity. *Spine* 2002;27:612-618.

The authors report the radiographic and clinical outcomes of 45 patients who underwent an eggshell pedicle subtraction osteotomy. The mean chin-brow angle improved from 32° to 0.9° and 38 of 45 patients were satisfied with the procedure. Forty-four patients returned to their previous occupations, and no vascular or permanent neurologic deficits were encountered.

Nakstad PH, Server A, Josefsen R: Traumatic cervical injuries in ankylosing spondylitis. *Acta Radiol* 2004;45: 222-226.

The authors of this study assessed the usefulness of MRI and CT for evaluation of 11 patients with ankylosing spondylitis and fractures of the cervical spine. They concluded that MRI is mandatory in the workup of all patients with cervical fractures for detecting the presence of epidural hematomas.

Reveille JD: The genetic basis of spondyloarthritis. *Curr Rheumatol Rep* 2004;6:117-125.

The author discusses the current literature as it pertains to the genetic basis of the spondyloarthropathies, particularly ankylosing spondylitis.

Simmons ED, Distefano RJ, Zheng Y, Simmons EH: Thirty-six years experience of cervical extension osteotomy in ankylosing spondylitis: Techniques and outcomes, in *Proceedings of the 32nd Annual Meeting*. Rosemont, IL, Cervical Spine Research Society, 2004. Available at: http://www.csrs.org/searchabstr/ 2004_papers_44.pdf. Accessed November 28, 2005.

The authors report on their experience with cervicothoracic osteotomy for the treatment of patients with ankylosing spondylitis. Clinical outcomes and potential adverse events are discussed.

Taggard DA, Traynelis VC: Management of cervical spinal fractures in ankylosing spondylitis with posterior fixation. *Spine* 2000;25:2035-2039.

The authors report the results of the surgical treatment of seven cervical fractures using posterior lateral mass/pedicular fixation with interspinous wiring and rib autograft. They report that stabilization involved at least two levels above and below the fractures and that postoperative collar support was adequate.

Ward MM: Decreases in rates of hospitalizations for manifestations of severe rheumatoid arthritis, 1983-2001. *Arthritis Rheum* 2004;50:1122-1131.

After reviewing data from the California hospitalization database for rheumatoid arthritis surgery, the author found decreases in rates of splenectomy and vasculitis. The author also found a 37% drop in spinal surgery, but this was not statistically significant because of the low number of patients.

## Classic Bibliography

Boden SD, Dodge LD, Bohlman HH, Rechtine GR: Rheumatoid arthritis of the cervical spine: A long-term analysis with predictors of paralysis and recovery. *J Bone Joint Surg Am* 1993;75:1282-1297.

Clark C, Goetz D, McNeles A: Arthrodesis of the cervical spine in rheumatoid arthritis. *J Bone Joint Surg Am* 1989;71:381-392.

Dvorak J, Grob D, Baumgartner H, et al: Functional evaluation of the spinal cord by magnetic resonance imaging in patients with rheumatoid arthritis and instability of upper cervical spine. *Spine* 1989;14:1057-1064.

Fujiwara K, Owaki H, Fujimoto M, Yonenobu K, Ochi T: A long-term follow-up study of cervical lesions in rheumatoid arthritis. *J Spinal Disord* 2000;13:519-526.

Kawaida H, Sakou T, Morizono Y, Yoshikuni N: Magnetic resonance imaging of upper cervical disorders in rheumatoid arthritis. *Spine* 1989;14:1144-1148.

Oda T, Fujiwara K, Yonenobu K, et al: Natural course of cervical spine lesions in rheumatoid arthritis. *Spine* 1995; 20:1128-1135.

Pellicci PM, Ranawat CS, Tsairis P, Bryan WJ: A prospective study of the progression of rheumatoid arthritis of the cervical spine. *J Bone Joint Surg Am* 1981;63:342-350.

Reiter MF, Boden SD: Inflammatory disorders of the cervical spine. *Spine* 1998;23:2755-2766.

Simmons EH: The surgical correction of flexion deformity of the cervical spine in ankylosing spondylitis. *Clin Orthop Relat Res* 1972;86:132-143.

Thomasen E: Vertebral osteotomy for the correction of kyphosis in ankylosing spondylitis. *Clin Orthop Relat Res* 1985;194:142-152.

Van Royen BJ, De Gast A: Lumbar osteotomy for the correction of thoracolumbar kyphotic deformity in ankylosing spondylitis: A structures review of three methods of treatment. *Ann Rheum Dis* 1999;58:399-406.

# Chapter 37

# Benign and Malignant Lesions of the Spine

Geoffrey A. Cronen, MD

Sanford E. Emery, MD, MBA

## Introduction

The diagnosis and management of spinal tumors has evolved considerably over the past few decades. Through advances in technology, development of classification schemes specific to the spine, and safer and more effective treatment regimens, significant improvements have been made in short- and long-term patient outcomes.

Tumors of the spine are relatively rare, and the related signs and symptoms are often similar to those of degenerative spinal disorders. A knowledgeable physician can prevent a delay in the diagnosis, which can have a tremendous effect on the patient's prognosis. With careful attention to detail, subtle clues may be extracted from the patient's history. Judicious use of imaging modalities, awareness of available nonsurgical protocols, an experienced multidisciplinary team and, most importantly, an informed patient and family are necessary to achieve the best outcomes.

## Incidence

Approximately 1.2 million Americans are diagnosed with cancer each year. Of these, approximately 600,000 will have bone metastases, whereas only 2,700 will have a primary bone sarcoma. The probability of bone metastases can be estimated by knowing the prevalence of the cancer and its predilection for bone. Breast, lung, renal, prostate, and thyroid tumors make up more than 60% of the lesions that invade bone. Women are most frequently affected by carcinoma of the breast, uterus, and colon, whereas men are most affected by carcinoma of the prostate, lung, and bladder. Up to 10% of newly diagnosed cancer patients will die without identification of the primary malignancy.

Metastatic lesions outnumber primary bone tumors by 25 to 40:1 and are the most common neoplasm affecting the spine. Bony metastases occur most commonly in the vertebral column. Of patients who die of cancer, 40% to 80% have evidence of skeletal metastases at autopsy. Spinal metastases are frequently asymptomatic, with estimates as high as 90%. The number of symptomatic metastases is highest in the thoracic spine. Seventy percent of spinal tumors are located in the thoracolumbar spine, 20% in the lumbosacral spine, and 10% in the cervical spine.

The overall incidence of primary bone tumors is 0.4%. Most benign spinal tumors occur during the second and third decades of life, whereas patients older than 30 years are more likely to have a malignant lesion. Benign lesions tend to favor the posterior elements, whereas malignant lesions are more commonly found in the vertebral body. Primary malignant tumors of the spine account for only 10% of the estimated 8,000 new sarcomas diagnosed each year.

## Evaluation

### History and Physical Examination

During the initial thorough patient history and physical examination, clues will be provided that should alert the physician to the presence of a tumor. Follow-up questions will help differentiate these symptoms from those not associated with a benign or malignant lesion. The age of the patient is important because it can limit the differential diagnosis. Primary benign tumors tend to occur in the first three decades of life, whereas primary malignant processes are more common in patients older than 21 years, with the exception of Ewing's sarcoma and osteosarcoma. More than 80% of spinal metastases occur in patients older than 40 years.

Approximately 85% of patients with spine tumors have a chief report of back pain, with or without antecedent trauma. This pain tends to be axial, have a slow onset, an unrelenting course, commonly occurs at night, and is often unrelated to activity. The pain timeline and the presence and rapidity of onset of neurologic insult are important determinants of prognosis. An acute onset of pain and/or associated radicular symptoms should raise the suspicion of a pathologic fracture. A neurologic deficit with an insidious onset carries a much better prognosis than a more acute onset. A high index of suspicion must be maintained in elderly patients and in those with chronic back pain; the temptation to at-

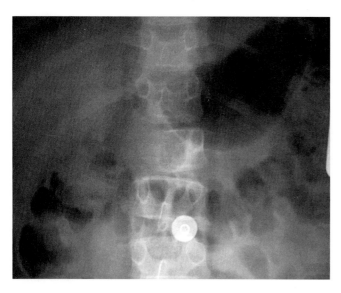

Figure 1  A radiograph showing the winking owl sign.

tribute their symptoms to degenerative changes or chronicity must be avoided. Any change in the quality of the underlying pain or the occurrence of new symptoms should be investigated.

A personal history of cancer, no matter how remote, should be ascertained. Patients with a history of breast cancer can have a disease-free interval of 10 to 20 years before a first episode of metastasis. The social history should include questions regarding occupational exposures to carcinogens, alcohol or tobacco use, sexual history, and transfusion history. A pertinent family history should be sought. A review of systems should address constitutional symptoms and whether the patient has had unintentional weight loss, anorexia, or fatigue. The physician should probe specifically for a personal history of cutaneous lesions, hematochezia, cough and/or shortness of breath, and whether a primary care physician has performed age-specific screening tests.

The physical examination in a patient with a suspected tumor should include a thorough evaluation of systems that may not be within the skill set of the surgeon; if this is the case, appropriate referrals should be made. The entire spine should be palpated for focal tenderness, which is more common in patients with tumors than in those with mechanical pain. Range of motion is usually severely limited in patients with pathologic fractures. The neurologic examination should assess muscular strength, reflexes, gait, and sensation. True weakness may be difficult to distinguish from weakness secondary to lethargy or guarding.

## Laboratory Evaluation

Laboratory screening tests can be helpful in narrowing the differential diagnosis. All patients with suspected tumors should have a complete blood cell count with dif-

ferential to assess for a previously unknown anemia. The erythrocyte sedimentation rate may be elevated in patients with malignancy, infection, and inflammation. The blood urea nitrogen level, creatinine level, and urinalysis results are frequently abnormal in patients with primary renal carcinoma. Patients with osteopenia and osteolytic lesions may have alterations of serum calcium, phosphate, and alkaline phosphatase levels. Urine calcium and phosphorous and serum parathyroid hormone levels also may need to be checked in these patients. Serum protein and urine protein electrophoresis will frequently show a monoclonal gammopathy in patients with multiple myeloma. Serum prostate specific antigen will be more than 4 ng/mL and acid phosphatase may be elevated in men with metastatic prostate cancer. If thyroid cancer is suspected, a thyroid panel should be performed. Liver function testing and carcinoembryonic antigen assays are important studies for patients with a history of gastrointestinal carcinoma.

## Imaging Modalities
### Plain Radiographs
Every patient suspected of having a spinal tumor, as well as those who have had back pain for longer than 6 weeks, should have AP and lateral plain radiographs of the area of interest. The overall alignment, bony integrity, location of the lesion within the vertebrae, quality of its appearance, and surrounding soft-tissue planes should be assessed. Vertebral body destruction is generally not visible until 30% to 50% of the trabeculae are involved.

Primary tumors tend to be associated with extension into the surrounding soft tissues. Metastatic lesions may have a lytic, blastic, or mixed appearance and are usually confined within the vertebral body. Early metastatic foci are most frequently found at the base of the pedicle; unilateral destruction of a pedicle may be seen on the AP radiograph as the so-called winking owl sign (Figure 1). Malignant tumors, both primary and metastatic, have a predilection for spread into the vertebral body, whereas tumors located in the posterior elements tend to be benign processes.

Plain radiographs have a low sensitivity for detecting early spinal tumors or infection. The usefulness of plain radiographic studies depends on the symptomatology and the tumor of origin. In patients who present with neurologic involvement, 90% will have abnormal plain radiographs, with 70% of lesions occurring in the vertebral body and 10% in the posterior elements. When back pain is the chief presenting symptom, radiographic abnormalities will be present in 94% of patients with breast metastases, 74% of those with lung metastases, and 40% of those with lymphoma. Negative plain radiographs, therefore, do not rule out the possibility of spinal involvement.

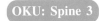 

It is frequently difficult to differentiate diskitis/vertebral osteomyelitis and spinal tumors based solely on plain radiographs. In general, metastatic tumors require a blood supply and will not affect the intervertebral disk. Infectious organisms prefer an avascular environment and after an initial seeding of the end plates will tend to rupture into the disk. These processes can be appreciated radiographically and are useful in the formulation of a differential diagnosis.

### Technetium Tc 99m Bone Scans
Technetium Tc 99m ($^{99m}$Tc) bone scans are used to identify amplified metabolic activity such as osteoblastic activity or areas of increased local blood flow. This test is used to qualify known, isolated lesions and to localize additional asymptomatic or unknown foci. Safe biopsy sites can frequently be determined from lesions seen on bone scans. Because of the sensitivity of $^{99m}$Tc bone scans, bony involvement may be overestimated and differentiation from traumatic, degenerative, or infectious lesions is difficult. Conversely, marrow-replacing tumors (such as multiple myeloma) may go undetected until cortical disruption occurs. A bone scan may remain 'hot' for up to 2 years after the initiation of a process.

### Single Photon Emission Computer-Assisted Tomography
Single photon emission computer-assisted tomography (SPECT) provides a higher resolution and more accurate localization of increased metabolic activity within a specific bone and requires no additional radiation exposure. In this regard, they are ideal for diagnosing benign painful lesions such as osteoid osteoma and osteoblastoma. SPECT more clearly defines pedicle involvement compared with planar bone scans and can lead to earlier recognition of spinal metastases. SPECT scans are more expensive than $^{99m}$Tc bone scans, but they have a higher sensitivity, specificity, positive predictive value, and negative predictive value. They have not been shown to detect pedicle involvement earlier than MRI.

### Positron Emission Tomography
Positron emission tomography (PET) uses fluorodeoxyglucose to define sites of increased metabolic activity. When PET scans and $^{99m}$Tc bone scans were compared for the detection of bone metastases in patients with newly diagnosed lung cancer, the sensitivities were 91% and 75% and the specificities were 96% and 95%, respectively. Another study showed the statistically significant inability of PET scans to differentiate between benign and low-grade malignant cartilage tumors. The higher-grade malignancies could be detected compared with the benign processes, but the low-grade cartilage malignancies were underestimated. Additional experience with PET scans and their usefulness with specific tumor types will be required to define the place of this imaging study in the care of patients with spinal tumors.

### Computed Tomography
CT, with or without intrathecal dye, is an important tool for direct evaluation of the bony architecture of the spine and indirect evaluation of canal compromise. CT is particularly helpful in evaluating vertebral integrity and stability. For example, when more than 50% of a vertebral body is affected along with any involvement of the posterior elements, further collapse is predicted to occur. When an MRI scan cannot be obtained, a CT myelogram is a suitable alternative. CT scanning is particularly useful during preoperative planning when identifying sites of fixation for reconstruction.

### Magnetic Resonance Imaging
MRI is a radiation-free study that should be used to evaluate most spinal tumors to define body and marrow involvement, evaluate paravertebral soft tissues, and assess canal encroachment. The number of protons within a tissue determines the signal that will be produced and interpreted during a pulse sequence. For this reason, MRI is superior to most other modalities with regard to the soft tissues, whereas CT provides better quality bone images. MRI is useful for the diagnosis of spinal tumors and for characterization of the lesion after diagnosis.

MRI may show obvious or subtle differences in pathologic fractures, infections, and benign compression fractures. Imaging of a pathologic fracture is typically isointense on T1-weighted and hyperintense on T2-weighted sequencing and often shows abnormal marrow signal in multiple vertebral bodies. Vertebral osteomyelitis/diskitis is characterized by isointense or hypointense T1-weighted sequencing signal and hyperintense T2-weighted sequencing signal. Soft-tissue abscesses of similar signal intensity are seen in patients with advanced disease, and the end plates are indistinct. Benign compression fractures have a normal marrow signal on T1-weighted sequencing and no soft-tissue mass. The T2-weighted sequencing signal may be isointense or have areas of slightly increased intensity. Metastases appear as areas of diminished signal on T1-weighted sequencing, whereas the surrounding fatty marrow is hyperintense. The addition of gadolinium can help to further delineate involved areas based on the surrounding vascularity.

### Angiography
Angiography is a useful additional study or treatment for the patient with a spinal tumor. However, in the era of CT and MRI, it has a limited role in the diagnosis and evaluation of bone metastases. Certain tumors, such as renal cell and thyroid carcinomas, may require preoperative embolization to reduce intraoperative bleeding. Angiography can define the local vascular anatomy, the blood supply to the spinal cord, or the vascularization of

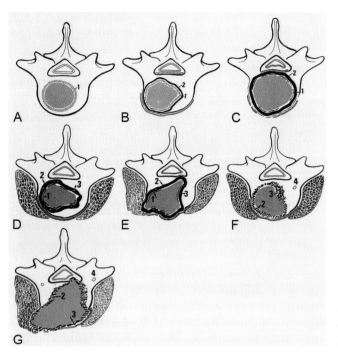

Figure 2    The Enneking staging system. **A,** Stage 1 benign tumor. The tumor is inactive and contained within its capsule (1). **B,** Stage 2 benign tumor. The tumor is growing, and the capsule (1) is thin and bordered by a pseudocapsule of reactive tissue (2). **C,** Stage 3 benign tumor. The aggressiveness of these tumors is evident by the wide reaction of healthy tissue (2), and the capsule (1) is thin and discontinued. **D,** Stage IA malignant tumor. The capsule, if any, is thin (1), and the pseudocapsule (2) is wide and contains an island of tumor (3). **E,** Stage IB malignant tumors. The capsule, if any, is thin (1), and the pseudocapsule (2) is wide and contains an island of tumor (3). The tumoral mass is growing outside the compartment of occurrence. **F,** Stage IIA malignant tumors. The pseudocapsule (2) is infiltrated by tumor (3), and the island of tumor can be found far from the main tumoral mass—the skip metastasis (4). **G,** Stage IIB malignant tumor. The pseudocapsule (2) is infiltrated by tumor (3), which is growing outside the vertebra. An island of tumor can be found far from the main tumoral mass—the skip metastasis (4). *(Reproduced with permission from Boriani S, Weinstein JN, Biagihi R: Spine Update. Primary bone tumors of the spine. Spine 1997;22:1036-1044.)*

the tumor, which can assist in preoperative planning. Angiography is particularly applicable in the cervical spine when the vertebral artery is enveloped by or in close proximity to the tumor.

## Diagnosis and Planning

The combined information provided by a complete history and physical examination, laboratory values, and various imaging modalities allow the physician to formulate a differential diagnosis and determine how to proceed. Before continuing to the next step, it is important to establish whether the lesion is primary or metastatic. Frequently this determination is made from the history, physical, and initial screening examination. When the primary tumor focus remains elusive, further workup should include a CT scan of the chest, abdomen, and pelvis with intravenous and oral contrast, and a mammogram when indicated. A $^{99m}$Tc bone scan can determine the presence of single or multiple lesions. Most primary tumors will be identified by this point, but a biopsy is frequently required.

If the primary diagnosis is still elusive at this point in the workup, the decision on how to proceed with the most appropriate and effective treatment depends on a histologic diagnosis. This strategy holds true for the patient with a remote history of cancer and a long disease-free interval because a second malignancy is not uncommon. The most accessible lesion should be biopsied, based on the imaging studies available, by the surgeon who will perform the definitive surgery. Important considerations for the selected biopsy site include minimal morbidity and the ability to include the biopsy tract with the resection. If the lesion is to be biopsied by a radiologist and a primary tumor of the spine is suspected, the tract can be tattooed to ensure appropriate removal at the time of surgery. CT-guided biopsy is safe, effective, and preferred in most circumstances. Little tissue contamination occurs with this technique, and no delays are required before initiation of chemotherapy or radiation. In some patients, needle biopsy is impossible or fails to yield an accurate diagnosis, necessitating an open biopsy. When benign tumors are suspected, the open biopsy can be the definitive procedure. Prior to completion of the surgical procedure, the initial microbiologic and pathologic results should be reviewed. Meticulous oncologic surgical principles should be observed at all times in the event that the histopathology determines an alternate course of treatment.

Once the diagnosis is firmly established, the appropriate treatment regimen should be initiated. This regimen may include chemotherapeutic and radiation treatments along with further surgical intervention.

## Primary Lesions
### Oncologic Staging

The information required for oncologic staging is obtained while achieving a diagnosis and includes the histopathologic grade, extent of local involvement, and regional or distant metastases. This information is an important part of disease management because it adds to the understanding of the tumor's biology and helps determine the most effective plan of treatment. Classification of patients based on tumor type is critical when determining the efficacy of specific treatment protocols.

The Enneking musculoskeletal staging system is useful for developing evaluation strategies, planning treatment, and predicting prognosis. According to Enneking's original text, the important aspects of a tumor's biology can be categorized as (1) localized, latent or static, inactive, and benign; (2) localized, active, and benign; (3) aggressive, invasive, but still benign; (4) indolent, invasive, malignant, and having a low risk of local, regional, and distant metastases; (5) rapidly destructive, malignant, and having a high risk of local, regional, and distant metastases; and (6) having regional and/or distant metastases. Enneking used one system for benign tumors and another for malignant tumors. Benign tumors are staged using Arabic numerals, whereas the staging of malignant lesions uses Roman numerals. Both systems require knowledge of the histologic grade, the anatomic location (intracompartmental or extracompartmental), and the presence of metastases (Figure 2).

The system and terminology developed by Enneking and the Musculoskeletal Tumor Society for the management of benign and malignant lesions works well for the appendicular skeleton; however, its application to the spine has been less useful because of differences between axial and appendicular anatomy. These limitations carry over to the terminology used for surgical margins required for tumor resection of the extremities. For example, radical resection in the thoracic spine would mean removing structures such as the spinal cord and aorta, which would be of obvious detriment to the patient. This system led to difficulties in the scientific evaluation of various types of spine tumor management.

Another staging system developed by Boriani, Weinstein, and Biagini applies Enneking's principles for classifying stages of tumors to the spine using a practical approach for surgical staging. Each involved vertebral body is divided into 12 segments in a clock face arrangement and into five layers from the paravertebral extraosseous area to dural involvement (Figure 3). Based on the results of the oncologic and surgical staging, one of three en bloc excisions ensues: vertebrectomy, sagittal resection, or resection of the posterior arch. Recent multicenter studies have shown that this system provides a standard with which to plan surgical approaches and evaluate the results of treatment.

### Benign Lesions

Benign primary lesions are much less common than malignant primary lesions. These lesions occur most commonly in the first two decades of life, whereas most lesions occurring after the age of 21 years are malignant. Tumors that occur in the posterior elements are usually benign, whereas those found in the body tend to be malignant. Pain is the most common presenting symptom, whereas neurologic compromise occurs much less frequently than in patients with malignant tumors.

Enneking classification of benign lesions applies to benign spinal tumors. Stage 1 lesions are latent, usually asymptomatic, and are discovered incidentally. Stage 2 lesions are active and usually present with symptoms (most commonly, pain in the area of the lesion). Stage 3 lesions are locally aggressive and can metastasize.

### Osteoid Osteoma

Osteoid osteomas represent 11% of all primary bone tumors and are one of the most common types of primary benign tumors. Patients range in age from the teens to the early 20s. Painful scoliosis or pain that is worse at

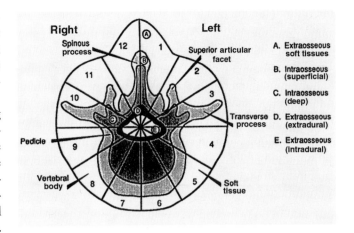

**Figure 3** The Boriani, Weinstein, Biagnini surgical staging system. The transverse extension of the vertebral tumor is described with reference to 12 radiating zones (numbered 1 to 12 in a clockwise order) and to five concentric layers (A to E, from the paravertebral extraosseous compartments to the dural involvement). The longitudinal extent of the tumor is recorded according to the levels involved. *(Reproduced with permission from Hart R, Boriani S, Biagini R, et al: A system for surgical staging and management of spine tumors. Spine 1997;22:1773-1782.)*

night and resolves with the use of nonsteroidal anti-inflammatory drugs should raise suspicion of this diagnosis. The lesions are found in the pedicles, transverse processes, laminae, and spinous processes. The lumbar spine is most frequently affected. Radiographs may show osteosclerosis surrounding a radiolucent nidus less than 2 cm in diameter. CT scans clearly define the lesion and are often required when plain radiographs are normal. An intense area of uptake will be seen on a bone scan and/or a SPECT scan.

The course of osteoid osteoma is typically benign and self-limiting over several years. If the patient's symptoms can be managed with nonsteroidal anti-inflammatory drugs, nonsurgical treatment is acceptable. However, if nonsurgical treatment is unsuccessful, patients require surgical treatment. En bloc excision is curative and provides excellent pain relief. Scoliosis associated with the lesion will resolve spontaneously if the resection is performed within 15 months of the onset of deformity.

### Osteoblastoma

Osteoblastomas are similar to osteoid osteomas in their histology and patient age of incidence but are differentiated based on size and clinical course (Figure 4). Grossly, these lesions are larger than 2 cm and associated pain is not as reliably controlled with anti-inflammatory drugs. Osteoblastomas account for 5% of all primary bone tumors, with approximately 40% found in the spine. As with osteoid osteoma, pain is the most frequently reported symptom, but unlike osteoid osteoma, neurologic compromise can occur as a result of neural impingement because associated soft-tissue involvement is common. Plain radiographs show an expansile, lytic lesion extending into the surrounding soft

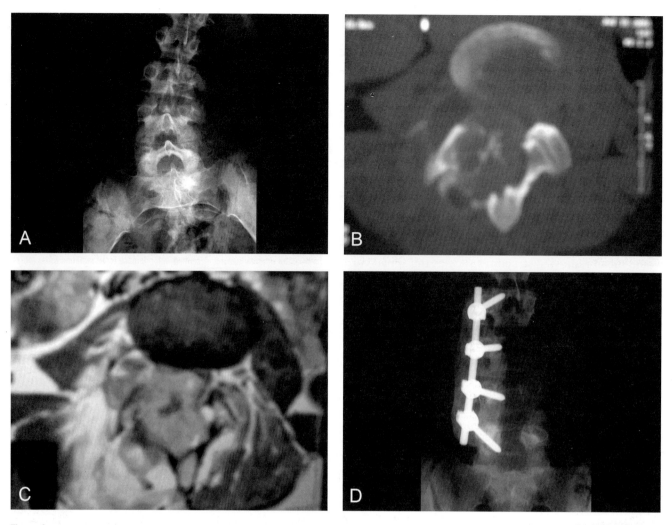

Figure 4  An AP radiograph (A), CT scan (B), and axial MRI scan (C) of the lumbosacral spine showing an osteoblastoma of the posterior elements of L3-4. D, AP radiograph after complete excision and unilateral reconstruction showing a solid fusion.

tissues. No septations are visualized within the lytic portion, which distinguishes it from an aneurysmal bone cyst. Treatment generally consists of a complete surgical excision, which achieves good local control with recurrences estimated at 10%. Radiation therapy is controversial, but has been successful used in patients with incomplete resection and recurrence.

*Aneurysmal Bone Cyst*
Aneurysmal bone cysts account for 1.4% of all primary bone tumors and approximately 20% occur in the spine (Figure 5). Peak incidence occurs in the second decade of life; these cysts are rare in patients older than 30 years. The most common location is the posterior elements of the cervical and thoracic spine, and males are affected more frequently than females. Most patients report pain and/or neurologic deficits resulting from nerve root or spinal cord compression. Larger lesions may be palpable in thin patients. Radiographs show an expansile, lytic lesion with a thin shell of reactive bone. Fine

bony septations give the lesion a soap-bubble appearance. MRI reveals fluid-fluid levels. Up to 40% of aneurysmal bone cysts will involve adjacent levels of the spine. Angiography and embolization can be used as a treatment or as a preoperative adjunct to minimize intraoperative blood loss. Surgical treatment includes intralesional curettage or excision. Recurrence is common, with rates as high as 25%. Radiation treatment has been described; however, there is a risk of late sarcomatous degeneration.

*Osteochondroma*
Osteochondromas are also known as osteocartilaginous exostoses and are the most common bone tumor, accounting for 20% to 50% of benign bone tumors and 15% of all bone tumors. The posterior elements of the cervicothoracic spine are the most frequent location for these tumors. These tumors do no represent true neoplasms, but rather a herniation of perichondrium. Osteochondromas are either diagnosed incidentally, can cause

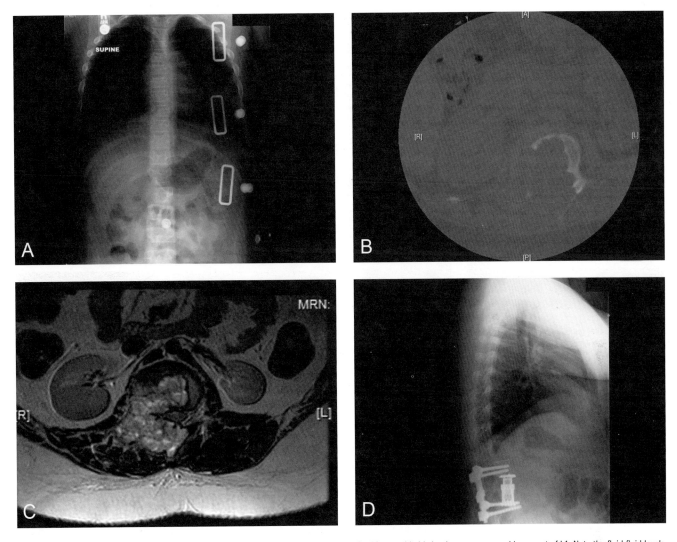

**Figure 5** An AP radiograph **(A)**, CT scan **(B)**, and MRI scan **(C)** of the thoracolumbar spine of a 10-year-old girl showing an aneurysmal bone cyst of L1. Note the fluid-fluid levels on the MRI scan. **D,** Lateral radiograph showing anterior reconstruction and posterior stabilization after curettage.

neurologic symptoms, or the patient may report a mass. Pain is an infrequent symptom and is associated with mass effect or malignant degeneration. Plain radiographs show a sessile or pedunculated mass, but are inadequate to evaluate the cartilage cap; therefore, a CT or MRI scan may be needed. Cartilage caps larger than 2 cm and enlarging lesions are prognostic signs of malignant degeneration. Persistently painful lesions or those causing neurologic symptoms can be excised, but asymptomatic lesions require no treatment. The risk of recurrence is low in children and is negligible in adults if the entire cartilage cap is excised. The risk of malignant degeneration to a chondrosarcoma may be as high as 25% to 30% in multiple hereditary exostoses; however, a solitary lesion carries a risk of about 1%.

### Neurofibroma
Neurofibromas of the spine can occur in isolation or in association with neurofibromatosis type I (von Reck-

linghausen disease) or type II and should be suspected when specific phenotypic traits (such as café au lait spots, cutaneous neurofibromas, and acoustic neuromas) are present. These lesions tend to arise from the nerve root sheath, with approximately 80% existing intradurally and in the immediate extradural space (Figure 6). When occurring within the neural foramen, they have a classic dumbbell shape.

Radiographically, sharp angular scoliosis, rib thinning, and enlarged neuroforamina may be seen. MRI and/or CT with myelography should be used to fully characterize the lesion. Symptomatic lesions should be excised en bloc when involved with noncritical structures. Otherwise, microsurgical procedures should be used to preserve uninvolved nerve fascicles. Malignant degeneration occurs in 20% of these lesions. Associated scoliosis should be treated aggressively because rapid curve progression occurs without treatment.

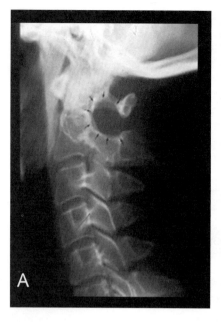 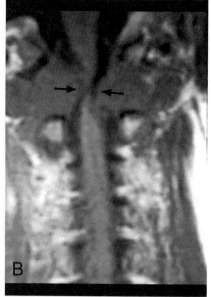 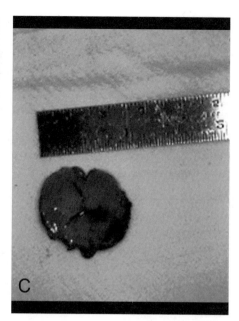

Figure 6 **A,** Lateral radiograph of the cervical spine showing enlargement of the C1-2 neural foramen by a neurofibroma. **B,** Coronal MRI scan showing compression of the upper cervical spinal cord. **C,** A gross specimen is shown.

### Giant Cell Tumors

Giant cell tumors account for up to 8% of all bone tumors, of which 3% occur in the spine. Patients are usually in the third to fifth decade of life, and females are affected twice as often as males. Any portion of the spine may be affected, but the sacrum is the most frequently affected area. The patient most commonly reports pain in the region of the tumor. Giant cell tumors have a predilection for the vertebral body rather than the posterior elements. They are usually benign but are locally aggressive tumors. Radiographically, these lesions are lytic and expansile in nature without septations. A variable amount of reactive bone is seen surrounding the lesion, and they are frequently associated with a soft-tissue mass. Preoperative embolization can minimize intraoperative blood loss. Successful surgical treatment requires complete excision, which can be complicated by the vital structures surrounding the spine. Adjuvant treatments include intralesional liquid nitrogen, phenol, and methylmethacrylate. Recurrence rates are reported to be as high as 40%; reexcision is required in these situations. Radiation therapy can be used with unresectable tumors; however, it is associated with a 15% risk of malignant degeneration. Metastases to the lungs occur in up to 3% of patients and follow a variable course.

### Eosinophilic Granuloma

Eosinophilic granuloma is also known as Langerhans' cell histiocytosis and is a member of a class of disorders that affects the reticuloendothelial system (Figure 7). These lesions tend to occur in patients who are younger than 10 years, are usually solitary, and affect the vertebral body, most commonly in the thoracic spine. The patient reports pain, and vertebra plana are seen on plain radiographs. Although probably unnecessary, bone scans are 'cold', and MRI reveals a flare that can be mistaken for malignancy. Immobilization and observation are usually sufficient because most of these lesions spontaneously regress and nearly complete reconstitution (72% to 97%) of vertebral body height occurs. Surgical indications include persistent pain or instability; however, surgery is rarely required. Low-dose radiation therapy has been used to treat patients with neurologic compromise.

### Hemangioma

The exact incidence of hemangiomas is unknown, but these lesions are seen in at least 12% of normal MRI scans. Most hemangiomas are clinically silent and are noted as incidental findings during studies performed for other reasons. Larger lesions can lead to pathologic fractures or can lead to cord compression. Pregnancy can induce symptoms in patients with previously asymptomatic lesions, and embolization may be required in severe cases. Radiographs are normal when small lesions are present, but may show coarse vertical striations (resembling corduroy) in larger lesions. Occasionally, hemangiomas are confused with Paget's disease, but the vertebral body enlargement typical of Paget's disease is not a characteristic of this entity. Coarse speckled trabeculae are seen on CT scans, sometimes referred to as a polka dot pattern. The findings on MRI scans are diagnostic; the lesions are hyperintense on T1- and T2-weighted MRI scans. Most patients do not require treatment. Surgical resection and reconstruction may be necessary in the presence of impending or actual pathologic fracture, impending or actual neurologic compromise, and/or persis-

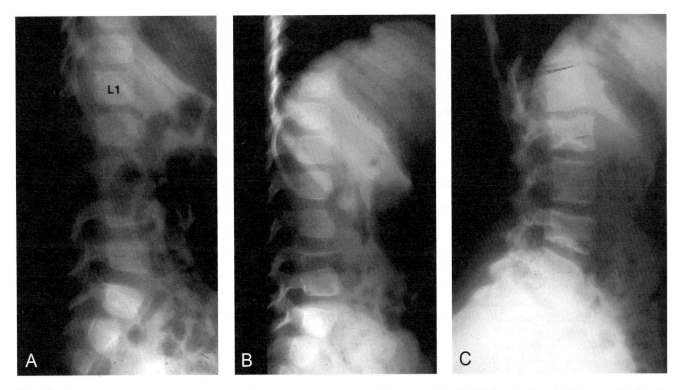

**Figure 7** **A,** Lateral radiograph of the lumbar spine in a young female with back pain. Note the disk space narrowing of L3-4. **B,** Lateral radiograph of the same patient 2 weeks later when she presented with an acute increase in pain. **C,** Radiograph taken 10 years after the initial fracture showing nearly complete reconstitution of vertebral body height.

tent pain. Embolization and/or radiation therapy can be used for a painful lesion without other indications for surgical intervention.

## Malignant Lesions

### Multiple Myeloma

The most common primary malignancy of bone is multiple myeloma. Most physicians believe that this lesion exists with solitary plasmacytoma on a spectrum of malignant B cell lines responsible for local destruction and aberrant immunoglobulin production. The incidence of multiple myeloma is estimated at 2.5 instances per 100,000 people. It occurs in older patients, most frequently in the seventh decade of life, and occurs twice as frequently in blacks as in whites. Approximately 75% of patients initially seek medical care for evaluation of a painful process, whereas approximately 20% present with a neurologic complaint. Frequently, the first sign of the disease will be a painful vertebral compression fracture. Continuous pain that is unrelenting and/or worse at night should raise the suspicion of a malignant process. A laboratory evaluation will reveal anemia, thrombocytopenia, hyperproteinemia, hypoalbuminemia, and an elevated erythrocyte sedimentation rate. A monoclonal gammopathy will be seen when serum and urine protein electrophoreses are performed; however, in 20% of patients, only the urine protein electrophoreses will be abnormal.

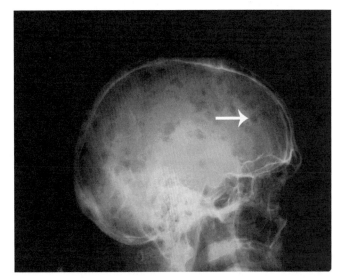

**Figure 8** Lateral skull radiograph showing classic punched-out lesions (*arrow*) in a multiple myeloma patient.

Initially, plain radiographs may be normal. When more than 30% of the vertebral body is involved, lytic lesions will become evident. A characteristic finding is multiple punched out lesions on a lateral skull radiograph (Figure 8). Compression fractures resulting from multiple myeloma can be difficult to differentiate from those resulting from osteoporosis based simply on radiographic findings; further testing should be guided by

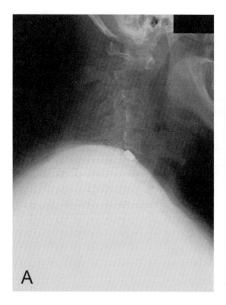 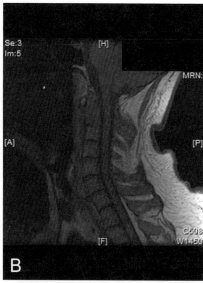 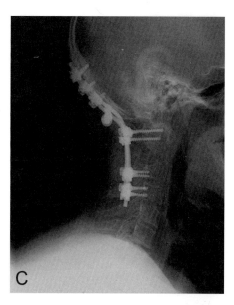

Figure 9  A lateral radiograph **(A)**, T1-weighted MRI scan **(B)**, and postoperative lateral radiograph **(C)** of a 62-year-old man who presented with an acute onset of pain after the tailgate of his truck struck the back of his head. The patient was diagnosed with a solitary plasmacytoma and underwent an occipitocervical fusion.

the patient's history and physical examination findings. CT scans are used to quantify the extent of vertebral body involvement and assess extension into the pedicles. Bone scans are routinely 'cold' as a result of a lack of bony reaction to the process. MRI will typically show diffuse marrow involvement at multiple levels with or without canal invasion.

Multiple myeloma is an exquisitely radiosensitive tumor; therefore, radiotherapy and pharmacologic pain management are the mainstays of treatment of spinal lesions. Chemotherapy is used to treat the systemic component. Bracing is indicated for lesions with less than 50% vertebral body involvement. Surgery is indicated in patients with impending or actual functionally significant neurologic compromise, in those with impending or actual pathologic fracture if a structural instability exists that is likely to persist after radiation therapy, and/or in patients with intractable pain despite radiation therapy. Surgery consists of posterior segmental instrumentation for lesions with suspected impending fracture. Anterior procedures may be indicated in patients with fracture, kyphosis, or neurologic involvement.

The clinical course is generally progressive and lethal, with an approximate 20% survival at 5 years. Patients who have neurologic involvement have a 75% rate of mortality at 1 year.

### Solitary Plasmacytoma

Solitary plasmacytomas are by definition isolated plasma cell lesions that affect a single vertebral body (Figure 9). These lesions account for only 3% of all plasma cell neoplasms and 50% of affected patients will develop multiple myeloma in their lifetime (usually within 3 to 4 years). The peak incidence of these lesions

occurs in the fifth to sixth decade of life, which is earlier than in patients with multiple myeloma. Most patients will present for evaluation of back pain, with or without a vertebral compression fracture. Because abnormal plasma protein levels are related to the total tumor mass, protein electrophoreses are usually normal. Radiographic abnormalities tend to appear as either advanced lytic areas, similar to those seen in multiple myeloma, or will appear as a straightforward compression fracture. Early on, however, radiographs are often normal. An apparent solitary plasmacytoma should stimulate an evaluation of the entire spine with MRI to rule out radiographically occult lesions. The diagnosis is confirmed with a biopsy. Histologically, solitary plasmacytoma may be confused with chronic osteomyelitis because of the abundance of plasma cells. Plasmacytoma cells, however, will produce monoclonal kappa or lambda light chains, whereas the plasma cells of chronic osteomyelitis will be polyclonal. As with multiple myeloma, plasmacytomas are highly sensitive to radiotherapy, making this modality the cornerstone of treatment. Surgery is indicated in rare instances for the same circumstances as in patients with multiple myeloma. There is a 10% incidence of local recurrence. The long-term prognosis is better than with multiple myeloma, but widespread dissemination may occur at any time; therefore, follow-up is indefinite. Serum protein electrophoresis is the most sensitive screening tool and is used to follow these patients. Chemotherapy is instituted when dissemination occurs.

### Osteosarcoma

Osteosarcoma is the second most common primary tumor of bone, and spinal involvement is rare, accounting for 3% of all osteosarcomas. It most frequently affects patients in their second decade of life; however, there is a second peak in the sixth decade. There is a slight preponderance of this lesion in males; no racial predilections have been observed. Osteosarcomas are more common in patients who are retinoblastoma gene carriers, in those with Rothmund-Thomson syndrome, or in those with Li-Fraumeni syndrome. Patients with a history of Paget's disease or prior radiation also have a higher risk for this lesion. Most patients present with a report of pain, with or without minor antecedent trauma. Night pain will be present in approximately 25% of patients, and up to 70% will have neurologic symptoms. Radiographically, a lytic, blastic, or mixed lesion with an ossifying matrix affects the vertebral body. Additional staging studies should include a whole body bone scan, CT of the chest, and MRI and CT of the lesion.

The biopsy is planned and/or performed by the surgeon who will perform the definitive procedure to ensure that the tract can be included with the final resection. Once the diagnosis is established, two cycles of neoadjuvant chemotherapy are administered. The resection proceeds in accordance with the principles of musculoskeletal surgical oncology. The margins of the resection must be carefully considered based on the preoperative studies and intraoperative findings, with careful attention given to the proximity of critical neurovascular structures. Every effort should be made to remove the tumor en bloc with a clear margin. It is well established that a resection with positive margins dramatically increases the rate of local recurrence. If the end plates are intact, the mass is removed with the disks above and below. Extension of the resection into surrounding vertebral bodies is based on preoperative evaluation so that contamination of the wound bed does not occur through inadvertent violation of the tumor. Anteriorly, the margin of resection should extend beyond the periosteum that can act as a barrier to local invasion and prevent disruption of the tumor while protecting the aorta and vena cava. Where possible, the posterior margin of the resection will be the posterior longitudinal ligament because this structure is frequently respected by sarcomas. Extension into the posterior elements may necessitate an en bloc spondylectomy. Lesions that only involve the posterior elements are less technically challenging to resect because the paraspinous muscles are used as the margin of resection. Anterior reconstruction of these lesions can be performed by a variety of implants, but most surgeons use a cage and/or allograft bone. A 6-week delay is allowed for initial bone healing before radiation or chemotherapy. Posterior stabilization is frequently required and generally consists of rod and screw constructs.

The percent of tumor kill, as determined by the pathologist, quantifies the response of the tumor to the neoadjuvant chemotherapy. A 90% tumor kill portends a 5-year survival rate of 85%, whereas a tumor kill of less than 90% indicates a 25% survival rate. The histopathologic specimen taken at resection determines the postoperative chemotherapy regimen. If the tumor kill is adequate, four cycles of the same preoperative agents are used. If, however, the response was inadequate, the regimen is altered to second-line agents.

Patients with a spinal osteosarcoma have a much poorer prognosis than those with an isolated extremity sarcoma. The prognosis for these patients has been improving steadily with the addition of new surgical and chemotherapeutic advances. The most optimistic mean survival has been reported to be 52 months for a primary spinal osteosarcoma, whereas the 5-year survival for secondary tumors is as low as 5%.

### Ewing's Sarcoma
Ewing's sarcoma is the most common primary malignancy of childhood, with a 75% incidence before 20 years of age and 90% of these lesions occurring before the age of 30 years. It is an exceedingly rare tumor in black and Asian populations. Patients with Ewing's sarcoma consistently have a translocation of chromosomes 11 and 22. Approximately 8% of Ewing's tumors occur in the spine, with the sacrum being the most common primary focus. Pain is a nearly universal symptom along with constitutional symptoms such as fever and malaise. Night pain was not a common symptom in a recent Swedish study in which the delay in diagnosis averaged 19 weeks. Palpable masses may be found on physical examination, and the laboratory evaluation reveals an elevated erythrocyte sedimentation rate. Neurologic deficits are reported to occur in as many as 83% of patients. Radiographic studies reveal a lytic, permeative process. This lesion may be confused with eosinophilic granuloma when pathologic fracture has resulted in a vertebra plana. Disk spaces are generally preserved until late in the disease. Plain radiographs are inadequate to make a diagnosis, and a CT-guided biopsy is commonly used to obtain a tissue diagnosis. Gadolinium-enhanced MRI is an excellent choice for evaluation of this tumor because of the almost universal presence of a soft-tissue extension. Bone scintigraphy is used for skeletal assessment, and a CT of the chest is required for evaluation of the lungs. Chemotherapy and radiation are effective for treating these tumors and are the mainstays of treatment. When there is actual or impending spinal instability or neurologic deficit, surgical resection and reconstruction are indicated. When possible, surgical intervention is delayed until a round of chemotherapy has been administered. This method allows the tumor to shrink and facilitates subsequent resection. It is often impossible to achieve a wide margin, resulting in intralesional curettage and violating the principles of musculoskeletal sarcoma surgery. If the margins remain positive, postoperative radiation therapy is recom-

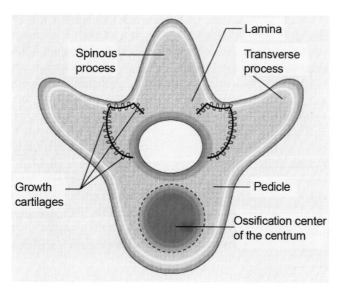

**Figure 10** Three cartilaginous growth centers of the vertebral body are shown. *(Reproduced with permission from Abeloff (ed): Clinical Oncology, ed 3. Churchill Livingstone, 2004, p 2542.)*

mended. The 5-year survival rate for all patients is estimated to be 50% to 60%, with a better prognosis for patients with tumors below the elbow and below the midcalf. Metastatic tumors have a poorer prognosis with a 25% survival rate at 5 years.

### Chondrosarcoma

Although chondrosarcomas are the second most common primary malignant tumor in adults, only 7% to 10% of chondrosarcomas are found in the spine. Unlike most other malignant spinal tumors, chondrosarcomas can originate in the anterior or posterior elements because there are three growth centers in each vertebral body from which the tumors originate (Figure 10). Nearly all patients present with a report of pain, and about half have neurologic symptoms. A new report of pain in a patient with a previously asymptomatic enchondroma or osteochondroma should heighten suspicion of malignant transformation. Radiographically, a poorly marginated, lytic lesion with stippled calcifications is seen. The true size of the lesion is often underestimated as the cartilage cap is poorly visualized. At least 90% of chondrosarcomas have associated soft-tissue masses; therefore, CT and MRI are both beneficial studies for characterizing the mass. Chemotherapy and radiation are generally not effective; thus, surgical extirpation is required, and outcomes are based on the margins achieved. The principles of en bloc excision and reconstruction are similar to those described previously for osteosarcoma.

### Chordoma

Chordomas are rare tumors accounting for 2% to 4% of all primary malignant bone tumors (Figure 11). With the exception of the lymphoproliferative disorders, they are the most common primary malignant spinal tumor in adults. They can occur at any time, but are most frequently seen in patients in the fifth and sixth decades of life. Remnants of the primitive notochord give rise to chordomas; therefore, they are found in the midline. The sacrum and coccyx are favored sites; however, chordomas have been described throughout the spine exclusive of the intervertebral disk. Males are affected three times more often than females. Slow, relentless growth characterizes these lesions, resulting in a gradual onset of symptoms that may initially be disregarded by the patient and/or the physician and is often the reason for a delay in the diagnosis. Patients frequently report pain, numbness, motor weakness, and constipation or incontinence.

Sacrococcygeal lesions are generally large and are readily palpable via a digital rectal examination. Plain radiographs show a lytic or mixed lytic/blastic picture, whereas CT and MRI clearly delineate the degree of bony destruction and soft-tissue extension. Of critical importance is a thorough evaluation of the involvement of surrounding structures. Sacrococcygeal lesions frequently involve the dura, roots, rectum, and local vessels, and necessitate the involvement of a team of surgeons for complete resection. Chordomas are highly resistant to radiation and chemotherapy. Radiation therapy, proton beam therapy, and brachytherapy have all been tried with few promising results. Anterior and posterior approaches are frequently required for lesions above S3. When possible, leaving S1 intact will provide stability to the pelvic girdle. Unilateral retention of all roots can provide near-normal bowel, bladder, and sexual function. Sacrificing the S2 nerve roots will render the patient incontinent. Sexual dysfunction also is a common complication of the resection, and these issues should be discussed with the patient early in the course of treatment. Reconstruction of sacral and lumbosacral defects created by the resection is often challenging and may require some creativity to establish a stable connection between the lumbar spine and the pelvis. En bloc excision is the rule, and survival is directly related to the quality of the margins achieved. Sacrococcygeal lesions portend a fair prognosis, with patients surviving an average of 8 to 10 years, whereas the survival rate for chordomas at other sites is 4 to 5 years. Metastases can occur and are found in the liver, lungs, regional lymph nodes, peritoneum, skin, and heart.

## Metastatic Disease

Metastatic tumors are by far the most common tumor found in the spine. The spine is the most frequent site of bony metastasis. Metastatic tumors are found in 40% to 80% of patients who die of cancer. Of patients with spinal metastases, up to 20% will develop neural compromise. As many as 75% of all bony metastases occur in

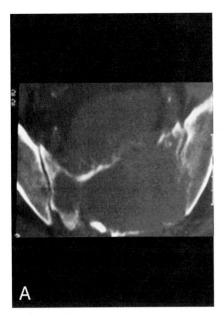 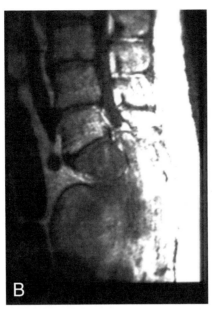 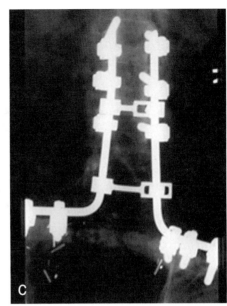

Figure 11 A CT scan **(A)**, MRI scan **(B)**, and radiograph **(C)** of a patient with a sacral chordoma that required total sacrectomy and iliolumbar reconstruction.

patients with carcinoma of the breast, lung, kidney, prostate, thyroid, and multiple myeloma.

The vertebral body is initially affected, whereas the disks are spared because of their relative hypovascularity. Several hypotheses have been proposed to explain the propensity of metastases to spinal foci. It is believed that tumor cells enter the bloodstream and come to rest in the filters of the vascular tree—the capillary beds of the liver, lungs, and bone marrow. They establish a foothold in the medullary sinusoids by a variety of direct and indirect routes. Batson's venous plexus is another potential direct route of spinal metastasis from the paired midline organs via retrograde venous flow. The contribution of this system to spinal metastases has been debated, and a variety of laboratory investigations directed at proving or disproving this theory have been performed without any definitive conclusions.

Patients who have spinal metastases generally can be categorized into one of two groups. The first group includes patients who have a known history of cancer or radiation therapy and develop new back pain. This group is assumed to have a spinal metastasis until proved otherwise. A thorough history related to the onset of pain, temporal factors, and any change in the use of pain medications will provide important information that will help guide further evaluation. The timing of onset of associated neural compromise has prognostic implications and will determine the urgency of any intervention. In the second group, metastatic lesions are found incidentally when the patient without a history of cancer or radiation exposure undergoes an evaluation. These patients may or may not have symptoms referable to the metastatic focus.

In these two groups, radiographs will show evidence of metastases if more than 30% to 50% of the vertebrae have been affected. All patients with a known history of cancer and new onset and/or focal back pain and patients with no history of cancer and symptoms lasting 6 weeks or more who have not responded to reasonable nonsurgical management should undergo plain radiographic imaging that centers on the area of interest. When plain radiographs show obvious destruction, CT and MRI will show the amount of vertebral body involvement and any neural structures at risk. CT-based predictors of stability were previously discussed and are useful in the planning stages of treatment. In a cancer patient who has normal radiographs, MRI should be obtained to localize or rule out new metastases. When there is no history of cancer or the known history is remote, staging should ensue. A bone scan; CT of the chest, abdomen and pelvis; and appropriate laboratory studies will accurately define the extent of the disease and guide further testing and treatment.

Patients with pain, nonprogressive neurologic involvement, and no suggestion of instability are candidates for medical and/or radiation therapy. Radiation therapy is effective in treating pain and neural element compression related to metastatic disease secondary to specific radiosensitive tumors. The timing of radiation therapy must be carefully considered when it is to be combined with surgical intervention. Animal studies suggest that radiation therapy should not be instituted until at least 3 weeks after surgery to improve the likelihood of a successful fusion. Many authors have shown that the rate of complications in patients who have preoperative or immediate postoperative radiotherapy is significantly higher. These complications include wound dehiscence, wound infection, and hardware failure.

Tremendous advances in radiation therapy have been made in recent years that have led to increased safety and improved local control of tumoral foci while minimizing the radiation dose to the spinal cord. Stereotactic radiosurgery, commonly known as the CyberKnife (Accuray, Sunnyvale, CA), holds significant promise for treating metastatic spinal tumors in medically inoperable patients, those with previously irradiated sites, and in those who are not amenable to open surgical techniques. Fiducials (small, gold, radiodense markers placed around the tumor for localization) are inserted under image intensification and local anesthesia 2 to 4 days before initiation of treatment. A CT scan is used by the surgeon to carefully outline the tumor and surrounding structures while the patient's body position is carefully maintained. Consultation between the surgeon and the radiation oncologist optimizes and finalizes the treatment plan. Outcome studies with significant power are currently lacking, but the early results are promising.

The Tokuhashi scoring system for patients with metastatic spinal tumors provides a method to guide treatment based on prognosis. Six parameters are used in this system and include (1) the patient's general condition, (2) the number of extraspinal bone metastases, (3) the number of vertebral body metastases, (4) the number of metastases to major visceral organs, (5) the primary cancer focus, and (6) and the presence of spinal cord palsy. Within each parameter, a score of 0 to 3 is given. Excisional procedures are indicated for patients with scores of 9 or greater, whereas a score of less than 5 is an indication for palliative methods. A 1997 study showed that with few exceptions, this scoring system was an excellent prognostic tool. The patients in the study with a score of 7 or less had an average survival of only 5.3 months, whereas patients with a score of 8 or more had an average survival of 23.6 months. Many authors suggest that a mean survival of approximately 3 months is a contraindication to aggressive surgical intervention.

Patients with a neurologic deficit resulting from metastatic disease present a special challenge. The timing of onset of the deficit is extremely important as has been shown in several studies. Rapid onset and complete paraplegia or dense anterior cord syndrome are poor prognostic signs because they suggest a vascular insult to the spinal cord. A more insidious onset of paraplegia resulting from epidural tumoral compression portends a more favorable prognosis. Any patient with a neural compression should undergo MRI of the entire spine to rule out multifocal compression. Up to one third of neurologic deficits are caused by multiple lesions, and the treatment of these patients may be less aggressive because their average period of survival is considerably shorter.

Patients with neurologic deficits who are not candidates for surgery or those with radiosensitive tumors can benefit from radiotherapy. Multiple myeloma and lymphoma are exquisitely radiosensitive, and the patient can have a rapid recovery of neurologic function when treated with radiation. Tumors such as renal cell, breast, prostate, and lung carcinoma respond less reliably. Intravenous dexamethasone administration to this group of patients has been shown to slow the progression of neurologic compromise by relieving spinal cord edema. Dosing regimens are variable, with initial boluses ranging from 10 to 100 mg followed by intermittent doses ranging from 12 to 96 mg on a daily to four times per day schedule. Most studies do not show added neurologic benefit from the higher dose regimens, and the associated complication rates are greater.

Surgery for patients with metastatic disease and a neurologic deficit can be controversial because several older studies comparing surgery with radiation suggest that outcomes are no better after surgery. These studies, however, focus on posterior procedures alone. As previously noted, most metastatic lesions occur anteriorly and laterally, whereas only 10% of metastases that cause neural compression arise from the posterior elements. Many studies have clearly demonstrated that anterior pathology is more reliably addressed by anterior procedures and that outcomes are clearly improved by this approach. Historically, the literature related to radiation therapy alone reported an average success rate of 73% (with success defined as retaining or regaining ambulatory status) and a rescue rate of approximately 30% (defined as those patients who regained ambulatory status). More recently, various studies have shown an average success rate of 85% and a rescue rate of 60%. One recent study clearly demonstrated the superiority of combining direct decompression and adjuvant radiation compared with radiation alone. Both groups were treated with the same steroid protocol and received the same total dose of radiation. Patients treated with surgery retained ambulatory and sphincter function significantly longer than patients in the radiation group. Additionally, 56% of nonambulators in the surgical group regained the ability to walk compared with 19% in the radiation group. As expected, length of survival was not significantly different between the two groups.

Percutaneous vertebroplasty and kyphoplasty are relatively new methods available for the treatment of painful vertebral body fractures resulting from metastases. Under fluoroscopic guidance, a trocar is introduced using a transpedicular or extrapedicular approach into the vertebral body, a biopsy is taken if required, and polymethylmethacrylate is injected. This procedure provides immediate stability, and pain relief can be dramatic. The minimally invasive nature of this procedure is attractive because no delay is required before institution of a chemotherapeutic or radiation regimen. Complication rates are as high as 10% (with 2% to 3% being clinically significant) and include cement extrusion into the foramen or spinal canal resulting in neurologic dysfunction and embolic events. A recent cadaveric study compared intravertebral pressures during vertebroplasty in normal and simulated metastatic vertebral bodies. Pressures in the metastatic vertebrae were significantly higher and were directly related to the amount of cement injected.

Advances in identifying metastatic disease have led to an increase in the diagnosis of solitary spinal metastases. In patients with a low tumor burden, biologically favorable tumors, and suitable general condition, the potential for long-term survival exists when these lesions are treated aggressively. Using the Tomita scoring system, which considers the grade of the malignancy, extent of metastatic disease, and extent of bone metastases, candidates for total vertebrectomy can be identified. The Boriani, Weinstein, and Biagini staging system is used for staging solitary spinal metastases, for surgical planning, and for comparison of surgical outcomes. A series of patients who underwent en bloc corpectomy experienced fewer local recurrences than those who had gross resection of the tumor alone. When used on appropriately selected patients by experienced surgeons, this technique provides significantly better neurologic outcome, pain relief, and local oncologic control than radiation with or without intralesional techniques.

## Summary

When treating a patient with a metastatic lesion of the spine, a tremendous amount of information must be acquired and presented to the patient and family. A realistic prognosis, goals of treatment, and potential outcomes should be clearly explained to allow a well informed decision to be reached. The treating surgeon should be well versed in the principles of conservative and aggressive management of these lesions and the oncologic principles that apply. Ultimately, the goals of treatment are enhanced quality of life, comfort, and continued independence of the patient.

## Annotated Bibliography

Cheran SK: Comparison of whole-body FDG-PET to bone scan for detection of bone metastases in patients with a new diagnosis of lung cancer. *Lung Cancer* 2004; 44:317-325.

The purpose of this study was to compare the accuracy and agreement of whole-body PET with bone scintigraphy for the detection of bony metastases in staging patients with newly diagnosed lung cancer. The accuracy of PET compared with bone scintigraphy was 94% and 85% ($P < 0.005$), sensitivity values were 91% and 75%, and specificity values were 96% and 95%, respectively. The authors concluded that the infor-

mation provided by the studies is redundant and that bone scanning should be eliminated from the workup at initial presentation.

Francis FY, Yu J, Chang SS, Fawwaz R, Parisien MV: Diagnostic value and limitations of fluorine-18 fluorodeoxyglucose positron emission tomography for cartilaginous tumors of bone. *J Bone Joint Surg Am* 2004;86:2677-2685.

The biologic activity of cartilaginous tumor measured by fluorodeoxyglucose PET scans was compared with the histopathologic grade to determine the prognostic capabilities of the scan. The authors concluded that PET scanning differentiated between high- and low-grade chondrosarcomas, but should not be used as a stand-alone test to rule out the presence of malignancy.

Gerszten PC, Germanwala A, Burton SA, Welch WC, Ozhasoglu C, Vogel WJ: Combination kyphoplasty and spinal radiosurgery: A new treatment paradigm for pathological fractures. *Neurosurg Focus* 2005;18:e8.

Twenty-six patients with painful vertebral compression fractures and no neurologic compromise secondary to metastatic disease underwent transpedicular kyphoplasty with placement of fiducial markers to allow image guidance for stereotactic radiosurgery. Patients then underwent single-fraction radiosurgery. This technique was found to be safe and clinically effective for patients with pathologic fractures without significant spinal canal compromise.

Masala S, Cesaroni A, Sergiacomi G, et al: Percutaneous kyphoplasty: New treatment for painful vertebral body fractures. *In Vivo* 2004;18:149-153.

Painful vertebral compression fractures were treated with percutaneous vertebroplasty. Excellent relief of symptoms was achieved, and no complications were noted. The authors determined that kyphoplasty was an effective, alternative, simple, and safe treatment for patients with vertebral collapse consequent to osteoporosis, aggressive hemangiomas, myelomas, and metastases.

Patchell R, Tibbs P, Regine W: A randomized trial of direct decompressive surgical resection in the treatment of spinal cord compression caused by metastasis. *J Clin Oncol* 2003;21:237s.

In this study, 101 patients with spinal metastases and neural compression were randomized into two groups to determine whether surgery and radiation or radiation alone provided a better outcome. Patients in the group treated with surgery and radiation maintained the ability to walk for a significantly longer period. Continence as well as American Spinal Injury Association and Frankel scores were significantly greater in the group treated with surgery. Length of survival was not significantly different, but a trend toward longer survival was found in the surgery group.

Reidy D, Ahn H, Mousavi P, Finkelstein J, Whyne C: A biomechanical analysis of intravertebral pressures during vertebroplasty of cadaveric spines with and without simulated metastases. *Spine* 2003;28:1534-1539.

Vertebroplasty was performed on normal and simulated metastatic cadaveric spines while pressures were recorded. Significantly higher intravertebral pressures were generated in the metastatic spines, and pressures generated were directly related to the amount of cement injected. The authors suggested that these pressures were sufficient to cause embolic phenomena.

Schoeggl A, Reddy M, Matula C: Neurological outcome following laminectomy in spinal metastases. *Spinal Cord* 2002;40:363-366.

Eighty-four patients with metastases to the vertebral column were treated with decompressive laminectomy alone. All preoperative ambulatory patients retained the ability to walk, whereas an additional 25% of patients regained mobility.

Tomita K, Kawahara N, Kobayashi T, Yoshida A, Murakami H, Akamaru T: Surgical strategy for spinal metastases. *Spine* 2001;26:298-306.

The authors present a new surgical strategy using a scoring system for the stratification and treatment of patients with spinal metastatic disease that considers the grade of the malignancy and visceral and bone metastases. Treatment is then recommended based on the patients score. The system guides selection of surgical procedures and provides prognostic information for individual patients.

Yao KC, Boriani S, Gokaslan ZL, Sundaresan N: En bloc spondylectomy for spinal metastases: A review of techniques. *Neurosurg Focus* 2003;15:1-6.

A series of patients with spinal metastases who were treated with en bloc spondylectomy were reviewed. The rationale for treatment, indications, and outcomes were critically analyzed. The authors provide a guideline for appropriate management of this patient population based on the Boriani, Weinstein, and Biagini surgical staging system.

## Classic Bibliography

Boriani S, Biagini R, De lure F, et al: En bloc resections of bone tumors of the thoracolumbar spine: A preliminary report on 29 patients. *Spine* 1996;21:1927-1931.

Boriani S, Weinstein JN, Biagini R: Primary bone tumors of the spine: Terminology and surgical staging. *Spine* 1997;22:1036-1044.

Bouchard JA, Koka A, Bensusan JS, Stevenson S, Emery SE: Effects of irradiation on posterior spinal fusions: A rabbit model. *Spine* 1994;19:1836-1841.

Byrne TN: Metastatic epidural spinal cord compression: Diagnosis and treatment. *N Engl J Med* 1992;327:614-619.

Chamberlain MC, Kormanik PA: Epidural spinal cord compression: A single institution's retrospective experience. *Neuro-oncol* 1999;1:120-123.

Constans JP, de Divitiis E, Donzelli R, Spaziante R, Meder JF, Haye C: Spinal metastases with neurological manifestations: Review of 600 cases. *J Neurosurg* 1983;59:111-118.

Emery SE, Brazinski MS, Koka A, Bensusan JS, Stevenson S: The biologic and biomechanical effects of irradiation on anterior bone grafts in a canine model. *J Bone Joint Surg* 1994;76:540-548.

Enkaoua E, Doursounian L, Chatellier G, Mabesoone F, Aimard T, Saillant G: Vertebral metastases: A critical appreciation of the preoperative prognostic Tokuhashi score in a series of 71 cases. *Spine* 1997;22:2293-2298.

Hammerberg KW: Surgical treatment of metastatic spine disease. *Spine* 1992;17:1148-1153.

Hart R, Boriani S, Biagini R, Currier B, Weinstein JN: A system for surgical staging and management of spine tumors: A clinical outcome study of giant cell tumors of the spine. *Spine* 1997;22:1773-1782.

Kienstra GE, Terwee CB, Dekker FW, et al: Prediction of spinal epidural metastases. *Arch Neurol* 2000;57:690-695.

Taneichi H, Kaneda K, Takeda N, Abumi K, Satoh S: Risk factors and probability of vertebral body collapse in metastases of the thoracic and lumbar spine. *Spine* 1997;22:239-245.

Whitehouse GH, Griffiths GJ: Roentgenologic aspects of spinal involvement by primary and metastatic Ewing's tumor. *J Can Assoc Radiol* 1976;27:290-297.

Yuh WT, Quets JP, Lee HJ, et al: Anatomic distribution of metastases in the vertebral body and modes of hematogenous spread. *Spine* 1996;21:2243-2250.

# Chapter 38

# Infections of the Spine

Darrel S. Brodke, MD

Daniel R. Fassett, MD

## Introduction

Spinal infections continue to be a formidable challenge to spinal surgeons despite significant advances in diagnostic imaging, laboratory tests, and antibiotics. These infections often have an early indolent course, and delay in diagnosis is quite common. New antibiotic-resistant strains of microorganisms are becoming more common and often require the use of novel antibiotic regimens. Failure to diagnose or effectively treat these infections can have dire consequences in terms of compromising spinal stability, injury to the neurologic elements, and even death.

## Pyogenic Vertebral Osteomyelitis

### Demographics

Pyogenic vertebral osteomyelitis, also known as diskitis, spondylitis, and spondylodiskitis, comprises less than 8% of all instances of pyogenic osteomyelitis. Spontaneous (not postoperative) diskitis can occur in any individual, but it is much more common in individuals with certain risk factors (Table 1). The median age for vertebral pyogenic osteomyelitis is 50 to 60 years, and a male gender predominance has been reported.

### Pathogenesis

The route of inoculation for spontaneous pyogenic diskitis has been greatly debated. Direct invasion from adjacent soft-tissue infections can occur, but it is generally agreed that a hematogenous seeding is usually the source, via either arterial or venous routes. An arterial route for the microbial seeding of these infections into the vertebral body end plates and intervertebral disks is currently thought to account for most infections. In the cartilaginous end plates of the vertebral bodies, there are small, low-flow, vascular anastomoses that, in theory, provide an ideal environment for hematogenous seeding of microorganisms. As the infection progresses, the end plate necroses and the pathogens can easily access the disk space via direct penetration. In the avascular environment of the disk space, infections thrive because of the lack of a direct immune response. According to this

**Table 1 | Risk Factors Associated With Pyogenic Vertebral Osteomyelitis**

Age > 50 years
Diabetes
Obesity
Malignancy
Immunodeficiency
Malnutrition
Intravenous drug abuse
Recent systemic infection
Trauma
Use of immunosuppressive medications
Tobacco use

theory, infections start on one end plate adjacent to the disk space, enter the disk space, and can eventually involve the other vertebral end plate via direct invasion.

Other early theories proposed that the microorganisms entered the vertebral bodies and intravertebral disk in a retrograde manner through venous channels. The rich network of valveless venous channels of the spinal epidural space (Batson's venous plexus) were thought to allow retrograde blood flow at times when pelvic and abdominal pressures are increased, such as during Valsalva maneuvers; however, it is now thought that extremely high, nonphysiologic, abdominal pressures are needed to produce retrograde flow.

### Diagnosis

#### Clinical History/Findings

Delay in diagnosis is common with all forms of vertebral osteomyelitis; most patients have symptoms for more than 3 months before the diagnosis is made. Patients often do not seek medical attention early in the infectious course or present with nonspecific complaints, such as back pain and muscle spasms that are misdiagnosed as other more common conditions, including degenerative spondylosis or muscle strain. Diskitis-associated back pain typically worsens with activity and is classically more severe and unremitting than typical

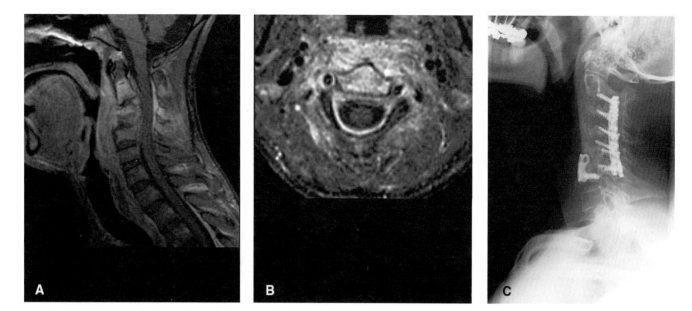

Figure 1  Sagittal **(A)** and axial **(B)** T1-weighted postgadolinium MRI scans of a 32-year-old man with insulin-dependent diabetes mellitus who spontaneously developed spondylodiskitis in his cervical spine show destruction of the C3 and C4 vertebral bodies with enhancement of C2, C3, C4, C5, and the surrounding soft tissues. A CT-guided biopsy was nondiagnostic, and the patient had open biopsy of the C3-4 disk space and surrounding end plates. Cultures grew methicillin-resistant *S aureus* that was treated for 6 weeks with intravenous vancomycin and rifampin. Despite apparent clearance of infection, based on normalization of inflammatory markers, the patient continued to have severe neck pain. **C,** The postoperative radiograph shows that the patient was treated with C3 to C5 corpectomies, allograft strut grafting, anterior plating, and supplementation with posterior instrumentation. Fusion was accomplished at 6 months, and the patient's pain was significantly reduced.

degenerative spondylosis. Pain that awakens patients at night should raise suspicion for sinister causes such as infections and malignancies. Unlike other systemic infections, pyogenic spinal osteomyelitis only causes fever in approximately one third of patients.

The lumbar spine is the most common site for pyogenic osteomyelitis in the spinal column, accounting for approximately 50% to 60% of all instances. The thoracic spine is involved in 30% to 40% of patients, and cervical spine osteomyelitis accounts for fewer than 10% of instances. Up to 17% of patients will present with neurologic deficits as a result of either direct infectious involvement of the neurologic elements, compression from epidural abscess formation, or neural compression caused by instability of the spinal column. Neurologic deficits are more common in patients older than 50 years; those with comorbidities such as diabetes, rheumatoid arthritis, and immunodeficiency; in the presence of *Staphylococcus aureus* infection or rapidly progressing infections; and when the cervical spine is involved. Up to 18% of patients with spondylodiskitis will have spinal epidural abscesses, and more than 50% of these will have neurologic deficits. Myelopathy is more common when the cervical and thoracic spine is involved, whereas radicular symptoms are more common when the cauda equina is compressed because of lumbar spine osteomyelitis.

### Diagnostic Imaging
Plain radiography, CT, MRI, and nuclear medicine studies may all help with the diagnosis of spinal infections

when advanced spondylodiskitis is present. Plain radiographs may show loss of disk height and erosion or sclerosis of the adjacent vertebral body end plates, but these findings are often delayed by weeks in comparison with the clinical history and thus are not extremely sensitive for the acute diagnosis of diskitis. CT has the advantage of providing better detail of the bony anatomy, and abscesses or phlegmon may be appreciated on the postcontrast CT scans, but early infections will often be missed. Air within the disk space (vacuum disk sign) as is most commonly seen on CT scans is not associated with infections, but more commonly with the vacuum disk effect of degenerative disks. In fact, the presence of air in the disk space is thought to preclude the presence of infection.

MRI is the most sensitive imaging modality for the diagnosis of spinal osteomyelitis (Figure 1). Paraspinal and epidural inflammation, disk and end-plate enhancement after gadolinium administration, T2-weighted hyperintensity in the disk and end plate, and end-plate erosion or destruction are all reported to have high sensitivity for spinal infections, but none are 100% sensitive or specific for infection. Isolated vertebral body involvement can occasionally be found in early infection, but this is uncommon. T1-weighted hypointensity and loss of disk height have both been reported in patients with spondylodiskitis, but they appear to be much less sensitive than the other MRI characteristics. Loss or effacement of the nuclear cleft, a hypointense band in the central portion of the intravertebral disk on T2-weighted

MRI scans, has also been reported to be associated with spinal infections, but does not appear to be as clinically reliable. Differentiating spondylodiskitis from spinal tumors using MRI can be difficult, but features such as disk space involvement, end-plate erosion, and paraspinous inflammation are much more likely with infections.

Nuclear medicine studies with technetium-99 bone scanning, gallium-67 scintigraphy, and indium-11-tagged white blood cell count studies have all been used to aid with the diagnosis of spondylodiskitis in patients in whom MRI scans are unobtainable or inconclusive. Bone scanning appears to be sensitive (90%), but not specific for diagnosing spondylodiskitis. Combining bone scintigraphy with gallium-67 scintigraphy appears to improve the specificity for diagnosing spinal infections. Indium scanning has poor sensitivity for detecting spinal infections and is not recommended as a diagnostic test for this indication.

### Laboratory Studies

The most commonly used laboratory studies are white blood cell count with differential, Westergren erythrocyte sedimentation rate (WESR), C-reactive protein (CRP) levels, and wound cultures. White blood cell count is often not elevated in patients with spondylodiskitis and thus is not a sensitive indicator for early infection. WESR and CRP level are both elevated in more than 90% of patients with pyogenic spinal infections. CRP level and WESR can both be monitored serially to help determine the effectiveness of treatment. Rapid responses (greater than 50% reduction in the first month) in WESR have been shown to correlate with an effective response to treatment. Other less dramatic responses in WESR are unreliable and should not be used to predict response or failure of treatment. CRP level tends to normalize more quickly than WESR and appears to be a more reliable monitoring tool for determining the effectiveness of medical therapy.

### Microbiology

The least invasive means of determining the infectious organism and antibiotic sensitivities is blood culture. Positive blood cultures are obtained in approximately one third of patients with spondylodiskitis and are 85% accurate in isolating the correct organism. Blood culture yield is improved by obtaining the cultures during a period when the patient is febrile, and all culture results are improved if antibiotics are withheld until all pertinent cultures are obtained.

CT-guided biopsy can provide a diagnosis in 50% to 75% of patients and should be used in those who do not have indications for open surgery. In patients in whom surgery is indicated or for whom CT-guided biopsies are nondiagnostic, blood cultures can be obtained at the time of surgical débridement. In 10% to 20% of patients, positive cultures are never obtained, presumably because of spontaneous resolution of the infection or masking by antibiotics administered before biopsy.

Cultures should include aerobic, anaerobic, fungal, and acid-fast cultures. In addition to standard cultures, antibiotic sensitivities should be performed on all positive cultures to help tailor the antibiotic regimen. *S aureus* is by far the most common pathogen (40% to 55% of patients), but a diverse group of other gram-positive, gram-negative, and mixed infections have been reported. In intravenous drug abusers, *Pseudomonas* osteomyelitis is particularly common, and *Salmonella* spondylolitis has been reported in patients with sickle cell disease.

### Management

### Medical Management

Nonsurgical management is successful in up to 80% of patients and includes antibiotics and bracing (Figure 2). Broad-spectrum antibiotics, with gram-positive and gram-negative coverage, should be used until antibiotic sensitivities are found. Vancomycin is advised for empiric coverage of penicillin-resistant, gram-positive bacteria, and a third-generation cephalosporin can provide gram-negative coverage. Once antibiotic sensitivities are obtained, antibiotic coverage should be narrowed for coverage of the infecting pathogen only.

New antibiotics are available to treat gram-positive bacteria that are resistant to conventional antibiotics. Quinupristin-dalfopristin, linezolid, and daptomycin (Table 2) all have been introduced over the past 4 years, and each is reported to have activity against methicillin-resistant *S aureus*, vancomycin-resistant *S aureus*, vancomycin-resistant *Enterococcus*, and other gram-positive pathogens. With resistance increasing among gram-positive bacteria, spinal surgeons should familiarize themselves with these new antibiotics and the clinical circumstances for which these antibiotics are appropriate. In addition, linezolid may be especially appropriate for the treatment of spinal infections because it is 100% bioavailable via an enteral route and can thus eliminate the need for expensive outpatient intravenous therapy.

A minimum of 6 weeks of intravenous antibiotics has traditionally been recommended to treat spondylodiskitis. Relapses have been reported in as many as 25% of patients who have received antibiotic treatment for less than 4 weeks. A supplemental course of oral antibiotics (up to 3 months) has been advocated by many clinicians, but this has not been sufficiently studied to determine whether it is beneficial. CRP level, WESR, and clinical symptoms may all help gauge the effectiveness of treatment and determine whether modifications to the treatment regimen should be made. Diagnostic imaging evidence of successful treatment often lags behind the actual response to treatment and should not be used to gauge treatment duration.

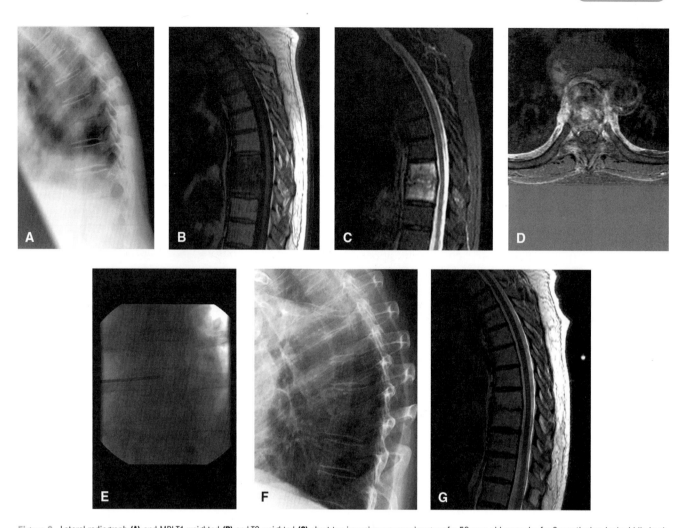

Figure 2  Lateral radiograph **(A)** and MRI T1-weighted **(B)** and T2-weighted **(C)** short tau inversion recovery images of a 58-year-old man who for 3 months has had middle back pain without radiating symptoms. Fever or other constitutional symptoms were not present. **D**, Axial gadolinium enhanced MRI scan confirmed diskitis/vertebral osteomyelitis. **E**, A fluoroscopic-guided biopsy revealed *S aureus*. The patient received intravenous antibiotics for 6 weeks and 2 months of oral rifampin. Three months later, the patient's pain had resolved and his white blood cell count, WESR, and CRP level were within normal ranges. Follow-up lateral radiograph **(F)** and MRI T2-weighted scan **(G)** show resolution of the infection.

**Table 2 | New Antibiotics Available to Treat Methicillin- and Vancomycin-Resistant Gram-Positive Bacterial Infections**

| Name | Quinupristin/Dalfopristin | Linezolid | Daptomycin |
|---|---|---|---|
| Class | Streptogramin | Oxazolidinone | Lipopeptide |
| Administration Route | Intravenous | Intravenous and enteral | Intravenous |

### Surgical Intervention

Surgical intervention is typically reserved for patients with neurologic deficits, progressive deformity, gross spinal instability, and persistent infection despite appropriate medical management. The indications for surgical intervention have not changed significantly over the past 50 years; however, new thoracoscopic and other minimally invasive approaches may reduce the morbidity and recovery time associated with these surgeries.

Spinal instrumentation in the setting of an active infection remains controversial. Some surgeons will place

bone grafts and hardware at the time of initial débridement in patients with gross purulence, whereas others will place hardware at the time of initial débridement only if no purulence is found. Others have an even more conservative philosophy of performing the débridement and then treating patients with antibiotics for a period before returning to the operating room for bone grafting and instrumentation. Cement impregnated with vancomycin or tobramycin may be used as a temporary strut to provide structural support and high local antibiotic concentrations. Retrospective studies support each

## Table 3 | Risk Factors Reported to Be Associated With an Increased Risk of Infection After Spinal Surgery

| Patient-Related | Pathology-Related | Surgery-Related | Postoperative |
|---|---|---|---|
| Obesity | Malignancy | Posterior approach | Urinary incontinence |
| Diabetes | Trauma | Fusion (number of levels fused) | Length of intensive care unit stay |
| Age | Use of corticosteroids | Duration of surgery | Wound seroma |
| Nutrition (albumin) | Previous spinal surgery | Blood loss | |
| Smoking | Extended preoperative admission | Instrumentation | |
| Alcohol abuse | Previous radiation therapy | Use of operating microscope | |

of these practices without a clear consensus regarding fusion rates and clearance of infection. Obviously, a single procedure with instrumentation provides the potential benefits of earlier mobilization without the need for bracing, reduced hospital stay, decreased cost of treatment, and elimination of potential complications associated with a second surgery, but it is unclear whether this practice is associated with an increased risk of treatment failure because of persistent infection. Recent reports suggest that a more aggressive approach with the use of allografts and metal implants does not impede the resolution of infection and is therefore warranted.

Titanium implants appear to be more appropriate than stainless steel implants in the setting of infection. Solid titanium and titanium alloys may be resistant to biofilm formation. In addition, the stability afforded by these implants plays an important role in the treatment of infection.

The surgical approach to the treatment of spondylodiskitis has not been studied sufficiently to favor anterior versus posterior approaches. The hallmark of surgical treatment includes successful débridement of infected tissues and abscesses as well as early stabilization to promote clearance of infection. Allograft, autograft, and vascularized bone grafts have all been successfully used for the treatment of these infections without a clear consensus as to the superiority of one particular treatment.

## Postoperative Spinal Infections
### Demographics
Although the overall rate of infection after spinal surgery is relatively low, certain procedures and patients are associated with a much higher risk of infection. More than 15 factors are cited in the literature in association with increased risk of postoperative spinal infection (Table 3). Risk factors may be patient-related, pathology-related, surgery-specific, or related to the postoperative course.

Posterior approaches, length of surgery, blood loss, fusion procedures, and implantation of instrumentation are infection risk factors related to the specific surgery. Infection rates for instrumented anterior spinal surgery appear to be less than 1%, whereas infection rates in large published series for posterior instrumented fusions approach 4% to 7%. Postoperative wound infection rates after simple diskectomy are less than 1%.

Patient-related risk factors such as obesity (body mass index > 35) have been reported to have a fivefold increased risk of infections, and patients with a poor nutritional status are 16 times more likely to have a postoperative infection. The infection rate in patients older than 65 years who receive posterior decompression and fusion has been reported to be as high as 10% to 15%. Malignancy appears to have the highest incidence of postoperative infections, with reported rates of approximately 20%.

### Pathogenesis
Postoperative wound infections from spinal surgery can result in severe osteomyelitis. The infecting organism is most commonly skin flora that contaminates the wound at the time of surgery.

### Diagnosis
#### Clinical History/Findings
Postoperative spinal infections typically present at least 7 days after surgery, and some have been reported months to years after surgery. Symptoms are similar to those of spontaneous pyogenic infections, with the addition of possible surgical wound breakdown and drainage. A significant early indicator of postoperative spinal infection is increased back pain and tenderness with or without recurrent neurologic symptoms.

#### Laboratory Studies
The only difference between postoperative infections and spontaneous infections is that the inflammatory markers are normally elevated for a period after surgery and, thus, an elevation in markers early after surgery is not specific for infection. CRP level appears to be a better indicator for diagnosis and monitoring for postoperative infections because it will normalize earlier after surgery than WESR. WESR peaks at approximately postoperative day 5 and is often elevated more than 40 days after surgery. CRP level typically peaks on post-

operative day 2 and will return to normal 5 to 14 days after surgery. Spinal instrumentation has been shown to increase the postoperative CRP level significantly in comparison with noninstrumented fusion procedures, but the CRP level still normalizes at approximately postoperative day 7. WESR greater than 45 mm/hr and CRP level greater than 2.5 mg/dL after postoperative day 5 have both been reported to be consistent with the presence of postoperative infection.

### Microbiology
Cultures are typically obtained via needle biopsy or open biopsy at the time of washout. Aerobic, anaerobic, and fungal cultures should be obtained. *S aureus* is the offending organism in most instances of postoperative spinal infection. Patients with diabetes and immuno-compromised patients may be at high risk for multimicrobial infections.

## Management
### Prevention
Preoperative prophylactic antibiotics appear to reduce postoperative spinal infections by 60% based on a meta-analysis of large surgical series. Preoperative antibiotics should be given 30 to 60 minutes before skin incision to allow for tissue penetration and should be of a spectrum to cover skin flora. Redosing of antibiotics every 2 hours in surgical procedures that last longer than 400 minutes has been shown to reduce postoperative infections in clinical studies. Although there have been no studies to support the use of postoperative antibiotic prophylaxis, this practice is continued by many.

### Medical Management
Medical management alone may be appropriate in patients with superficial postoperative spinal infections without abscess or fluid collection. A CT scan may aid in detecting the presence of abscess or fluid, although it is common to have a small amount of fluid present (seroma) even in the normal healing wound. Antibiotic treatment is similar to that of spontaneous pyogenic spinal infections.

### Surgical Intervention
The management of postoperative spinal infections results in some of the same dilemmas as the management of spontaneous pyogenic infections. Management in the presence of infection, without hardware removal, is common, as the implants provide ongoing stability and aid in the treatment of the infection. Some surgeons will remove all hardware at the time of surgical débridement, which can be problematic and slow or inhibit recovery. Other management approaches include multiple washouts until no pyogenic material is found and wound cultures are negative, use of antibiotic irrigation/sump

systems, and prolonged antibiotic use for months until fusion is achieved. If hardware is loose, it is not providing structural support and should be removed. Several retrospective studies have evaluated treatments for postoperative spinal infections, but there are insufficient data to support one treatment over another.

## Nonpyogenic Vertebral Osteomyelitis
### Pathogenesis
Nonpyogenic vertebral osteomyelitis includes bacterial and fungal infections that cause a granulomatous immune response. The most common form of nonpyogenic spinal osteomyelitis is spinal tuberculosis (Pott's disease). The incidence of tuberculosis was on a decline, but it has made a resurgence over the past decade because of a larger immunocompromised and elderly population. These infections (tuberculosis and other bacterial granulomatous infections) are thought to spread mainly via a hematogenous seeding, most commonly from a pulmonary source with tuberculosis. Direct extension and lymphatic spread have also been theorized. Fungal spinal infections can occur as a result of hematogenous seeding from a distant infection, local extension from adjacent fungal infection, or postoperatively from surgery.

### Demographics
Most patients with nonpyogenic spinal osteomyelitis (bacterial and fungal) are immunocompromised. In patients with tuberculosis, a large percentage live or have lived in developing countries. The median age of patients with spinal tuberculosis is between 40 and 50 years, and there may be a slight male predominance. Up to one third of these patients will have active extraskeletal tuberculosis at the time of diagnosis.

### Diagnosis
#### Clinical Presentation
Patients with nonpyogenic forms of spinal osteomyelitis typically have an indolent disease course, possibly lasting years, with most presenting with gradually worsening back pain. In patients with tuberculosis, constitutional symptoms such as weight loss and night sweats are reported in 50%. Neurologic deficits appear to be more common in patients with spinal tuberculosis (40% to 75% with deficits) and fungal forms of osteomyelitis than in pyogenic spondylodiskitis.

#### Diagnostic Imaging
Spinal tuberculosis may appear identical to pyogenic infections, but some MRI characteristics may help differentiate these infections. Heterogenous signal intensity in the vertebral body marrow, more extensive paraspinal involvement, and isolated posterior element involvement have all been reported in patients with spinal tuberculo-

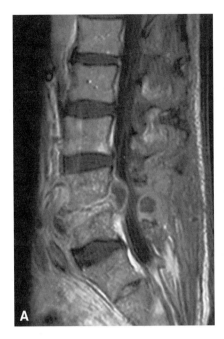
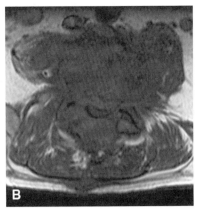
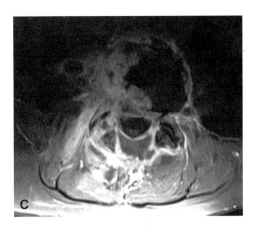

**Figure 3** Sagittal T1-weighted postgadolinium **(A)** and axial T1-weighted MRI scans without **(B)** and with **(C)** gadolinium of a 62-year-old man with tuberculous spondylolitis at L4-5 show extensive paraspinous inflammation and abscesses and extensive enhancement of the vertebral bodies, disk space, and adjacent soft tissues with abscess formation.

sis (Figure 3). Relative sparing of the intravertebral disk is much more consistent with nonpyogenic than pyogenic infections. Spinal tuberculosis has a propensity for the thoracic spine, followed by the lumbar spine, and rarely the cervical spine. Multiple contiguous vertebral involvement via abscess formation spread along the anterior longitudinal ligament may be seen. There are no specific MRI characteristics reported to be helpful in delineating fungal infections of the spine from other forms of spinal osteomyelitis. Nuclear medicine studies can be sensitive for nonpyogenic spondylodiskitis and can serve as an alternative when MRI is unavailable.

### Laboratory Studies
With nonpyogenic infections of the spine, inflammatory markers, such as WESR and CRP level, are more reliably elevated in comparison with white blood cell count, which is only elevated in approximately one third of patients.

### Microbiology
Cultures for nonpyogenic organisms can be obtained via needle biopsy or open biopsy. Needle aspirate from paraspinous abscesses has been reported to have a higher yield than core samples taken from vertebral bodies. Culturing these organisms can be difficult and result in a high rate of false-negative cultures and long periods (weeks) before cultures become positive. Acid-fast smears can provide a yield comparable to that of cultures and are available much sooner. Histologic evidence of granuloma formation can also aid in the diagnosis of these infections.

*Mycobacterium tuberculosis* is the most common pathogen causing nonpyogenic spondylitis. Other bacterial organisms causing granulomatous spondylitis include

*Mycobacterium avium-intracellulare*, *Nocardia*, and *Brucella*. *Candida* (*albicans*, *tropicalis*, *paratropicalis*, *parapsilosis*) appears to be the most common pathogen implicated in fungal spondylitis, but others such as *Aspergillus*, *Coccidioides*, and *Petriellidium* have been reported.

### Management
#### Medical Management
Treatment of spinal tuberculosis usually involves administration of isoniazid, ethambutol, rifampin, and pyrazinamide for the first 2 to 3 months of therapy. If antibiotic sensitivities are unavailable, then isoniazid, ethambutol, and rifampin are continued for a total of 12 months. If sensitivities are available, two antibiotics, isoniazid and rifampin preferably, are used for a total of 12 months. If combinations other than isoniazid and rifampin are used, the duration of these regimens is often extended to 18 months. Streptomycin and ciprofloxacin can be used in patients with multidrug-resistant organisms. Medical management of tuberculosis and other nonpyogenic spinal infections should be managed under the guidance of infectious disease experts. Approximately 90% of patients will respond to medical management.

Amphotericin B is the most common antibiotic treatment of most fungal infections. Ketoconazole and miconazole can be used as alternatives or adjuncts to amphotericin B depending on the respective sensitivity of the organism. Rifampin and 5-fluorocytosine are also used as adjuncts for certain organisms.

#### Surgical Management
Alternatives for surgical treatment include anterior débridement and bone grafting without instrumenta-

tion, anterior débridement and bone grafting with anterior instrumentation, anterior approaches supplemented by posterior instrumentation, and posterior approaches that can address anterior pathology. Transpedicular and costotransversectomy are posterior approaches that can address anterior pathology and have been reported to be especially useful in the treatment of patients with spinal tuberculosis. Although these approaches avoid thoracotomy and issues associated with performing surgery in the pleural cavity of patients with infection, they can be technically challenging.

Kyphosis and other spinal deformities are particularly common in patients with tuberculosis. Destabilizing procedures such as laminectomy may promote deformity progression and should be avoided. The use of spinal instrumentation will aid in deformity correction and preservation of alignment and is especially important in the setting of multisegmental fusion. Anterior instrumentation has been used and may allow for earlier mobilization without bracing. Others prefer posterior instrumentation, especially in the setting of significant kyphotic deformity. Placing instrumentation in the setting of infection remains controversial, but many report that tuberculosis and other granulomatous infections are less problematic with hardware because of the inability of the bacteria to form a biofilm.

Based on the limited number of reports in the literature, it appears that there is a high propensity for patients with fungal spinal infections to fail to respond to medical management and require surgical débridement. Most surgical débridements for fungal spondylitis have been performed through an anterior approach.

## Summary

Spondylodiskitis and vertebral osteomyelitis, although uncommon, usually occur via hematogenous spread or direct inoculation as a complication of surgery. The white blood cell count can be normal, but the WESR and C-reactive protein level are usually elevated. In neurologically intact patients, without instability or abscess formation, long-term medical management (antibiotic administration of 6 weeks or longer) may be appropriate. If surgical management is required, the hallmarks of treatment are thorough débridement, decompression of neural elements, realignment of deformity, and immediate stability. These methods are followed by antibiotic treatment and are usually successful in eradicating the disease.

## Annotated Bibliography

### Pyogenic Vertebral Osteomyelitis

Dimar JR, Carreon LY, Glassman SD, Campbell MJ, Hartman MJ, Johnson JR: Treatment of pyogenic vertebral osteomyelitis with anterior debridement and fusion followed by delayed posterior spinal fusion. *Spine* 2004; 29:326-332.

The authors treated 42 patients with vertebral osteomyelitis with staged surgical procedures. An anterior débridement and noninstrumented fusion was performed followed by 2 weeks of intravenous antibiotics and a second-stage operation with an instrumented posterior fusion. There were no recurrences of infection and no instrumentation failures.

Klockner C, Valencia R: Sagittal alignment after anterior débridement and fusion with or without additional posterior instrumentation in the treatment of pyogenic and tuberculous spondylolitis. *Spine* 2003;28:1036-1042.

The authors retrospectively reviewed the surgical results of 71 patients with spondylodiskitis who were treated with anterior débridement and bone grafting, including 22 patients who received supplemental posterior instrumentation. They found no benefit of supplemental posterior instrumentation in the 53 patients who underwent monosegmental fusion. In the 19 patients who underwent multisegmental fusions, the authors found better correction of the deformity with supplemental posterior instrumentation.

Ledermann HP, Schweitzer ME, Morrison WB, Carrino JA: MR imaging findings in spinal infections: Rules and myths? *Radiology* 2003;228:506-514.

The authors studied the MRI characteristics of 44 patients with spontaneous pyogenic osteomyelitis. They found that paraspinal or epidural inflammation had the highest sensitivity (97.7%), followed by disk enhancement (95.4%), disk space T2-weighted hyperintensity (93.2%), and erosion of at least one vertebral end plate (84.1%). Loss of disk height and T1-weighted disk space hypointensity had much lower sensitivity.

Muckley T, Schutz T, Schmidt MH, Potulski M, Buhren V, Biesse R: The role of thoracoscopic spinal surgery in the management of pyogenic vertebral osteomyelitis. *Spine* 2004;29:E227-E233.

The authors describe a minimally invasive thoracoscopic approach to treat thoracic vertebral osteomyelitis with débridement and reconstruction of the anterior column. In their small series (three patients), they report no complications and suggest that this approach results in less morbidity than open thoracotomy.

### Postoperative Spinal Infections

Barker FG: Efficacy of prophylactic antibiotic therapy in spinal surgery: A meta-analysis. *Neurosurgery* 2002; 51:391-401.

The author performed a meta-analysis evaluating the effectiveness of prophylactic antibiotics for patients undergoing spinal surgery. The pooled infection rate with antibiotic prophylaxis was 2.2% (10 of 451 patients) and 5.9% (23 of 392 patients) without antibiotics. The pooled odds ratio was 0.37 ($P < 0.01$) in favor of preincisional, prophylactic antibiotics.

Fassett DR, Brodke DS: Antibiotics in the management of spinal postoperative wound infections. *Semin Spine Surg* 2004;16:174-181.

The authors reviewed new antibiotics that are available to treat spinal infections.

Olsen MA, Mayfield J, Lauryssen C, et al: Risk factors for surgical site infection in spinal surgery. *J Neurosurg* 2003;98:149-155.

The authors performed a retrospective case-control study of patients undergoing laminectomy or spinal fusion. Independent risk factors for postoperative wound infections were identified using multivariate analysis. Postoperative incontinence (odds ratio = 8.2), posterior approach (odd ratio = 8.2), procedure for tumor resection (odd ratio = 6.2), and morbid obesity (odd ratio = 5.2) were identified as independent risk factors.

Takahashi J, Kamimura M, Kinoshita T, et al: Pro-inflammatory and anti-inflammatory cytokine increases after spinal instrumentation surgery. *J Spinal Disord Tech* 2002;15:294-300.

The authors serially studied inflammatory markers after posterior spinal fusion with and without instrumentation and found that instrumentation results in a significantly higher elevation in CRP levels on postoperative day 2 compared with noninstrumented fusions. The instrumented and noninstrumented patients all had a normalization of CRP levels by postoperative day 7.

*Nonpyogenic Vertebral Osteomyelitis*

Frazier DD, Campbell DR, Garvey TA, Wiesel S, Bohlman HH, Eismont FJ: Fungal infections of the spine. *J Bone Joint Surg Am* 2001;83:560-565.

The authors retrospectively reviewed 11 patients who were treated for fungal infections of the spine. An average delay in diagnosis of more than 3 months was noted. Nine of the 11 patients were immunocompromised. Ten patients failed to respond to medical management and were treated with surgical débridement. One patient died of general sepsis, and one patient died of another cause. Infection resolved in the remaining nine patients.

Ozdemir HM, US AK, Ogun T: The role of anterior spinal instrumentation and allograft fibula for the treatment of Pott disease. *Spine* 2003;28:474-479.

The authors retrospectively reviewed 28 patients who underwent anterior débridement and fusion with fibular allograft and anterior spinal instrumentation. They reported one instrumentation failure and no graft-related problems. The overall fusion rate was 96%, and the authors maintained segmental correction in all patients, with only 6° of correction loss in follow-up.

Schimmer RC, Jeanneret C, Nunley PD, Jeanneret B: Osteomyelitis of the cervical spine: A potentially dramatic disease. *J Spinal Disord Tech* 2002;15:110-117.

The authors reviewed the clinical course, treatment, and outcome of 15 patients with cervical spine osteomyelitis. Sixty percent of patients had neurologic deficits at presentation. With aggressive débridement, decompression, and stabilization, 50% of the patients with neurologic deficits had a complete resolution of their deficits, and 14 of 15 patients had evidence of fusion in follow-up.

## Classic Bibliography

An HS, Vaccaro AR, Dolinskas CA, Colter JM, Balderston RA, Bauerle WB: Differentiation between spinal tumors and infections with magnetic resonance imaging. *Spine* 1991;16(suppl 8):S334-S338.

Dietze D, Fessler G, Jacob R: Primary reconstruction for spinal infections. *J Neurosurg* 1997;86:981-989.

Krodel A, Kruger A, Lohscheidt K, Pfahler M, Refior HJ: Anterior debridement, fusion, and extrafocal stabilization in the treatment of osteomyelitis of the spine. *J Spinal Disord* 1999;12:17-26.

Levi AD, Dickman CA, Sonntag VK: Management of postoperative spinal infections after spinal instrumentation. *J Neurosurg* 1997;86:975-980.

Lifeso RM, Weaver P, Harder EH: Tuberculous spondylitis in adults. *J Bone Joint Surg Am* 1985;67:1405-1413.

Modic MT, Feiglin DH, Piraino DW, et al: Vertebral osteomyelitis: Assessment using MR. *Radiology* 1985;157:157-166.

Moon MS: Tuberculosis of the spine: Controversies and a new challenge. *Spine* 1997;22:1791-1797.

Rezai AR, Woo HH, Errico TJ, Cooper PR: Contemporary management of spinal osteomyelitis. *Neurosurgery* 1999;44:1018-1026.

Wimmer C, Gluch H, Franzreb, Ogon M: Predisposing factors for infection in spine surgery: A survey of 850 spinal procedures. *J Spinal Disord* 1998;11:124-128.

Chapter 39

# Management of Osteoporotic Vertebral Compression Fractures

Tom Faciszewski, MD

Fergus E. McKiernan, MD

Raj Rao, MD

## Introduction

The management of osteoporosis and osteoporotic vertebral compression fractures is a relatively new opportunity for orthopaedic surgeons. Orthopaedists with vast experience in treating high-energy spine fractures should exercise caution in transferring that experience directly to the management of patients with osteoporosis. Recent application of high-energy fracture classification schemes and treatment principles to low-energy osteoporotic vertebral compression fractures has generated confusion within the orthopaedic literature.

Osteoporotic vertebral compression fractures will occur with increasing frequency as the size of the geriatric population increases; currently 700,000 vertebral compression fractures occur annually in the United States. The estimated national direct expenditure (hospitals and nursing homes) for osteoporosis and related fractures was $17 billion in 2001 ($47 million each day) and this cost is rising. Additional economic burden results from lost productivity, earlier transition to functional dependency, and aggravation of underlying medical conditions.

## Pathogenesis of the Osteoporotic Fracture

Osteoporotic bone has a reduced number, thickness, and connectivity of trabecular plates and rods, resulting in increased fragility and predisposing patients to fracture with relatively minor trauma. Peak bone mass is achieved by the third decade of life and remains stable until perimenopause in women and until a slightly older age in men. In the absence of additional skeletal threats, the rate of subsequent annual bone loss in men is less than 1% to 2% and relatively linear, whereas female menopause can be followed by a transient (4- to 8-year) accelerated bone loss, resulting in a 5% to 10% loss of cortical bone and a 20% to 30% loss of trabecular bone mass. The metabolic state of bone and the rate of subsequent bone loss are influenced by numerous hormonal, hereditary, medical, and lifestyle factors.

For research and epidemiologic purposes, osteoporotic vertebral fracture is generally defined as the reduction of any vertebral body height (anterior, mid-dle, or posterior) by 20% from the nonfractured height and by at least 4 mm. Osteoporotic vertebral compression fractures are distributed bimodally in the spine and cluster at the midthorax and at the thoracolumbar junction. Although fracture morphology is usually characterized as wedge, crush, or biconcave (Figure 1), in reality, fracture configuration may not conform to these simple, descriptive morphologies and fracture configuration may change over time. Nevertheless, wedge and crush fractures occur more commonly in the midthoracic and thoracolumbar regions. Biconcave fractures are more common in the lumbar region. Fracture severity is graded as mild (20% to 25% reduction in any anterior, middle or posterior height), moderate (25% to 40% reduction), or severe (> 40% reduction). Acute fractures of the thoracolumbar junction (T11-L1) are more likely to be severe, contain intravertebral clefts, and demonstrate the property of dynamic mobility. Increasing fracture severity and the number of prevalent fractures is correlated with an increased risk of future fracture.

## Consequences of Fracture

About one fourth of patients with osteoporotic vertebral compression fractures become sufficiently symptomatic to seek medical attention. Annually, osteoporotic vertebral compression fractures account for 66,000 physician office visits and as many as 70,000 hospitalizations in the United States. Some form of continuing care in a skilled nursing facility is required after half of these hospitalizations. The 2-year mortality rate for patients with osteoporotic vertebral compression fractures is 1.5 times greater than that of age-matched controls and equals that of patients with hip fractures. Most of these patients have multiple medical comorbidities; a vertebral compression fracture may, therefore, be a surrogate marker for frailty.

Although acute vertebral compression fracture pain can be severe and functionally incapacitating, it is self-limited and responds to simple measures such as analgesia, modification, or temporary restriction of physical activity and bracing in most patients. Acute fracture pain usually resolves within several months, but the more in-

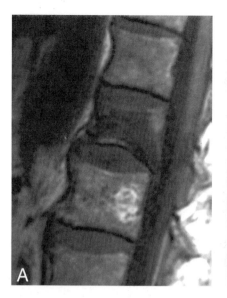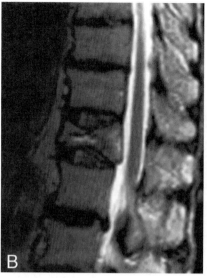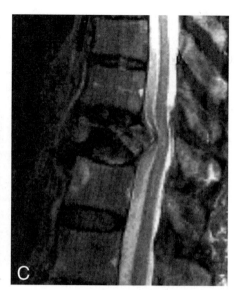

**Figure 1**    MRI scans showing inferior wedge **(A)**, biconcave **(B)**, and crush **(C)** osteoporotic vertebral fractures.

sidious effects of vertebral fracture may persist indefi-
nitely. Lost vertebral height and increased local spinal
kyphosis contribute to a reduction in standing height,
compression of abdominal viscera, early satiety, and
weight loss. As a general rule, a 9% reduction in predicted forced vital capacity can be expected for each
thoracic vertebral compression fracture. Fortunately,
neurologic deficits are rarely associated with these low-
energy fractures, even when bone is retropulsed into the
spinal canal. Psychosocial effects of vertebral compression fracture include loss of functional independence, reduction in quality of life, depression, and anxiety.

As occurs with fractures in other locations, acute
vertebral compression fracture pain is generally believed to result from motion at the fracture site. Parox-
ysms of intense muscle spasm may complicate early
fracture pain, particularly with motion of the trunk.
Transient wraparound pain is not uncommon early. The
mechanism of chronic pain with vertebral compression
fractures is more complex. Patients with persistent nonunion continue to have fracture pain because of microscopic or macroscopic motion at the fracture site.
Chronic back pain that persists after fracture healing
may be related to muscle fatigue of a kyphotic postural
deficit and sagittal trunk imbalance. Secondary facet
joint arthrosis, recurring vertebral microfracture, and
neural irritation are also postulated mechanisms of
chronic back pain associated with vertebral compression
fractures. Impingement of the anterior rib cage on the
pelvis (costopelvic friction) may cause significant pain
anterolaterally to the fracture site.

## Forces

The spine transmits forces from the upper extremities
and torso through the pelvis into the lower extremities.

In the surgical trauma literature, the vertebrae is divided into three columns for biomechanical purposes:
anterior (ventral half of the vertebral body), middle
(dorsal half of the vertebral body to the midpoint of the
pedicle), and posterior (midpoint of the pedicle dorsally). The medical literature on osteoporosis frequently
refers to only two columns: anterior (vertebral body)
and posterior (bone dorsal to the base of the pedicle).
Anterior compressive forces are borne by the anterior
and middle columns. The middle column serves as a fulcrum by which posterior tensile forces mitigate compressive forces on the anterior column. During spinal
flexion, the center of gravity moves ventrally, increasing
the bending moment while displacing the axis of rotation dorsally. Increased loads thereby lead to failure of
the anterior and middle columns in osteoporotic vertebrae. Degenerative changes of the disk result in uneven
transmission of load to the vertebral end plates. Loss of
disk height and kyphotic posture further increase compressive loads on the vertebral body.

## Dynamic Mobility

There is increasing recognition that some osteoporotic
vertebral compression fractures change configuration
under different loading conditions and in different body
positions. This fracture property has been termed "dynamic mobility" and has been identified in as many as
one third of patients referred for vertebroplasty. In
these patients, a supine cross-table lateral radiograph
centered on the index vertebra will demonstrate an increase in vertebral height when compared with a standing lateral radiograph. Dynamic mobility is most common at the thoracolumbar junction (T11-L1) and
implies complete disruption of cortical and cancellous
bone. The radiographic correlate of this disruption is the

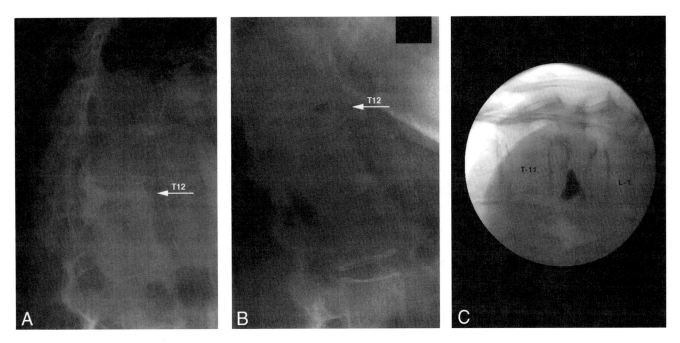

Figure 2  **A,** Standing lateral radiograph showing severe compression fracture of T12 (vertebra plana). **B,** Supine cross-table radiograph showing remarkable dynamic mobility and restoration of anterior column height. Evidence of an intravertebral cleft is visible in the anterosuperior aspect of the vertebrae. **C,** Prone intraoperative fluoroscopic view showing the restoration of height and PMMA filled intravertebral cleft.

intravertebral cleft. Clefts occur primarily beneath the superior end plate near the anterior margin of the vertebra (Figure 2). Cleft margins appear increasingly sclerotic over time, and persistent nonunion may result in true intravertebral pseudarthrosis.

## General Management of Patients With Osteoporosis

Osteoporosis is a skeletal disorder characterized by compromised bone strength that predisposes patients to an increased risk of fracture. Osteoporosis can be primary or, in approximately one third of women and one half of men, secondary to an underlying medical condition or skeletal toxin (Table 1). Both forms of osteoporosis commonly occur in the context of other medical comorbidities and frailty. In practice, the diagnosis of osteoporosis is either based on (1) the presence of a fragility fracture (typically the distal forearm, hip, or vertebra) or (2) low bone mineral density. Fragility is the clinical judgment that the fracture resulted from energy that should be insufficient to cause structural failure of healthy bone. Fractures resulting from a fall from stationary standing height are usually considered fragility fractures. Bone mineral density is most commonly measured by dual energy x-ray absorptiometry at the lumbar spine (L1-L4) and hips and is reported as the number of standard deviations above or below the mean of a young, healthy, gender-matched Caucasian population (T-score). Each standard deviation point above or below this young, normal mean is equivalent

to a T-score of +1.0 or –1.0, respectively. According to World Health Organization guidelines, osteoporosis may be diagnosed in women with a T-score ≤ –2.5 and severe osteoporosis in women with a T-score ≤ –2.5 in the presence of a fragility fracture. Osteopenia may be diagnosed in patients with a T-score > –2.5 and < –1.0. These diagnostic cut-points were chosen so that the prevalence of osteoporosis as defined by bone mineral density testing would be similar to the prevalence of osteoporosis estimated from large, population-based radiographic surveys. Fracture risk is strongly, continuously, and inversely correlated with T-score such that site-specific fracture incidence at least doubles with each integer decline in the site-specific T-score. Because substantially more women are osteopenic than osteoporotic, the absolute number of osteopenic women who experience fracture is greater than the number of osteoporotic women who experience fracture. The diagnostic criteria of the World Health Organization have been validated for predicting fracture risk in postmenopausal Caucasian women. Nevertheless, because the general relationship between bone mineral density and fracture risk is similar among other ethnic groups, men, and younger premenopausal women, bone mineral density is often measured to assess fracture risk and monitor antiosteoporosis therapy in these patient groups.

The goal of osteoporosis treatment is to prevent fragility fracture and mitigate fracture-related morbidity and mortality. This is accomplished by achieving and maintaining a healthy peak skeletal mass, identifying all causes of skeletal fragility, treating established os-

## Table 1 | Conditions Affecting Bone Turnover and Predisposing to Osteoporosis

| Genetic Disorders | Endocrine Disorders | Rheumatic and Autoimmune Diseases |
|---|---|---|
| Cystic fibrosis | Acromegaly | Ankylosing spondylitis |
| Imperfecta | Adrenal insufficiency | Lupus |
| Ehlers-Danlos syndrome | Cushing syndrome | Rheumatoid arthritis |
| Glycogen storage diseases | Diabetes mellitus (type 1) | **Miscellaneous** |
| Gaucher disease | Hyperparathyroidism | Alcoholism |
| Hemochromatosis | Thyrotoxicosis | Amyloidosis |
| Homocystinuria | **Gastrointestinal Diseases** | Chronic metabolic acidosis |
| Hypophosphatasia | Celiac disease | Congestive heart failure |
| Marfan syndrome | Cirrhosis | Depression |
| Idiopathic hypercalciuria | Gastrectomy | Emphysema |
| Menkes steely hair syndrome | Inflammatory bowel disease | End-stage renal disease |
| Osteogenesis | Malabsorption | Epilepsy |
| Porphyria | Primary biliary cirrhosis | Idiopathic scoliosis |
| Riley-Day syndrome | **Hematologic Disorders** | Immbolization |
| **Hypogonadal States** | Hemophilia | Multiple sclerosis |
| Androgen insensitivity | Leukemia and lymphomas | Muscular dystrophy |
| Anorexia nervosa | Multiple myeloma | Posttransplant bone disease |
| Athletic amenorrhea | Sickle cell disease | Sarcoidosis |
| Hyperprolactinemia | Systemic mastocytosis | |
| Panhypopituitarism syndrome | Thalassemia | |
| Premature ovarian failure | | |
| Turner and Klinefelter disease | | |

*(Reproduced with permission from United States Department of Health and Human Services: Bone Health and Osteoporosis: A Report of the Surgeon General, 2004. Available at: http://www.surgeongeneral.gov/library/bonehealth/content.html. Accessed November 23, 2005.)*

teoporosis and preventing skeletal trauma, particularly falls. Fifty percent to 70% of variance in peak bone mass is genetically determined, which makes the remaining portion of variance subject to environmental conditioning. Optimal peak bone mass requires nutritional sufficiency (adequate calcium, phosphorus, and vitamin D intake), healthy hormonal milieu, regular physical activity, and avoidance of smoking and excessive alcohol use, all of which constitute the so-called "foundational therapies" of osteoporosis. Nutritional and medical threats to skeletal health need to be identified and rectified. Secondary causes of osteoporosis should be considered in the presence of unexpectedly low bone mineral density or unusual skeletal fragility (Table 1). Most secondary causes of osteoporosis involve premature or iatrogenic hypogonadism and use of systemic glucocorticoids.

Pharmacotherapy for established osteoporosis reduces osteoporotic fracture incidence by approximately 50%. The risk of multiple fractures is reduced even further with pharmacotherapy. Current antiosteoporosis therapies consist of either anticatabolic therapies (hormone replacement therapy, calcitonin, raloxifene, and the aminobisphosphonates [alendronate, ibandronate, and risedronate]) or anabolic therapy (teriparatide).

Calcitonin and raloxifene are relatively weak anticatabolic therapies and have only proven to reduce the vertebral fracture rate. The aminobisphosphonates also have been proven to reduce the incidence of hip fracture, although it is widely believed that the profound anabolic effect of teriparatide will be shown to share this benefit once an appropriately powered study has been conducted. Optimal antifracture efficacy occurs when these medicines are used in populations that are at highest risk of fracture (Caucasian, Asian, or Hispanic women and patients with lower bone mineral density, increasing age, lower bone mass index, and maternal hip fracture) even into the ninth decade of life. With the exception of aminobisphosphonates, bone mineral density and the antifracture efficacy of antiosteoporosis therapies begin to wane soon after drug discontinuation. Emerging data suggest that because of the lengthy half-life of aminobisphosphonates in bone a discontinuation of drug therapy may be possible in some patients after at least 5 years of skeletal saturation with these compounds. When the dominant fracture risk is nonskeletal (patients who fall, have seizures, have hypotension, and those who abuse alcohol) or nutritional (patients with hypovitaminosis D), the primary therapeutic intervention should be directed toward rectifying these issues.

The period immediately after experiencing a fracture is one of considerable physiologic vulnerability and accelerated fracture risk and provides an opportune time for a collaborative intervention among orthopaedists, primary care physicians, specialists in metabolic bone diseases, physiatrists, physical therapists, and nutritionists.

## Clinical Evaluation

Only about 40% of patients with painful vertebral compression fractures recall a specific inciting event to which they ascribe the fracture. Fracture pain is typically posterior and felt approximately at the anatomic level of the vertebral compression fracture. Pain may wrap around the trunk or radiate caudally and can be mistaken for pain emanating from a more anterior, caudal, or visceral structure. Although pain intensity is variable, it typically worsens with movements of the trunk and may be excruciating when moving to and from the supine position. Patients can usually identify some position of reasonable comfort. Surprisingly, approximately one fifth of patients with vertebral compression fractures are most comfortable standing. Findings on the physical examination are often nonspecific. The spinous process of the fractured vertebra may be painful with deep pressure, but this is not an infallible indicator of the presence, absence, or level of fracture. Palpation of the entire spine and rib cage should be performed to search for unexpected synchronous vertebral and rib fractures. Neurologic symptoms and deficits resulting from vertebral compression fractures are rare, but they must be carefully sought and excluded in all patients.

The presence of a malignant neoplasm is always of concern in elderly patients with nontraumatic spine fractures, and concern should be heightened when fracture occurs cephalad to T5, have atypical radiographic features, or occur in the setting of significant constitutional symptoms or failing health. Because this patient population is prone to multiple complex health issues, a comprehensive medical history and general physical examination is mandatory. A complete blood count, comprehensive metabolic panel, erythrocyte sedimentation rate, and serum and urine protein electrophoresis will assist in the initial detection of an underlying infectious, metabolic, or malignant process.

## Diagnostic Imaging

Plain radiography is the usual initial imaging modality used to diagnose vertebral compression fractures. Osteoporotic vertebral compression fractures are typically seen in the context of diffuse skeletal demineralization. Ironically, a collapsed vertebra may appear more dense as bone is compacted into a smaller space. A new fracture is suggested by radiographic evidence of sharp cortical breaks, a change in vertebral configuration compared with recent radiographs, and the presence of

dynamic mobility. An older fracture is suggested by radiographic evidence of remodeled fracture margins, osteophytic vertebral bridging, lack of dynamic mobility, and the absence of change compared with recent radiographs. Vigilance is warranted when vertebral compression fracture is clinically suspected, but radiographically unapparent because conformational changes of the fracturing vertebra typically lag behind the clinical event.

MRI is the single most useful imaging modality in the evaluation of osteoporotic vertebral compression fractures. MRI will identify intravertebral edema acutely, define intravertebral clefts, and assist in the evaluation of vertebral malignant neoplasms. Evidence of a high-intensity signal on T2-weighted and fat suppression or short tau inversion recovery sequences signifies fracture edema. Involvement of the pedicle or posterior elements by signal abnormality or the presence of soft tissue in the epidural or paraspinal area should alert the clinician to the presence of an underlying malignant neoplasm or infection. Nuclear scintigraphic bone scanning is a sensitive indicator of fracture and is a readily accessible, inexpensive means of detecting the location and extent of a fracture, provided it is performed at least 48 to 72 hours after the fracture event. Scintigraphic uptake, however, can be nonspecific and may persist for as long as 2 years after fracture, thereby reducing diagnostic specificity. Multiple skeletal lesions suggest metastasis. Single photon emission CT, when combined with nuclear scintigraphy, can more accurately localize the anatomic site of radionuclide concentration when location is in doubt. Positron emission tomography can assist the discrimination of malignant from nonmalignant fractures when standard uptake values are greater than 2.5. Low specificity within the first month after fracture limits the usefulness of positron emission tomography acutely. Both MRI and bone scanning have the additional value of revealing synchronous, otherwise unsuspected fragility fractures in the pelvis and spine.

## Surgical Treatment of Osteoporotic Vertebral Fractures

### Open Surgical Treatment

Patients with osteoporotic vertebral compression fractures rarely develop neurologic indications that mandate open surgical intervention. Surgeons performing such procedures must be experienced in treating patients with deformities of the spine and familiar with the altered biomechanical behavior of osteoporotic bone. Instrumentation in osteoporotic bone necessitates multiple points of fixation proximal and distal to the fractured level, use of larger pedicle screws, potential pedicle screw augmentation with polymethylmethacrylate (PMMA), and consideration of the concomitant need for sublaminar wires. Open surgery involves large dissections, prolonged anesthetic times, and a high inci-

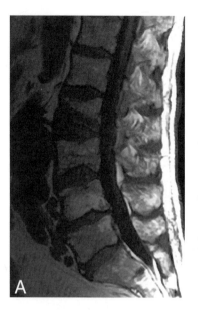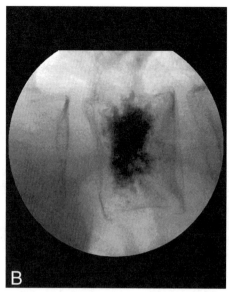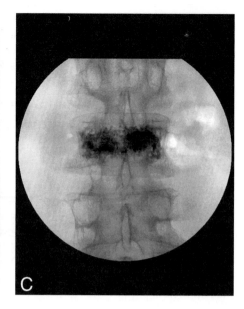

Figure 3　**A,** MRI scan showing an inferior concave fracture of L2. **B,** Lateral intraoperative fluoroscopic view of a vertebral body at completion of vertebroplasty procedure. **C,** Posteroanterior intraoperative fluoroscopic view of a vertebral body at completion of vertebroplasty procedure.

dence of complications. Recent reports of complication rates in this patient population are as high as 80%. Preoperative dual energy x-ray absorptiometry may indicate the degree of skeletal fragility and facilitate surgical planning. Early engagement of medical specialists with expertise in the management of osteoporosis and the medical complexities of frail elderly patients may expedite recovery from open surgery.

## Percutaneous Vertebral Augmentation

Vertebroplasty and kyphoplasty (Figures 3 and 4) are percutaneous vertebral augmentation procedures that have experienced rapid growth in recent years. Both procedures consist of the percutaneous cannulation of the fracturing vertebral body followed by intravertebral installation of PMMA for fracture stabilization and relief of fracture pain. In kyphoplasty, before cement injection, a balloon tamp is introduced into the vertebral body through a large cannula and subsequently inflated, deflated, and withdrawn, leaving a cavity into which PMMA is injected. The intent of balloon inflation is to effect vertebral height restoration and improve spinal alignment. Claims that creation of an intravertebral cavity results in a safer, low-pressure PMMA injection have been challenged. The results of an appropriately designed head-to-head comparison of vertebroplasty and kyphoplasty have not yet been published. The benefit of any form of percutaneous vertebral augmentation over initial nonsurgical management in early osteoporotic vertebral compression fracture has never been demonstrated. When patients remain intolerably symptomatic in spite of comprehensive nonsurgical management, percutaneous vertebral augmentation can safely result in

dramatic pain relief and functional improvement. Percutaneous vertebral augmentation is contraindicated in the presence of local spinal or uncontrolled systemic infection, uncorrectable coagulopathy, or when extensive vertebral disruption or technical factors preclude safe augmentation.

The mechanism of pain relief in percutaneous vertebral augmentation is unproven, but it is generally believed to result from the stabilization of the fractured vertebra and the elimination of microscopic and/or macroscopic motion at the fracture site. Other postulated mechanisms of pain relief include a chemical neurolytic effect of PMMA and the thermal neurolytic effect of the PMMA exotherm. Vertebroplasty and kyphoplasty result in immediate pain relief in most patients. Pain from pathologic fracture is usually substantially relieved after percutaneous vertebral augmentation, but relief may be less dramatic than that achieved in patients with osteoporosis. Patients must be specifically counseled that back, trunk, and limb pain of nonfracture origin, which is nearly ubiquitous in this age group, will not be directly affected by percutaneous vertebral augmentation.

As a general rule, a 9% decrease in predicted forced vital capacity can be expected for each thoracic vertebral compression fracture. Subjective improvement in pulmonary capacity after percutaneous vertebral augmentation is common. Rigorous documentation of improved pulmonary mechanics after percutaneous vertebral augmentation does not yet exist.

## Height Restoration

Dynamic mobility can be harnessed to achieve significant vertebral height restoration through careful surgi-

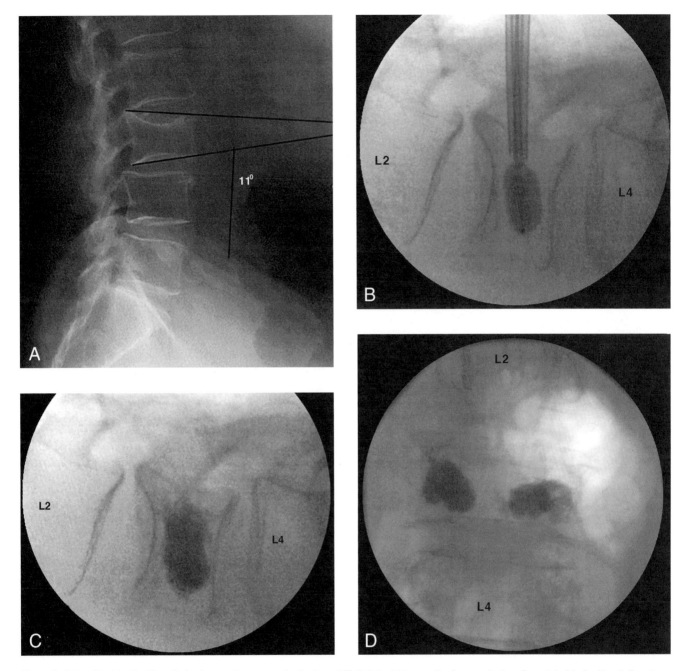

Figure 4  **A,** Standing lateral radiograph showing a wedge compression fracture of L3. **B,** Lateral intraoperative fluoroscopic view of a vertebral body with a balloon tamp inflated. Lateral **(C)** and AP **(D)** intraoperative fluoroscopic views of L3 after removal of the balloon and after PMMA has been injected into the created cavity.

cal patient positioning. Vertebral height restoration attributable to balloon inflation beyond what can be ascribed to dynamic mobility alone has not been convincingly demonstrated. Vertebral height restoration may help improve sagittal alignment and reduce the postural deficit associated with vertebral compression fracture. Although these anatomic derangements contribute to the chronic morbidity and economic burden of osteoporosis, the corollary assumption that vertebral height restoration will reduce morbidity and cost remains unproven.

## Surgical Anatomy

The preferred percutaneous vertebral augmentation technique will depend on the vertebral level being treated. This is because of anatomic differences between thoracic and lumbar vertebrae. In the axial plane, thoracic vertebrae are more conical or bullet-shaped. In the sagittal plane, thoracic pedicles are located more cephalad and are often narrower than those of the lumbar spine. Thus, in thoracic vertebrae, the parapedicular approach is more commonly used, PMMA can often be injected into the center of the vertebral body using a unilateral approach, and the injected volume of PMMA is usually smaller. In lumbar vertebrae and at T12, the approach will more likely be transpedicular, adequate vertebral fill is more likely to require bipedicular instrumentation, and the volume of injected PMMA is greater. The pattern and severity of fracture must be taken into account when determining the anatomic course of the needle. For instance, bipedicular instrumentation may be necessary in patients with severe biconcave deformities in whom navigation of the needle across the midline should not be attempted. In patients with fractures with an axial cleft, precise needle placement is required to enter the cleft and render the vertebra stable by filling this potential space.

## Radiologic Issues

Biplanar fluoroscopy is preferred because it allows for the nearly instantaneous and simultaneous visualization of needle placement and PMMA flow. Fluoroscopic visualization of critical anatomic landmarks can be challenging in patients with osteoporosis, and when visualization is inadequate, percutaneous vertebral augmentation should not be attempted. Fluoroscopy exposes the percutaneous vertebral augmentation operator to high levels of ionizing radiation. The use of protective wear and surgical strategies that minimize radiation exposure is mandatory.

## Strength, Stiffness, and Durability

Two milliliters of PMMA can restore prefracture strength to fractured osteoporotic vertebral bodies ex vivo. Larger volumes (4 to 8 mL) are required to restore prefracture stiffness. The optimal balance of stiffness and strength needed for fracture stability, pain relief, and healing is unknown. Although a specific volume of injected PMMA has not been correlated with clinical success in percutaneous vertebral augmentation, voluminous PMMA injection has been associated with increased incidence of adjacent level vertebral fracture, possibly as a result of excessive stiffness. The biomechanical performance of PMMA-impregnated vertebral bone probably reflects the volume, distribution, and geometry of the fill and may differ between static, dynamic, and repetitive load-bearing circumstances. Cyclical loading of osteoporotic vertebrae in which kyphoplasty or vertebroplasty had been performed ex vivo has been reported to have resulted in late vertebral failure after the former but not the latter procedure, suggesting that vertebral integrity may have been compromised by the destruction of native trabecular scaffolding during balloon inflation. Substantial shortcomings in basic and clinical research within this field should serve as a cautionary restraint on unbridled proliferation of percutaneous vertebral augmentation.

The durability of PMMA within the vertebral body is uncertain, although no reports of mechanical failure after percutaneous vertebral augmentation have yet been published. It seems unlikely that fatigue failure will result given the magnitude of stress and number of cycles to which PMMA is likely to be exposed during activities of daily living in frail elderly patients. The vertebral tissue response to injected PMMA is not completely understood. Percutaneous vertebral augmentation using other cements and incorporating skeletal anabolic agents is under investigation.

## Complications

Complications associated with vertebroplasty and kyphoplasty are infrequent, generally avoidable, and often relate to inaccurate needle placement or inattention to PMMA flow during fluoroscopically guided injection. A thorough understanding of spinal anatomy, careful patient selection, and high-quality fluoroscopic imaging capability are essential for a successful outcome. The symptomatic complication rate in patients with osteoporotic fractures should be less than 1%, but this rate can be expected to be greater in patients with pathologic fractures. Extreme care must be exercised during sedated intraoperative positioning of these patients to avoid complications related to soft-tissue and skeletal fragility. Serious harm and even death have been reported as the result of spinal cord and radicular injury, hemothorax, hypotensive methacrylate monomer reaction, and massive PMMA embolism.

### PMMA Leak

The PMMA leak rate from osteoporotic vertebral compression fractures has been reported in 7% to 70% of patients, but this wide range reflects considerable ascertainment and reporting bias. Most contemporary studies report radiographic leak rates of approximately 10% and symptomatic leak rates of less than 1%. The location and extent of PMMA leak will determine the presence and nature of clinical symptoms. Paravertebral soft-tissue leaks may occur through osteoporotic, pathologic, or iatrogenic cortical breach when PMMA filling volumes and rates exceed intravertebral (volume and pressure) capacity. Small paravertebral venous leakage is not uncommon. Because vigilance during high-resolution biplanar imaging is usually sufficient to abort azygous or caval propagation, pulmonary embolism has been rare. Epidural venous leak can be avoided by ceasing injection once PMMA reaches the junction of the middle and posterior one third of the vertebral body during fluoroscopic monitoring with the patient in the lateral position. Symptomatic foraminal venous leak may be problematic because the volume of PMMA necessary to compress the foraminal nerve root is relatively small.

PMMA leak into the disk may be anticipated by the presence of coronal and sagittal splits through the vertebral end plate observed on preoperative imaging. Disk space leaks are not symptomatic, but they have been implicated in adjacent vertebral fracture when injected cement volumes are high. CT with three-dimensional reconstructions accurately shows the location and degree of PMMA leakage and will assist in the evaluation of those suspected to have symptomatic PMMA leaks.

## Refracture

Considerable attention has been given to determining whether percutaneous vertebral augmentation increases the risk of subsequent vertebral fractures. Determining whether the observed vertebral fracture incidence after percutaneous vertebral augmentation is excessive is a complex undertaking. Factors that must take into consideration include the anticipated fracture rate of a specific study population with osteoporosis, fracture definition (clinical versus morphometric), definition of methods (semiquantitative versus quantitative) and fracture definition cut points (15% versus 20% vertebral height loss), the integrity of fracture ascertainment, and the period of observation. In general, fracture after percutaneous vertebral augmentation is more common in patients with malignancy and multiple myeloma than in those with osteoporosis. Published vertebral fracture rates after percutaneous vertebral augmentation in patients with osteoporosis range from 0 to 52% over periods ranging from 6 weeks to 5 years and generally seem to be declining as vertebral augmentation experience increases. Subsequent fracture rate may be attenuated by comprehensive postoperative medical and rehabilitative care that is osteoporosis-specific. One study reported that 20% of women with osteoporosis experience one new morphometric vertebral fracture within 1 year of an incident vertebral fracture; however, only about one fourth of these fractures were symptomatic. Vertebral fracture incidence is reportedly increased with increasing age, multiple medical comorbidities, a greater number of prevalent fractures, greater severity of prevalent vertebral fractures, the degree of spinal kyphosis, the rate of falling, and glucocorticoid therapy. The occasional temporal and spatial clustering of osteoporotic vertebral fractures further confounds estimation of the expected incident vertebral fracture rate. Powering a prospective vertebral augmentation trial to determine whether subsequent vertebral fracture incidence is excessive compared with continued nonsurgical therapy would require a large series of patients that controls for all of the previously enumerated variables and, therefore, is unlikely to be undertaken.

## Summary

Skeletal health is centered on foundational therapies that should be instituted early and continued throughout life. Management of patients with osteoporosis involves an appreciation of the roles of physiotherapy, pharmacotherapy, and surgical intervention. Management of vertebral compression fractures is an evolving, multidisciplinary clinical science that is of increasing interest in part because of the introduction of minimal access vertebral augmentation procedures. Orthopaedists should be cautious when transferring high-energy spine fracture experience to the care of patients with osteoporosis and be mindful of the multiple medical comorbidities in the frail, elderly, osteoporotic population. Osteoporosis fracture care should be viewed as a multidisciplinary collaboration and existing and emerging surgical interventions subjected to rigorous scrutiny.

## Annotated Bibliography

### Pathogenesis of the Osteoporotic Fracture

Rao RD, Singrakhia MD: Painful osteoporotic vertebral fracture: Pathogenesis, evaluation, and roles of vertebroplasty and kyphoplasty in its management. *J Bone Joint Surg Am* 2003;85-A:2010-2022.

A comprehensive review of the pathophysiology of osteoporosis and osteoporotic fracture is presented, along with a discussion of evaluation of management of patients with vertebral fracture and summary evaluation of evidence regarding vertebral augmentation procedures.

### Consequences of Fracture

Lindsay R, Silverman SL, Cooper C, et al: Risk of new vertebral fracture in the year following a fracture. *JAMA* 2001;285:320-323.

A post-hoc analysis of 2,725 postmenopausal women with osteoporosis assigned to placebo in the large multinational trials of oral weekly risedronate is presented. Overall, 19.2% of women experienced a second radiographic vertebral fracture within 1 year of an incident vertebral fracture; however, only 23% of these fractures were clinically apparent as fracture events.

### Dynamic Mobility

McKiernan F, Jensen R, Faciszewski T: The dynamic mobility of vertebral compression fractures. *J Bone Miner Res* 2003;18:24-29.

The initial definition and systematic description of dynamic mobility in osteoporotic vertebral compression fractures is presented. The authors demonstrate that dynamic mobility is the permissive property allowing vertebral height restoration at vertebroplasty.

### General Management of Patients With Osteoporosis

United States Department of Health and Human Services: *Bone Health and Osteoporosis: A Report of the Surgeon General, 2004.* Available at: http://

www.surgeongeneral.gov/library/bonehealth/content.html. Accessed November 23, 2005.

This article focuses on bone health and osteoporosis information multiauthored by leaders in the field of osteoporosis and metabolic bone disease. A concise summary and patient-friendly synopsis are available.

## Surgical Treatment of Osteoporotic Vertebral Fractures

Lieberman IH, Dudeney S, Reinhardt MK, Bell G: Initial outcome and efficacy of "kyphoplasty" in the treatment of painful osteoporotic vertebral compression fractures. *Spine* 2001;26:1631-1638.

This initial peer review article is the most widely referenced detailing experience with kyphoplasty and is suggested reading for anyone performing vertebral augmentation procedures.

Mathis J, Deramond H, Belkoff S: *Percutaneous Vertebroplasty*. New York, NY, Springer, 2002.

This book addresses the clinical context in which to consider vertebroplasty and details technical aspects of vertebroplasty.

McKiernan F, Faciszewski T, Jensen R: Quality of life following vertebroplasty. *J Bone Joint Surg Am* 2004;86-A:2600-2606.

In a prospective, consecutive case series, a visual analog scale and an osteoporosis-specific health-related quality of life outcome instrument were used to measure outcomes of vertebroplasty. After vertebroplasty, quality of life and pain relief rapidly and significantly improve and remain improved for at least 6 months. PMMA leak rate and subsequent vertebral fracture rate were very low.

## Radiologic Issues

Kruger R, Faciszewski T: Radiation dose reduction to medical staff during vertebroplasty: A review of techniques and methods to mitigate occupational dose. *Spine* 2003;28(14):1608-1613.

This article discusses a case crossover study of a single operator implementing radiation exposure reduction strategies. Reductions in whole-body and hand radiation dose ranged from 42.9% to 86.1% following implementation of behavioral and shielding interventions. Operators performing vertebroplasty should implement radiation protection strategies.

## Strength, Stiffness, and Durability

Alamin T, Kim M, Carragee E, Stevens K, Lindsey D: Kyphoplasty vs vertebroplasty behavior under repetitive loading conditions. *Spine J* 2004;4(5S):47S.

Sixteen cadaveric thoracic vertebrae from eight elderly women were treated ex vivo with vertebroplasty or kyphoplasty and subjected to repetitive loading. Those treated with kyphoplasty were more likely to show progressive loss of height under these experienced conditions.

## Complications

Liebschner MA, Rosenberg WS, Keaveny TM: Effects of bone cement volume and distribution on vertebral stiffness after vertebroplasty. *Spine* 2001;26:1547-1554.

This article presents an ex vivo biomechanical analysis of osteoporotic vertebral strength and stiffness after being subjected to various PMMA fill volumes and distributions. The results suggest that symmetric intravertebral placement of approximately 15% volume fraction PMMA is the optimal biomechanical configuration for vertebral augmentation.

# Chapter 40

# Complications of Spinal Surgery

Hargovind DeWal, MD

Robert F. McLain, MD

## Introduction

Prior to undertaking a surgical procedure, the surgeon and patient should discuss the surgery and possible complications. Because the patient should make an informed decision, the surgeon must have a thorough understanding of the possible complications of the intended procedure. An in-depth understanding of potential complications is needed to adequately anticipate and prevent such events. Complications of spinal surgery may result from errors or events occurring preoperatively, intraoperatively, or postoperatively.

## Intubation and Patient Positioning Prior to the Incision

Patients with cervical instability must be handled carefully during intubation, whether the instability is acute, chronic, or caused by trauma, tumor, or degenerative or rheumatoid disease. When cord compression is clinically apparent, intubation should be performed on an awake patient to provide maximal safety. Because the patient has muscular control of the neck, instability is lessened and increasing impairment can be signaled by the patient if it occurs. Hyperextension of the neck increases cord impingement and should be avoided.

Correct patient positioning is of prime importance before beginning any surgical procedure. Two specific forms of injury, from pressure and traction, must be anticipated and prevented. Adequately padding bony prominences and superficial nerves is necessary, especially when surgery is performed on the prone patient. Pressure on the eyes should be avoided. Ophthalmic complications are uncommon, but can be devastating. In a study of 3,450 spinal procedures, the incidence of loss of visual function was 0.20%. Although visual complications were traditionally believed to result from improper positioning, this study showed that hypertension and peripheral vascular disease also contribute to the development of this complication. Smoking, diabetes, chronic hypertension, intraoperative hypotension, and low flow states may all contribute to the risks for ischemic ocular complications. Pressure on the eyes should be assiduously avoided and a minimum systolic blood pressure should be established preoperatively to avoid excessive hypotension.

Excessive traction should not be placed on the arms. The patient's elbows should be kept flexed at 90° and the ulnar nerve at the elbow should be free from any compression. Knees should be flexed to reduce traction on the sciatic nerve. Bony prominences of the knees and feet should be padded. When the patient is prone, the abdomen should be allowed to hang freely to avoid excessive intra-abdominal pressure, which can interfere with normal excursion of the diaphragm and with venous return from the lower extremities. Pressure on the abdominal contents can be transmitted to the epidural venous system and may therefore increase bleeding. In one study, patients were randomized to one of two groups with different support widths on a Wilson frame to determine its effect on intraoperative estimated blood loss. The narrow pad support widths of the Wilson frame produced higher intra-abdominal pressure than the wide pad support widths. The group with the higher intra-abdominal pressure had significantly more blood loss than the group with a lower intra-abdominal pressure.

Some thoracic and thoracolumbar procedures require patient positioning in the lateral decubitus position. Adequate chest padding must be provided to prevent injury to the brachial plexus in the axilla. It should be remembered that the axillary roll is placed under the chest wall, not in the axilla. The common peroneal nerve should be padded in the region of the fibular head to prevent peroneal nerve palsy. During anterior lumbar surgery, the extreme Trendelenburg position can lead to decreased diaphragm excursion because of the pressure of the abdominal contents.

## Preventing Intraoperative Complications
### Localizing the Surgical Level

Localizing the correct surgical spinal level is essential. Anatomic landmarks are unreliable and radiographic confirmation is always recommended. Localizing radiographs should include an unequivocal landmark (such as the odontoid or lumbosacral junction), as well as a surgical marker (such as a spinal needle or Penfield elevator). Using both AP and lateral radiographs may be necessary, particularly in obese patients or those with segmental anomaly. In other patients, fluoroscopy may be preferred. Image guidance may be helpful in patients with severe deformity or altered anatomy. Repeat radiographs are advised whenever the surgical findings fail to show the expected pathology.

### Vascular Injuries

Vascular injuries can occur during any aspect of a spinal procedure, from any approach. The most common areas for vascular injury include: injury to the vertebral artery during anterior cervical diskectomy, or placement of posterior cervical lateral mass screws; injury of the iliac vessels during anterior fusion or disk arthroplasty placement or by penetration of a screw or probe during pedicle screw instrumentation; perforation of the aorta, vena cava, or iliac vessel by pituitary or curet during lumbar diskectomy surgery, and direct injury to the aorta or vena cava during anterior thoracolumbar reconstruction and instrumentation.

Prevention is crucial in the management of vascular injury during spinal surgery. The surgeon must be knowledgeable about anatomy and its variations, and should know the pattern of vascular supply of the specific patient. The surgeon must be certain of the location of the surgical instrument at all times. It is crucial that no cutting instrument is inserted into the disk space without knowing the exact length of the instrument within the disk.

### Incidental Durotomy

Incidental durotomy is a tear of the dura mater that occurs during a surgical procedure. Cerebrospinal fluid (CSF) leaks may also persist after invasive procedures such as myelography or epidural injection. Incidental durotomy is more likely to occur during revision surgery at spinal levels with scarring and adhesions. In the cervical spine, ossification of the posterior longitudinal ligament is a condition that carries a higher incidence of durotomy because of either an adherent posterior longitudinal ligament or the absence of dura mater in the involved region.

Lumbar durotomy is more likely to occur in areas of severe stenosis, where epidural fat has been displaced and where the dura may have become adherent to the lamina or facet capsule. Lumbar durotomy is also likely in any area of scar tissue. Folds of redundant dura may become trapped by the Kerrison rongeur in the lateral recess or under the rim of the lowermost lumbar lamina (Figure 1). The reported incidence of durotomy varies. One review of 641 patients who underwent lumbar de-

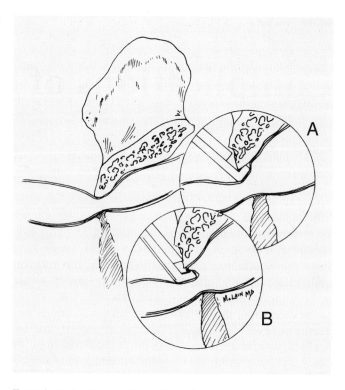

**Figure 1** A potential cause of an incidental durotomy during laminectomy is illustrated. Inset (A) shows that angling the Kerrison rongeur properly adjacent to bone or using a 90°-angled Kerrison rongeur may help to avoid entrapment of dura. Inset (B) shows how a Kerrison rongeur that is improperly angled may allow dura to become entrapped in the rongeur and thus lead to a durotomy.

compression reported that 14% of patients had intraoperative durotomies. A separate review of 450 patients who had lumbar surgery reported a 4% rate of durotomy recognized at surgery, whereas a more recent review of 2,144 patients reported a 3.1% overall incidence. The incidence of unrecognized clinically significant durotomies was 0.28%. Adequate repair of the durotomy during surgery allows early mobilization with rare clinical symptoms. Persistent dural leaks can lead to several sequelae, including persistent recurrent headaches, pseudomeningocele, cutaneous fistula, neurologic deficit, or meningitis. In one study, five of six patients with unrecognized durotomy developed pseudomeningocele and all had subsequent repair of dural defects after nonsurgical treatment failed. Reoperation was successful and no long-term sequelae were encountered.

Small durotomies recognized intraoperatively should be repaired primarily. Repairs for larger defects may be augmented with muscle, fascia, or fat grafts, fibrin patches, fibrin glue, or a hemostatic gelatin sponge. The Valsalva maneuver should be used to confirm the adequacy of repair. A lumbar subarachnoid drain may be used with larger defects or complex tears that defy direct repair.

The use of subfascial drains in patients with a durotomy is controversial. Some authors believe a subfascial postoperative drain may be used if an adequate dural repair is achieved. However, the risk associated with such drainage devices, including durocutaneous fistula and cerebellar herniation, must be weighed against any benefit derived from the use of a drain. A recent study showed no adverse events associated with the use of subfascial drains in patients with durotomies when adequate repair of the dura was achieved.

An incidental durotomy may not be recognized until the postoperative period. Patients may report headaches that worsen on elevation of the head. Clear drainage from the incision site should raise the suspicion of a CSF leak. Beta-2-transferrin can be tested in wound drainage to determine the presence of CSF. An MRI scan or CT myelogram may show a dural defect. If a CSF leak is detected, reexploration and another repair or patching may be performed. A lumbar drain also may be used for management. The patient is kept at bed rest; drainage rates of 50 to 100 mL every 8 hours for 4 to 6 days should be maintained. The drained fluid should be monitored for white blood cells to prevent infection. If drainage is not effective, surgical treatment should ensue.

Extended bed rest is not necessary in patients who undergo standard dural repair techniques following a durotomy. There is little consensus concerning the proper period of bed rest after durotomy; therefore, patients may be mobilized according to the individual surgeon's postoperative protocol. Although patients with a small durotomy and a water-tight repair may be mobilized the day of surgery, patients with more extensive tears and/or a tenuous repair may benefit from 48 to 72 hours of bed rest before mobilization. If symptoms of postural headache or photophobia recur, further bed rest would be indicated, and placement of a subarachnoid drain may be considered.

### Neural Element Injury

Neural element injury can involve the spinal cord or the nerve roots and can result from direct trauma, indirect trauma, traction, or from spinal cord ischemia. Patients with preexisting cord compression are at higher risk of injury, as are patients with previous cord injuries, extensive spondylosis, or impaired vascular perfusion.

In the cervical spine, nerve root injury has been reported with both the anterior and posterior approaches. Most root injuries are transient. Permanent spinal cord injury is rare. The risk of cord injury is increased in patients with myelopathy. This increased risk may be the result of decreased physiologic reserve of an already injured spinal cord. Quadriplegia may result from injudicious manipulation of the neck during intubation or positioning in any patient with segmental instability. Excessive traction or manipulation during surgical treatment can have the same effect. Any graft placed for cer-

vical fusion, either an interbody or segmental strut, must be contoured and positioned carefully to avoid impingement or extrusion into the spinal canal.

During laminectomy, the risks of neural element injury vary with the level of laminectomy performed. Nerve roots can in general tolerate more manipulation and retraction than the spinal cord or the conus medullaris. Vigorous manipulation of the spinal cord or conus medullaris is unwise, and will likely lead to permanent neurologic injury.

During decompression, nerve roots may be injured with a high-speed burr or a Kerrison rongeur. The neural elements should be protected with an intermediate barrier such as a cottonoid while using a high-speed burr. In the lumbar spine, it is sometimes difficult to distinguish the contour of the nerve root that is stretched tightly across an extruded disk fragment, or to be sure that the thecal sac has been mobilized free from the fragment or scar. Time should be taken to identify the lateral edge of the thecal sac and retract it medially over the large extrusion and to extend the laminotomy enough to isolate the nerve root before incising the annulus for diskectomy.

A large footplate of a Kerrison rongeur may produce further compression in an already stenotic spinal canal. The use of a rongeur with a thin footplate is recommended when decompressing stenotic spinal segments.

Electrocautery can injure neural elements as well. Monopolar electrocautery should not be used near nerve roots. It is recommended that bipolar electrocautery be used near nerve roots on a minimal setting. Moreover, it is essential to limit contact between the bipolar and the neural elements. When possible, cottonoid, sterile hemostatic gelatin sponge, or topical hemostatic fabric should be used to limit the use of electrocautery.

### Pedicle Screw Placement

Nerve injury can result from errant pedicle screw placement or inaccurate pedicle sizing. Nerve root injury is more likely at the inferomedial aspect of the pedicle in the thoracic and lumbar spine. Nerve damage can occur from direct screw contact or from pedicle fracture fragments resulting from screw penetration.

Meticulous preoperative planning is vital when planning pedicle screw fixation. Preoperative radiographs and CT scans should be examined to check for pedicle size, angle, and length. CT scans are more accurate than radiographs in planning the correct placement of pedicle screws. Computer-guided stereotactic systems may be useful in decreasing the pedicle perforation rate, but cost and time demands associated with these systems have limited their widespread use. Fluoroscopy is the most commonly used method for confirming both the starting point for screw insertion and for checking the alignment and depth of placement during screw insertion.

Electrical stimulation of screws while recording electromyographic (EMG) activity intraoperatively has been studied to help increase the accuracy of screw placement. In one study of 90 patients in which 512 pedicle screws were placed in the lumbosacral spine, intraoperative EMG was performed. Postoperative CT scans were checked to determine the accuracy of the EMG readings with regard to pedicle screw placement. The authors reported that a stimulation threshold of 15 mA provides a 98% confidence that the screw was well positioned within the pedicle. A threshold between 10 and 15 mA provided an 87% confidence of accurate screw positioning; exploration is recommended to rule out a cortical breach. In 9% of patients, EMG detected screw malposition that was not identifiable on the lateral radiograph.

A recent study examined the use of EMG for determining the accuracy of placement of pedicle screws in the thoracic spine. EMG recordings were compared with a postoperative CT scan. Eighty-seven screws were examined in 22 patients. In this study, a stimulation threshold of 11 mA provided a 97.5% negative predictive value, indicating the screw was within the pedicle.

## Complications of the Anterior Surgical Approach

### Cervical Surgery

There are numerous complications associated with the anterior approach to the subaxial spine. Infection, dysphagia, esophageal perforation, vascular injury, hardware-related complications, tracheal injury, and bone graft dislodgement have all been reported. A review of 4,589 cases to examine complications related to surgery of the cervical spine showed a total complication rate of 5.3%. The authors noted that the use of the anterior approach was involved in 65% of cases. Hoarseness can occur in 51% of patients and is related to elevated cuff pressures and prolonged intubation. It has been shown that vocal cord paralysis can occur in up to 5% of patients.

The transoral approach is used to gain anterior exposure to the upper cervical spine. Difficulties associated with this approach include exposure, infection, and wound closure. Because the approach is through the oral cavity, adequate antibiotic prophylaxis is warranted. Broad-spectrum antibiotics should be given preoperatively and continued for 3 days postoperatively. Retractors should be placed carefully to prevent pinching of the upper lip, and the tongue blade should be periodically relaxed to limit tongue swelling.

The sympathetic chain lies lateral and ventral to the longus colli musculature. Injury to this structure may produce a Horner syndrome. Prevention of sympathetic chain injury is best achieved by avoiding lateral dissection of the longus colli musculature and by careful placement of retractors medial and deep to the longus colli musculature.

Postoperative difficulty in swallowing is common and can occur in 60% of patients with symptoms lasting for more than 6 months in 12% of patients. A recent study prospectively evaluated 23 patients undergoing anterior cervical diskectomy and fusion with a preoperative and postoperative modified barium swallow study and videolaryngoendoscopy. The objective of this study was to determine the incidence and risk factors for swallowing and voice difficulties following anterior cervical diskectomy and fusion. Patients undergoing multilevel surgery were more likely to experience increased soft-tissue swelling; this swelling was more frequent in patients whose swallowing function was worse postoperatively.

With prolonged and unrelieved pressure, or with direct trauma caused by surgical instruments or power instruments, either the carotid artery or the esophagus may sustain a significant injury.

To limit the risk of tissue injury during anterior cervical procedures, precautions must be taken. The endotracheal cuff should be released and reinflated after exposure to avoid excessive pressure. Prolonged retraction should be avoided and self-retaining retractors should be frequently repositioned. Scarred tissue should be carefully dissected, the esophagus should be identified (place an esophageal stethoscope for palpation), and the thoracic duct (low, left-sided approach) and recurrent laryngeal nerve (right-sided approach) should be avoided. An attempt at revision surgery from the side opposite the first approach should not be made without performing a careful examination of vocal cord function. Voice disturbance (dysphonia) is one of the possible complications of any anterior approach to the cervical spine. Voice and swallowing difficulties may each occur after inadvertent injury to the recurrent laryngeal and/or superior laryngeal nerve (a recognized and potentially preventable complication of the anterior approach to the cervical spine). This complication occurs in 1% to 2% of right-sided cervical approaches and is characterized by distinctive hoarseness that is unrelated to inflammation or intubation trauma. On the left side, the nerve is protected in the tracheoesophageal groove. On the right, however, the nerve crosses the field and may be injured by stretch or sectioning. Recurrent laryngeal nerve injury is confirmed by direct visualization of the vocal cords, showing paralysis of the cord ipsilateral to the nerve injury.

### Thoracolumbar Surgery

Anterior approaches in the thoracic and lumbar spine can be associated with serious vascular injury. The particular vascular structures that are at risk depend on the level of the spine being exposed and whether a left- or right-sided approach is used. A left-sided approach is more commonly used; in the lumbar spine it involves mobilization of the iliac vein, which typically overlies the L4-L5 disk. The L5-S1 disk lies between the iliac vessels, which are at less risk at this level. The aorta lies on the left side in the upper lumbar and thoracic regions and is rarely injured. However, the aorta can be quite tortuous in some patients and the degree of retraction required is variable. Right-sided procedures place the vena cava and its tributaries at more risk than the arteries. A recent study of 207 patients undergoing anterior thoracic and lumbar spinal reconstructive surgeries examined the incidence, causes, and treatment of vascular complications. The incidence of vascular complications was 5.8% and the mortality rate was 1%.

Vascular injuries can occur through inadvertent sectioning of a segmental or vascular branch, through avulsion of the segmental artery or vein during dissection, or by direct perforation of a major vessel. Segmental vessels are usually well controlled with a tie or a clip, but avulsions must be repaired at the wall of the aorta or vena cava. Similarly, any perforation of a major vessel must be isolated, controlled, and carefully oversewn to provide a water-tight repair without compromising the patency of the vessel. In the thoracic spine, particularly in the lower thoracic segments, large caliber segmental arteries should not be ligated. To avoid ischemic injury to the cord, segmental arteries should be spared whenever possible, and should only be ligated unilaterally.

The thoracic duct is at risk during left-sided approaches to the thoracic spine. The thoracic duct typically lies posterior to the esophagus and empties into the left jugular and subclavian veins. If the thoracic duct is injured, it should be ligated and then oversewn. The patient should be placed on a low-fat diet postoperatively to reduce the risk of chylothorax.

Neurologic injury to the lumbar plexus can occur during anterior surgical approaches. Injury to the parasympathetic plexus at the L4-5 or L5-S1 levels can result in retrograde ejaculation. Disruption of the sympathetic chain will result in a lower extremity sympathectomy. The incidence of retrograde ejaculation is reported to be 2% and the incidence of lower extremity sympathectomy is reported to be 10%. To minimize injury to the parasympathetic plexus, monopolar electrocautery should not be used directly anterior to the L5-S1 disk. Blunt dissection is encouraged in this region.

Visceral injury is another anterior approach-related complication that may occur. The ureters, which lie on the psoas muscle, may be injured during the anterior approach to the lumbar spine. Clear fluid may be seen intraoperatively; however, the injury diagnosis may also occur postoperatively. Signs and symptoms of ureteral injury may include abdominal or flank pain, fever, and hematuria. A urinoma, a mass of encapsulated urine, may form in the abdomen producing abdominal disten-

tion. Ultrasound or CT should be used in conjunction with a urinalysis to help arrive at a diagnosis.

### Anterior Hardware-Related Complications

Neurologic and vascular injuries have occurred following interbody cage placement. Erosion of vascular structures by anteriorly placed hardware has been reported and can cause catastrophic hemorrhage. When placing screws into the vertebral bodies, bicortical placement increases the force required for screw pullout. However, it is important to measure the vertebral body depth and width during screw placement. In a recent study, CT scan evaluation of anterior vertebral body screws placed thoracoscopically was performed to determine screw position relative to the spinal canal and the aorta. The average distance from the posterior aspect of the screw to the spinal canal was 5.3 mm. When screws were analyzed in relationship to the aorta, 12.3% of screws were noted to create a contour deformity of the aorta.

Complications of disk replacement surgery have recently been reported in the literature. In a study of 27 patients who underwent disk replacement surgery with unsatisfactory results, early complications included prosthesis dislocation, abdominal wall hematoma, and retrograde ejaculation. Late complications included prosthesis subsidence, prosthesis displacement, and the occurrence of polyethylene wear. Errors in patient selection, choice of implant size, and inaccurate positioning of the implant greatly increase the risk of these complications.

### Bone Graft Complications

Complications related to bone graft harvest from the ilium are common. Reported complications include pain, nerve injury, arterial injury, hematoma, gait abnormalities, stress fracture, peritoneal perforation, and herniation of abdominal contents. Corticocancellous graft harvest may result in chronic graft-site pain. Superior gluteal artery injury may occur if the sciatic notch is entered inadvertently. Control of bleeding may require ligation of the vessel, embolization, or emergent laparotomy because the severed end of the vessel tends to retract into the pelvis where it may not tamponade. Neurologic injuries occur in 8% of patients undergoing iliac crest bone graft harvest. The lateral femoral cutaneous nerve is at risk during an anterior harvest, whereas the cluneal nerve is more commonly injured with a posterior bone graft harvest. After harvest, fractures may occur through the wing of the ilium, or there may be an avulsion of the anterior superior iliac spine.

## Postoperative Complications
### Airway
A recent review of 311 anterior cervical procedures examined the incidence and risk factors associated with

airway complications following surgery. The overall airway complication rate was 6%, with one third of patients requiring reintubation. Risk factors for airway complications included surgical time of more than 5 hours and exposure of four or more vertebral bodies involving C4 or higher. Pulmonary disease, smoking, absence of drainage, and myelopathy were not related to the development of postoperative airway complications. Airway obstruction resulting from a hematoma can occur, although rarely, and is treated with emergent decompression. For the first 24 hours following anterior cervical surgery, it is sound practice to have a suture set available at the bedside of the patient.

## Ischemic Cord Injury

Although few articles have appeared in the literature regarding cord injury caused by postoperative ischemia, the poor outcome associated with this uncommon complication warrants discussion. The spinal cord compromised by prolonged stenosis, compression, tumor, or infection may be stressed when its tenuous blood supply is further impaired by surgical dissection. When postoperative hypotension is superimposed, irreversible injury or cord-stroke can occur. This complication may occur more than 24 hours after surgery.

Hypertensive patients allowed to languish with a low systolic and mean arterial pressure have sustained permanent cord injuries despite normal initial cord function. Patients at risk should be treated promptly for episodes of postoperative hypotension, and attention should be given to careful neurologic checks if circulation is impaired for any length of time.

## Wound Infections

Estimates of the incidence of spinal wound infections vary from 1% to 11%. Instrumented fusions are associated with higher rates of infection than noninstrumented fusions. A recent study showed that the risk of infection after instrumented fusion is higher in trauma patients than in patients undergoing elective spinal surgery. Moreover, patients with a complete neurologic deficit are also at a greater risk for developing a postoperative wound infection. Postoperative infection can be difficult to diagnose because the erythrocyte sedimentation rates are naturally elevated, as is the white blood cell count, and the wound rarely shows much evidence of a deep infection. The most reliable signs of infection are the presence of progressively worsening pain and pain unrelated to activity. The most helpful laboratory study is the C-reactive protein level.

Postoperative wound infections should be treated aggressively with surgical irrigation and débridement. Serial débridements may be necessary; however, many patients may be successfully managed with suction-drainage systems after initial débridement. Long-term

antibiotic treatment should be initiated with the choice of antibiotic dependent on the culture results.

## Thromboembolism

A prospective study of 116 patients was undertaken to determine the incidence of deep venous thrombosis (DVT) and symptomatic pulmonary embolism (PE) in patients undergoing spinal surgery. Duplex scans revealed an asymptomatic DVT rate of 0.9%. A 2.6% rate of symptomatic PE was found, with six PEs occurring in patients undergoing combined anterior-posterior surgeries and one PE occurring in a patient who had only posterior surgery. All patients in this study were prophylactically treated with thigh-length compression stockings and mechanical compression devices. The authors suggested that simple mechanical prophylaxis may provide inadequate treatment in patients undergoing combined anterior-posterior procedures. Patients with a history of, or risk factors for DVT or PE should be treated with an effective antithrombotic regimen after surgery.

## Ileus

Adynamic ileus is a complication seen with both anterior and posterior lumbar spinal surgery. Adynamic ileus can involve the small intestine, large intestine (Ogilvie's syndrome), or both. Signs and symptoms of an ileus include abdominal pain and distention, nausea, vomiting, and absent/hypoactive bowel sounds. Most patients with adynamic ileus can be treated with nasogastric tube decompression, withdrawal of narcotics, and supplemental intravenous fluid hydration. Other causes for adynamic ileus should be sought, such as electrolyte imbalance or retroperitoneal hematoma.

## Epidural Hematoma

Spinal epidural hematoma can occur following any spinal surgery. Although most spinal epidural hematomas that develop are clinically insignificant, a small subset of patients can develop large hematomas that can cause pain and neurologic deficit, requiring surgical decompression. Early diagnosis and rapid surgical decompression are crucial in successfully reversing neurologic impairments. A recent study was done to identify risk factors for the development of a spinal epidural hematoma. Patients undergoing multilevel lumbar procedures and/or those patients with a preoperative coagulopathy were found to be at significantly higher risk for developing a postoperative epidural hematoma. Compressive hematoma should be considered in any patient who has neurologic deterioration in the postoperative period.

## Late Graft Complications

Bone graft and hardware-related complication in anterior thoracolumbar surgery are not uncommon. Bone graft collapse, resorption, fracture, and dislodgment have been reported. Between 26% and 30% of patients who have had a corticocancellous graft harvest from the iliac crest will develop a significant complication. Typical wound complications include wound infection, hematoma formation, skin necrosis, and scar formation. Infection of the pelvis can occur. Most commonly, patients report persistent pain at the graft site, sometimes years after the harvest.

## Summary

Spine surgery is never minor surgery. The surgical team must always prepare to prevent the varied and potentially devastating complications that can occur as a result of patient positioning, surgical technique, planning, and simple postoperative ill-fortune. Careful preparation and constant vigilance during treatment can maintain complication rates at an acceptable level even in patients undergoing complex surgical procedures.

## Annotated Bibliography

### Preventing Intraoperative Complications

Frempong-Boadu A, Houten JK, Osborn B, et al: Swallowing and speech dysfunction in patients undergoing anterior cervical discectomy and fusion: A prospective, objective preoperative and postoperative assessment. *J Spinal Disord Tech* 2002;15:362-368.

This prospective study was undertaken to identify patients with swallowing and speech dysfunction before and after anterior cervical diskectomy and fusion.

Perez-Cruet MJ, Fessler RG, Perin NI: Review: Complications of minimally invasive spinal surgery. *Neurosurgery* 2002;51:S26-36.

This article is a comprehensive review of complications specifically associated with minimally invasive spinal surgery.

Shi Y, Binette M, Martin WH: Electrical stimulation for intraoperative evaluation of thoracic pedicle screw placement. *Spine* 2003;28:595-601.

In this study, thoracic pedicle screws were stimulated intraoperatively while recording EMG activity in associated muscle groups. Postoperatively, a CT scan was used to analyze screw placement and these results were compared with intraoperative EMG recordings.

### Complications of the Anterior Cervical Approach

Ohnishi T, Neo M, Matsushita M, et al: Delayed aortic rupture caused by an implanted anterior spinal device: Case report. *J Neurosurg* 2001;95:253-256.

This case report describes a patient with an aortic rupture that occurred 20 months after the placement of a smooth-rod Kaneda instrument.

Oskouian RJ, Johnson JP: Vascular complications in anterior thoracolumbar spinal reconstruction. *J Neurosurg* 2002;96:1-5.

The medical records of 207 patients who underwent anterior thoracic and lumbar spinal surgery were retrospectively reviewed. The incidence and causes of vascular complications occurring in this patient population were identified.

Sagi H, Beutler W, Carroll E, Connolly PJ: Airway complications associated with surgery on the anterior cervical spine. *Spine* 2002;27:949-953.

This retrospective chart review of 311 anterior cervical procedures attempted to determine the incidence and risk factors for the development of airway complications following anterior cervical surgery.

Sucato DJ, Kassab F, Dempsey M: Analysis of screw placement relative to the aorta and spinal canal following anterior instrumentation for thoracic idiopathic scoliosis. *Spine* 2004;29:554-559.

In this study, CT was used to analyze thorascopically-placed screws to determine screw location relative to the spinal canal and the aorta. These scans were performed following screw placement for anterior instrumentation in patients with thoracic idiopathic scoliosis.

Van Ooij A, Oner FC, Verbout AJ: Complications of artificial disc replacment: A report of 27 patients with the SB charite disc. *J Spinal Disord Tech* 2003;16:369-383.

This article describes the possible short- and long-term unsatisfactory results of disk replacement surgery.

### Postoperative Complications

Banco SP, Vaccaro AR, Blam O, et al: Spine infections: Variations in incidence during the academic year. *Spine* 2002;27:962-965.

This study is a prospective analysis of variations in monthly spinal infection rates at a spinal cord injury center.

Kou J, Fischgrund J, Biddinger A, Herkowitz H: Risk factors for spinal epidural hematoma after spinal surgery. *Spine* 2002;27:1670-1673.

This retrospective study compared patients who developed a postoperative epidural hematoma with those who did not develop this complication following spinal surgery. Risk factors for development of an epidural hematoma were sought in the group of patients developing this complication.

### Classic Bibliography

Cammisa FP, Girardi FP, Sangani PK, et al: Incidental durotomy in spine surgery. *Spine* 2000;25:2663-2667.

Daniels SK, Mahoney MC, Lyons GD: Persistent dysphagia and dysphonia following cervical spine surgery. *Ear Nose Throat J* 1998;77:470.

Dearborn JT, Hu SS, Tribus CB, Bradford DS: Thromboembolic complications after major thoracolumbar spine surgery. *Spine* 1999;24:1471-1476.

Eismont FJ, Wiesel SW, Rothman RH: Treatment of dural tears associated with spinal surgery. *J Bone Joint Surg Am* 1981;63:1132-1136.

Farber GL, Place HM, Mazur RA, et al: Accuracy of pedicle screw placement in lumbar fusions by plain radiographs and computed tomography. *Spine* 1995;20: 1494-1499.

Jones AA, Stambough JL, Balderston RA, et al: Long-term results of lumbar spine surgery complicated by unintended incidental durotomy. *Spine* 1989;14:443-446.

Park CK: The effect of patient positioning on intraabdominal pressure and blood loss in spinal surgery. *Anesth Analg* 2000;91:552-557.

Schwarzenbach O, Berlemann U, Jost B, et al: Accuracy of computer-assisted pedicle screw placement: An in vivo computed tomography analysis. *Spine* 1997;22:452-458.

Stevens WR, Glazer PA, Kelley SD, Lietman TM, Bradford DS: Ophthalmic complications after spinal surgery. *Spine* 1997;22:1319-1324.

Wang JC, Bohlman HH, Riew DK: Dural tears secondary to operations on the lumbar spine: Management and results after a two-year-minimum follow-up of eighty-eight patients. *J Bone Joint Surg Am* 1998;80:1728-1732.

Zeidman SM, Ducker TB, Raycroft J: Trends and complications in cervical spine surgery: 1989-1993. *J Spinal Disord* 1997;10:523-526.

# Section 4

# Pediatric Topics

Section Editor:
Denis S. Drummond, MD

# Chapter 41

# Pediatric Cervical Spine Trauma

Joshua D. Auerbach, MD

John M. Flynn, MD

## Introduction

Cervical spinal trauma in the pediatric population is relatively uncommon but potentially life-threatening. Children differ from adults in aspects of cervical spine anatomy, communication ability, healing rates, body proportions, and treatment options. An understanding of the unique cervical spine anatomic considerations in children forms the basis for diagnosis and treatment.

## Anatomic Considerations

The pediatric cervical spine is more mobile than the adult cervical spine for several reasons. Children demonstrate increased ligamentous laxity and have facet joints that are more horizontally oriented. Until approximately 8 years of age, the synchondroses and the polar growth plates (epiphyses) are potentially weak areas that determine the location of fractures. Children also have relatively poor head control as a result of a higher head-to-body mass ratio and relatively weak paraspinal musculature. This increased spinal laxity and motion, coupled with decreased head control and the more proximally located biomechanical fulcrum of cervical spine motion around the C2-C3 level, predispose infants and young children to upper cervical spine injuries.

As the spine matures, the biomechanical fulcrum of cervical spinal motion gradually descends caudally, reaching C5-C6 by approximately 10 years of age. With maturity, reduced head-to-body ratio, increased muscular control over head movements, a shift toward more vertically oriented facets, and a general increased resistance to physiologic motion in the upper cervical spine lead to proportionately lower rates of upper cervical spine injury.

## Epidemiology

Pediatric cervical spine trauma accounts for approximately 1.5% of traumatic injuries in children. From 60% to 80% of pediatric spinal injuries occur in the cervical spine, with nearly 70% of these in the upper cervical spine. Children are more likely than adults to sustain concomitant head injury with cervical spinal trauma, a factor contributing to the higher cervical spine injury mortality rates than in adults. Associated traumatic brain injury has been reported to occur in up to 37% of children with cervical spine injuries, with mortality rates exceeding 50%. One third of all cervical spine injuries in children are associated with a neurologic deficit, 76% of which are incomplete. In the largest published series of pediatric cervical spinal trauma to date, spinal cord injury (SCI) was present in 35% of children, 50% of whom had no radiographic abnormalities. Mortality is higher in patients with upper cervical spine injuries than with lower cervical spine injuries, and is highest in patients with atlanto-occipital dislocation.

## Injury Mechanisms

Regardless of age group, motor vehicle accidents (MVAs) account for most cervical spine injuries in children. Birth injuries to the bony column of the cervical spine and spinal cord injuries have been identified in up to 50% of neonatal deaths. Forceps delivery and breech presentation can lead to rotation and traction forces to the newborn cervical spine. Child abuse can occur at any age, but it most commonly occurs in children younger than 2 years. The injury mechanism may be a whiplash-type motion, inflicting excessive rotational, flexion, and extension forces on an already hypermobile spinal column. In young children, MVAs (passenger, pedestrian, and bicyclist) and falls are the most common mechanisms of injury. In older children, MVAs are the most common mechanism of injury, followed by sports-related injuries (particularly football, diving, wrestling, ice hockey, and gymnastics).

Sports-related quadriplegia, most commonly seen in football players, typically results from a large and sudden axial load to the top or crown of the helmet with the neck in approximately 30° of flexion, thereby producing a straight spine that transmits the axial load directly to the spinal structures. With the spine straight and immobile, the paraspinal musculature can no longer aid in the dissipation of loading forces. As a result, spinal column buckling or catastrophic failure can occur in the form of fractures and dislocations (Figures 1 and 2).

## Motor Vehicle Accidents

Some mechanisms of injury that occur as a result of MVAs lend themselves more easily to prevention than others. It is well documented that car restraint systems

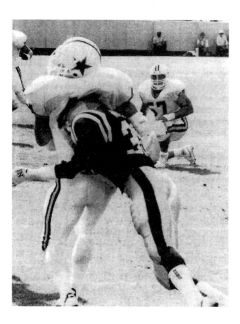

Figure 1 Spearing injury. The defensive back (dark jersey) is using an improper tackling technique by ramming the ball carrier with the crown of his helmet. The defensive player was rendered quadriplegic as a result of C4-C6 fractures. *(Reproduced with permission from Torg JS, Guille TT, Jaffe S: Injuries to the cervical spine in American football players. J Bone Joint Surg 2002;84: 112-122.)*

significantly reduce cervical spine injuries. When properly installed, safety seats or booster seats reduce fatal injuries in up to 69% of young children. Up to 80% of patients with pediatric cervical spine trauma from MVAs are improperly restrained. Studies have documented the danger of air bag systems to the front-seat child passenger which, when deployed, can directly propel the head of the child into hyperextension and cause fatal craniocervical injuries. The safest position for child restraint devices is the rear seat of the car. No child should be placed in a seat within the deployment trajectory of an airbag.

## Birth Injuries

Birth injuries can occur if the infant's cervical spine is subjected to traction and torsional forces. Neonatal high cervical SCI is sometimes the result of rotational forceps delivery exerting torsional forces that can cause quadriparesis, areflexia, and diaphragmatic paralysis. Other risk factors include breech position, which can place traction forces on the neonate's spine and cause injury, typically at the cervicothoracic junction. Given the limitations of plain film assessment in the newborn, both MRI and bedside ultrasound have proved to be useful in detecting spinal injuries in this population, although the latter precludes the need for sedation and patient transport and may therefore be preferred in most circumstances.

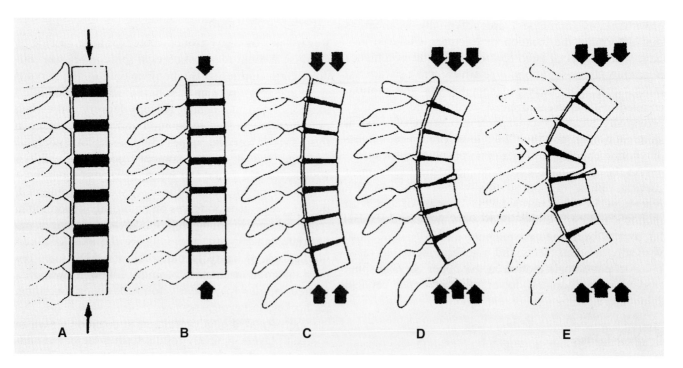

Figure 2 With the neck flexed 30°, the cervical spine becomes straight and dissipates axial loading forces like a segmented column. Axially-loaded forces (A) initially cause compressive deformation of the intervertebral disks (B). Once maximum compressive deformation is reached, angular deformation and buckling occur (C). Ultimately, the spine fails in a flexion mode, with resulting fracture, subluxation, or dislocation (D and E). The sequence of events from initial compressive load to ultimate failure in the form of fracture, dislocation, or subluxation, occurs in as little as 8.4 ms. *(Reproduced with the permission from: Torg JS, Vegso JJ, O'Neill MJ, Sennett B: The epidemiologic, pathologic, biomechanical, and cinematographic analysis of football-induced cervical spine trauma. Am J Sports Med 1990;18:53.)*

## Child Abuse

In shaken baby syndrome, the spine is exposed to potentially violent flexion, distraction, and rotational forces. Presenting signs include nonspecific symptoms, decreased level of consciousness, or respiratory difficulty. In one study, a previous history of maltreatment was present in up to 60% of patients. The mortality from direct effects of shaken baby syndrome is 19%. Because concomitant head or brain stem injury can mask cervical spinal injury, the evaluation of the patient suspected of being abused should include a comprehensive history and physical examination, a low threshold for full skeletal survey, ophthalmologic examination, CT or MRI, and social intervention.

## Sports-Related Injuries

Sports-related activities account for approximately 5% to 10% of the 10,000 cervical spine injuries that occur each year in the United States. Diving injuries, although completely preventable, are one of the leading causes of sports-related quadriplegia. Reckless behavior and alcohol are involved in up to 40% of patients. It is estimated that diving accidents account for 8.5% of SCIs in the United States. The injury sustained is usually the result of head impact directly onto the bottom surface of the pool. These injuries typically result in a complete SCI picture, most commonly at the C4-C6 levels. A recent study evaluated the long-term efficacy of a safe diving skills intervention program aimed at recreational swimmers with poor diving skills. At over 600 days follow-up without any subsequent training, divers demonstrated safer arm and hand positions and performed dives with a shallower and presumably safer trajectory. This highlights the potential efficacy of an intervention program in preventing disastrous cervical spinal injuries.

The potential for spine injury in football players has received significant attention throughout the years and has led to the implementation of injury prevention programs and significant reductions in incidence of injury. Better protective equipment, proper tackling techniques, and rule changes penalizing spear tackling or helmet-to-helmet initial contact have decreased the rate of quadriplegia from 13 cases per 1,000,000 players to 3 cases per 1,000,000 players.

Attention has recently been focused on preventing head and neck injuries during skiing and snowboarding. One study found that the use of a helmet for snowboarders and skiers reduced the incidence of head injury in children younger than 13 years. Another study demonstrated that snowboarding was associated with a fourfold higher incidence of spinal injury compared with skiing, and that 77% of injuries were caused by jumping from heights greater than 2 m. Because jumping is required in snowboarding, the authors suggest that injury prevention programs that restrict jumping areas will be

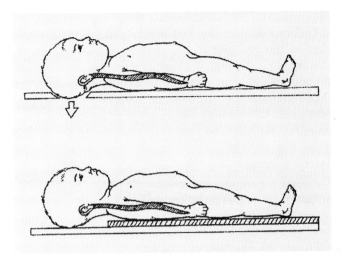

**Figure 3**  Safe immobilization of young children can be accomplished by using either a modified backboard with an occipital recess (top) or a mattress pad to raise the chest (bottom). *(Reproduced from Copley LA, Dormans JP: Cervical spine disorders in infants and children.* J Am Acad Orthop Surg *1998;6:204-214.)*

ineffective and instead the focus should be on teaching safe jumping techniques while making children aware of the great potential danger associated with this popular sport.

## Initial Management and Evaluation

Children suspected of having cervical spinal trauma or SCI should be immobilized in the neutral position to prevent possible further damage to the spinal cord. Children younger than 8 years have disproportionately large heads compared with the torso. When these children are positioned flat onto a spinal immobilization board, this may place the neck into flexion. A neutral position of the head can be obtained by placing blankets underneath the child's shoulders and trunk, or by using a half spine-board with occipital recess (Figure 3). Current recommendations for immobilizing the pediatric cervical spine include a half-spine board with occipital recess with the external auditory meatus in line with the shoulder to avoid placing the neck into kyphosis, a rigid collar, and possibly tape across the torso in patients without respiratory compromise. A recent study found that children brought to the emergency department with precautions to immobilize the spine were immobilized with the cervical spine in a position other than neutral up to 37% of the time.

Once the patient is safely immobilized and Advanced Trauma and Life Support protocol has been instituted, a comprehensive physical examination should be conducted. Examination findings suggestive of cervical spinal injury include head injury, neurologic deficit (including transient deficits possibly indicating instability), torticollis, cervical guarding, tenderness, palpable step-off between contiguous spinous processes, and multiple trauma. The "shoulder-belt sign," characterized by skin abrasions over the neck area, should alert the clinician to the possibility of underlying cervical spine or vertebral artery injury. Combinations of examination findings can help to successfully identify cervical spinal injury in about 85% of patients. It may be necessary to perform serial examinations in uncooperative children.

## Imaging

The history and physical examination findings dictate the need for subsequent imaging. If history or physical examination suggests the possibility of a cervical spinal injury, or if the patient exhibits unexplained hypotension, an AP, lateral, and open-mouth odontoid view of the cervical spine should be obtained. The value of open-mouth odontoid views has recently been called into question. Several studies cited inconsistent usage as part of the trauma series and low diagnostic yield as limitations of this study. In awake and alert patients, voluntary flexion and extension views may be performed to assess spinal stability, provided there are no abnormalities seen on static films. Some authors have recently suggested, however, that flexion and extension views contribute little new information in the setting of a normal trauma series.

In older high-risk children, CT may serve as an adjunct to the radiographic evaluation of the bony cervical spine to reduce the incidence of missed fractures from plain radiographic evaluation alone. Helical CT is recommended for the evaluation of high-risk older children or adults who have sustained multisystem trauma after significant blunt injuries. Performance of a CT of the cervical spine, at the same time it is performed for the evaluation of potential head injuries, has been suggested as a method to increase the accuracy and efficiency of cervical spine clearance protocols. In children younger than 5 years, however, plain radiography evaluation is usually adequate and the additional yield of CT is extremely low.

Evaluation of the unconscious patient begins with strict immobilization for presumptive cervical spinal trauma. In these patients, plain radiographic imaging should be performed but has some limitations in its ability to consistently detect spinal injury. Although the false-negative rates for a single cross-table lateral cervical spine film range from 21% to 26%, the complete plain film radiographic evaluation has a sensitivity of 94%. The assessment of instability should never include flexion and extension radiographs in the unconscious or uncooperative patient. Alternatively, MRI has been shown to be highly effective in ruling out injury to the cervical spine in patients who are obtunded and intubated, as well as in alert children with persistent pain or neurologic symptoms without radiographic abnormalities. Injuries to the soft tissue and ligamentous structures, vertebral growth centers, intervertebral disks, and

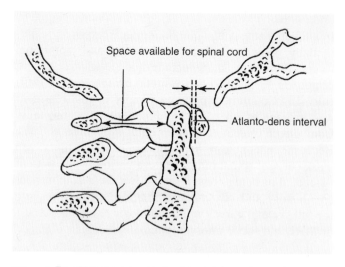

**Figure 4** The atlanto-dens interval is the distance between the anterior aspect of the dens and the posterior aspect of the anterior ring of the atlas. The space available for the cord is divided into thirds among the odontoid process, the spinal cord, and the subarachnoid space. *(Reproduced with permission from Hensinger RN, Fielding JW: The cervical spine, in Morissy RT (ed): Lovell and Winter's Pediatric Orthopaedics, ed 3. Philadelphia, PA, JB Lippincott, 1990, pp 703-740.)*

spinal cord without radiographic findings (which account for approximately 40% to 70% of pediatric spinal injuries) can be effectively evaluated using MRI. Using an MRI protocol to evaluate the cervical spine in patients unable to be cleared after 72 hours, one children's trauma center reported a decrease in time spent in the intensive care unit (ICU), time to clearance, length of hospital stay, and total cost when compared with the "preprotocol" group. Using this same clearance protocol, MRI altered the diagnosis in 34% of patients.

## Normal Radiographic Variants in the Pediatric Cervical Spine

Accurate interpretation of pediatric cervical spine plain radiographs requires consideration of the age and skeletal maturity of the patient. An atlanto-dens interval greater than 5 mm in children may indicate ligamentous disruption and instability. Occasionally, connective tissue disorders or inflammatory arthritides are associated with chronic instability and an increased atlanto-dens interval at baseline. In these instances, use of the space available for the cord, which is shared equally among the odontoid, spinal cord, and subarachnoid space, may provide a more useful measurement in detecting instability (Figure 4).

In up to 46% of normal children, there is pseudosubluxation of C2 on C3, with sagittal plane translation of 4 mm during flexion and extension radiography. Use of Swischuk's line will differentiate between pseudosubluxation and true injury, such as a hangman's fracture or traumatic subluxation (Figure 5). Other radiographic findings of potential concern include the absence of lordosis (may be present up to age 16 years), ossification

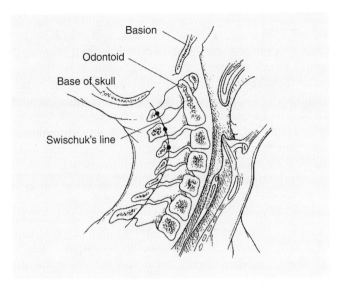

Figure 5  Swischuk's line is drawn along the posterior arch (spinolaminar line) from C1 to C3. If this line does not pass within 1.5 mm of the anterior cortex of the posterior arch of C2, a true injury is suspected. (*Reproduced from Copley LA, Dormans JP: Cervical spine disorders in infants and children. J Am Acad Orthop Surg 1998;6:204-214.*)

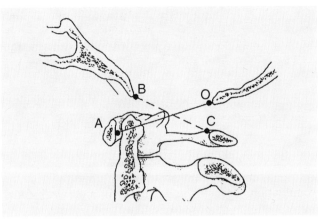

Figure 6  The Power's ratio is the distance from the basion, or tip of the clivus, to the posterior aspect of the spinolaminar line of the atlas (BC) divided by the distance from the anterior tubercle of the atlas to the rim of the foramen magnum (OA). A ratio of > 1.0 is diagnostic of anterior occipitoatlantal dislocation. (*Reproduced from Copley LA, Dormans JP: Cervical spine disorders in infants and children. J Am Acad Orthop Surg 1998;6:204-214.*)

centers in the spinous processes and unfused ring apophyses, pseudo-Jefferson fractures (physiologic lateral displacement of the lateral masses up to 6 mm seen on the odontoid view), overriding of the anterior arch of the atlas on the odontoid (present in up to 20% of children younger than 8 years), anterior vertebral body wedging (most pronounced at C3), and prominence of prevertebral soft tissues.

## Treatment of Specific Injuries
### Atlanto-Occipital Dislocation
Anatomic and biomechanical factors such as a large head, small occipital condyles, horizontally oriented atlanto-occipital joints, ligamentous laxity, and a higher biomechanical fulcrum predispose young children to these often fatal injuries in the upper cervical spine when subjected to rapid deceleration. Traumatic atlanto-occipital dislocations have been reported in up to 25% of fatal pediatric trauma cases and have a mortality rate exceeding 50%. Recent studies have shown that the diagnosis is frequently missed on initial radiographic evaluation because of low clinical suspicion and spontaneous reduction. A worsening neurologic examination may call attention to the injury. Among survivors, it is estimated that 20% have no neurologic deficits upon presentation. Limitations of traditional diagnostic radiographic methods, such as the Powers ratio (Figure 6), have led to the increased use of MRI and CT, which have sensitivities of 0.84 and 0.86, respectively. The ability of MRI to differentiate partial from complete ligamentous rupture may help identify patients who may be successfully treated nonsurgically.

The preferred initial management of atlanto-occipital dislocations consists of halo immobilization, or, less preferably, a Minerva cast. One recent study demonstrated two instances of atlanto-occipital dislocation successfully treated nonsurgically with halo immobilization, augmented by dual straps to maintain the reduction. Generally, unstable injuries should be managed by posterior occipitoatlantal fusion with internal fixation, possibly in combination with postoperative immobilization in a halo device.

## Atlantoaxial Rotatory Subluxation
Atlantoaxial rotatory subluxation is a rotational disorder of the atlantoaxial joint that typically presents as painful torticollis and limited neck rotation, usually without neurologic deficits. The etiology of atlantoaxial rotatory subluxation is major or minor trauma, ligamentous laxity (Marfan syndrome or rheumatoid arthritis), congenital abnormalities within the sternocleidomastoid muscle, and is postinfectious or postsurgical (for example, following tonsillectomy). Grisel's syndrome refers to atlantoaxial rotatory subluxation resulting from inflammation-induced ligamentous laxity that occurs as a result of hematogenous communication among the periodontoidal venous plexus, the suboccipital epidural sinuses, and the pharyngovertebral veins. The diagnosis of atlantoaxial rotatory subluxation is confirmed with dynamic CT scanning to identify malrotation of C1 on C2 (Figure 7). A recent dynamic CT classification was described that correlated degree of rotation with duration of symptoms and intensity of treatment.

If the patient has had symptoms for only a few days, a period of soft-collar immobilization and the use of nonsteroidal anti-inflammatory drugs is often effective. If symptoms persist for more than 1 or 2 weeks, the

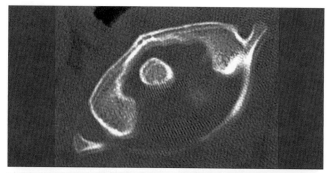
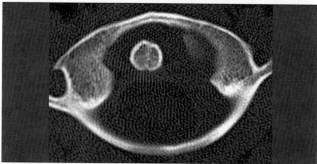
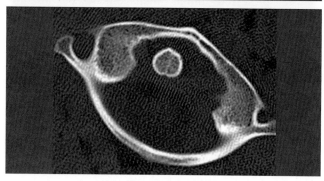

Figure 7  CT scans showing atlantoaxial rotatory subluxation in an 8-year-old boy with Grisel's syndrome who presented in the cock-robin position with right-sided lateral bending and rotation. CT scans demonstrates the head maximally rotated to the right (top), neutral (middle), and left (bottom). In all views, the odontoid is located to the right of the midline but is able to rotate past the midline, indicating atlantoaxial rotatory subluxation. In atlantoaxial rotatory fixation (not seen here), the patient is unable to rotate the head past the midline position.

child is typically admitted to the hospital for cervical traction, with administration of a muscle relaxant. The neck spasms usually resolve in a few days, then a brace or cervical collar is applied and the patient is sent home. The patient is weaned from the collar or brace at 4 to 6 weeks. At some centers, a dynamic CT protocol (CT of C1-C2 in neutral, maximum right cervical rotation and maximum left cervical rotation) is used to evaluate the C1-C2 articulation, defining it as either limited motion, rotatory subluxation, or rotatory fixation. Should symptoms persist beyond 1 to 2 months, or if the rotational deformity is fixed, C1-C2 fusion may be indicated. The potential for neurologic compromise as a result of manipulative reduction before cervical fusion has led some authors to recommend in situ fusion alone, even if a reduction is not achieved.

### Atlantoaxial Instability

Detailed evaluation of atlantoaxial instability is discussed in chapter 42. Up to 10% of pediatric cervical spinal injuries involve atlantoaxial instability. Sagittal plane translation of 5 mm or more on the lateral radiograph suggests rupture of the transverse ligament and instability. In one recent study, a traumatic etiology of atlantoaxial instability was identified in 4 of 10 patients; the other 6 patients had congenital abnormalities. MRI allowed visualization of the ruptured ligaments. Surgical stabilization was required in half of these patients.

### Odontoid Fractures

Odontoid fractures represent 75% of all childhood cervical spinal fractures. In children younger than 7 years, odontoid fractures usually occur through the cartilaginous synchondrosis between the odontoid process and the body of C2. A recent study emphasized the occasional need to use CT, MRI, or bone scans to distinguish between fractures through the synchondrosis and C2 pedicle fractures in patients with equivocal plain radiographs. Because fractures through the C2 synchondrosis generally do not interrupt blood supply to the lower dens, these fractures have a high propensity toward healing without the complications seen in the adult population.

Reduction of the anteriorly displaced odontoid is performed with gentle extension, followed by halo immobilization. Approximately 80% of children treated initially with halo immobilization achieve a stable fusion at an average of 13 weeks. In one study, complications were noted in all three patients with surgically-treated odontoid fractures, compared with the nonsurgical group that experienced no complications and 100% fracture healing.

### Lower Cervical Spine Injuries

By approximately 8 years of age, the patterns of injury become similar to those of adults, reflected by a higher incidence of lower cervical spine fractures and dislocations. One recent case report described a 4-year-old child who was a restrained back-seat passenger involved in an MVA who sustained a simultaneous noncontiguous fracture through the C2 synchondrosis and traumatic dislocation of the spine at C6-C7. This case report highlights the possibility of multilevel injury and the need for vigilance in assessment of the lower cervical spine in young children, despite the infrequency of injuries in this location.

### Spinal Cord Injury Without Radiographic Abnormality

Spinal cord injury without radiographic abnormality (SCIWORA) represents a subgroup of SCIs that produce abnormalities on MRI without evidence of skeletal injury or instability on radiographic plain films or CT.

The most common causes of injury include MVAs, falls, sports activity, and birth-related injuries. Children are affected most often and may be predisposed to this injury pattern because of elasticity of the immature spinal column, which can undergo distractive forces up to 5 cm before failing, in combination with the inelasticity of the spinal cord, which can safely undergo only 5 to 6 mm of traction because of its attachments to the brachial plexus and cauda equina. Other proposed mechanisms of injury include transient disk herniation, vascular insufficiency with cord infarction, and transient subluxation (followed by spontaneous reduction) and occult segmental spinal instability, not demonstrable on dynamic radiographs. Incomplete SCIs have a better prognosis than complete SCIs.

MRI often reveals the underlying spinal cord insult and offers prognostic value. One author recently described five classes of post-SCIWORA spinal changes that occur and showed that patients with no abnormality made a full recovery, whereas patients with neural transection and major hemorrhage had the worst prognosis. Other common findings on MRI include cord swelling or edema, minor hemorrhage, and traumatic disk herniation.

Potential spinal column instability may predispose to recurrent SCIWORA. Patients are typically immobilized using a rigid cervical orthosis for 3 months, despite lack of radiographic evidence of instability, followed by another 3 months of activity modification. The authors of one recent study have suggested that bracing may not be necessary in patients with transient deficits and normal MRI and/or somatosensory-evoked potentials. More studies will be needed, however, to evaluate whether or not bracing has any protective role.

## Halo Application

Advantages of halo vest application over Minerva casting in children include ease of application, more rigid immobilization, better positioning, fewer skin and chewing problems, and the ability for earlier mobilization, which may be important to minimize the risk of respiratory compromise in the multiple-trauma patient. A pre-application CT of the skull or cranium is valuable to assess the areas with thickest bone density. For younger patients, typical pediatric halo constructs include 8 to 12 pins placed with low insertional torque (1 to 5 in-lb), compared with adolescents and adults where 4 pins are used with higher insertional torque (6 to 8 in-lb). It was recently shown that certain torque wrenches are more reliable than others in achieving the desired low torque values in children and that variability among different wrenches from the same manufacturers may exist. Complications from halo vest application are pin site infection and anterior pin placement.

## Summary

The evaluation of a child with a potential injury to the cervical spine begins with the recognition of the unique anatomy, physiology, and social setting in which these injuries occur. Prevention efforts that can reduce the incidence of pediatric spinal injury include the proper use of seat belts, education on safe participation in sport activities, and early recognition of the signs of child abuse. Although advanced imaging techniques can be useful in the evaluation of subtle spinal injuries, a thorough knowledge of normal anatomic variants is essential to identify true spinal pathology and to help direct proper treatment.

## Annotated Bibliography
### Epidemiology
Ghatan S, Ellenbogen RG: Pediatric spine and spinal cord injury after inflicted trauma. *Neurosurg Clin North Am* 2002;13:227-233.

The authors report a case and literature review with emphasis on the epidemiology, mechanisms of injury, developmental and radiographical anatomy, and neuropathology of inflicted spine and SCI in children.

Patel JC, Tepas JJ, Mollitt DL, Pieper P: Pediatric cervical spine injuries: Defining the disease. *J Pediatr Surg* 2001;36:373-376.

The authors of this review of 75,000 trauma patients conclude that upper cervical spine injuries occur across all pediatric age groups and are not limited to younger children. Mortality is sixfold higher with upper cervical injuries.

### Injury Mechanisms
Blitvich JD, McElroy GK, Blanksby BA, Parker HE: Long term retention of safe diving skills. *J Sci Med Sport* 2003;6:348-354.

This study evaluated the long-term efficacy of a safe diving skills intervention program aimed at recreational swimmers with poor diving skills. At over 600 days follow-up without any subsequent training, divers demonstrated safer arm and hand positions and had shallower dives.

Kim DH, Vaccaro AR, Berta SC: Acute sports-related spinal cord injury: Contemporary management principles. *Clin Sports Med* 2003;22:501-512.

A concise review of epidemiology, mechanisms of injury, and treatment rationale for sports-related SCIs is presented.

King WJ, MacKay M, Sirnick A: with the Canadian Shaken Baby Study Group: Shaken baby syndrome in Canada: Clinical characteristics and outcomes of hospital cases. *CMAJ* 2003;168:155-159.

A retrospective review from 11 pediatric tertiary hospitals in Canada identified 364 patients with shaken baby syndrome.

Previous maltreatment was noted in 60% of cases, and 22% of families had previous involvement with child welfare authorities.

Kokoska ER, Keller MS, Rallo MC, Weber TR: Characteristics of pediatric cervical spine injuries. *J Pediatr Surg* 2001;36:100-105.

In this review of 408 cases of pediatric cervical spine trauma, the authors describe different mechanisms of injury and outcomes across age groups, and highlight the fact that 80% of children involved in MVAs were improperly restrained.

Macnab AJ, Smith T, Gagnon FA, Macnab M: Effect of helmet wear on the incidence of head/face and cervical spine injuries in young skiers and snowboarders. *Inj Prev* 2002;8:324-327.

The authors studied young skiers and snowboarders under age 13 years at one ski resort between 1998-1999 who had sustained injuries to the head/face and cervical spine. The authors conclude that wearing a helmet reduces the incidence of these injuries.

Management of pediatric cervical spine and spinal cord injuries. *Neurosurgery* 2002;50(suppl 3):S85-S99.

The authors review 58 articles from 1966-2001 to establish guidelines for the management and treatment of pediatric cervical spinal injuries.

Torg JS, Guille JT, Jaffe S: Current concepts review: Injuries to the cervical spine in American football players. *J Bone Joint Surg Am* 2002;84:112-122.

A concise literature review of cervical spine injuries in American football players is presented, with an emphasis on mechanism of injury.

Zuckerbraun BS, Morrison K, Gaines B, Ford HR, Hackam DJ: Effect of age on cervical spine injuries in children after motor vehicle collisions: Effectiveness of restraint devices. *J Pediatr Surg* 2004;39:483-486.

Despite being properly restrained, younger children had a higher incidence of head and cervical spine injuries than older children, suggesting that current restraint devices are inadequate for young children and that design modifications may be necessary.

## Initial Management and Evaluation

Boswell HB, Dietrich A, Shiels WE, et al: Accuracy of visual determination of neutral position of the immobilized pediatric cervical spine. *Pediatr Emerg Care* 2001; 17:10-14.

Of 59 children presenting to the emergency department in full spinal immobilization, 37% of children were immobilized in a position other than neutral.

## Imaging

Flynn JM, Closkey RF, Mahboubi S, Dormans JP: Role of magnetic resonance imaging in the assessment of pediatric cervical spine injuries. *J Pediatr Orthop* 2002;22: 573-577.

In an obtunded, nonverbal child with suspected cervical spine injury, equivocal plain films, neurologic symptoms without radiographic abnormalities, and inability to clear the spine within 3 days, MRI confirmed the diagnosis in 66% of patients and altered the diagnosis in 34%.

Frank JB, Lim CK, Flynn JM, Dormans JP: The efficacy of magnetic resonance imaging in pediatric cervical spine clearance. *Spine* 2002;27:1176-1179.

The authors propose an MRI clearance protocol for obtunded, nonverbal patients with an inability to clear the spine within 3 days. Application of the protocol led to decreased length of stay in the ICU, hospital stay, time to clearance, and cost when compared to the "preprotocol" group.

Hernandez JA, Chupik C, Swischuk LE: Cervical spine trauma in children under 5 years: Productivity of CT. *Emerg Radiol* 2004;10:176-178.

Twenty-four percent of 606 pediatric trauma patients younger than age 5 years underwent CT evaluation for clearing of the cervical spine. CT scan detected cervical spinal injury in 4 patients (3%), each of whom had the same findings on plain radiographs.

McGuire KJ, Silber J, Flynn JM, Levine ML, Dormans JP: Torticollis in children: Can dynamic computed tomography help determine severity and treatment? *J Pediatr Orthop* 2002;22:766-770.

This retrospective review of 50 children with torticollis describes a new classification system using dynamic CT scanning in the evaluation of atlantoaxial rotatory subluxation which correlates higher stage with duration of symptoms and severity of treatment.

## Treatment of Specific Injuries

Heilman CB, Riesenburger RI: Simultaneous noncontiguous cervical spine injuries in a pediatric patient: Case report. *Neurosurgery* 2001;49:1017-1020.

The authors present the case of a 4-year-old boy with simultaneous traumatic cervical spinal injuries, highlighting the need for vigilance in assessment of the lower cervical spine in young children, despite the infrequency of injuries in this location.

Pang D: Spinal cord injury without radiographic abnormality in children, 2 decades later. *Neurosurgery* 2004; 55:1325-1343.

The author reports 5 classes of post-SCIWORA spinal changes that occur and show that patients with no abnormality made a full recovery, while patients with neural transection and major hemorrhage had the worst prognosis.

Steinmetz MP, Verrees M, Anderson JS, Lechner RM: Dual-strap augmentation of a halo orthosis in the treatment of atlantooccipital dislocation in infants and young children: Technical note. *J Neurosurg* 2002;96:346-349.

The authors report the successful nonsurgical treatment of two patients with atlanto-occipital dislocation using halo immobilization augmented with dual straps to improve the fit of the vest.

### *Halo Application*

Copley LA, Dormans JP, Pepe MD, Tan V, Browne RH: Accuracy and reliability of torque wrenches used for halo application in children. *J Bone Joint Surg Am* 2003; 85:2199-2204.

Safe halo application in children requires lower insertional torque than in adults. The authors of this study demonstrate that certain torque wrenches available are more accurate than others. The authors also report variability among different wrenches from the same manufacturer.

## Classic Bibliography

Birney TJ, Hanley EN Jr: Traumatic cervical spine injuries in childhood and adolescence. *Spine* 1989;14:1277-1282.

Cattell HS, Filtzer DL: Pseudosubluxation and other normal variations in the cervical spine in children: A study of one hundred and sixty children. *J Bone Joint Surg Am* 1965;47:1295-1309.

Dormans JP: Evaluation of children with suspected cervical spine injury. *J Bone Joint Surg Am* 2002;84:124-132.

Dormans JP, Criscitiello AA, Drummond DS, Davidson RS: Complications in children managed with immobilization in a halo vest. *J Bone Joint Surg Am* 1995;77:1370-1373.

Herzenberg JE, Hensinger RN, Dedrick DK, Phillips WA: Emergency transport and positioning of young children who have an injury of the cervical spine: The standard backboard may be dangerous. *J Bone Joint Surg Am* 1989;71:15-22.

Khanna AJ, Wasserman BA, Sponseller PD: Magnetic resonance imaging of the pediatric spine. *J Am Acad Orthop Surg* 2003;11:248-259.

Mackinnon JA, Perlman M, Kirpalani H, et al: Spinal cord injury at birth: Diagnostic and prognostic data in 22 patients. *J Pediatr* 1993;122:431-437.

Mubarak SJ, Camp JF, Vuletich W, Wenger DR, Garfin SR: Halo application in the infant. *J Pediatr Orthop* 1989;9:612-614.

Smith MD, Phillips WA, Hensinger RN: Fusion of the upper cervical spine in children and adolescents: An analysis of 17 patients. *Spine* 1991;16:695-701.

Swischuk LE: Anterior displacement of C2 in children: physiologic or pathologic. *Radiology* 1977;122:759-763.

# Chapter 42

# Pediatric Cervical Spine

Harish S. Hosalkar, MD

Denis S. Drummond, MD

## Introduction

The evaluation and management of pediatric cervical spine disorders requires an understanding of anatomic and developmental features that are unique to the pediatric spine. Congenital and developmental alterations can affect evaluation and treatment. This chapter examines the developmental anatomy of the cervical spine and discusses the nontraumatic conditions leading to cervical instability in the pediatric population along with epidemiology, presentation, evaluation, and management of congenital anomalies, and other conditions leading to instability.

## Developmental Anatomy of the Cervical Spine

The notochord is formed by the second week of intrauterine life (IUL) and is in close proximity to the paraxial mesoderm, which becomes segmented into four occipital and eight cervical somites at weeks two and three. The notochord constitutes the framework around which the vertebral column, the basiocciput, and basisphenoid are formed. The somites each differentiate into cranial and caudal halves that subsequently unite with the cranial and caudal halves of the adjacent somites forming each provertebra. The notochord eventually forms the apical and alar ligaments as well as the nucleus pulposus of each intervertebral disk (Figure 1). During the fifth and sixth week of IUL, chondrification takes place in each half of the vertebral body and neural arch. Ossification then follows in each body and lateral mass.

The contributions of the first three sclerotome segments to the atlantoaxial complex and its ligaments are outlined in Figure 2. Diagrammatic representation of the primary and secondary ossification centers in the cervical vertebrae is presented in Figure 3.

### The Atlas

The atlas arises from the fourth occipital and the first cervical somites. There are three centers of ossification; two (one for each of the two lateral masses) that appear about the seventh week of fetal life, and one (located in

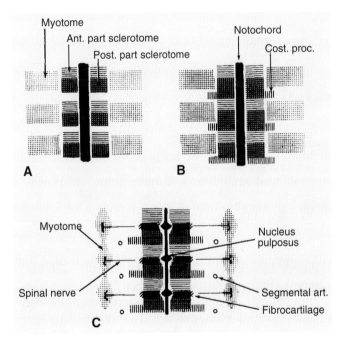

Figure 1 Schematic representation of the resegmentation of the vertebral primordial and their eventual relation with other segmented structures. (*Reproduced with permission from Sherk HH: Developmental anatomy of the normal cervical spine, in Clark CR (ed): The Cervical Spine, ed 4. Philadelphia, PA, Lippincott Williams and Wilkins, 2005, pp 37-45.*)

the anterior arch) that ossifies at approximately 1 year of age. The posterior arch ossifies from the lateral masses by two extensions that fuse by the age of 3 to 4 years either directly or through an additional midline center of ossification. The synchondroses between the lateral masses and the body fuse at approximately 6 to 8 years of age.

### The Axis

The axis arises from the first and second cervical somites. It is derived from five primary ossification centers including two lateral masses, an odontoid process (two longitudinal halves at birth), and a body or centrum. There are two secondary ossification centers; the ossiculum terminale at the tip of the odontoid and the

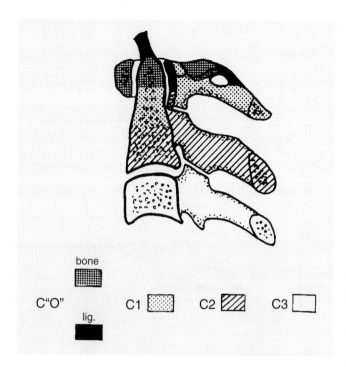

Figure 2 The hemisclerotome C0 provides the upper part of the odontoid process, the hypochordal anterior arch, and the dorsal part of the superior atlas facet, as well as the alar, transverse (upper part), and retroarticular ligaments (shown in black). The conventionally designated C1 sclerotome then provides the remainder of the posterior arch and the inferior part of the odontoid process. (*Reproduced with permission from Sherk HH: Developmental anatomy of the normal cervical spine, in Clark CR (ed): The Cervical Spine, ed 4. Philadelphia, PA, Lippincott Williams and Wilkins, 2005, pp 37-45.*)

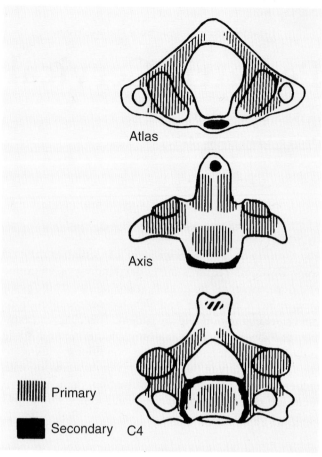

Figure 3 Diagrammatic representation of the primary and secondary ossification centers in the cervical vertebrae. (*Reproduced with permission from Sherk HH: Developmental anatomy of the normal cervical spine, in Clark CR (ed): The Cervical Spine, ed 4. Philadelphia, PA, Lippincott Williams and Wilkins, 2005, pp 37-45.*)

inferior ring apophysis. The two halves of the odontoid may sometimes persist as two centers known as dens bicornis. The odontoid process is separated from the body by dentocentral synchondrosis. The synchondrosis remains open in most instances until the age of 3 years and is fused by approximately 6 years. The tip of the odontoid appears around the age of 3 years and fuses to the odontoid by the age of 12 years. It may sometimes remain unfused and is then termed as ossiculum terminale persistens.

### The Subaxial Spine

The subaxial vertebrae arise from the cervical somites. Each subaxial vertebra is composed of three primary ossification centers, one for the body and one each for the two neural arches. The ring apophyses ossify during late childhood and fuse late in the second decade of life. Neural arches fuse posteriorly by the age of 2 or 3 years and the neurocentral synchondroses fuse between the ages of 3 and 6 years.

## Evaluation

Evaluation of the cervical spine is more difficult in children than in adults. The proper approach to a case of traumatic cervical instability is outlined in chapter 41.

A thorough physical examination of the child should be performed with particular attention to the upper cervical spine. The patient may have more than one level of involvement. Localizing pain or symptoms to a precise point may be difficult in children. Therefore, clinical signs are important. Torticollis, spasm, and pain on motion are useful signs that can help to identify instability. Detailed neurologic examination is essential and should include assessment of active flexion-extension and muscle power at all major joints.

The approach for evaluation of an alert (conscious) child with nontraumatic cervical spine instability is outlined in Figure 4.

General examination should include assessment of associated presenting features in patients with an insidious onset of instability. Multiple joint involvement as well as systemic involvement should be assessed in patients suspected of having juvenile rheumatoid arthritis. A thorough assessment for associated anomalies should be done in patients with Down syndrome or Klippel-Feil syndrome. A mental status examination should be performed with specific evaluation of the features of

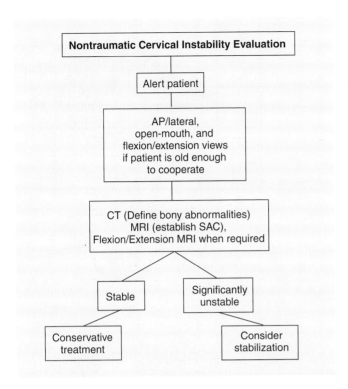

**Nontraumatic Cervical Instability Evaluation**

Alert patient

AP/lateral, open-mouth, and flexion/extension views if patient is old enough to cooperate

CT (Define bony abnormalities) MRI (establish SAC), Flexion/Extension MRI when required

Stable

Significantly unstable

Conservative treatment

Consider stabilization

Figure 4   Approach to nontraumatic cervical instability in children. *(Reproduced with permission from Drummond DS, Hosalkar HS: Treatment of cervical spine instability in the pediatric patient, in Clark CR (ed): The Cervical Spine, ed 4. Philadelphia, PA, Lippincott Williams and Wilkins, , 2005, pp 427-447.)*

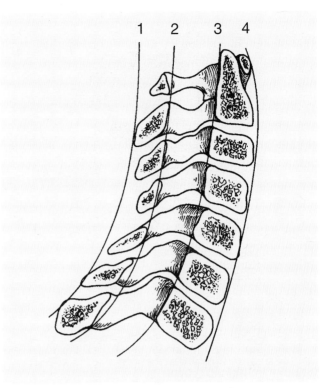

Figure 5   Four-line analysis of the cervical spine. These are lines connecting the (1) tips of the spinous processes; (2) spinolaminar line; (3) posterior margins; and (4) anterior margins of the vertebral bodies. All of these lines should follow a smooth, even contour. *(Reproduced from Copley LA, Dormans JP: Cervical spine disorders in infants and children. J Am Acad Orthop Surg 1998;6;205.)*

storage diseases in patients with mucopolysaccharidoses. Examination of sclera and dentition with thorough evaluation for multiple fractures is important in assessment of osteogenesis imperfecta.

## Diagnosis of Instability

In all patients suspected of having an element of cervical instability, initial evaluation should include a cervical spine radiograph (AP and lateral). An initial four-line analysis of the radiograph is useful in evaluation of irregular contour (Figure 5). Flexion-extension lateral views are extremely informative and should be performed when possible (when there is no contraindication to the study). CT may help elaborate the nature of instability and document fixed subluxation. MRI with or without dynamic stress applied to the cervical spine in flexion or extension should be performed only if the patient is old enough to cooperate and can help to detect any impending neurologic compromise.

### Unique Pediatric Diagnostic Features

Variability of the radiographic appearance of the pediatric cervical spine, especially in children younger than 8 years, makes interpretation of imaging difficult at times for the clinician not accustomed to evaluating the pediatric spine. Unique features of the pediatric spine have been outlined in chapter 41.

### Atlanto-occipital Instability

Plain radiographs (AP and lateral along with flexion/extension views when feasible) help in the primary evaluation. CT is useful to demonstrate the exact location of the occipital condyles and can offer a sagittal reconstruction. MRI is helpful in imaging the atlanto-occipital interval and can assess the edema in occipitocervical facet capsules, basicervical ligaments, and cervicomedullary angulation.

The occipital-C1 level often is difficult to observe because reliable cranial reference points frequently are hard to discern. The occipital condyles normally should rest in the depressions of the atlas facets and the facet-condyle interval should be less than 5 mm. The interval between the basion (anterior cortical margin of the foramen magnum) and the tip of the dens should be less than 10 mm. A widely used method for diagnosis of atlanto-occipital instability is the Powers ratio, the ratio of a segment drawn from the basion to the posterior arch of the atlas, and the opisthion to the anterior arch of the atlas. Several other methods of measuring potential occipitocervical instability have been described.

The published norm for the upper limit for atlanto-occipital translation is 1 mm in adults. Two millimeters of translation or less is considered normal for children,

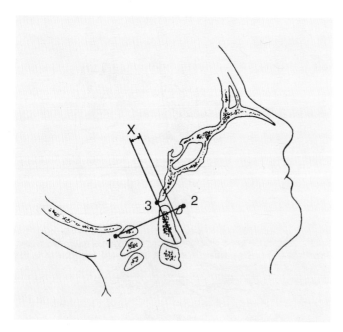

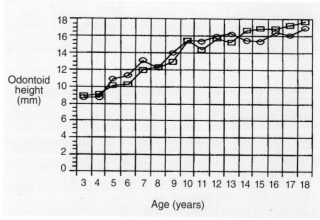

Figure 7 Graph demonstrating the expected age-related ossification as measured from lateral radiographs. Early examination can lead to an erroneous impression of hypoplasia. *(Reproduced with permission from Drummond DS: Pediatric cervical instability, in Weisel SW, Boden SD, Wisneski RJ (eds): Seminars in Spine Surgery. Philadelphia, WB Saunders, 1996: pp 292-309.)*

Figure 6 The Rothman-Weisel method of measuring occipitoatlantal instability. The atlantal line is drawn connecting points 1 and 2. A line is drawn perpendicular to the atlantal line at the posterior margin of the anterior arch of the atlas. A second perpendicular line is drawn intersecting the basion (point 3). The distance (x) between these lines should not vary more than 1 mm in flexion and extension. *(Reproduced from Copley LA, Dormans JP: Cervical spine disorders in infants and children. J Am Acad Orthop Surg 1998;6:204-214.)*

and 4 mm is accepted in patients with Down syndrome. Measurements outside these ranges are suggestive of atlanto-occipital instability (Figure 6).

It is necessary to determine the space available for the cord (SAC) in patients with an atlanto-occipital translation of 5 mm or more. The SAC is measured from the posterior margin of the odontoid to the anterior margin of the posterior ring of C1. It has been observed that a good rule of thumb is that one third of the space of the cross-sectional diameter can be available for the dens, one third for the spinal cord, and one third is needed as available space. An absolute SAC less than 13 mm indicates insufficient space for the spinal cord and serves as an indirect measurement of encroachment on the neurologic structures. A relatively narrow canal is associated with greater risk for injury than a capacious one. It is important to observe any pathologic motion, such as a hinged motion or opening at the atlanto-occipital articulation. This suggests defective development of the condyle articulation.

### Atlantoaxial Instability

Flexion-extension lateral radiographs of the cervical spine are helpful in defining atlantoaxial instability. The growth of odontoid is sometimes underestimated because only the ossified part is detected on standard radiographs. Figure 7 shows the progressive ossification process of the odontoid. The tip of the dens does not

reach the upper edge of the ring of the atlas until an average age of 9 years in normal children. Odontoid hypoplasia may, therefore, be overdiagnosed.

### Atlanto-Dens Interval

The important radiographic test for instability is the lateral flexion-extension radiograph where translation can be measured by the atlanto-dens interval (ADI). The ADI is greater in children than in adults; up to 4.5 mm is considered normal for children. This interval should be measured from the posterior–inferior cortex of the body of the atlas along a line perpendicular to its posterior surface. MRI is helpful to evaluate the SAC, and flexion and extension MRI can reveal a more dynamic appreciation of the space at this level.

The most frequently encountered causes of cervical spine instability in children can be categorized etiologically (Table 1).

### Congenital Anomalies

Congenital anomalies have a varied spectrum ranging from benign asymptomatic conditions to those with a potential for fatal instability. Congenital causes of cervical spine instability are complex because congenital vertebral anomalies of the cervical spine arise from defective somatogenesis. Congenital anomalies of the cervical spine often occur in clusters, which further complicates these cases because more than one congenital anomaly frequently exists in the same patient. Additionally, the radiographic examination is often difficult to interpret in children because of the dynamic process of growth and ossification of the developing spine.

Because the identification of congenital cervical spine instability is often delayed, neurologic sequelae can occur insidiously and progressively. Thus, myelopa-

**Table 1 | Classification of Cervical Instability**

| Causes | Subtypes |
|---|---|
| Congenital | Vertebral (bony anomalies) |
| |    Cranio-occipital defects (occipital vertebrae, basilar impression, occipital dysplasias, condylar hypoplasia, occipitalized atlas) |
| |    Atlantoaxial defects (aplasia of atlas arch, aplasia of odontoid process) |
| |    Subaxial anomalies (failure of segmentation and/or fusion, spina bifida, spondylolisthesis) |
| | Ligamentous, or |
| | Combined anomalies found at birth as an element of somatogenic aberration |
| | Syndromic disorders (ie, Down syndrome, Klippel-Feil syndrome, 22q11.2 deletion syndrome, Marfan syndrome, Ehlers-Danlos syndrome) |
| Acquired | Trauma |
| | Infection (pyogenic/granulomatous) |
| | Tumor |
| | Inflammatory conditions (ie, juvenile rheumatoid arthritis) |
| | Osteochondrodysplasias (ie, achondroplasia, spondyloepiphyseal dysplasia) |
| | Storage disorders (ie, mucopolysaccharidoses) |
| | Miscellaneous (ie, postsurgery) |

*(Adapted with permission from Drummond DS, Hosalkar HS: Treatment of cervical spine instability in the pediatric patient, in Clark CR (ed): The Cervical Spine, ed 4. Philadelphia, PA, Lippincott Williams and Wilkins, 2005, pp 427-447.)*

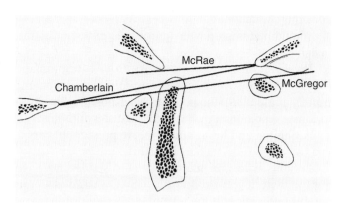

**Figure 8** Methods of determining basilar invagination. McGregor's line is drawn from the hard palate to the lowest point of the occiput. Protrusion of the tip of the dens greater than 4.5 mm above this line is abnormal. Chamberlain's line extends from the dorsal margin of the hard palate to the dorsal lip of the foramen magnum. The normal position of the dens is between 1 mm below this line and as much as 0.6 mm above it. McRae's line extends from the basion to the posterior lip of the foramen magnum. Protrusion of the tip of the dens above McRae's line is indicative of basilar invagination.

thy may not be evident initially. Although an insidious course is more frequent, acute-onset quadriparesis has been reported in the literature.

Abnormal development of cervical vertebrae is frequently associated with anomalies of the brain stem, such as the Arnold-Chiari I malformations. Caudally displaced brain stem and cerebellar tonsils through the foramen magnum characterize these malformations. The Chiari I malformation may disturb the flow of cerebrospinal fluid and lead to an obstructive hydromyelia; this situation frequently causes progressive scoliosis.

Congenital anomalies may also be observed elsewhere in the spine and spinal cord. Vertebral anomalies and neural tube defects may also occur in the thoracic spine. Defective development may also be observed in other parts of the musculoskeletal system as well as in other organ systems. Therefore, the need for a thorough investigation in search of associated conditions is necessary.

## Basilar Impression
Basilar impression is one of the most common developmental malformations of the upper cervical spine. With this anomaly the dens is displaced cranially through the foramen magnum to encroach on the brain stem. It is commonly associated with other anomalies such as Klippel-Feil syndrome, hypoplastic atlas, and occipitocervical synostosis. It may also accompany systemic disorders such as achondroplasia, osteogenesis imperfecta, and Morquio-Brailsford syndrome.

Most patients remain asymptomatic until the second or third decade of life, when they may present with headache, neck pain, and neurologic compromise. Motor and sensory loss has been noted in 85% of the patients with symptoms. Cerebellar ataxia and lower cranial nerve involvement may occur with dysarthria, dysphagia, nystagmus, and bizarre respiratory patterns caused by respiratory center compression.

Evaluation should include plain radiographs and MRI. McGregor's line, drawn from the upper surface of the posterior edge of the hard palate to the most caudal point of the occipital curve, is a commonly used measurement. McGregor's line and other methods of determining basilar invagination are shown in Figure 8. CT can more precisely define the osseous deformity. Treatment may require neurosurgical assistance. Anterior impingement may need fusion in extension or anterior odontoid excision (transoral approach), and stabilization in extension. Posterior impingement may require suboccipital craniectomy and decompression of the posterior ring of C1 and possibly C2 followed by fusion at appropriate levels.

## Occipitalization of the Atlas
There is a bony union between the skull and the atlas. Fusion is usually anterior between the anterior arch of the atlas and the rim of foramen magnum. This may be commonly associated with fusion of the C2-3 vertebrae and basilar impression. Fifty percent of patients with occipitalization of the atlas are known to have atlantoaxial

instability, which may be progressive. Hence, this anomaly should be assessed with appropriate radiographs and imaging.

Presentation ranges in severity from asymptomatic to potential for severe neural compromise. Neck pain is usually present as is a peculiar head posture. Intracranial manifestations are headache, visual symptoms and signs, tinnitus, and lower cranial nerve pressure phenomena causing dysphagia and dysarthria.

Patients who are neurologically unstable and have high activity levels or decreased SAC should undergo careful restoration of the atlantoaxial relationship in extension and occiput-cervical arthrodesis, usually to C2. In case of neural impairment, decompression (suboccipital craniectomy and upper cervical laminectomy) with fusion is often also required.

## Odontoid Anomalies

Odontoid anomalies have a varied spectrum of presentation from aplasia through varying degrees of hypoplasia. These anomalies may lead to atlantoaxial instability, because the odontoid is no longer a functioning peg. Ossification of the odontoid occurs through three centers of ossification, one on either side of the midline and one at the tip. Os odontoideum, currently believed to be traumatic in origin, has features similar to aplasia or hypoplasia of the odontoid. It is important to remember that in the young patient with an incompletely ossified odontoid, a diagnosis of hypoplasia may be made in error (Figure 7).

Clinical presentation may vary from neck pain and discomfort to frank neural compromise and occasionally sudden quadriparesis or death caused by minor trauma. Surgical stabilization is indicated when there is neurologic involvement, documented instability on flexion-extension radiographs (supervised) with reduced SAC, or persistent symptoms of neck pain and discomfort. Atlantoaxial stabilization and arthrodesis is required in these patients.

Congenital muscular torticollis is the most common cause of wryneck in an infant. It is believed to be secondary to a "packing syndrome" and is therefore more common in first-born children. Familial basis and hereditary muscle aplasia have also been suggested in the etiogenesis of congenital muscular torticollis. There is some evidence that the process may be caused by a compartment syndrome involving the sternocleidomastoid muscle, in some cases, with subsequent intramuscular fibrosis. In almost three fourths of patients, the abnormally tight sternocleidomastoid muscle is on the left side. This condition is known to coexist with developmental dysplasia of the hip in 5% of patients.

It is important to evaluate and rule out ocular dysfunction, spinal cord and cerebellar tumors, infection and inflammation, traumatic causes, and atlantoaxial rotatory displacement.

Passive stretching exercises are known to give excellent results especially when started early. If the limitation of range of motion is more than 30° or if the patient's condition persists beyond 1 year, surgical release of the sternocleidomastoid may be necessary. Unipolar or bipolar release may be decided based on the severity.

## Syndromes

The most common syndromes giving rise to cervical instability in children are Down syndrome, Klippel-Feil syndrome, and the 22q11.2 deletion syndrome.

Down syndrome, or trisomy 21, is a genetic disorder that occurs in 1 of 700 live births. Common clinical features include characteristic facies, congenital heart disease, ligamentous laxity, and mental retardation. Instability of the C1-C2 level is found in up to 40% of children with Down syndrome (Figure 9). Atlantooccipital instability is now believed to be as common as atlantoaxial instability in this population and is reported to be as high as 61% in one study.

Children with progressive cervical instability typically present with gait abnormalities, diminished exercise tolerance, and neck pain. An ADI of greater than 5 mm occurs in up to 15% of asymptomatic patients. MRI is indicated to detect neurologic compromise in patients with radiologic instability. Recommendations in the literature for surveillance of potential cervical instability in children with Down syndrome are still unclear. Plain radiographs of the cervical spine, including flexion-extension views, are one option for children with Down syndrome. Follow-up neurologic examination with flexion-extension views should be performed to monitor patients with potential instability.

Stressful activities including tumbling and diving should be avoided if possible by asymptomatic children with ADI greater than 5 mm. Prophylactic fusion at this point is not recommended. Surgery is indicated for neurologic symptoms, intermittent torticollis, excessive translation and a reduction in the SAC.

Klippel-Feil syndrome was first described in the early 20th century and is now recognized to be associated with a variety of anomalies in the spine and other organ systems. The syndrome results from defective development of the cervical spine and in its most complete form is marked by a short neck, low hairline, and limited range of motion in the cervical spine. The lesion is present at birth but the radiographic findings may be delayed and slowly progressive (Figure 10). Both sexes are equally affected but the severity of involvement is highly variable. There are three types described; (1) vertebrae massively fused into blocks, giving the patient a grossly abnormal appearance, a stiff neck, and severe disability; (2) fusions involving only one or two inter-

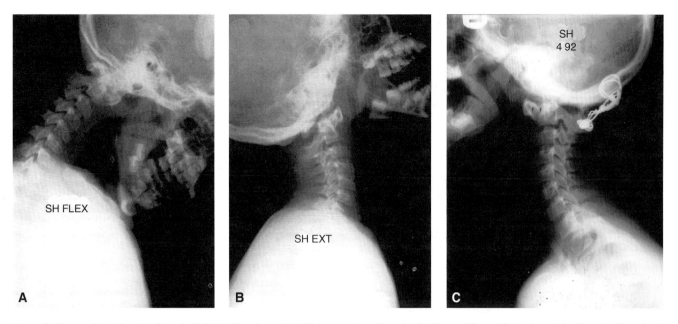

Figure 9   Down syndrome. Lateral radiographs in flexion **(A)** and extension **(B)** demonstrating atlanto-occipital hypermobility and fixed atlantoaxial subluxation. *(Reproduced with permission from Drummond DS: Pediatric cervical instability, in Weisel SW, Boden SD, Wisneski RJ, (eds): Seminars in Spine Surgery. Philadelphia, PA, WB Saunders, 1996, pp 292-309.)*

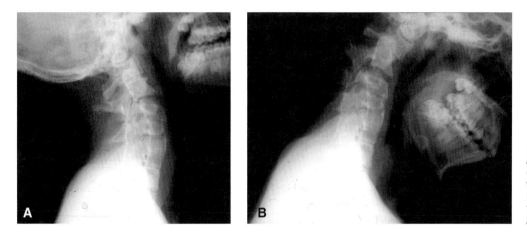

Figure 10 Klippel-Feil syndrome. **A** and **B,** Lateral radiographs of the cervical spine (flexion-extension views) showing multiply fused vertebrae, decreased range of cervical motion, and an abnormally increased ADI.

spaces; and (3) deformity including cervical fusion, with coexisting fusion or segmental failure in the lumbar or thoracic spine, inherited as an autosomal dominant trait. Also, occipitalization of the atlas may coexist.

Clinically, there may be associated facial asymmetry, torticollis, and webbing of the neck. Limitation of neck motion is the most consistent and constant clinical manifestation. Occasionally, Sprengel's deformity and scoliosis may also be associated with this syndrome.

Instability in Klippel-Feil syndrome may occur at the interface between the normal spine and fused segments or between two fused segments. There are three high-risk patterns that commonly produce instability and require early recognition: (1) fusion of C2 to C3 with occipitocervical synostosis; (2) long fusion with an abnormal occipitocervical junction; and (3) a single open interface between two fused segments.

With each of these patterns increased motion may be focused at one segmental level, with the abnormal biomechanics producing increased translation of one vertebra on an adjacent caudal one, producing instability. Nonsurgical treatment such as activity modification and bracing may be attempted before offering surgical stabilization.

The chromosome abnormality, deletion of 22q11.2, is one of the most common genetic syndromes and encompasses a wide spectrum of abnormalities including cardiac, palate, and immunologic anomalies. Anomalies of the upper cervical spine are also common (Figure 11). At least one vertebral anomaly is seen in most patients and usually two or more can be observed. The most common anomalies noted are incomplete closure of the arch of the atlas, C2-3 fusion, dysmorphic dens, and occasionally segmental instability.

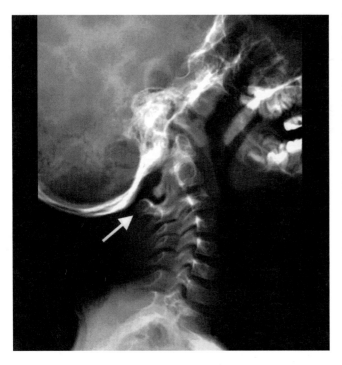

Figure 11  In a 13-year-old girl with 22q11.2 deletion syndrome, a lateral radiograph of the cervical spine shows hypoplastic odontoid, platybasia, and C2 swoosh.

Although upper cervical spine variations in the 22q11.2 deletion syndrome occur frequently, it is premature to predict the clinical implications of these radiographic findings. Advanced imaging and regular follow-up can help clarify the clinical course.

## Other Congenital Conditions Leading to Instability

### Osteochondrodysplasias

These are a heterogeneous group of heritable disorders characterized by an intrinsic abnormality of bone and cartilage growth and remodeling. There is a generalized disturbance of skeletal growth that manifests as disproportionately short stature. Angular deformities of limbs and premature degenerative joint disease, spinal disorders including cervical spine instability with potentially serious sequelae are common.

Achondroplasia is the most common variant of short limb disproportionate dwarfism and is inherited as an autosomal dominant trait. Common characteristics include enlarged neurocranium with frontal bossing, midface hypoplasia and flattened nasal bridge, rhizomelic extremities with normal trunk length, thoracolumbar kyphosis, and exaggerated lumbar lordosis. Foramen magnum stenosis and spinal stenosis are the most common cervical anomalies and may be associated with sleep apnea or sudden death. CT can better define the anatomy, and MRI with somatosensory-evoked potentials best defines the brain stem and spinal cord anoma-

lies. Foramen magnum decompression with or without occipitocervical fusion is occasionally necessary for repeated apneic episodes or neurologic compromise.

Spondyloepiphyseal dysplasia (SED) is characterized by primary epiphyseal and vertebral involvement resulting in a short-trunk disproportionate dwarfism. SED congenital, SED tarda, spondylometaphyseal dysplasia, and spondyloepimetaphyseal dysplasia are the subtypes of SED.

SED congenita is commonly associated with involvement of the upper cervical spine and up to 40% of children have C1-2 instability. Odontoid hypoplasia and os odontoideum are common features that predispose patients to this instability. Persistent hypotonia and delay in motor milestones may be the only early manifestations of neurologic involvement.

Lateral flexion-extension radiographs are recommended at presentation for all types of SED. MRI will help outline any spinal cord involvement. Surgical stabilization is recommended for instability greater than 5 mm and for instability with evidence of abnormal neurologic involvement either clinically or by diagnostic workup.

### Storage Diseases

Children with storage diseases, such as Morquio's syndrome, may present with atlantoaxial instability. Odontoid hypoplasia, rather than transverse ligament incompetency, usually is the cause of instability. Myelopathy secondary to instability is also common in these patients.

### Miscellaneous

Posterior column resection (postlaminectomy) can proceed to give rise to spinal instability. Similarly, other skeletal dysplasias such as osteogenesis imperfecta and neurofibromatosis may be associated with spinal instability on rare occasions.

## Summary

Cervical spine disorders in children differ significantly than those of adults. A clear and comprehensive understanding of the anatomy, physiology, and biomechanics of the pediatric cervical spine, particularly for the segment between the occiput and C3, is of paramount importance in managing these patients. A careful and thorough clinical and neurologic evaluation and appropriate radiographic assessment are essential to make an accurate diagnosis, understand the pathogenesis, and outline the appropriate management. Surgical treatment of cervical spine instability in children may be indicated to protect the neural structures (axis and nerve roots) from insult or damage and arthrodesis may be needed to stabilize a segment of the spine.

## Annotated Bibliography

Drummond DS, Hosalkar HS: Treatment of cervical spine instability in the pediatric patient, in Clark CR (ed): *The Cervical Spine*, ed 4. Philadelphia, PA, Lippincott Williams and Wilkins, 2005, pp 427-447.

A detailed review of presentation, classification, evaluation and management of traumatic and nontraumatic cervical instability in children is presented.

Pizzutillo PD: Klippel-Feil syndrome, in Clark CR (ed): *The Cervical Spine*, ed 4. Philadelphia, PA, Lippincott Williams and Wilkins, 2005, pp 448-458.

Historical aspects, clinical features, radiology, embryology, natural history, associated problems, and management of Klippel-Feil syndrome are discussed.

Ricchetti ET, States L, Hosalkar HS, et al: Radiographic study of the upper cervical spine in the 22q11.2 deletion syndrome. *J Bone Joint Surg Am* 2004;86:1751-1760.

The authors present 79 consecutive patients with the 22q11.2 deletion who underwent clinical and radiographic evaluation of the occiput and cervical spine. The authors attempts to define and determine the frequency of variations of the occiput and cervical spine on plain radiographs in patients with the 22q11.2 deletion syndrome and postulate the potential clinical importance of these variations.

Warner WC: Torticollis in children, in Clark CR (ed): *The Cervical Spine*, ed 4. Philadelphia, PA, Lippincott Williams and Wilkins, 2005, pp 551-560.

The multiple causes and clinical presentations as well as management of congenital muscular torticollis and acquired torticollis in children are outlined.

## Classic Bibliography

Adams SB Jr, Flynn JM, Hosalkar HS, Hunter J, Finkel R: Torticollis in an infant caused by hereditary muscle aplasia. *Am J Orthop* 2003;32:556-558.

Cattell HS, Filtzer DL: Pseudosubluxation and other normal variations in the cervical spine in children: A study of one hundred and sixty children. *J Bone Joint Surg Am* 1965;47:1295-1309.

David KM, Crockard A: Congenital malformations of the base of the skull, atlas and dens, in Clark CR (ed): *The Cervical Spine*, ed 4. Philadelphia, PA, Lippincott Williams and Wilkins, 2005, pp 415-426.

Dormans JP: Evaluation of children with suspected cervical spine injury. *Instr Course Lect* 2002;51:401-410.

Drummond DS: Pediatric cervical instability: Diagnosis and treatment concepts. *Semin Spine Surg* 1996;8:292-309.

Hosalkar HS, Gerardi JA, Shaw BA: Combined asymptomatic congenital anterior and posterior deficiency of the atlas. *Pediatr Radiol* 2001;31:810-813.

Hosalkar H, Gill IS, Gujar P, Shaw BA: Familial torticollis with polydactyly: Manifestation in three generations. *Am J Orthop* 2001;30:656-658.

Khanna AJ, Wasserman BA, Sponseller PD: Magnetic resonance imaging of the cervical spine: Current techniques and spectrum of disease. *J Bone Joint Surg Am* 2002;84-A(suppl 2):70-80.

Kornblum M, Stanitki DF: Spinal manifestations of skeletal dysplasias. *Orthop Clin North Am* 1999;30:501-520.

Lachman RS: The cervical spine in the skeletal dysplasias and associated disorders. *Pediatr Radiol* 1997;27:402-408.

Lustrin ES, Karakas SP, Ortiz AO, et al: Pediatric cervical spine: Normal anatomy, variants, and trauma. *Radiographics* 2003;23:539-560.

Mackenzie WG, Shah SA, Takemitsu M: The cervical spine in skeletal dysplasia, in Clark CR (ed): *The Cervical Spine*, ed 4. Philadelphia, PA, Lippincott Williams and Wilkins, 2005, pp 459-480.

Pizzutillo PD, Herman MJ: Cervical spine disorders in children. *Orthop Clin North Am* 1999;30:457-466.

Spranger JW, Langer LO Jr: Spondyloepiphyseal dysplasia congenita. *Radiology* 1970;94:313-322.

Ulmer JL, Elster AD, Ginsberg LE, Williams DW: Klippel-Feil syndrome: CT and MR of acquired and congenital abnormalities of cervical spine and cord. *J Comput Assist Tomogr* 1993;17:215-224.

Wang H, Rosenbaum AE, Reid CS, Zinreich SJ, Pyeritz RE: Pediatric patients with achondroplasia: CT evaluation of the craniocervical junction. *Radiology* 1987;164:515-519.

# Chapter 43

# Back Pain in Children and Adolescents

Martin J. Herman, MD

Peter D. Pizzutillo, MD

## Epidemiology

Back pain is common in children and adolescents. More than 30,000 children and adolescents each year present to an emergency department or primary care provider with a report of back pain. Recent epidemiologic evidence suggests that the lifetime prevalence of low back pain in children and adolescents is 30% to 50%. Most adolescents report episodes of back pain in general health surveys. Female gender, parental history of back pain, smoking, heavy school backpacks, and increased television viewing are some associated factors. One long-term follow-up survey of adults with a history of back pain showed a higher rate of hospital admissions and decreased work capacity in those adults who reported frequent low back pain as adolescents.

Classic teaching regarding back pain in children and adolescents supported the belief that a specific etiology is identifiable in most children. Recent studies report evidence to the contrary. In a 2000 study of 226 children and adolescents who underwent bone scans for back pain, only 22% of patients had identifiable pathology including spondylolysis, disk herniation, neoplasia, and infections; the others had nonspecific musculoskeletal back pain. Thus, the physician's challenge is to separate those patients with nonspecific sources of back pain from those with identifiable spinal conditions. This may be particularly difficult for the physician unaccustomed to evaluating children and adolescents with back pain because the common etiologies of back pain are different than those for adults. Boys and younger children, competitive athletes, individuals with constant progressive back pain or pain at night, and children and adolescents with back pain associated with systemic signs and symptoms or neurologic dysfunction are most likely to have serious spinal conditions.

## History and Physical Examination

A thorough history is the most useful tool to effectively diagnose children and adolescents with back pain. The specific location and type of pain, time of onset, frequency and intensity of pain, and those measures that relieve the pain must be determined. A recent history of trauma, participation in sports or other physical activities, and backpack use at school are also pertinent information. Specific inquiries about limitation of activities because of the pain and the presence of night pain, fever, chills, or other systemic signs and symptoms are necessary for all patients. Patterns of radiation of the back pain to the buttock or lower extremity, extremity numbness or weakness, and bowel and bladder dysfunction must also be discussed. For younger children, questioning parents about changes in gait or balance and toileting skills or bedwetting may reveal subtle signs of neurologic abnormalities.

The physical examination is best performed with the child or adolescent in a gown. The skin of the back, torso, and extremities is inspected for lesions such as ecchymoses or abrasions and café-au-lait spots. The spinal midline is assessed for signs of spinal dysraphism including hemangiomata, sinus tracts, and hairy patches. Spinal alignment is assessed with the child standing; signs of scoliosis, including asymmetry of shoulder heights and hip creases and torso shift, are noted. Viewing the child from the side, excessive kyphosis or lordosis of the thoracic and lumbar spine is recorded. The spinal midline is palpated for defects of the posterior elements and tenderness. Paraspinal muscles are palpated for tenderness and spasm. Range of motion of the spine is evaluated including flexion, extension, lateral bending and rotation; specific limitations of motions or those movements that elicit discomfort are recorded.

A careful neurologic examination is mandatory when evaluating children and adolescents with back pain. Observation of gait and motor and sensory testing are routinely performed. Deep tendon reflexes of the knee and ankle, as well as abdominal reflexes, are elicited; asymmetry is recorded as abnormal. The presence of sustained clonus and an abnormal Babinski reflex correlate with upper motor neuron pathology. Hamstring tightness as reflected by popliteal angle measurement and straight-leg raise testing for sciatic nerve irritation complete the examination.

## Diagnostic Tests

Plain radiography of the spine is the primary diagnostic tool to evaluate back pain. Standing PA and lateral radiographs of the spine are useful to assess overall alignment and abnormalities of the vertebral bodies and disk spaces. Coned-down views of the lumbosacral junction or specific areas of concern along the spine provide a higher quality image and may reveal more subtle findings. Supine oblique views of the lumbosacral junction are necessary only for those individuals with suspected spondylolysis.

Single photon emission CT (SPECT), a technetium bone scan that provides axial, coronal, and sagittal spinal images of the spine, is the best test for children and adolescents whose radiographs are normal. Infections, neoplasia (both benign and malignant), fractures, and spondylolysis may be detected by increased uptake of technetium at the affected site. Because SPECT is sensitive but not specific, other tests are often necessary to confirm the specific diagnosis. MRI is used for assessing spinal cord pathology and nerve root compression from a herniated disk or other pathologies. MRI is also useful to define the extent of vertebral body and paravertebral soft-tissue involvement from infections and neoplasms. CT is the most reliable study for defining bony morphology of spinal pathology.

## Differential Diagnosis

### Traumatic

#### Sprain and Strain

Spinal ligamentous and fascial sprains and paraspinal muscle strains are the most common etiologies of back pain and are likely the source of nonspecific back pain in the older child and adolescent. Often the patient describes a localized spasm or ache of the low back associated with an acute event or a strenuous repetitive activity or sport. Night pain and radicular symptoms are not present. On physical examination, the paraspinal muscles and midline may be tender. Paraspinal muscle spasm may be present. The neurologic examination is normal. The differential diagnosis includes herniated lumbar disk, vertebral end-plate fracture, and spondylolysis.

Plain radiographs may show abnormal spinal alignment secondary to guarding or spasm but are otherwise normal. Treatment of nonspecific back pain is always nonsurgical. A period of rest from activities, use of nonsteroidal anti-inflammatory drugs (NSAIDs), stretching of the paraspinal muscles and hamstrings, and strengthening of paraspinal and abdominal muscles are successful in improving back pain in most individuals. Gradual return to activities and modifications in training or technique may be necessary in those patients whose pain is secondary to overuse or repetitive injury.

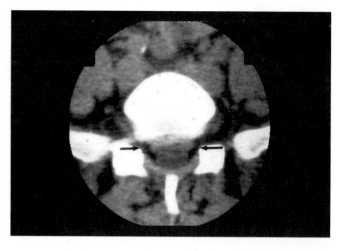

**Figure 1** CT scan of an adolescent female gymnast with severe back pain after a fall from the balance beam reveals a large, central disk herniation.

### Herniated Lumbar Disk

Back pain secondary to a herniated lumbar disk is uncommon in older children and adolescents. The history usually includes a specific episode of trauma and pain is predominantly localized to the back and buttocks without radiation to the leg in many instances. The child or adolescent may walk with an antalgic list. The mobility of the lumbar spine is often severely limited because of pain and paraspinal spasm. Most affected individuals will demonstrate a positive straight-leg raise test. Decreased or asymmetric deep tendon reflexes, motor weakness, and sensory changes are less common findings in the child or adolescent compared with the adult with a herniated disk. Differential diagnosis includes lumbar sprain/strain and vertebral end-plate fracture.

Plain radiographs are typically normal with the exception of loss of a normal lumbar lordosis or mild scoliosis secondary to spasm. CT (Figure 1) or MRI confirm the presence of a herniated disk and nerve root compression. Overdiagnosis of disk pathology by MRI is common in older children and adolescents. MRI findings must correlate with the clinical evaluation before definitive diagnosis of a herniated disk.

Nonsurgical treatment is successful in alleviating signs and symptoms of a herniated disk in many children and adolescents. Activity restriction, NSAIDs, and judicious use of muscle relaxants combined with a structured physical therapy regimen are recommended. Only those children without improvement after 3 months of conservative therapy and those with significant neurologic dysfunction are treated with surgical diskectomy. Although favorable short-term outcomes may be expected, long-term studies of children and adolescents who undergo disk surgery show an increased need for repeat surgery in comparison with adults who undergo diskecetomy.

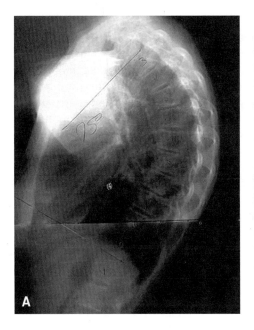
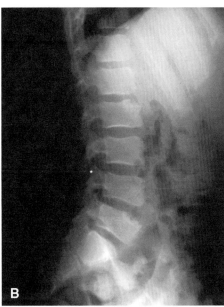

**Figure 2** **A,** Lateral standing radiograph of a teenager with back pain and "poor posture" reveals findings consistent with thoracic Scheuermann's disease. Note hyperkyphosis, apical vertebral body wedging, and end-plate irregularities. **B,** Lateral standing radiograph of an adolescent with chronic low back pain. Note end-plate irregularities, Schmorl's nodes, and L5 megavertebra consistent with lumbar Scheuermann's disease.

### Vertebral End-Plate Fracture

Acute separation of the vertebral end plate with protrusion into the spinal canal is a rare entity that occurs in the older adolescent. The clinical history often includes participation in weight-lifting or other strenuous sports during which an acute flexion injury of the spine occurs. The onset of low back pain with occasional radicular symptoms is acute. The physical examination mimics that of the adolescent with a herniated disk. The differential diagnosis is a herniated lumbar disk.

Plain radiographs may reveal evidence of end-plate separation with posterior protrusion, most commonly at L4. CT is most useful to assess the size of the bony fragment and the degree of spinal canal encroachment. Initial treatment is nonsurgical and similar to that prescribed for a herniated disk. Some adolescents will show improved symptoms over time as some diminution of canal compromise occurs with healing and resorption of the end-plate fragment. Surgical excision of the end plate is frequently necessary for those adolescents without improvement of symptoms after nonsurgical treatment or for those with acute, severe, or unremitting neurologic dysfunction.

### Developmental

#### Scheuermann's Kyphosis

Scheuermann's kyphosis is believed to be a developmental growth disturbance of the vertebral end plates, occurring most frequently in the thoracic spine, and is the most common cause of thoracic back pain in the older child and adolescent. Typically the pain is localized to the middle or low thoracic spine and is incited by prolonged periods of standing or sitting. Occasionally the diagnosis is made because of parental concerns about "poor posture." The physical examination is nota-

ble for pronounced thoracic kyphosis and compensatory lumbar lordosis. Some children have associated mild scoliosis. Palpation of the spinal midline at the apex of the deformity and adjacent thoracic paraspinal musculature may elicit discomfort. Overall spinal motion is usually normal, except for partial or complete inflexibility of the kyphotic segment. The neurologic examination is normal. The differential diagnosis is postural kyphosis, congenital kyphosis, compression fracture, neoplasia, and lumbar sprain/strain in those with mild deformity.

Standing coronal images reveal mild scoliosis in approximately 30% of patients. Thoracic kyphosis is increased compared with normal (normal is 20° to 40°). Apical vertebral body end-plate irregularities and anterior wedging of vertebral bodies at several adjacent levels confirm the diagnosis (Figure 2, *A*); the apex is most commonly at T8 or T9 but may be as caudad as the thoracolumbar junction. Younger patients with at least 2 years of growth remaining and flexible deformity as documented by hyperextension radiographs may benefit from bracing. A modified low profile orthosis or a Milwaukee brace are best for applying appropriate corrective forces. A period of serial casting may be useful before bracing for those whose kyphosis is initially inflexible. Maintenance of the initial amount of kyphosis or improvement in some instances may be expected. A minimum of 18 months of bracing is necessary. For older adolescents, an exercise regimen of spinal stretching and strengthening, abdominal strengthening, and hamstring stretching improves pain, but will not significantly improve deformity.

Indications for surgical treatment of Scheuermann's kyphosis are few. The natural history of Scheuermann's thoracic kyphosis is that deformity progression and chronic pain are uncommon in adulthood. Patients with chronic pain despite nonsurgical treatment and deformity greater than 70° that is cosmetically unacceptable are candidates for surgery. Instrumentation and spinal fusion either by a combined anterior-posterior approach or posterior-only surgery is the treatment of choice. Surgical complications are higher in this group than in children and adolescents who undergo spinal fusions for idiopathic scoliosis.

Lumbar Scheuermann's disease is less common than thoracic disease. This entity typically occurs in adolescents with low back pain and stiffness. Radiographs reveal characteristic changes (Figure 2, *B*). Treatment is nonsugical and according to symptoms.

### Spondylolysis and Spondylolisthesis

Spondylolysis is the most common identifiable etiology of lumbar back pain in children and adolescents. Athletes who participate in activities that involve spinal hyperextension or loading with torsion such as gymnastics or football are most susceptible to developing this condition. Spondylolysis most commonly describes a defect of the pars interarticularis of L5. Spondylolisthesis describes the anterior translation of the lumbar vertebral bodies relative to its adjacent caudad vertebral segment. In children and adolescents this translation is most commonly seen in association with a pars defect (isthmic spondylolisthesis) or dysplasia of the posterior elements at the L5-S1 vertebral segment (dysplastic spondylolisthesis).

The child or adolescent with spondylolysis and spondylolisthesis presents with low back pain, occasionally with radiation to the buttocks. Radicular symptoms occur infrequently. The pain worsens with activity and is often relieved by rest. Physical examination in patients with spondylolysis reveals no deformity; patients with spondylolisthesis may have an exaggerated lumbar lordosis or a flattening of the buttocks. The low lumbar paraspinal muscles and lumbopelvic fascia are often tender to palpation. Lumbosacral hyperextension is limited and elicits discomfort. Hamstring tightness as reflected by an increase in popliteal angles is a frequent associated finding. Differential diagnosis includes a lumbar sprain/strain and herniated lumbar disk.

Standing radiographs of the lumbosacral spine may reveal a pars defect or spondylolisthesis. Oblique views improve visualization of smaller pars defects not seen on the lateral view. Hypoplasia of the posterior elements or elongation of the pars without a defect may be seen in dysplastic spondylolisthesis. SPECT bone scan is the best test to diagnose spondylolysis in those individuals with suspicious clinical findings but with normal radiographs. CT is useful to define the morphology of the pars defect or dysplastic posterior elements. MRI may also be used to diagnose spondylolysis but is best indicated for patients with back pain and radiculopathy to differentiate spondylolysis from disk disease or other pathology.

Nonsurgical treatment of spondylolysis and low-grade spondylolisthesis (less than 50% slip) includes activity restriction combined with physical therapy that emphasizes hamstring stretching, spinal flexibility, and strengthening. Improvement of symptoms may be expected in most patients. Bracing may be used as an adjunct in patients initially unresponsive to this treatment regimen. Although the pars defect may heal in a small percentage of patients with spondylolysis, radiographs show persistence of the pars defect in most patients, despite improvement of symptoms.

In situ posterolateral L5 to sacrum fusion is indicated for children and adolescents with L5 spondylolysis and low-grade spondylolisthesis that do not respond to nonsurgical treatment. Repair of the pars defect is indicated for unresponsive individuals with spondylolysis at L4 or more cephalad vertebral levels. Surgical treatment is indicated for most children and adolescents with high-grade spondylolisthesis (greater than 50% slip) regardless of symptoms. In situ L4-S1 fusion and hyperextension casting or instrumented partial reduction and fusion are options. The best method of surgical fusion for high-grade spondylolisthesis remains a controversial topic.

### Infectious

### Pyogenic Spondylitis

Diskitis and vertebral osteomyelitis, known collectively as pyogenic spondylitis, are the most common etiologies of back pain in children younger than 8 years of age. Because of common blood flow between the vertebral body and disk in younger children, the entities are sometimes indistinct and likely represent a spectrum of disease from bacterial diskitis to the more involved vertebral osteomyelitis. Pyogenic spondylitis occurs most commonly in the cervical and lumbar spine. The typical child presents with fever, refusal to walk, or has a limp or back pain. The child appears ill. Examination is significant for spinal tenderness and guarded range of motion, especially lumbar extension. Neurologic examination is normal. Because of the child's young age and inability to cooperate with a complete examination, the differential diagnosis is broad and includes appendicitis and abdominal conditions, psoas abscess, septic arthritis of the sacroiliac joint or hip, osteomyelitis of the pelvis, and neoplasia.

Blood tests aid in the diagnosis. Typically the white blood cell count, erythrocyte sedimentation rate (ESR) and C-reactive protein (CRP) are elevated. Plain radiographs reveal disk space narrowing, vertebral end-plate irregularities, or deep soft-tissue swelling in more than half of patients. SPECT of the spine shows increased technetium uptake at the involved disk and the adjacent vertebral bodies. MRI defines the extent of vertebral body involvement by osteomyelitis and paravertebral soft-tissue abscesses.

Treatment is mostly nonsurgical. *Staphylococcus aureus* is the most common bacteriologic etiology. Intravenous antibiotic therapy that empirically covers *S aureus*, including resistant strains, is recommended for 2 to 6 weeks. Duration is determined by the initial extent of vertebral body involvement, clinical response to treatment, and normalization of blood work. A spinal orthosis or cast may be useful to alleviate symptoms of back pain and spasm, but is not always necessary. Tuberculous osteomyelitis is often associated with greater vertebral body disruption and requires different empiric therapy and a longer course of treatment.

Surgical management is indicated only for those children and adolescents unresponsive to antibiotic therapy. Image-guided percutaneous aspiration or laparoscopic biopsy may be necessary to obtain culture. Débridement is rarely necessary. Reconstitution of the disk space is seen after treatment within 2 years in most children. Spontaneous fusion, while uncommon, may occur at the involved vertebral levels.

### Neoplastic-Benign

### Langerhans Cell Histiocytosis

Langerhans cell histiocytosis of the spine occurs most commonly in children between the ages of 5 and 10 years. Cervical and lumbar spine lesions are seen more frequently in those with multifocal disease. The child typically presents with focal constant back pain and tenderness, mild scoliosis or kyphosis, and no neurologic dysfunction. The classic radiographic finding is a lytic lesion of the vertebral body with complete vertebral flattening (vertebra plana). New evidence shows that asymmetric collapse of the vertebral body is more common (Figure 3). The differential diagnosis includes compression fracture, vertebral osteomyelitis, and other neoplasms of the spine.

Treatment is generally nonsurgical and symptomatic, including activity restriction and bracing. Chemotherapy may be necessary for those patients with extraskeletal disease. Vertebral body biopsy is necessary only for those children with an uncertain diagnosis. Vertebrectomy for decompression of neural elements and fusion for secondary deformity are rarely indicated.

### Osteoid Osteoma and Osteoblastoma

Osteoid osteomas are the most common benign bone lesions of the posterior spinal elements that occur in older children and adolescents. The typical presentation is back pain, sometimes relieved by NSAIDs and worse at night, or new onset of painful scoliosis. Examination is notable for spinal tenderness, guarded range of motion, and coronal plane deformity. Differential diagnosis includes osteoblastoma, aneurysmal bone cyst, pyogenic spondylitis, spondylolysis, and other neoplasms.

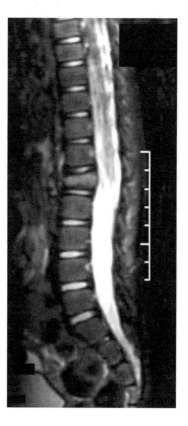

Figure 3 Sagittal MRI scan of the spine in a child with new onset of back pain reveals asymmetric vertebral collapse secondary to biopsy-proven Langerhans cell histiocytosis.

Radiographs are usually normal, but may reveal a localized area of sclerosis, frequently in the pedicle or posterior elements. SPECT shows intense focal increased technetium uptake at the affected site. A thin-cut CT scan of the abnormal area identifies the focal, lytic nidus surrounded by sclerotic bone; this finding is diagnostic for osteoid osteoma (Figure 4). NSAIDs may provide symptomatic relief in some patients. Surgical excision of the nidus is often necessary.

Osteoblastoma is pathologically similar to osteoid osteoma but is associated with a larger area of sclerosis without a definable nidus in some instances. Almost half of the osteoblastomas diagnosed in children and adolescents occur in the spine. The clinical presentation is similar to that for patients with an osteoid osteoma except that associated neurologic findings may be seen in those with osteoblastoma. Excision is indicated in most instances and is associated with a 10% recurrence rate.

### Aneurysmal Bone Cyst

Aneurysmal bone cysts (ABCs) are lesions of the spinal posterior elements and occur occasionally in the vertebral body; they are diagnosed most commonly in adolescents. The clinical history and examination is similar to that for patients with an osteoblastoma. Radiographs reveal a characteristic focal, expansile, lytic lesion of the posterior elements and body; contiguous vertebral bodies may be involved. CT best delineates the extent of the cyst and its loculations. T2-weighted MRI reveals

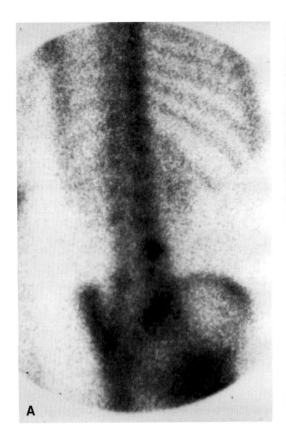

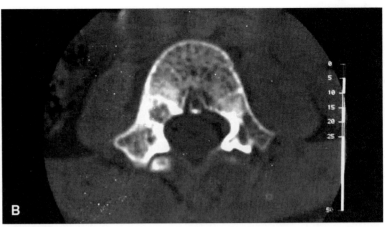

Figure 4 **A,** Bone scan of an adolescent with scoliosis and back pain reveals focal increased uptake at L4. **B,** CT scan of the affected area shows a focal area of lysis with surrounding sclerosis consistent with an osteoid osteoma.

fluid-fluid levels within the cyst cavity that are diagnostic of an ABC. Differential diagnosis includes other spinal column neoplasms.

Small, minimally symptomatic ABCs may be observed. Curettage and bone grafting are necessary for most ABCs of the spine. Preoperative embolization may reduce intraoperative blood loss but care must be taken to avoid diminution of normal spinal cord blood flow. Recurrence rate after excision is 10%.

### Neoplastic-Malignant

Malignancies of the spinal column are rare. Children and adolescents with constant, progressively worsening back pain, pain at night, neurologic dysfunction, and systemic complaints associated with back pain including weight loss, lethargy, and fever must be suspected of having a malignancy. Typically the clinical presentation evolves over weeks and delay in diagnosis is not uncommon.

In patients with acute lymphocytic leukemia, 6% first seek medical care because of back pain. Other symptoms of acute lymphocytic leukemia include increased bruising, fatigue, and extremity pain. At presentation, the child appears ill with generalized paraspinal muscle tenderness, limited spinal range of motion, and occasional tenderness at the metaphyses of long bones. The neurologic examination is generally normal. The differential diagnosis includes systemic inflammatory disease, pyogenic spondylitis, and other neoplasms.

Spinal radiographs may reveal diffuse osteopenia and minimal compression fractures at several vertebral body levels. Osteopenia and lytic areas may be seen in the metaphyses of long bones. Bone scan shows diffuse increased technetium uptake throughout the spine and metaphyses. Laboratory studies are significant for an elevated white blood cell count, ESR, and CRP; anemia and a decreased platelet count assist in establishing the diagnosis. Approximately 10% of children with leukemia will have normal white blood cell counts. Bone marrow aspiration that reveals a proliferation of lymphoblasts confirms the diagnosis.

Systemic chemotherapy is the treatment for acute lymphocytic leukemia in children and adolescents. Management of vertebral compression fractures is mostly nonsugical and includes activity restriction and bracing. Surgical treatment of spinal lesions in patients with acute lymphocytic leukemia is reserved for those with neurologic compromise or severe deformity.

Other primary malignancies of the spine include lymphoma, osteosarcoma, Ewing's sarcoma, and chordoma. Metastatic disease of the spine from neuroblastoma occurs in younger children. Malignancies of the spinal cord and neural elements are rare. These conditions often are associated with a history of constant, progressively worsening back pain and neurologic abnormalities including lower extremity weakness or alteration of gait, unexplained hamstring spasm, and changes in bowel or bladder functions. The most common malignancies of the neural elements are astrocytoma and ependymoma. Malignant degeneration of spinal neurofibromatosis into neurofibrosarcoma is exceedingly rare. Spinal cord anomalies may present similarly. Syringomyelia, a cause of left thoracic scoliosis and painful adolescent idiopathic scoliosis, and spinal cord tethering are the most common of these rare conditions.

### Other Etiologies
#### Inflammatory Arthritis
Juvenile rheumatoid arthritis may cause back pain. Many patients with this type of arthritis, however, have cervical spine complaints; spontaneous cervical fusion can occur. Other etiologies of thoracic and lumbar back pain must be ruled out before attributing back pain in these patients to juvenile rheumatoid arthritis.

Ankylosing spondylitis is often first diagnosed in adolescence and is more common in boys than girls. The presenting symptom is frequently thoracic and lumbar diffuse back pain. On examination, spinal motion is limited globally and thoracic excursion with inspiration is limited. Radiographs of the sacroiliac joints may reveal sclerosis, narrowing, or fusion. A positive blood test for HLA-B27 has been linked to ankylosing spondylitis. Treatment in this age group is nonsurgical and as symptoms occur.

#### Adolescent Idiopathic Scoliosis
Almost one third of individuals with adolescent idiopathic scoliosis report back pain. Although classic teaching was that painful scoliosis demands a thorough diagnostic evaluation to identify a pathologic condition such as a spinal syrinx or neoplasm, fewer than 10% of these patients have an identifiable etiology of back pain. If radiographs reveal no abnormalities other than scoliosis, only those adolescents with painful left thoracic scoliosis, painful rapidly progressive curvature, or neurologic abnormalities require further testing.

#### Sickle Cell Disease
In one large series of children who presented to a pediatric emergency department with back pain, 13% were diagnosed with sickle cell crisis. Twenty-six percent of children with sickle cell crises have spinal involvement and pain. The physician must be aware that sickle cell anemia may be a cause of back pain in African American children and adolescents.

#### Visceral Etiologies
Pneumonia is an uncommon cause of thoracic back pain. Urinary tract infections, renal calculi, inflammatory bowel disease, and other intra-abdominal conditions, and pelvic etiologies such as ovarian cysts may also be associated with back pain. A careful history and physical examination are most helpful to establish these diagnoses.

#### Psychosomatic Back Pain
Conversion reactions and psychosomatic disorders may manifest as back pain in the older adolescent. These etiologies are diagnosed by exclusion of other more common spinal pathologies. A family history of chronic back pain is a risk factor. A multidisciplinary approach that includes psychological and psychiatric support for patients with these conditions is most successful in improving symptoms.

## Summary
Back pain is common in children and adolescents. A specific etiology is identified in fewer than 25% of patients. A careful history and thorough physical examination are most useful for narrowing the differential diagnosis of back pain. Constant or progressive pain, night pain, pain associated with systemic signs and symptoms, and pain with neurologic dysfunction are findings suggestive of a serious spinal condition. Plain radiography is the primary diagnostic test for evaluating the spinal column. SPECT is useful for children and adolescents with normal radiographs. CT defines bone morphology, and MRI is best for assessment of the spinal cord and nerve roots and neoplasms. Traumatic etiologies, such as soft-tissue sprains and strains and disk herniations, and developmental etiologies, such as spondylolysis/spondylolisthesis and Scheurmann's kyphosis, are most common in adolescents. Pyogenic spondylitis occurs in children. Benign and malignant neoplasms of the spine are uncommon. Unusual causes of back pain, such as inflammatory arthritis and psychosomatic pain, are identified after other common etiologies have been ruled out.

## Annotated Bibliography
### Epidemiology
Brattberg G: Do pain problems in young school children persist into early adulthood: A 13-year-follow-up. *Eur J Pain* 2004;8:187-199.
This Swedish study suggests that children with nonspecific back pain continue to have pain into adulthood.

Siambanes D, Martinez J, Butler E, Haider T: Influence of school backpacks on adolescent back pain. *J Pediatr Orthop* 2004;24:211-217.
The authors of this large American series report a high prevalence of nonspecific back pain and conclude that heavy backpacks may be a cause.

### Differential Diagnosis
Early SD, Kay RM, Tolo VT: Childhood diskitis. *J Am Acad Orthop Surg* 2003;11:413-420.
This article discusses current concepts.

Garg S, Mehta S, Dormans JP: Langerhans cell histiocytosis of the spine in children: Long-term follow-up. *J Bone Joint Surg Am* 2004;86:1740-1750.

Asymmetric collapse of vertebral bodies is more common than vertebra plana and spinal deformity rarely results from vertebral histiocytosis.

Parisini P, Di Silvestre M, Greggi T, Miglietta A, Paderni S: Lumbar disc excision in children and adolescents. *Spine* 2001;26:1997-2000.

Deterioration of outcomes of diskectomy is seen in long-term follow-up; 10% of patients require repeat intervention.

## Classic Bibliography

Balague F, Troussier B, Salimen J: Non-specific low back pain in children and adolescents: Risk factors. *Eur Spine J* 1999;8:429-438.

De Kleuver M, van der Heul RO, Veraart BE: Aneurysmal bone cyst of the spine: 31 cases and the importance of the surgical approach. *J Pediatr Orthop B* 1998;7:286-292.

Feldman DS, Hedden DM, Wright JG: The use of bone scan to investigate back pain in children and adolescents. *J Pediatr Orthop* 2000;20:790-795.

Fernandez M, Carrol CL, Baker CJ: Discitis and vertebral osteomyelitis in children: An 18-year review. *Pediatrics* 2000;105:1299-1304.

Kayser R, Mahlfeld K, Nebelung W, Grasshoff H: Vertebral collapse and normal peripheral blood cell count at the onset of acute lymphatic leukemia in childhood. *J Pediatr Orthop B* 2000;9:55-57.

Lowe TG: Scheuermann's disease. *Orthop Clin North Am* 1999;30:475-487.

Micheli L, Wood R: Back pain in young athletes: Significant differences from adults in causes and patterns. Arch Pediatr Adolesc Med 1995;149:15-18.

Papagelopoulos PJ, Currier BL, Shaughnessy WJ, et al: Aneurysmal bone cyst of the spine: Management and outcome. *Spine* 1998;23:621-628.

Ramirez N, Johnston C, Browne R: The prevalence of back pain in children who have idiopathic scoliosis. *J Bone Joint Surg Am* 1997;79:364-368.

Richards BS, McCarthy RE, Akbarnia BA: Back pain in childhood and adolescence. *Instr Course Lect* 1999;48:525-542.

Roger E, Letts M: Sickle cell disease of the spine in children. *Can J Surg* 1999;42:289-292.

Saifuddin A, White J, Sherazi Z, Shaikh MI, Natali C, Ransford AO: Osteoid osteoma and osteoblastoma of the spine: Factors associated with the presence of scoliosis. *Spine* 1998;23:47-53.

Selbst SM, Lavelle JM, Soyupak SK, Markowitz RI: Back pain in children who present to the emergency department. *Clin Pediatr (Phila)* 1999;38:401-406.

Shaikh MI, Saifuddin A, Pringle J, Natali C, Sherazi Z: Spinal osteoblastoma: CT and MR imaging with pathological correlation. *Skeletal Radiol* 1999;28:33-40.

Song K, Ogden J, Ganey T, Guidera K: Contiguous discitis and osteomyelitis in children. *J Pediatr Orthop* 1997;17:470-477.

Tribus CB: Scheuermann's kyphosis in adolescents and adults: Diagnosis and management. *J Am Acad Orthop Surg* 1998;6:36-43.

# Chapter 44

# Spondylolysis and Spondylolisthesis in Children and Adolescents

Richard E. McCarthy, MD

## Introduction

Spondylolisthesis is the forward displacement of one vertebra with reference to the one below. Derived from Greek roots spondylos (vertebra) and lysis (break of defect), spondylolysis is the antecedent to the development of anterior displacement. Spondylolysis refers to a defect in the pars interarticularis of the vertebra allowing for forward slippage. This forward translation was first described in 1782 by Herbiniaux, a Belgian obstetrician who noted its effect on the birth canal. In addition to its localized effect, spondylolysis affects the overall trunk via forward slippage. In the sagittal plane, the human posture of a standing subject can be analyzed as a combination of articulating body sections. The head is balanced on the trunk by the cervical spine, the trunk articulates on the pelvis, and the pelvis articulates with the lower limbs at the hip joints. The function of each of these sections is to maintain a stable and balanced posture with a minimal amount of energy expended. The disruption of this stable relationship is evident in patients with spondylolisthesis. Because of its position at the last mobile segment articulating with the stability of the sacrum, L5 becomes the focal point for forces from above; L5 is therefore the most commonly affected level in patients with spondylolysis and spondylolisthesis. The biomechanics of the lumbosacral joint can be enhanced by environmental influences, such as those resulting from the repetitive hyperextension maneuvers of a gymnast. In an individual who has a genetic predisposition for developing this deformity, repeated stresses on the pars interarticularis may lead to spondylolysis.

## Classification

Multiple classification systems have been used to describe spondylolisthesis. Marchetti and Bartholozzi proposed a classification system dividing this deformity into two major groups: developmental or acquired. These are further divided into subgroups that distinguish the different origins of this disorder. Developmental spondylolisthesis (type 1) has two subtypes: highly dysplastic spondylolisthesis (rounding of the sacral dome and an-

terior translation more than 50%) and low dysplastic (less than 50% translation without secondary changes in the sacrum). Each subtype can be seen with lysis of the pars interarticularis or with elongation of the pars interarticularis. This category encompasses what has been described by Wiltse as type 1 or type 2 deformity, which characteristically occur most commonly in children and adolescents. Acquired spondylolisthesis (type 2A) is traumatic in origin, either acute or stress related. Acquired spondylolisthesis (type 2B) typically occurs postoperatively and is either directly or indirectly related to surgery. Acquired spondylolisthesis (type 2C) is pathologic in etiology (either local or systemic). Acquired spondylolisthesis (type 2D) is degenerative in nature (either primary or secondary).

## Incidence

Despite the developmental nature of this disorder in children, a defect in the pars interarticularis has never been identified at birth and spondylolisthesis has not been observed in children before walking. The earliest reported instances have occurred in a few patients younger than 1 year; however, by age 5 to 7 years, the incidence is 4.4% to 5% and increases to 6% by age 18 years. The incidence of spondylolisthesis associated with spondylolysis increases during the juvenile years (age < 10 years) and has been noted to be as high as 74% by age 18 years. In a 20-year review of 255 patients with spondylolysis and spondylolisthesis, an 81% prevalence of spondylolisthesis was reported on initial examination. The prevalence of spondylolysis based on gender and race in the United States has been reported to be 6.4% in Caucasian males, 2.8% in African-American males, 2.3% in Caucasian women, and 1.1% in African-American women. It has also been noted that although pars interarticularis defects are half as common in girls as in boys, high-grade slippage is four times more common in girls. One study noted the incidence of spondylolysis to be 11% (which is four times higher than normal) in female gymnasts. The highest reported incidence of spondylolisthesis occurs in Alaskan Eskimos (26%).

Familial studies have reflected a high incidence of this deformity in first-degree relatives of children with these conditions as well as a higher incidence in relatives with spina bifida occulta of S1.

## Slippage

The Meyerding grading system is the most commonly used to describe the amount of forward translation. With this classification, slippage is defined as the percent of anterior translation of one vertebra on another adjacent vertebra. For example, with an L5-S1 spondylolisthesis, the translation is described relative to the superior surface of S1 as observed on a weight-bearing lateral radiograph of the lumbosacral junction. Grade I refers to a forward slippage of L5 of 1% to 25%; grade II refers to a forward slippage of 26% to 50%; grade III refers to a forward slippage of 51% to 75%; and grade IV refers to a forward slippage of 76% to 100%. Forward slippage greater than 100% is called spondyloptosis (grade V spondylolisthesis). Grade III or higher (forward slippage > 50%) is defined as a high-grade slip.

Growth seems to play a role in the development of spondylolisthesis, with an increase in anterior translation occurring during the adolescent growth spurt. Consequently, spondylolisthesis is observed earlier in girls because of the earlier onset of maturity. Because most individuals with lytic pars defects are asymptomatic and delay seeking medical attention, it has been noted that in most instances 90% of the slippage has already occurred by the time of the initial presentation. Additionally, most of the patients included in treatment or population reviews have a slippage of less than 30%. High-grade spondylolisthesis is rare, but it can occur during the growing years.

## Biomechanics

Compression at the L5-S1 junction is biomechanically resisted by the disk and the vertebral body. In contrast, shear forces are resisted by the disk and posterior bony elements. Because the pars interarticularis represents the bony bridge between these two regions, it can be identified as the weak link once the posterior tension band is lost either as the result of fracture or dysplastic posterior elements. This can allow the anterior vertebral column to migrate forward on the sacrum in which instance increased shear forces bear upon the disk.

With spondylolysis, trauma plays a role, especially with activities that result in repetitive hypertension forces on the pars interarticularis, such as gymnastics and football. In particular, the squatting posture of weight lifters has been noted to concentrate stress forces on the L5 pars interarticularis, which is the lowest functional mobile segment of the spine, and result in stress fractures.

As a result of these biomechanical forces coming to bear on the lumbosacral junction, predisposing defects in the morphology of the pelvis may act as precursors to the development of spondylolysis and spondylolisthesis. The pelvic incidence angle, which is a measurement of pelvic morphology that is not dependent on the position of the hips or stance, can help identify some of the underlying predisposing factors of this disorder. Because the pelvic incidence angle is not an assessment of pelvic orientation but rather morphology, it is correlated with lumbar lordosis: the larger the pelvic incidence angle, the larger the lumbar lordosis. Although the pelvic incidence angle remains constant after adolescence in normal individuals, it can be altered by pathologic conditions that modify the shape of the sacrum or the position of the acetabuli within the pelvis. A Salter iliac osteotomy, for instance, can alter the pelvic incidence angle as can developmental spondylolisthesis with rounding or doming of the sacral end plate and anterior lipping of S1 or morphologic changes associated with highly dysplastic spondylolisthesis. The doming of the sacrum is believed to be a secondary change occurring through the growth plate with adaptive changes in the upper sacrum secondary to the high-grade forward slippage of L5. If the L5-S1 disk is vertical because of the morphology of the pelvis, more shear forces are present, and progression of the slippage will be promoted with worsening of the slip angle (noted as a more vertical position to L5). It has been postulated that pelvic and sacral morphology are the most important predisposing factors for the development of spondylolisthesis. Depending on the shape and orientation of the sacral-pelvic foundation, the lumbosacral junction will experience a combination of normal and shear forces. When occurring with dysplastic changes at L5, asymmetric forces can occur at the upper S1 growth plate and subsequently produce doming of the sacrum promoting slippage. This disrupts the spinal-pelvic balance in patients with high-grade spondylolisthesis. As a result, additional lumbar lordosis cannot be achieved, and the body attempts to compensate by increasing pelvic retroversion and flexing the hips, producing the characteristic waddle gait of patients with high-grade spondylolisthesis. The entire spine remains decompensated and tilted forward. Interestingly, the effects of lordosis on spondylolisthesis have been noted in patients with Scheuermann's kyphosis, which is compensated by an equal degree of lordosis and leads to spondylolisthesis in 32% to 50% of patients.

## Symptoms

Back pain is the usual presenting symptom in patients with spondylolysis. The pattern of the pain is commonly localized to the low back region and occasionally radiates into the posterior thighs and rarely into the feet when there is a radicular component to the spondylolisthesis. Patients often report a positive family history of back pain, which is not surprising, considering the strong family history of spondylolysis. The adult incidence of spondylolysis is 5%. Clinically, the pain is most often reproduced by hyperextension maneuvers and can be reproduced in the physician's office either with double-leg hyperextension with the patient in the standing position or with single-leg hyperextension by bringing the opposite leg up to the abdomen. This maneuver recreates the hyperextension cyclic loading that often occurs in athletes who participate in gymnastics, cheerleading, or weightlifting.

The clinical presentation depends on the severity of the spondylolisthesis. With grade I or II spondylolisthesis, mild slippage is present with little or no pain and normal gait. With high-grade slippage (grade III or higher), self-restriction in activity and a characteristic crouched knee gait will often be evident, which are signs of hamstring spasm that may be accompanied by nerve root irritation. A careful neurologic examination is essential to detect signs of nerve root impingement or, more importantly, cauda equina syndrome with sacral anesthesia and bladder dysfunction. Motor weakness during physical examination is an important radicular sign that is occasionally present, particularly with involvement of the L5 nerve root. The muscles most commonly affected by this radiculopathy include the extensor hallucis longus and peroneal muscles. Tightness in the hamstrings may be so extreme that the patient may not be able to bend forward, in which instance a positive straight-leg raising test result will be elicited. In patients with high-grade slippage, palpable step-off between the spinous processes may be evident in the low back region between the anterior position of the L4 spinous process and the posteriorly placed spinous process of L5.

## Radiographic Studies
The correct identification of the etiology of low back pain in young patients is essential to treat the disorder appropriately. For instance, although radiographs may clearly show evidence of grade I spondylolisthesis, the source of the patient's leg pain on MRI may be demonstrated secondary to nerve root compression from disk protrusion. Early identification of spondylolisthesis can help halt progression of the slippage to a higher grade.

In approximately 20% of patients, the spondylolytic defect occurs in the pars interarticularis unilaterally and can be easily missed on initial presentation. Weight-bearing AP and lateral radiographs of the lumbar spine and left and right oblique radiographs obtained with the patient supine are often necessary to appropriately view these structures unobstructed by overlying osseous elements and in their functional positions. In the radio-

graphs of patients with spondylolysis, the Scottie dog sign can be observed. In some instances, the gap may be wide with rounded edges, which implies the presence of a long-standing lesion and suggests a pseudarthrosis of the pars interarticularis. In patients with more acute injuries, the gap may be narrower and have irregular edges, which implies that the lesion may be more amenable to immobilization and eventual healing without surgical intervention. Approximately one third of symptomatic patients have spondylolisthesis with no evidence of spondylolysis because of dysplasia and elongation of the pars interarticularis neck region. In younger patients (those in the first decade of life), the elongation of the neck may become attenuated.

Bone scanning can help confirm the presence of spondylolysis, especially in the early phases when the stress reaction is acute and sometimes even before the fracture occurs. Single photon emission CT is a sensitive method for confirming the diagnosis in patients with this disorder. These studies can demonstrate areas of increased bone turnover at the site of healing fractures. Bone scanning is especially helpful in identifying patients who are still in a phase of healing before the establishment of a nonunion, in which instance a period of brace immobilization would likely be beneficial. Bone scanning is not recommended for asymptomatic patients or those whose symptoms have been present for more than 1 year. Bone scanning, however, can be used to assess recovery and facilitate return to activity following a period of treatment.

## Radiographic Measurements
The radiographs required to assess the pelvic incidence angle can be obtained with the patient either standing or supine and usually include the femoral heads superimposed as much as possible onto each other. The sacral end plate must also be clearly visualized. The pelvic incidence angle is measured from the hip axis line (a line drawn from the center of the femoral heads) to the center of a line drawn across the top of the sacrum; the perpendicular at this point forms the other arm of the angle (Figure 1). For radiographs on which the femoral heads are not superimposed, the center of each femoral head is marked and a line segment will connect the centers of the femoral heads. The pelvic radius is then drawn from the center of this line to the center of the sacral end plate. The sacral end plate is defined by the line constructed between the posterior corner of the sacrum and the anterior tip of the S1 end plate at the sacral promontory. This angle represents pelvic morphology; it increases during adolescence, but once it reaches its maximum, it remains constant throughout adulthood. Meyerding classification is used to define the degree or percentage of anterior translation of L5 forward on the sacrum; greater than 50% slippage typically requires surgical intervention. The

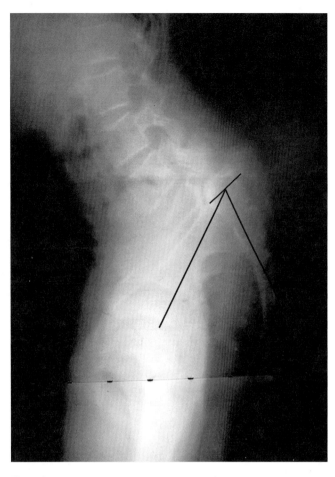

**Figure 1** Radiograph showing how the pelvic incidence reflects pelvic morphology—the larger the incidence, the larger the lumbar lordosis, leading to a greater chance of forward slippage. The angle is formed by a line drawn perpendicular to the top of S1 joined to a line drawn from the center of the femoral heads.

angle of the L5 vertebral body changes with increased percentages of forward migration. The slip angle reflects this change because it is subtended by a line across the top of L5 meeting a somewhat vertical line along the posterior margin of the sacrum. As the L5 vertebra progresses forward and angles downward, the slip angle decreases and becomes more acute (Figure 2). The ultimate forward translation occurs when L5 is anterior to S1, a condition known as spondyloptosis. This condition can be compensated or decompensated, depending on the slip angle reflecting the rotation of L5.

MRI has been used with increased frequency for identifying pars interarticularis defects and offers reduced radiation exposure to the patient. Short TI inversion recovery images can reveal changes in the pars interarticularis areas as well as edema in the adjacent pedicles. The best diagnostic modality for spondylolytic defects is CT; CT is also the best diagnostic modality for assessing bony healing after nonsurgical treatment.

## Treatment

Slippage of less than 50% in a symptomatic child typically warrants nonsurgical intervention. Use of a Boston overlap brace with physiologic lordosis built into the brace has been proposed for immobilization of young athletes. Return to participation in athletic activities is eventually allowed provided the patient avoids the particular activity that precipitated the problem. A 24-hours a day/7 days a week immobilization schedule that allows the patient out of the brace only for bathing seems to offer the best outcome, with 35% of patients experiencing healing of the pars interarticularis defect

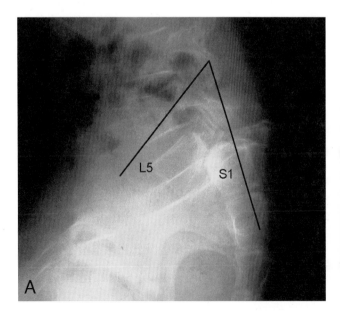

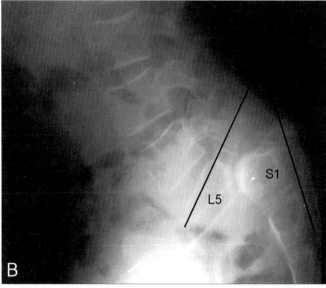

**Figure 2** Radiographs showing how the slip angle reflects the forward rotation of L5 as it falls off the top of S1. A line is drawn vertically along the posterior edge of the sacrum and across the top of L5. The angle of intersection is the slip angle. As the spondylolisthesis increases, the slip angle decreases. **A,** Weight-bearing lateral radiograph of a 14-year-old boy with a slip angle of 60°. **B,** Weight-bearing lateral radiograph of the same patient 3 months later showing progression of spondylolisthesis and decrease of the slip angle to 50°.

noted on follow-up studies 6 months after initiation of the treatment. Another study reported a high success rate using a brace, whereas others have not supported this treatment modality. The brace may be worn for relapses. Once brace immobilization is concluded, a series of exercises emphasizing trunk stabilization and hamstring stretching is instituted. This course of therapy has been reported to be successful in the relief of pain in most patients with low-grade slippages, whereas those with higher grades of spondylolisthesis have been shown to be less responsive to bracing.

## Direct Repair of Spondylolysis

Direct repair of the pars interarticularis defect has been proposed. The indications for direct surgical repair include a 6-month history of activity-limiting low back pain that has been unresponsive to nonsurgical measures, a minimal amount of spondylolisthesis (< 2-mm gap), and absence of transitional pathology. Disks and facets must be normal on MRI. Some studies have advocated using pars interarticularis injections to test for the origin of pain in the pars interarticularis area. The goal of direct treatment is to preserve motion segments. The initial results of grafting of the pars defect without instrumentation have been mixed. Other techniques using surgical implants have been attempted, including translaminar screws and transverse process wiring; more recently, however, the combination of a pedicle screw and a wire or a laminar hook has been advocated. These techniques involve removal of the fibrous nonunion in the pars interarticularis area, with insertion of autogenous bone graft and compression across the pars interarticularis area. This treatment is followed by a period of immobilization to promote healing in the pars interarticularis. A small number of published studies have reported generally good results in a selectively chosen patient population. The pars interarticularis repair procedure has been recommended by some to treat lesions at L4 or above to avoid a floating fusion of lumbar segments.

## Fusion

In adolescent and adult patients with spondylolysis and less than 50% of slippage, the recommended treatment has been intertransverse posterolateral fusion with or without instrumentation. The single-incision bilateral direct approach of Wiltse has been most commonly used in younger patients for a bilateral intertransverse fusion, with autogenous bone graft harvested through the same incision. In older patients, pedicle instrumentation has been recommended. In adult patients with wide disk spaces, the use of posterior lumbar interbody fusion or transforaminal lumbar interbody fusion bone grafts has been recommended to increase the incidence of successful fusion by providing anterior bony column support.

The treatment of patients with high-grade spondylolysis is somewhat controversial and is best accomplished by highly experienced surgeons. The difference between a well-balanced and an unbalanced high-grade spondylolisthesis is an important distinction. The well-balanced high-grade spondylolisthesis is associated with a good adaptation of the lumbar lordosis and a well-balanced sagittal contour overall. The treatment of high-grade L5 spondylolisthesis in this context may simply involve an in situ fusion coupled with a fibular strut graft and possibly supplemented with posterior interbody screws. An unbalanced high-grade spondylolisthesis requires a reduction maneuver. When the spinal pelvic balance is compromised by the extreme tilt of L5 with a high slippage angle, this leads to an exaggerated lordotic response in the lumbar spine. The goal of reduction in this situation is to decrease the slippage and, more importantly, the tilt of L5. This reduction can be achieved by placing pedicle screws into L4, the gradual posterior approximation of L4 toward a rod fixed to the sacrum, introduction of screws into the L5 vertebral body, and gradual realignment of L5 with or without an interbody fusion at L5-S1. This procedure produces a lengthening of the trunk and correction of the deformity that has been reported to lead to an L5 radiculopathy in approximately 20% of patients. Most often the foot drop will be transient, but the presence of this complication emphasizes the need for a careful decompression of the roots bilaterally and reduction under direct vision. In addition, loss of reduction, pseudarthrosis, and implant failure have also been reported with this procedure. One study recommended the use of an L5 excision for patients with spondyloptosis in a staged anterior-posterior procedure. This procedure places L4 onto the dome of the sacrum, where it is fused and undergoes instrumentation. Decompression of the L5 nerve root is an essential part of any of these procedures to minimize neurologic defects.

## Summary

Spondylolysis is characterized by a defect in the pars interarticularis that is most often seen in the lower lumbar spine. This condition can lead to forward slippage of one vertebral body onto the subjacent one (spondylolisthesis). Spondylolysis occurs in approximately 5% of the population. Spondylolisthesis has both developmental and acquired types and occurs as a consequence of the forward curvature of the lumbar segments coupled with the disassociation between the posterior elements and the vertebral body because of the pars defect. The slippage can be severe and can be graded radiographically. Treatment can be nonsurgical, with bracing and exercises, or surgical, with fusion either of posterolateral elements or the anterior and posterior columns, depending on the severity of the slippage.

## Annotated Bibliography
### Classification

Hammerberg KW: New concepts on the pathogenesis and classification of spondylolisthesis. *Spine* 2005;30:S4-S11.

The author reviews the literature pertaining to pathogenesis and classification of spondylolisthesis, reviewing the morphology and biomechanics of the lumbosacral junction. The Marchetti-Bartolozzi classification system is found to be applicable to all forms of spondylolisthesis and clinically relevant.

Herman MJ, Pizzutillo PD: Spondylolysis and spondylolisthesis in the child and adolescent: A new classification. *Clin Orthop Relat Res* 2005;434:46-54.

The authors present a classification system based on clinical presentation and spinal morphology designed specifically for the child and adolescent. Algorithms for evaluation and treatment based on this classification are also presented.

Timon SJ, Gardner JM, Wanich T, Poynton A, et al: Not all spondylolisthesis grading instruments are reliable. *Clin Orthop Relat Res* 2005;434:157-162.

Eight radiographic measurement instruments described to predict progression and need for intervention in spondylolisthesis were evaluated by four raters. Of the eight, three measurements (Meyerding's grade, slip percent, and sacral inclination) had excellent interobserver and intraobserver agreement.

### Incidence

Logroscion G, Mazza O, Aulisa G, et al: Spondylolysis and spondylolisthesis in the pediatric and adolescent population. *Childs Nerv Syst* 2001;17:644-655.

A review of spondylolysis and spondylolisthesis including incidence, etiologies, pathogenesis, and diagnostic and therapeutic approaches is presented.

### Slippage

Beutler WJ, Fredrickson BE, Murtland A, et al: The natural history of spondylolysis and spondylolisthesis: A 45-year follow-up evaluation. *Spine* 2003;28:1027-1035.

A prospective study of 500 first-grade children followed to document the natural history of spondylolysis and spondylolisthesis is presented.

Jackson RP, Phipps T, Hales C, Surber J: Pelvic lordosis and alignment in spondylolisthesis. *Spine* 2003;28:151-160.

Pelvic morphology and lumbopelvic lordosis were measured on standing radiographs of 75 patients with greater than 10% L5-S1 spondylolytic spondylolisthesis and compared with 75 volunteers. Radiographic angles for pelvic morphology were measured by two observers. There were differences between the two groups, suggesting that pelvic morphology may play a role in the development of spondylolisthesis.

Sairyo K, Katoh S, Ikata T, et al: Development of spondylolytic olisthesis in adolescents. *Spine J* 2001;3:171-175.

The authors retrospectively studied 46 athletes in an attempt to clarify when slippage in pediatric spondylolyis starts and stops. Their conclusion was that slippage was more common with skeletal immaturity and halted when growth was completed.

Whitesides TE Jr, Horton WC, Hutton WC, Hodges L: Spondylolitic spondylolisthesis: A study of pelvic and lumbosacral parameters of possible etiologic effect in two genetically and geographically distinct groups with high occurrence. *Spine* 2005;30:S12-S21.

The authors performed an anatomic and radiographic study of archaeological skeletal remains from two genetically and geographically distinct groups with high occurrence rates of spondylolytic spondylolisthesis.

### Biomechanics

DeWald RE: Classification, epidemiology, and natural history, in *Spondylolysis and Spondylolisthesis: A Review of Current Trends and Controversies*. Milwaukee, WI, Scoliosis Research Society, 2003.

This article presents a discussion of the classification, epidemiology, and natural history of spondylolysis and spondylolisthesis with reference to the Marchetti and Bartolozzi classification system and with emphasis on the importance of understanding the pelvic morphology, pelvic incidence, and forces on the disk.

Sairyo K, Katoh S, Sasa T, et al: Athletes with unilateral spondylolysis are at risk of stress fracture at the contralateral pedicle and pars interarticularis: A clinical and biomechanical study. *Am J Sports Med* 2005;33:583-590.

Patients with unilateral spondylolysis were studied to determine the effect on the contralateral side with the conclusion that there was risk of stress fracture on the contralateral side because of increased stress in that region.

Sakamaki T, Katoh S, Sairyo K: Normal and spondylolytic pediatric spine movements with reference to instantaneous axis of rotation. *Spine* 2002;27:141-145.

To clarify the kinematic alteration in the pediatric spine with pars defects, a radiologic study measuring the location of the instantaneous axis of rotation was done by the authors. They concluded that the axis of rotation deviated cranially as the stage of pars defect advanced and as the wedge deformity increased.

### Radiographic Studies

Campbell RS, Grainger AJ, Hide IG, et al: Juvenile spondylolysis: A comparative analysis of CT, Single photon emission computed tomography, and MRI. *Skeletal Radiol* 2005;34:63-73.

The authors evaluate, compare, and correlate CT, Single photon emission computed tomography, and MRI for the diagnosis of juvenile spondylolysis, concluding that MRI can be used as an effective and reliable first-line imaging modality. Localized CT is recommended as a supplementary examination for assessment of healing and evaluation of indeterminate cases.

Hollenberg GM, Beattie PF, Meyers SP, Weinberg EP, Adams MJ: Stress reactions of the lumbar pars interarticularis: The development of a new MRI classification system. *Spine* 2002;27:181-186.

The authors of this retrospective study assessed the MRI scans of 55 young athletic patients with low back pain. The MRI scans were given one of five grades based on the bone stress reactivity of the pars interarticularis. High-field strength MRI using fat saturation techniques and dedicated coil technology was used. The authors reported that both intraobserver and interobserver reliability coefficients were high.

Van der Wall H, Storey G, Magnussen J, et al: Distinguishing scintigraphic features of spondylolysis. *J Pediatr Orthop* 2002;22:308-311.

A unique pattern of uptake is described in spondylolysis not found in other causes of back pain.

## Radiographic Measurements

Berthonnaud E, Dimnet J, Labelle H, Kuklo T, O'Brien M, Roussouly P: Spondylolisthesis, in O'Brien M, Kuklo T, Blanke K, Lenke L (eds): *Radiographic Measurement Manual*. Memphis, TN, Medtronic Sofamor Danek, 2004, pp 95-108.

This chapter on spondylolisthesis illustrates many of the methods of measuring spondylolisthesis with diagrams and correlated with radiographic studies.

Huang RP, Bohlman HH, Thompson GH, Peo-Kochert C: Predictive value of pelvic incidence in progression of spondylolisthesis. *Spine* 2003;28:2381-2385.

The authors performed a retrospective analysis of pelvic incidence and other radiographic parameters to evaluate their value as predictors of progression of isthmic spondylolisthesis. Their conclusions were that pelvic incidence did not adequately predict progression but that slip percentage and high-grade spondylolisthesis were the most positive predictors of progression.

Labelle H, Roussouly P, Berthounnaud E, et al: Spondylolisthesis, pelvic incidence, and spinopelvic balance: A correlation study. *Spine* 2004;29:2049-2054.

A retrospective study was performed to investigate the role of pelvic anatomy and its effect on the global balance of the trunk in developmental spondylolisthesis. The authors concluded that pelvic anatomy has a direct influence on both the development and progression of developmental spondylolisthesis.

## Treatment

Debnath UK, Freeman BJ, Gregory P, et al: Clinical outcome and return to sport after the surgical treatment of spondylolysis in young athletes. *J Bone Joint Surg Br* 2003;85:244-249.

Twenty-two athletes who had undergone surgical treatment were studied prospectively. After rehabilitation, 82% were able to return to their previous sports activity.

D'Hemecourt PA, Zurakowski D, Kriemler S, Micheli LJ: Spondylolysis: Returning the athlete to sports participation with brace treatment. *Orthopedics* 2002;25:653-657.

The results of treatment of 73 adolescent athletes with a brace are discussed. Eighty percent achieved a favorable clinical outcome, with those participating in low-risk sports activity being more likely to have favorable results.

Fujii K, Katoh S, Sairyo K, Ikata T, Yasui N: Union of defects in the pars interarticularis of the lumbar spine in children and adolescents: The radiological outcome after conservative treatment. *J Bone Joint Surg Br* 2004;86:225-231.

The authors attempt to retrospectively identify factors that affect healing of the pars interarticularis in conservative treatment.

## Direct Repair of Spondylolysis

Aksar Z, Wardlaw D, Koti M: Scott wiring for direct repair of lumbar spondylolysis. *Spine* 2003;28:354-357.

A retrospective study was done to assess the clinical outcome of the Scott wiring technique after a mean follow-up period of more than 10 years. The result was good or excellent in 86% or patients, all of whom were younger than 25 years at the time of surgery.

Ivanic GM, Pink TP, Achatz W, et al: Direct stabilization of lumbar spondylolysis with a hook screw: 11-year follow-up period for 113 patients. *Spine* 2003;28:255-259.

A retrospective study of 113 patients who underwent direct repair with a hook screw was conducted. The conclusion was that this procedure is best for a select group of patients and can save a functional segment.

Lundin DA, Wiseman D, Ellengoben RG, Shaffrey CI: Direct repair of the pars interarticularis for spondylolysis and spondylolisthesis. *Pediatr Neurosurg* 2003;39:195-200.

The authors discuss their experience with five patients managed by direct repair after failure of nonsurgical treatment.

## Fusion

Bartolozzi P, Sandri A, Cassini M, Ricci M: One-stage posterior decompression-stabilization and trans-sacral interbody fusion after partial reduction for severe L5-S1 spondylolisthesis. *Spine* 2003;28:1135-1141.

A retrospective study of 15 patients who were treated with the stabilization and fusion procedure was done. The procedure was determined to be a safe and effective technique for managing severe spondylolisthesis.

Helenius I, Lambert T, Osterman K: Posterolateral, anterior, or circumferential fusion in situ for high-grade spondylolisthesis in young patients: A long-term evaluation using the Scoliosis Research Society questionnaire. *Spine* 2006;31:190-196.

The authors carried out a retrospective, comparative study looking at clinical and radiographic outcomes of posterolateral, anterior, and circumferential fusion in situ for high-grade spondylolisthesis in adolescents. Their conclusion was that circumferential fusion provided better clinical and radiographic results and a better total score on the Scoliosis Research Society questionnaire than posterolateral or anterior fusion.

Lamberg TS, Remes VM, Helenius IJ, et al: Long-term clinical, functional, and radiological outcome 21 years after posterior or posterolateral fusion in childhood and adolescent isthmic spondylolisthesis. *Eur Spine J* 2005; 14:639-644.

The authors reviewed 129 patients radiologically and functionally (spinal mobility, trunk strength measurements, Oswestry disability index scores). All patients had undergone either a posterior or posterolateral fusion. Spinal mobility and trunk strength were compared with that of a reference population. Although the overall long-term clinical outcome was good, the clinical and radiologic outcomes did not appear to correlate with each other.

## Classic Bibliography

Gaines R, Nichols W: Treatment of spondyloptosis by two stage L5 vertebrectomy and reduction of L4 onto S1. *Spine* 1985;10:680-686.

Hensinger RN: Acute back pain in children. *Instr Course Lect* 1995;44:111-126.

Jackson DW: Low back pain in young athletes: Evaluation of stress reaction and discogenic problems. *Am J Sports Med* 1979;7:364-366.

Kakiuchi M: Repair of the defect in spondylolysis: Durable fixation with pedicle screws and laminar hooks. *J Bone Joint Surg Am* 1997;79:818-825.

Lonstein JE: Spondylolisthesis in children: Cause, natural history, and management. *Spine* 1999;24:2640-2648.

Marchetti PC, Bartolozzi P: Classification of spondylolisthesis as a guideline for treatment, in Bridwell KH, DeWald RL, Hammerberg KW, et al (eds): *The Textbook of Spinal Surgery*, ed 2. Philadelphia, PA, Lippincott-Raven, 1997, pp 1211-1254.

Meyerding H: Low backache and sciatic pain associated with spondylolisthesis and protruded disc: Incidence, significance, and treatment. *J Bone Joint Surg* 1947;23:461-470.

Salib RM, Pettine KA: Modified repair of a defect in spondylolysis or minimal spondylolisthesis by pedicle screw, segmental wire fixation, and bone grafting. *Spine* 1993;18:440-443.

Smith JA, Hu SS: Management of spondylolysis and spondylolisthesis in the pediatric and adolescent population. *Orthop Clin North Am* 1999;30:487-499.

Steiner M, Micheli L: Treatment of symptomatic spondylolysis and spondylolisthesis with the modified Boston brace. *Spine* 1985;10:937-943.

Wiltse LL: Spondylolisthesis: Classification and etiology, in *Symposium on the Spine*. Rosemont, IL, American Academy of Orthopaedic Surgeons, 1969, pp 143-166.

# Chapter 45

# Congenital Scoliosis

John P. Dormans, MD

Leslie Moroz

## Introduction

Anomalies in the formation and segmentation of vertebrae and ribs can lead to asymmetric growth of the spine and progressive deformity. Although some deformities have little effect on patients and do not require treatment, the natural history of the anomaly should be considered and carefully monitored for signs of progression with the goal of maintaining spinal balance and stability throughout growth. Surgical intervention is sometimes indicated to prevent curve progression or to reestablish alignment and balance in patients with established deformities.

Estimates of the incidence of congenital scoliosis in the general population range from 1% to 4%. Interestingly, a higher incidence of idiopathic scoliosis has been reported in families of children with congenital scoliosis. In a study of 237 children with congenital scoliosis, a 3.4% rate (8 of 237) of familial congenital scoliosis and a 20.7% rate (41 of 237) of familial idiopathic scoliosis were reported. These observations have led investigators to explore the role of genetic defects as a predisposing factor for spinal deformities.

One condition involving congenital vertebral defects for which the genetic etiology is known is spondylocostal dysostosis. Spondylocostal dysostosis is the association of vertebral anomalies with rib or sternal abnormalities (sometimes also associated with diastematomyelia, meningocoele, or underlying cardiovascular abnormalities) that has been mapped to chromosome 19q13.1-q13.3. Sequencing and analysis of the gene encoding the notch ligand delta-like 3 (DLL3) in families with spondylocostal dysostosis has provided evidence of the importance of the notch signaling pathway and its components in patterning the mammalian axial skeleton. A recent study on mice with an induced mutation of the notch ligand *DLL3* gene has shown that the mutation has different effects on the expression of cycling and stage-specific genes involved in somite formation. These findings suggest that the deformities seen in human spondylocostal dysostosis may arise from unique and specific disruptions of genes expressed during somatogenesis, the process by which the axial skeleton is formed during embryogenesis.

Although the genetic and developmental etiology of most congenital spine deformities remains largely unknown, progress is being made. There is evidence that congenital vertebral anomalies arise from disruptions in somatogenesis. Defects can arise from the disruption of genes involved in development, environmental insults during gestation, or a combination of both factors. A radiographic analysis of vertebral anomalies reported that 70% of patients with vertebral anomalies (57 of 81) had multiple adjacent vertebral defects. The authors suggested that this pattern is consistent with the continuous process of somite formation such that multiple, contiguous vertebral defects would be distributed along the craniocaudal axis of the spine. In this same series, 54% of the patients with nonsyndromatic congenital vertebral defects (13 of 24) also had rib malformations, which was consistent with the developmental progression of both ribs and vertebrae from somites. Neurologic and vertebral anomalies associated with congenital scoliosis may share a common etiology or could be secondary to disruptions in somatogenesis.

## History and Physical Examination

Most children with congenital scoliosis present at an early age. Some mild deformities in young children are noted by parents or pediatricians, and many anomalies are found incidentally on radiographs. A careful history should be taken, with particular attention given to a family history of spine deformities, spina bifida, dysraphic problems, and maternal exposure to teratogens. Assessment should include evaluation of spine and shoulder symmetry; rib or lumbar prominences; head tilt; cervical, thoracic, and lumbar range of motion and flexibility; pelvic tilt; limb-length differences; and calf and thigh circumference differences.

Congenital anomalies are frequently associated with other organ system disorders. In a recent series of 110 children with congenital scoliosis, it was reported that 55 (50%) had associated organ defects (Table 1). In this se-

**Table 1 | Summary of the Incidence of Organ Defects by Type of Vertebral Anomaly for a Series of Patients With Congenital Scoliosis**

| | Number of Patients (%) With Organ Defects (N = 110) |
|---|---|
| Failure of formation | 30 (47%) |
| Failure of segmentation | 3 (37%) |
| Mixed defects | 22 (73%) |

*(Adapted with permission from Basu PS, Elsebaie H, Noordeen MH: Congenital spinal deformity. Spine 2002;27:2255-2259.)*

**Table 2 | Congenital Segmental Vertebral Syndromes**

Spondylocostal dysostosis types 1 and 2 (Jarcho-Levin syndrome)

Alagille syndrome

Vertebral agenesis/caudal regression/limb-body wall defect/axial mesoderm

Dysplasia

Klippel-Feil syndrome

Facioauriculovertebral spectrum (Goldenhar's and Wildervanck syndromes)

Vertebral anomalies, anorectal anomalies, tracheoesophageal fistula, and renal and vascular anomalies (VATER syndrome)

Vertebral anomalies, anorectal anomalies, tracheoesophageal fistula, renal and vascular anomalies, and cardiac and limb defects (VACTERL syndrome)

Mullerian, renal, cervicothoracic, and somite abnormalities (MURCS association)

ries, the incidence of congenital heart disease (particularly atrial and ventricle septal defects and patent ductus arteriosus) was 18% among patients with failure of formation, 10% among those with failure of segmentation, and 37% among those with mixed defects. Estimates of the frequency of genitourinary anomalies (most often renal hypoplasia, horseshoe kidney, and single kidney) range from 21% to 34% of patients with congenital vertebral anomalies. Although symptoms of other system involvement are not always present in patients who present with spine deformity, the high incidence of associated disorders warrants a thorough examination to detect other anomalies. Patients undergoing surgery for congenital scoliosis should have a screening renal ultrasound and cardiac evaluation and/or echocardiogram.

Careful neurologic examination is also indicated in infants and children with congenital scoliosis. Neurologic deficits may be associated with vertebral anomalies or secondary to the spine deformity. Current estimates indicate that between 20% and 40% of patients with congenital spine deformities also have a congenital anomaly of the neural axis. Signs of associated intraspinal anomalies are sometimes apparent on physical examination. The presence of hair patches, dimples, nevi, tumors, and absent or asymmetric abdominal reflexes may be indicative of spinal dysraphism.

Although anomalies of other systems can occur independently in patients with congenital scoliosis, they are also often seen together as part of a syndrome. Abnormalities noted in one system indicate the need to evaluate others. Recent studies indicate that between 38% and 55% of patients with vertebral anomalies have a constellation of defects that comprise a syndrome. The presence of vertebral anomalies, anorectal anomalies, tracheoesophageal fistula, and renal and vascular anomalies (the VATER syndrome) and Goldenhar's syndrome are most frequent among infants and children with congenital scoliosis. (The presence of vertebral anomalies, anorectal anomalies, tracheoesophageal fistula, and renal and vascular anomalies together with

cardiac and limb defects are known as the VACTERL syndrome.) The spectrum of oculoauriculovertebral defects that comprise Goldenhar's syndrome include partially formed or completely absent ears, eye growths or an absent eye, and an asymmetric mouth or chin, usually affecting one side of the face only (hemifacial microsomia). Children with Goldenhar's syndrome may have hearing loss, weakness in the smaller side of the face, a shift in the soft palate to the unaffected side of the face, or a tongue that is smaller on the affected side of the face. A more complete overview of the syndromes for which scoliosis associated with congenital vertebral anomalies has been reported is provided in Table 2.

Careful evaluation of pulmonary function is important in this patient population. Thoracic insufficiency syndrome is defined as the inability of the thorax to support normal respiration or lung growth. Patients with thoracic insufficiency syndrome comprise a small subset of patients with congenital anomalies of vertebrae and ribs, although the exact incidence is unknown. Thoracic volume in these patients is restricted by the physical limitations of the thorax. The rib anomalies include congenital rib fusions or, less commonly, the absence of ribs. Both of these anomalies contribute to a reduction of thoracic size, motion, and compliance, leading to impaired respiratory function. Patients usually present with a history of respiratory symptoms (such as fatigability, frequent respiratory infection, increased respiratory rate, or the need for supplemental oxygen). Thoracic hypoplasia can be evaluated by measuring the circumference of the chest. Loss of chest wall mobility is determined by the thumb excursion test, a measure of the expansion of the chest during a deep breath (Figure 1). Pulmonary function testing can quantify the amount of lung volume in infants and children with rib anomalies. Thoracic insufficiency is diagnosed based on de-

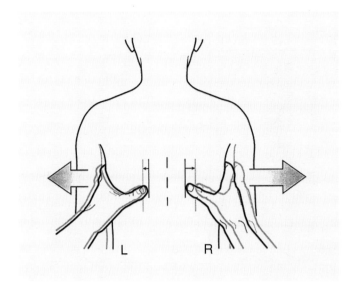

Figure 1 Schematic illustration of how the thumb excursion test can be used to determine the degree of unilateral loss of secondary breathing. The examiner encircles the base of the chest with fingers anterior to the anterior axillary line and thumbs equidistant from the spine. Motion of the thumbs away from the spine upon inhalation is an indication of the secondary breathing mechanism. *(Reproduced with permission from Campbell R, Smith M, Mayes T, et al: The characteristics of thoracic insufficiency syndrome associated with fused ribs and congenital scoliosis. J Bone Joint Surg Am 2003;85A(3):399-408.)*

creased vital capacity noted on pulmonary function tests and the restriction of space available for the lung as seen on diagnostic imaging studies. The condition may be progressive, and patients suspected of having decreased thoracic volume should be closely monitored.

## Diagnostic Imaging

Plain PA radiographs that include the lateral margins of the thoracic cage and lateral radiographs that show the entire spine from the head to the pelvis are essential for evaluating vertebral anomalies and Cobb angle in patients with congenital scoliosis. There is variation in the reproducibility of angle measurement on radiographs. Recent analyses of Cobb angle measurements made on radiographs of children with congenital scoliosis indicate that intraobserver variability ranges 3° to 10°. In patients with severe congenital scoliosis and fused or absent ribs, the evolution of three-dimensional deformity can be monitored with plain radiographs: an increasing Cobb angle usually corresponds to decreasing height of the hemithorax. The relationship between the center of the body and the outside of the rib cage is indicative of trunk shift. Lateral radiographs are also useful for evaluating sagittal plane deformity, the lumbosacral junction, and ruling out spondylolysis/ spondylolisthesis as the underlying cause of the curve. Anomalies in the posterior elements of the spine may also be present, but are difficult to evaluate on plain radiographs. Bending films (active, passive, fulcrum, or traction) are essential for evaluating the flexibility of

the curve and assessing each potential motion segment. The Stagnara view is obtained perpendicular to the rib prominence and is useful for making measurements of large curves with severe rotational components.

When evaluating patients with proved or suspected congenital scoliosis, the first step is to characterize bony abnormalities with high-quality radiographs. It is important to carefully evaluate the vertebrae and disk spaces and define the exact type and natural history of the given anomaly. Congenital vertebral anomalies have been classified as defects of formation and defects of segmentation (Figure 2). Incomplete failure of formation results in a wedge vertebra in which height asymmetry is noted, but both pedicles are present. Failure of formation leading to hemivertebra results in one of three types of abnormality: a fully segmented vertebra with growth cartilage and disk spaces above and below, a partially segmented vertebra with the hemivertebra partially fused to one adjacent vertebra and separated by growth cartilage and a disk space between the other adjacent vertebra, or an unsegmented hemivertebra that is partially fused to both adjacent vertebra. A butterfly vertebra is characterized by a central defect in the vertebral body that results in two hemivertebrae at the same level. Hemimetameric segmental displacement or shift is a multilevel pattern of vertebral anomalies characterized by two contralateral hemivertebrae separated by at least one normal vertebra. This pattern of vertebral anomalies has been reported to occur in 5% to 15% of patients with congenital scoliosis. Contralateral hemivertebrae, either at different levels or the same level, can result in a relatively balanced spine and favorable natural history depending on the location of the deformity.

Examples of failures of segmentation include bilateral or unilateral unsegmented fibrous or bony bars between adjacent vertebrae. Bilateral failure of segmentation results in a block vertebra. Unilateral defects in segmentation result in a unilateral fusion bar on the concave side of the curve. This occurs occasionally opposite a hemivertebra and results in particularly aggressive progression. The risk associated with each of these types of vertebral anomalies is asymmetric growth and progressive deformity.

Primary thoracic deformity may also result from anomalies of the ribs (fusion or absence of ribs). Thoracic deformity resulting from unilateral unsegmented vertebral bar and congenitally fused ribs can be classified as unilateral failure of thoracic segmentation with an unsegmented vertebral bar or as a unilateral failure of thoracic formation with hemivertebrae and absent ribs (Figure 3). The tethering effect exerted on the spine from rib anomalies can produce a secondary deformity of the rib cage. In patients with severe primary thoracic deformities, a windswept thorax results from the combination of severe lordosis and rotation.

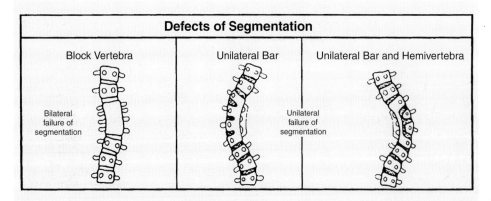

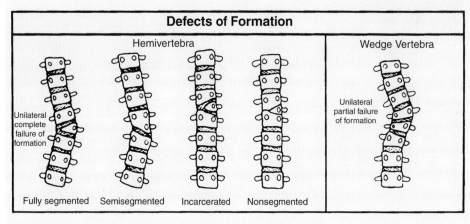

Figure 2 Classification of congenital vertebral anomalies. Defects of segmentation include block vertebra, unilateral bar, and unilateral bar with contralateral hemivertebra. Defects of formation include unilateral complete or partial failures of formation. *(Reproduced with permission from McMaster MJ: Congenital scoliosis, in Weinstein SL (ed): The Pediatric Spine: Principles and Practices. New York, NY, Raven Press, 1994, pp 227-244.)*

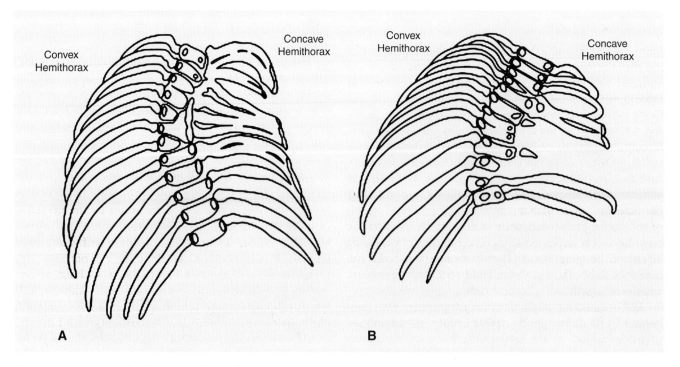

Figure 3 Schematic illustration of the unilateral failure of thoracic segmentation **(A)** and thoracic formation **(B)**. *(Reproduced with permission from Campbell R, Smith M, Mayes T, et al: The characteristics of thoracic insufficiency syndrome associated with fused ribs and congenital scoliosis. J Bone Joint Surg Am 2003;85A(3):399-408.)*

| Site of Curvature | Type of Congenital Anomaly | | | | | |
|---|---|---|---|---|---|---|
| | Block Vertebra | Wedged Vertebra | Hemivertebra | | Unilateral Unsegmented Bar | Unilateral Unsegmented Bar and Contralateral Hemivertebrae |
| | | | Single | Double | | |
| Upper thoracic | <1° – 1° | * – 2° | 1° – 2° | 2° – 2.5° | 2° – 4° | 5° – 6° |
| Lower thoracic | <1° – 1° | 2° – 2° | 2° – 2.5° | 2° – 3° | 5° – 6.5° | 6° – 7° |
| Thoracolumbar | <1° – 1° | 1.5° – 2° | 2° – 3.5° | 5° – * | 6° – 9° | >10° – * |
| Lumbar | <1° – * | <1° – * | <1° – 1° | * | >5° – * | * |
| Lumbosacral | * | * | <1° – 1.5° | * | * | * |

No treatment required    May require spinal fusion    Require special fusion

\* Too few or no curves

Figure 4   Summarization of the natural history of deterioration for congenital curves by type of vertebral anomaly and curve location for a series of 251 patients. Median yearly deterioration is given for children younger than 10 years on the left and for children 10 years and older on the right of each cell in the table. *(Reproduced with permission from McMaster MJ, Ohtsuka K: The natural history of congenital scoliosis: A study of two hundred and fifty-one patients. J Bone Joint Surg Am 1982;64(8):1128-1147.)*

Advanced CT can help determine the full extent of vertebral anomalies, particularly in young children whose vertebrae are still largely cartilaginous, and is an essential part of preoperative planning. In a series of 31 patients, assessment of plain radiographs and three-dimensional CT scans revealed that additional abnormalities were detected in more than 50% of the patients when advanced CT images were examined. Another study compared preoperative three-dimensional CT reconstructions with intraoperative findings and reported that anterior and posterior anomalies corresponded in each of the 15 patients assessed. For patients with thoracic deformity, changes in the width and depth of the rib cage can be appreciated using CT scans. The milliampere-second settings for CT should be decreased to an appropriate level for children to decrease exposure to effective radiation. The results of recent studies suggest that the lifetime radiation risk of children may be increased, even with a single axial CT study, because of the young age of the patients at the time of exposure and also organ radiosensitivity. The benefits of obtaining advanced imaging usually far outweigh the risks, but care should be taken to minimize the radiation exposure whenever possible.

MRI should be performed for all patients with congenital spine deformity to detect intraspinal anomalies. Diastematomyelia, tethered cord, low conus, syringomyelia, and intradural lipoma occur most often. Diastematomyelia in particular has been noted to occur more often in patients with scoliosis because of an unsegmented bar with a contralateral hemivertebra. A recent advance

in diagnostic imaging technology with potential applications in the evaluation of congenital spine deformities is the use of periodically rotated overlapping parallel lines with enhanced reconstruction MRI. This technology uses multiple shots to disperse motion artifacts and has the potential to eliminate the need for using general anesthesia.

## Nonsurgical Management

The risk associated with vertebral malformations is asymmetric spine growth. The natural history of congenital scoliosis depends on the type and location of the vertebral anomalies. The presence of fused ribs or a unilateral unsegmented bony bar on one side of the vertebra can exert compression forces and produce tension forces on the other side, creating a tethering effect. Longitudinal growth may be inhibited on one side, for example, by the absence of growth cartilage in an unsegmented bar and promoted on the other by the presence of extra growth cartilage associated with a hemivertebra. In a classic series of 251 patients with congenital scoliosis, it was reported that the curves of patients with a unilateral unsegmented bar (with or without a contralateral hemivertebra) progressed most rapidly, followed by patients with a hemivertebra, wedge vertebra, and block vertebra (Figure 4). In patients with bilateral failure of segmentation (block vertebra), butterfly vertebrae, and hemimetameric shifts, the spine usually remains balanced.

The natural history of the global deformity of the thorax associated with thoracic insufficiency syndrome is uncertain. In a report of experience with more than 500 children with severe spine and rib deformities, it was proposed that the concave hemithorax acts as a lateral tether, promoting the unbalanced growth of the spine already underway because of vertebral deformities. In a series of 16 patients, it was reported that patients with fused ribs tended to have a higher curve progression index for each of the five types of congenital spinal deformities, except unilateral bar with contralateral hemivertebra. Progression of thoracic deformity can correspond to progression of thoracic insufficiency, resulting in apparent or occult severe restrictive lung disease and ventilator dependency early in life or once compensatory mechanisms are no longer sustainable.

According to the results of a study reporting Pediatric Outcomes Data Collection Instrument scores, patients with congenital scoliosis differed from children without orthopaedic conditions with respect to their activity performance, comfort, and possibly self-image. Responses from 26 patients with congenital scoliosis to questions about upper extremity function, transfers and mobility, sports and physical function, comfort/pain, and global function (an average of the previous scores) yielded scores that were significantly lower than those in the patient group without spine deformity. The scores of the patients with congenital scoliosis were similar to those of patients with idiopathic scoliosis.

The most appropriate treatment is determined by the natural history of the particular type or types of anomalies present, an assessment of the potential for asymmetric growth, and the extent of loss of spine balance. Children with mild congenital scoliosis with a favorable natural history may not require treatment, but children with vertebral anomalies that are prone to progression should be closely monitored with radiographs until they are skeletally mature. Likewise, surgical correction may not be indicated for patients with mild thoracic insufficiency syndrome, but pulmonary function testing should be performed along with diagnostic imaging studies to quantify existing thoracic insufficiency and detect progression. The frequency of radiographic assessment should correspond to suspicion of progression (natural history) based on the type and location of the deformity and patient age.

The potential for growth in a particular region can be estimated by assessing the growth cartilage on either side of an abnormal vertebra. Curves progress more quickly during times of rapid growth, particularly between 2 and 3 years of age and during adolescence. An increased rate of deterioration after age 10 years that is consistent with earlier findings has been reported. Radiographic measurement of the deformity every 4 to 6 months during these critical periods enables surgeons to detect the rate of progression and plan appropriate surgical intervention if necessary.

Because curves produced by congenital anomalies progress as a result of asymmetric vertebral growth and are generally less flexible than idiopathic curves, bracing is rarely used to manage the primary curve. Orthotic management may be used in some patients with long flexible curves to achieve spinal balance through the normal vertebrae adjacent to the pathologic vertebrae at the apex of the curve. Compensatory or secondary curves are also occasionally managed with bracing. However, long-term bracing during active growth can have a deleterious effect on the growth of the thoracic cavity and can result in chest wall deformities in young children.

## Surgical Management

The goals of surgical treatment are to halt asymmetric growth, achieve spinal balance, or correct existing deformity. Prophylactic surgery can be used to prevent curve progression; in situ anterior and/or posterior hemiepiphysiodesis is a surgical option for addressing a deformity that is likely to result in imbalanced growth. The use of more aggressive surgical approaches to manage congenital scoliosis has been more widely described, particularly for patients who have not reached skeletal maturity. Hemivertebra excision and anterior-posterior osteotomy/vertebrectomy with or without instrumentation are indicated in some patients, particularly at the thoracolumbar and lumbosacral junctions. Although most of these approaches appear to be safe when performed by experienced surgeons, the risks and benefits should be carefully assessed, especially when excellent results have been achieved with more conservative surgical procedures.

All surgical procedures carry the risk of affecting overall spine length. Although trunk height may be further reduced by progression of deformity and the development of a secondary curve, surgical intervention may also limit growth potential. Depending on the type and location of the vertebral anomaly and pattern and flexibility of the curve, it may be possible to surgically reduce the degree of deformity. However, a correction that lengthens the spine tends to increase the risk of neurologic injury. The use of MRI to detect intraspinal anomalies before surgery is essential. Intraspinal anomalies should be addressed before fusion if neurologic symptoms are present. High-quality neuromonitoring, including somatosensory-evoked potentials, transcranial motor-evoked potentials, and electromyography, should be conducted during surgery.

Early in situ arthrodesis is usually indicated for infants or children with unilateral unsegmented bars. For younger children, fusion of the involved segment of the spine should often be anterior and posterior. One of the risks associated with posterior fusion alone in skeletally immature patients is the crankshaft phenomenon, defined as a greater than 10° progression in Cobb angle resulting from continuing anterior growth of the spine. One study reported that the crankshaft phenomenon was observed in 8 patients (15%) in a series of 54 skeletally immature patients during 12 years of follow-up (until skeletal maturity). The crankshaft phenomenon was more likely to occur in patients who were younger at the time of surgery and with curves with an initial measurement of greater than 50°. Postoperative immobilization with a cast, orthotic device, or more rarely in a halo vest may be used for noninstrumented patients. Instrumentation is sometimes used to stabilize fusions in older patients with flexible or less severe curves. However, the neurologic risks (overdistraction or direct injury to the cord or roots) are greater for posterior instrumentation in patients with congenital scoliosis than in those with idiopathic scoliosis. The risk of spinal cord ischemia can be reduced in anterior procedures by preserving the segmental vessels and by avoiding excess lengthening of the spine with distraction maneuvers.

For children with a fully segmented hemivertebra who are 5 years of age or younger, convex anterior and posterior hemiepiphysiodesis and fusion may allow for continued growth on the concave side of the curve, thus preventing the progression of deformity and in some patients resulting in a gradual correction of the deformity. Preoperative imaging of the three dimensions of the anomalous vertebra is an integral part of surgical planning. Sagittal plane deformity has been considered to be a contraindication for hemiepiphysiodesis. One study of 11 children with congenital scoliosis and sagittal plane deformity who were treated with hemiepiphysiodesis reported that at an average 40-month follow-up the sagittal Cobb angle had progressed in 4 patients.

Anterior or posterior osteotomy or vertebrectomy with or without instrumentation and fusion may be indicated for patients with severe rigidity, fixed pelvic obliquity, or decompensated deformities. However, the neurologic risks to patients are greater with these procedures. Transpedicular eggshell osteotomy has also been described as a potential approach to treating older patients with multiple anomalies and multiplanar deformities. Screws or hooks are placed above and below the osteotomy site, transpedicular decancellation of the body is performed as close to the end plates as possible, and the correction is maintained by means of internal fixation. One study reported obtaining an average correction of 38° in the sagittal plane and 28.7° in the coronal plane in three patients who were treated with this specific technique. If this technique is used, excess growth cartilage associated with the hemivertebra must be removed.

Reports of hemivertebra excision are appearing more frequently in the literature. The goal of hemivertebra excision is to directly address spinal imbalance. Ideally, correction can be achieved and future asymmetric growth can be prevented using this technique. Hemivertebra excision should be reserved for patients who are at high risk for progression if the more traditional in situ fusion or hemiepiphysiodesis and fusion techniques have already been attempted. The best indication for excision is the presence of a fully segmented hemivertebra at the lumbosacral junction. Resection may be posterior, anterior, or combined, and approaches to instrumentation vary.

Reports of combined anterior and posterior hemivertebra excision have shown good postoperative correction with little deterioration. Estimates of the mean postoperative curve correction obtained in hemivertebra resections in all parts of the spine range from of 59% to 67% of the initial curve with little loss of correction at least 24 months postoperatively. Hemivertebra resection via a posterior approach minimizes surgical exposure with similar potential for correction, but may be a more difficult and higher-risk procedure. Correction with single-stage posterior thoracolumbar hemivertebra excision and instrumentation has been reported to be between 23° to 36°, with an average total of 3.7° loss of correction at last follow-up. The neurologic risks of hemivertebra excision are greater than those of hemiepiphysiodesis, and reoperation is sometimes necessary to correct implant failures or to address progressing asymmetric growth.

The correction achieved with lumbosacral hemivertebra resection has been reported to be less than that which can be achieved with hemivertebra excision in other regions of the spine, ranging from 10° to 12° of correction with similar rates of deterioration. One technique involves pelvic fixation following anterior and posterior excision of a hemivertebra at the lumbosacral junction. A cable construct connects the adjacent normal vertebra to the ilium with screws and provides an alternative construct for achieving fixation in the smaller and more porous bones of young children (Figure 5). One study reported that correction was achieved and maintained throughout a follow-up period of at least 3 years in each of the three patients managed with hemivertebra excision, pelvic fixation, and bilateral posterior fusion.

For children with thoracic insufficiency syndrome associated with fused ribs and congenital scoliosis, thoracoplasty and opening wedge thoracostomy with instrumentation for longitudinal lengthening can enable growth and provide increased thoracic spinal height, depth, and width. One study reported an average thoracic spine growth rate of 8 mm/yr over an average 4.2-year follow-up in 21 patients with congenital scoliosis and fused ribs following expansion thoracoplasty with vertical, expandable prosthetic titanium rib implants (Figure 6). The growth rate on the concave side averaged 7.9 mm/yr and 8.3 mm/yr on the convex side. In a subsequent series, the results of management with

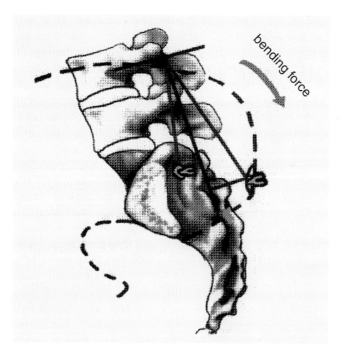

Figure 5 Schematic representation showing corrective forces applied by pelvic fixation to maintain correction following lumbosacral hemivertebra excision. *(Reproduced with permission from Hosalkar H, Luedtke L, Drummond DS: New technique in congenital scoliosis involving fixation to the pelvis after hemivertebra excision. Spine 2004; 29:2581-2587.)*

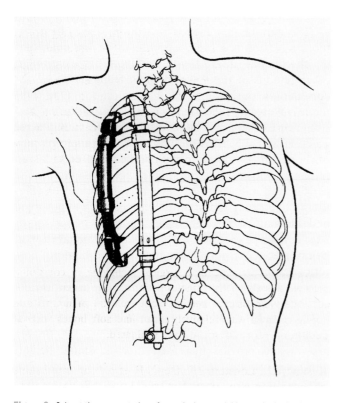

Figure 6 Schematic representation of a vertical, expandable prosthetic titanium rib. This device is implanted after opening wedge thoracostomy in patients with congenital vertebral anomalies and fused ribs. Gradual correction promotes thoracic growth to increase height, depth, and width. *(Reproduced with permission from Campbell RM, Smith MD, Mayes TC, et al: The effect of opening wedge thoracostomy on thoracic insufficiency syndrome associated with fused ribs and congenital scoliosis. J Bone Joint Surg Am 2004;86A:1659-1674.)*

vertical, expandable prosthetic titanium rib implants on scoliosis and thoracic insufficiency were reported in 27 patients (average age, 3.2 years; range, 0.6 to 12.5 years) with fused ribs and congenital scoliosis that was progressing at an average rate of 15° per year. In this series, scoliosis decreased from an average 74° to 49° at the time of last follow-up (mean, 5.7 years), and statistically significant increases in the volume of vital capacity were reported in all patients. Although the long-term pulmonary function of children treated with the vertical, expandable prosthetic titanium rib technique remains unknown, the early results are encouraging.

## Summary

The understanding of the etiology and natural history of congenital scoliosis continues to improve. Based on this new knowledge, treatment methods also continue to advance. The addition of new techniques to avoid pulmonary compromise in very young children with congenital scoliosis is an important area of such improvements.

## Annotated Bibliography
### General

Erol B, Tracy MR, Dormans JP, et al: Congenital scoliosis and vertebral malformations: Characterization of segmental defects for genetic analysis. *J Pediatr Orthop* 2004;24:674-682.

The authors evaluated and classified patients with congenital vertebral defects into groups based on developmental etiology. Eighty-four patients with vertebral segmentation disorders were evaluated radiologically and genetic analysis was done on 39 patients. The extent of contiguous defects was quantified and patients were organized by craniocaudal localization.

Purkiss SB, Driscoll B, Cole WG, Alman B: Idiopathic scoliosis in families of children with congenital scoliosis. *Clin Orthop Relat Res* 2002;401:27-31.

The authors of this study reported that 49 of 237 children (20.7%) with congenital scoliosis reported a family history of spinal deformity, and pedigrees of 17.3% of the patients showed a history of idiopathic scoliosis.

### History and Physical Examination

Basu PS, Elsebaie H, Noordeen MH: Congenital spinal deformity: A comprehensive assessment at presentation. *Spine* 2002;27:2255-2259.

In this study of 126 consecutive patients with congenital spinal deformity, intraspinal abnormalities were found in 47 patients (37%). Patients with scoliosis and cervical and thoracic hemivertebrae had significantly more intraspinal abnormalities ($P = 0.0253$) than those with lumbar hemivertebrae. In 64 patients (55%), other organic defects were found. These defects were more common in patients with congenital scoliosis resulting from mixed defects (*P* = 0.002). Cardiac defects were detected in 26% of patients and urogenital anomalies in 21%.

Belmont PJ Jr, Kuklo TR, Taylor KF, Freedman BA, Prahinski JR, Kruse RW: Intraspinal anomalies associated with isolated congenital hemivertebra: The role of routine magnetic resonance imaging. *J Bone Joint Surg Am* 2004;86-A:1704-1710.

Of 76 patients studied, 29 patients had an isolated hemivertebra and 47 had a complex hemivertebral pattern. Overall, an abnormal finding on the history or physical examination demonstrated an accuracy of 71%, a sensitivity of 56%, a specificity of 76%, a positive predictive value of 42%, and a negative predictive value of 85% for the diagnosis of an intraspinal anomaly.

Campbell RM Jr, Smith MD, Mayes TC, et al: The characteristics of thoracic insufficiency syndrome associated with fused ribs and congenital scoliosis. *J Bone Joint Surg Am* 2003;85-A:399-408.

The authors of this article describe the clinical and radiographic characteristics of thoracic insufficiency syndrome and the prognosis and treatment options for patients with this disorder.

## Nonsurgical Management

Lerman JA, Sullivan E, Haynes RJ: The Pediatric Outcomes Data Collection Instrument (PODCI) and functional assessment in patients with adolescent or juvenile idiopathic scoliosis and congenital scoliosis or kyphosis. *Spine* 2002;27:2052-2057.

In this study, 47 patients with congenital scoliosis completed the Pediatric Outcomes Data Collection Instrument. Responses were compared with those from a normal population. In patients with congenital scoliosis, scores in all categories except happiness were significantly lower (*P* < 0.05) than in the normal group.

Shahcheraghi GH, Hobbi MH: Patterns and progression in congenital scoliosis. *J Pediatr Orthop* 1999;19:766-775.

The authors reviewed 60 patients who had congenital scoliosis over a 13-year period. Anomalies were classified and rates of progression calculated.

## Surgical Management

Campbell RM Jr, Hell-Vocke AK: Growth of the thoracic spine in congenital scoliosis after expansion thoracoplasty. *J Bone Joint Surg Am* 2003;85-A:409-420.

Results of this study showed that children with congenital thoracic scoliosis associated with fused ribs with a unilateral unsegmented bar adjacent to convex hemivertebrae have curve progression without treatment. Results indicate that there is a 0.6 cm per year longitudinal growth of the thoracic spine in a normal child between the ages of 5 and 9 years, whereas after expansion thoracoplasty, there is an 8 mm per year growth of the thoracic spine in children with congenital scoliosis and fused ribs.

Campbell RM Jr, Smith MD, Mayes TC, et al: The effect of opening wedge thoracostomy on thoracic insufficiency syndrome associated with fused ribs and congenital scoliosis. *J Bone Joint Surg Am* 2004;86-A:1659-1674.

In this study of 27 patients, an opening wedge thoracostomy was performed by using a chest-wall distractor that directly treats segmental hypoplasia of the hemithorax resulting from fused ribs associated with congenital scoliosis. It was shown that the scoliosis decreased from a mean of 74° preoperatively to a mean of 49° at the time of the last follow-up.

Cil A, Yazici M, Alanay A, Acaroglu RE, Uzumcugil A, Surat A: The course of sagittal plane abnormality in the patients with congenital scoliosis managed with convex growth arrest. *Spine* 2004;29:547-552.

In this study of 38 patients, the authors found that sagittal segmental abnormality did not have a negative effect on the control of congenital scoliosis managed with convex growth arrest in 11 of 13 patients (84.6%). Also, if the coronal curve stabilizes or improves, the sagittal segmental abnormality could be stabilized in 7 of 11 patients (63.6%).

Deviren V, Berven S, Smith JA, Emami A, Hu SS, Bradford DS: Excision of hemivertebrae in the management of congenital scoliosis involving the thoracic and thoracolumbar spine. *J Bone Joint Surg Br* 2001;83:496-500.

In this study of 10 patients, a mean preoperative coronal curve of 78.2° (range, 30° to 115°) and a postoperative coronal curve of 33.9° (range, 7° to 58°) was found, which indicated a 59% correction for those who had excision of thoracic or thoracolumbar hemivertebrae for either angular deformity in the coronal plane or both coronal and sagittal deformity. Preoperative coronal decompensation of 35 mm improved to 11 mm postoperatively.

Hosalkar HS, Luedtke LM, Drummond DS: New technique in congenital scoliosis involving fixation to the pelvis after hemivertebra excision. *Spine* 2004;29:2581-2587.

In this article, the new surgical technique in congenital scoliosis to stabilize the spine of patients with congenital scoliosis after lumbosacral hemivertebra excision in infants and young children with relatively small and soft bones without pedicle screws was described and evaluated.

Kesling KL, Lonstein JE, Denis F, et al: The crankshaft phenomenon after posterior spinal arthrodesis for congenital scoliosis: A review of 54 patients. *Spine* 2003;28:267-271.

The incidence of and any possible risk factors for the crankshaft phenomenon after posterior spinal arthrodesis for congenital scoliosis were discussed in this article. The authors found a Cobb angle increase of more than 10° in 15% of the

54 patients studied, and found a positive correlation with earlier surgery and larger (> 50°) curves.

Klemme WR, Polly DW Jr, Orchowski JR: Hemivertebral excision for congenital scoliosis in very young children. *J Pediatr Orthop* 2001;21:761-764.

In this study of a consecutive series of six very young patients, the authors found single-anesthetic sequential anterior and posterior hemivertebral excision to be a safe and efficacious treatment. The mean postoperative curve correction of 67% (range, 52% to 84%) compared favorably with the average correction at final follow-up of 70% (range, 50% to 85%).

Mikles MR, Graziano GP, Hensinger AR: Transpedicular eggshell osteotomies for congenital scoliosis using frameless stereotactic guidance. *Spine* 2001;26:2289-2296.

In this study of three patients, the authors found that the transpedicular eggshell osteotomy with frameless stereotactic guidance can be used to correct a sagittal and/or coronal congenital spinal curve.

Nakamura H, Matsuda H, Konishi S, Yamano Y: Single-stage excision of hemivertebrae via the posterior approach alone for congenital spine deformity: Follow-up period longer than ten years. *Spine* 2002;27:110-115.

The long-term results for single, fully-segmented hemivertebrae that were treated with single-stage excision via the posterior approach alone were evaluated in this study. For patients with a thoracolumbar hemivertebra, scoliosis improved from 49° ± 6° to 22.3° ± 3.5°, accounting for a 54.3% correction. The correction ratio for kyphosis was 67.4%.

Ruf M, Harms J: Posterior hemivertebra resection with transpedicular instrumentation: Early correction in children aged 1 to 6 years. *Spine* 2003;28:2132-2138.

In this study of 28 consecutive very young patients with congenital scoliosis, the use of posterior hemivertebra resection with transpedicular instrumentation was evaluated. The mean Cobb angle of the main curve was 45° before and 14° after surgery. Compensatory cranial curve also improved from 17° to 5° and compensatory caudal curve improved from 17° to 5°. The angle of kyphosis was 22° before surgery and 10° after surgery.

Shono Y, Abumi K, Kaneda K: One-stage posterior hemivertebra resection and correction using segmental posterior instrumentation. *Spine* 2001;26:752-757.

This study presents the results of 12 patients with congenital kyphoscoliosis caused by a single hemivertebra who underwent one-stage posterior hemivertebra resection and correction by posterior segmental instrumentation. Excellent results were found in all patients. Preoperative scoliosis averaging 49° was corrected to 18° (correction rate, 64%). Preoperative kyphosis of 40° was corrected to 17°. Trunk shift improved from 23 mm to 3 mm.

## Classic Bibliography

McMaster MJ, Ohtsuka K: The natural history of congenital scoliosis: A study of two hundred and fifty-one patients. *J Bone Joint Surg Am* 1982;64:1128-1147.

# Chapter 46

# Infantile, Juvenile, and Adolescent Idiopathic Scoliosis

Behrooz A. Akbarnia, MD

Lee S. Segal, MD

## Introduction

There are three types of idiopathic scoliosis based on the age of onset: infantile, juvenile, and adolescent. Infantile idiopathic scoliosis is diagnosed in patients with spinal curves who present before the age of 3 years, juvenile idiopathic scoliosis is diagnosed in those with curves who present between the ages of 4 to 9 years, and adolescent idiopathic scoliosis is diagnosed in those with curves who present after age 10 years or until the end of growth. These three types of idiopathic scoliosis correspond to distinct periods of growth during childhood and adolescence. The infantile and adolescent periods are marked by an increased growth velocity, whereas the juvenile period correlates with a deceleration of spinal growth and the onset of scoliosis is relatively uncommon. In addition, the term "early onset" is used to reflect the presence of scoliosis by age 5 years and late onset reflects the appearance of scoliosis after the age of 5 years. These age groups represent an important treatment factor because patients with a significant spinal deformity before age 5 years will have a higher likelihood of developing cardiopulmonary abnormalities such as restrictive lung disease, pulmonary hypertension, or cor pulmonale.

## Infantile and Juvenile Idiopathic Scoliosis

The treatment of children with progressive infantile or juvenile scoliosis has proved to be difficult. Standard modalities used to treat older patients with scoliosis, such as orthotic devices or spinal fusion, have limited roles in the treatment of young children because they may adversely affect the growth and function of the immature spine, lungs, and thoracic cage. There are many etiologies for scoliosis in this age group. Only after eliminating all other possible causes of deformity should a child be diagnosed with infantile or juvenile idiopathic scoliosis.

### Epidemiology

#### Infantile Scoliosis

Infantile idiopathic scoliosis comprises less than 1% of all instances of idiopathic scoliosis in the United States.

Although rare, it is more common in males, with a ratio of 3:2. The spinal curves also tend to be left-sided (75% to 90% of patients). These deformities may be associated with other anomalies such as hip dysplasia, congenital heart disease, and mental retardation.

Fortunately, the prognosis for patients with infantile scoliosis also differs from that for juvenile or adolescent scoliosis. In one study, it was shown that more than 90% of patients experienced spontaneous resolution of their symptoms without the need for treatment. Nonetheless, girls presenting with right-sided thoracic infantile curves have been noted to have a poor prognosis and do not typically experience spontaneous resolution.

Multiple hypotheses have been put forth to explain infantile scoliosis. Intrauterine molding was believed to be responsible for infantile scoliosis as well as associated crowding deformities such as plagiocephaly, plagiopelvy, decreased hip abduction, or rib molding. However, hypotheses involving intrauterine molding and crowding have subsequently been refuted because of the absence of scoliosis at birth. Another hypothesis that has been postulated is infant positioning while sleeping. It was believed that prolonged oblique supine positioning in the crib was responsible for infantile scoliosis. The postnatal pressure theory was believed to explain the higher incidence (approximately 72%) of plagiocephaly and infantile scoliosis observed in children within the first 6 months of life (the period during which children are unable to reposition independently). The rate of plagiocephaly in children without scoliosis is 28%.

The genetics of infantile scoliosis have been noted to be similar to those of juvenile and adolescent scoliosis in which parents or siblings of affected children are 30 times more likely than control subjects to have scoliosis. One study reported that 13% of male infants with progressive curves were mentally retarded, and 7% also had concomitant inguinal hernias. It was noted that infants with hypotonia were unable to resist deformation compared with children with normal tone. In addition, it was believed that children with congenital malformations, including hiatal hernia, were at increased risk of scoliosis progression.

Although several factors, such as age of onset, location, type and magnitude of the curve, associated anomalies, gender, and family history were proposed as predictors of spinal curve progression, the most reliable indicator has become the rib-vertebra angle difference.

### Juvenile Scoliosis

Juvenile idiopathic scoliosis accounts for 12% to 21% of reported instances of idiopathic scoliosis. Juvenile scoliosis is more prevalent in females than males, with a 2:1 to 4:1 ratio per different reports. However, between the ages of 3 and 6 years, males are equally as likely to be affected by juvenile onset scoliosis as females (1:1 ratio). After 10 years of age, the ratio of females to males affected is 8:1, which is more in line with the female to male ratio for adolescent idiopathic scoliosis.

Right-sided thoracic and double major curves are the principal curve patterns associated with juvenile idiopathic scoliosis. Slow to moderate progression of the deformity is usually seen in patients with juvenile idiopathic scoliosis. Reports indicate that approximately 70% of spinal curves progress and necessitate some type of treatment. One study demonstrated a 50% rate of spontaneous resolution of curves that were less than 25° at presentation and left untreated. Although spontaneous resolution has been reported in patients with juvenile scoliosis, it is more frequently observed in those with infantile idiopathic scoliosis.

Eight percent to 21% of children with juvenile scoliosis are less likely to respond to the nonsurgical treatments available and experience retardation of their curve progression compared with those who are diagnosed with adolescent scoliosis. Children with juvenile scoliosis are also more likely to require surgery than children with adolescent scoliosis. Unlike adolescent idiopathic scoliosis, there is an increased risk of death in this age group if the scoliosis is left untreated.

Results again suggest that juvenile scoliosis is often more progressive, unresponsive to bracing, and predisposed to surgical treatment than adolescent idiopathic scoliosis.

### History

The clinical evaluation of a young child with a spinal deformity must proceed in a thorough, systematic fashion, and a complete history must be obtained before a physical examination is performed. A prenatal history of the mother, including all health problems, previous pregnancies, and medications, should be recorded. Birth history of the child should include length of gestation, type of delivery (vaginal or caesarean), birth weight, and complications.

The developmental history should include both motor and cognitive milestones. Because the presence of cognitive delay has been shown to correlate with curve progression, particular attention should be given to whether the child has appropriately reached the developmental milestones. As with developmental dysplasia of the hip, infantile scoliosis can be associated with a breech presentation. However unlike developmental dysplasia of the hip, infantile scoliosis occurs more commonly in males of low birth weight than females.

### Physical Examination

The spinal deformity should be assessed during the physical examination, and associated conditions should be eliminated from the potential diagnosis. The skin, the entire spine, the head, the pelvis, and the extremities should all be assessed during the initial inspection. The skin must be examined for cutaneous stigmata such as café au lait spots or axillary freckles associated with neurofibromatosis, midline patches of hair associated with spinal dysraphism, or bruising associated with trauma. The spine examination should include inspection and palpation of the spine. For patients in the infantile age group, some aspects of the standard physical examination are more difficult to perform; therefore, different techniques must be used. In young children, the Adams forward bend test (which assesses patients for prominence of the ribs in the thoracic spine or transverse processes in the lumbar spine) cannot be performed, but it can be simulated by laying the child over the examiner's knee in a prone position. Curve flexibility can be assessed by placing the child in a lateral position on the convex side of the curve over the knee or suspending the infant under the arms.

The physical examination must also include notation of chest or flank asymmetry, chest excursion, and abdominal reflexes. Limitation in chest excursion may indicate syndromic scoliosis and thoracic insufficiency syndrome. Abdominal reflex abnormalities should initiate a thorough neurologic evaluation. The absence of an abdominal reflex has been the only objective finding observed in some patients with an Arnold-Chiari malformation. When abnormal, the absent reflex is usually on the convex side of the curve.

The head must also be thoroughly examined. Plagiocephaly commonly occurs in patients with infantile scoliosis and typically responds well to therapy. Other conditions affecting the head that are associated with infantile scoliosis include bat-ear deformity and congenital muscular torticollis. Although these conditions frequently occur without scoliosis, it is important to be aware of the association. A pelvic examination should be done to rule out plagiopelvy and developmental hip dysplasia, both of which are associated with infantile scoliosis. The lower extremity examination must exclude limb-length inequality as the etiology of scoliosis. When scoliosis is secondary to a limb-length inequality, the lumbar prominence is found on the side of the longer limb. Functional scoliosis caused by limb-length inequality may be negated by performing a sitting forward bend or placing a lift under the short limb to equalize the limb lengths.

## Differential Diagnosis

The diagnosis of infantile and juvenile idiopathic scoliosis is primarily based on the radiologic examination and by ruling out all other potential etiologies. If developmental delay is present, a neuromuscular etiology such as hypotonia or other myopathic conditions should be ruled out. Occasionally, congenital anomalies of the spine such as a unilateral unsegmented bar do not appear in the initial screening radiographs and instead are found in subsequent radiographs once the bar has ossified. Other diagnoses to be considered are trauma or tumors. Syndromic scoliosis is usually associated with other anomalies and often requires a genetic workup.

## Diagnostic Imaging

### Magnetic Resonance Imaging

Even in the presence of normal physical examination findings, total spine MRI is indicated in patients with moderate or progressive infantile scoliosis because of the high incidence of neural axis abnormalities such as Arnold-Chiari type I malformation and syringomyelia. The reported incidence of positive MRI findings indicative of neural axis abnormalities in patients with infantile scoliosis has been reported to range from 21% to 50%. The current recommendation is to perform MRI on patients with infantile scoliosis and a Cobb angle greater than 20°.

Studies have been conducted with respect to neural axis abnormalities seen in patients with juvenile onset scoliosis. The reported incidence of Arnold-Chiari type I malformation and syringomyelia ranges from 15% to 26% of patients with juvenile scoliosis as evaluated in various prospective and retrospective case series. From these studies, no clinical parameters have been determined to prognosticate a positive MRI finding. As with patients with infantile scoliosis, MRI is recommended as part of a routine evaluation for all patients presenting with juvenile onset scoliosis and a Cobb angle greater than 20°.

### Radiologic Evaluation

Initial evaluation of a patient with suspected scoliosis should consist of AP and lateral radiographs of the entire spine (including the cervical spine and pelvis). In children who are too young to stand, the radiographs should be taken with the patients in the supine position. Cervical spine abnormalities should be evaluated. Similarly, the lumbosacral junction, pelvis, and hips should be carefully examined to rule out congenital anomalies or developmental dysplasia of the hip.

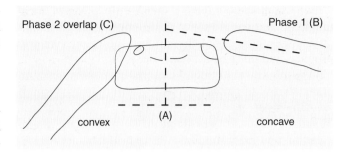

**Figure 1** Schematic representation of the rib-vertebra angle difference measurement and phase 1 and 2 relationships. To measure the rib-vertebra angle difference, a dotted line is drawn parallel to the end plate and another is drawn down the middle of the apical vertebra, perpendicular to the end plate. A dotted line is then drawn down the center of the concave and convex ribs that intersects the midpoint of the ribs. The rib-vertebra angle difference is the difference between the angles that the concave and convex ribs make with the line perpendicular to the end plate (A). The phase 1 relationship to the apical vertebra, normally occurring bilaterally, is depicted by the nonoverlapping rib head shown on the concave side (B). The phase 2 relationship is observed by an overlapping rib head on the convex side only (C). *(Adapted with permission from the Mehta MH: The rib-vertebra angle in the early diagnosis between resolving and progressive infantile scoliosis. J Bone Joint Surg Br 1972;54:230-243.)*

Scoliosis measurement is done using the Cobb angle, which is used to monitor the progression of the curve. Unlike juvenile or adolescent scoliosis, infantile scoliosis frequently resolves spontaneously. The rib-vertebra angle difference method is available to predict progression or resolution of the curve. The rib-vertebra angle difference method measures the angle of a line drawn perpendicular to the apical thoracic vertebra end plate and a line drawn down the center of the concave and convex ribs (Figure 1). The actual difference is calculated by subtracting the convex from the concave angles. A rib-vertebra angle difference of less than 20° indicates a curve that is likely to resolve (in 85% to 90% of patients), whereas a rib-vertebra angle difference of greater than 20° is frequently associated with curves that will progress. An additional tool, known as the phase of the rib head, has also been described for prognostication of infantile scoliosis. The phase of the rib head notes the position of the convex rib head on the apical vertebra. A phase 1 relationship indicates no overlap of the rib head or neck on the apical vertebra. In patients with a phase 1 relationship, the rib-vertebra angle difference may be calculated and used to determine likelihood of progression. In a phase 2 relationship, the head of the rib on the convex side of the apical vertebra overlaps with the vertebra, and the rib-vertebra angle difference is not measured because the curve is certain to progress. In the initial description of the rib-vertebra angle difference and phase of the rib head, an 83% rate of resolution in phase 1 relationships was reported in patients with a rib-vertebra angle difference less than 20°. Conversely, the group that progressed included 84% of the patients with a rib-vertebra angle difference of greater than 20°.

One final radiographic element to help assess curve progression is the presence of a lumbar curve. In addition, it should be noted that double curves are likely to progress and must be followed closely.

The rib-vertebra angle difference has been used in other studies to predict and monitor the progression of juvenile onset scoliosis. A rib-vertebra angle difference of greater than 10° was found to be indicative of progression and poor response to nonsurgical treatment. However, the use of rib-vertebra angle difference in patients with juvenile scoliosis has not been effectively validated. Another study reported that an apical vertebra of T8, T9, or T10 was the most reliable factor for predicting progression and the need for surgical intervention.

## Nonsurgical Treatment

The treatment of children with infantile and juvenile scoliosis is based on anticipated or actual curve progression. As discussed, established prognostic criteria have proved to be helpful in differentiating between resolving and progressive curves. Patients with infantile curves with Cobb angles less than 25° and a rib-vertebra angle difference of less than 20° are at low risk for progression. These patients may be observed and should be re-evaluated with serial radiographs every 4 to 6 months. Active treatment should be initiated if curve progression of greater than 10° occurs. If the curve resolves, it is prudent to follow the patient at 1- to 2-year intervals until maturity to ensure that there is no recurrence during the adolescent growth spurt. Similar guidelines should be followed in managing patients with a juvenile curve. Observation with regular follow-up to monitor for progression is indicated for patients with curves less than 20° to 25°.

A recent long-term study of resolving curves validated the use of the rib-vertebra angle difference and demonstrated that there was no advantage of plaster bed treatment over physiotherapy with regard to either the time to resolution or functional outcomes. Infants with a high likelihood of progression are those with a rib-vertebra angle difference of greater than 20° or a phase II rib-vertebra relationship and a Cobb angle between 20° and 35°. These patients should also be followed closely at 4- to 6-month intervals with the initiation of active treatment if progression occurs. An initial curve of greater than 25° to 30° or a rib-vertebra angle difference of greater than 10° has been associated with a higher probability of progression in patients with juvenile onset scoliosis.

Traditional nonsurgical treatment approaches to infantile and juvenile scoliosis include casting and bracing. Casting is more effective than orthotic device treatment for patients with rigid curves. Treatment usually begins with a molded body cast application with the patient un-

der anesthesia. The cast is changed at 6- to 12-week intervals until maximum correction is achieved. Following this, the cast may be replaced by a Milwaukee brace with full-time implementation (23 hours per day). Milwaukee braces are more often preferred for patients with more flexible type curves. Milwaukee braces have been preferred over thoracolumbar orthotic devices because of the distortion of the rib cage and reduction of pulmonary function that may occur with the circumferentially fitting thoracolumbar braces. In addition, the immature rib cage often deforms before significant correction is transmitted to the spine. Bracing is generally continued for a minimum of 2 years or until there is no evidence or potential for curve progression. When total correction is obtained before the prepubertal growth spurt, no relapse occurs during adolescence. However, without full correction, small relapses may occur, in which instance surgery may be required if further progression is observed during the adolescent growth spurt. The patient should be followed until skeletal maturity.

## Surgical Treatment

The ultimate goal of surgical treatment of patients with infantile or juvenile scoliosis is to stop progression of the curve while allowing maximum growth of the spine, lungs, and thoracic cage. Surgical treatment of infantile scoliosis is recommended for patients with progressive curves greater than 45°. There is a current trend toward less tolerance of curve progression before surgical management. The age of the patient at the time of curve progression will frequently dictate the type of surgical procedure chosen. There are no definitive guidelines for recommending surgical intervention for patients with juvenile onset scoliosis because of the broad age range of patients being treated. However, generally speaking, patients with juvenile curves respond less favorably to nonsurgical treatment and are more likely to require surgery than those with adolescent idiopathic scoliosis.

### *Definitive Spinal Fusion*

Surgical techniques have traditionally focused on spinal fusion as the primary method to halt curve progression. Isolated posterior spinal fusion with or without instrumentation in young children may lead to the crankshaft phenomenon because of continued anterior growth of the spine. Patients who have open triradiate cartilages and are Risser stage 0 have a high likelihood of curve progression because of the crankshaft phenomenon if an isolated posterior fusion is performed.

To prevent the crankshaft phenomenon in this age group, anterior arthrodesis is combined with posterior fusion. Because there are two stages of maximal spinal growth velocity (0 to 5 years and 10 to 15 years), it can be concluded that early anterior and posterior fusion for infantile and early juvenile scoliosis will result in substantial loss of expected trunk height. In addition to the detrimental effects on spinal growth, premature fusion has potential deleterious repercussions for the developing thoracic cage and lungs. This has prompted attempts to devise other methods of treatment. Current research has focused on fusionless techniques for the treatment of infantile and juvenile scoliosis.

### Fusionless Techniques

Spinal deformity in infantile and juvenile scoliosis was once believed to result from asymmetric growth of the convex (faster growing) and concave (inhibited) side of the curve. Because of the success of treating angular growth deformities in the extremities of growing children with hemiepiphysiodesis, a similar approach to the spine was recommended that involved ablation of the convex epiphyseal cartilage of the vertebrae and the adjacent disks near the apex of the curve. Although 23% of patients treated with this technique showed improvement in the Cobb angle, 40% had little or no improvement ($< 10°$ change). More recently, convex epiphysiodesis with or without Harrington instrumentation was examined. The current recommendations suggest the use of instrumentation at the time of convex epiphysiodesis as a viable option to control but not reverse the progression of the curve.

The concept of convex growth retardation continues to have supporters in the treatment of idiopathic scoliosis. The latest attempts to control curvature involve intervertebral stapling or tethering via a minimally invasive anterior thoracoscopic approach. Staples similar to those used to treat angular deformity of the lower extremities are placed on the convex side of the vertebrae at the apex of the curve. The technique avoids fusion and may allow for future growth. Long-term results of these techniques are not available for patients with early onset scoliosis, but the technique may become a treatment option in the future.

Use of a vertical expandable prosthetic titanium rib is another nonfusion technique that is aimed at correcting the thoracic deformity and improving lung function. It is used in patients with thoracic insufficiency syndrome and congenital scoliosis with associated fused ribs. No data are yet available for its use in treating patients with infantile or juvenile idiopathic scoliosis.

### Posterior Growing Rod Techniques

The goal of this type of treatment is preservation of spinal growth in concert with correction of the deformity. This technique was initially reported in 1962 by Harrington for the treatment of scoliosis. A fusionless approach was described with a distraction rod attached to laminar hooks placed at each end of the concave side of the deformity. Subsequently, this technique for instrumented spinal fusion altered the course of modern scoliosis surgery and has continued to be modified. This tech-

nique was later modified by Moe and since then, single submuscular or subcutaneous growing rods with and without apical fusion have been used over the past three decades. Complications often included implant-related problems such as hook displacement, rod breakage, and superficial wound infections. Despite the complications, the technique became particularly useful in the treatment of significant spinal deformity in young children.

The aim of current treatment efforts continues to be the promotion of spinal growth while maintaining deformity correction and minimizing complications. The most recent endeavor has involved the introduction of the dual growing rod technique that can be used submuscularly or subcutaneously.

### Dual Growing Rod Technique

With the dual growing rod technique, subperiosteal dissection is performed only at the upper and lower anchor sites of the implant. At the upper end of the curve, hooks or screws are placed in a claw pattern spanning two or three levels. A similar pedicle screw or hook pattern is used at the lower end of the construct. These sites are called the foundations of the construct. A transverse connector is preloaded at the level of each foundation, especially when hooks are used. A limited fusion is performed at the site of the foundations with the use of local bone or synthetic graft. Contoured rods are placed on each side of the spine, and the upper and lower rods are linked by way of a tandem connector placed at the thoracolumbar junction. Bracing is used on all patients until a solid fusion is achieved.

After the initial placement of the construct, lengthening procedures are performed at 6-month intervals (Figure 2). Lengthening of the construct is performed via the tandem connector. Somatosensory-evoked potential monitoring is used at the time of lengthening to monitor spinal cord response to the correction. Patients who undergo lengthening procedures more frequently (6-month intervals or less) have better correction of scoliosis and greater increase in T1-S1 length than those who undergo lengthening procedures less frequently (6-month intervals or more). When it is determined that the patient has reached skeletal maturity or is no longer benefiting from the treatment, definitive fusion or final fusion is performed. The final arthrodesis usually involves the removal of implants and reinstrumentation of the spine.

Minimum 2-year follow-up data have been reported on the use of dual growing rod treatment. The age at the time of initial surgery averaged 5.4 years, and patients underwent an average of 6.6 lengthenings. The Cobb angle averaged 82° and initially improved to 36° at the most recent follow-up or after final fusion. Growth of the spine approached normal spinal growth, with an average of 1.21 cm per year. Patients who were followed to final fusion averaged 11.8 cm of total spine growth

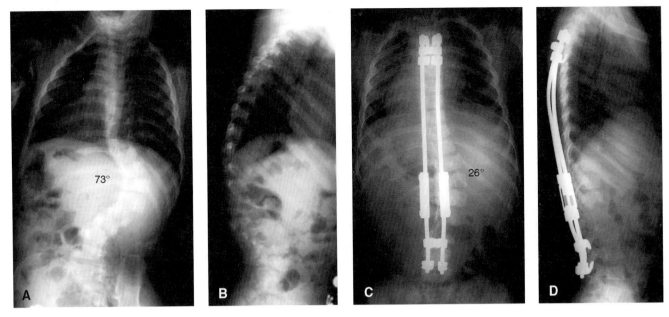

**Figure 2** Radiographs of a 20-month-old girl with infantile idiopathic scoliosis whose curve progressed, despite orthotic treatment, from 21° at 8 months of age to 73° before surgery. Preoperative AP **(A)** and lateral **(B)** radiographs of the spine taken at age 20 months. Scoliosis curve magnitude was 73°. Postoperative AP **(C)** and lateral **(D)** radiographs taken following the first lengthening procedure. The curve was measured to be 26°.

during the time of treatment. Complications occurring in the series included anchor (hook or screw) displacements (three), rod breakages (two), deep wound infections (two), and superficial wound problems (four). The crankshaft phenomenon and junctional kyphosis were observed less frequently in patients who underwent dual growing rod treatment compared with those who had single rod treatment.

More recent data on the dual growing rod technique again support the use of dual growing rod instrumentation. In one study, 28 patients were divided into three groups: single rod with anterior and posterior apical fusion (5 patients), single rod without apical fusion (16 patients), and dual rod without apical fusion (7 patients). At the time of final fusion, although it was determined that the single or dual growing rod technique was equally effective in controlling curve correction and allowing spinal growth, the dual growing rod technique not only improved curves, but maintained initial correction better and facilitated increased spinal growth. In this series, short apical fusion was associated with curve stiffening, the crankshaft phenomenon, and a higher incidence of complications. As a result, the effect of combining apical fusion with the dual and single growing rod techniques in treating patients with infantile and juvenile scoliosis has been brought into question.

### Discussion

The treatment of infantile and juvenile scoliosis is one of the most challenging aspects of pediatric spine surgery. Historical data have demonstrated that untreated curves have the potential for causing serious cardiopul-

monary and skeletal complications. Observation, casting, orthotic devices, traction, and surgical treatment are the currently available options for the treatment of infantile and juvenile scoliosis. Surgical treatment should be reserved for patients who do not meet the criteria for observation and fail or do not meet the criteria for orthotic device management.

Although current surgical techniques attempt to allow continuing spinal growth and prevent curve progression, patients require numerous surgical procedures before definitive spinal fusion is achieved. Reducing the frequency of repeat surgery or removing the need for it altogether without sacrificing the growth or correction achieved by the fusionless techniques should be one of the goals in the development of new treatment methods. Future research and long-term follow-up data will help to achieve this objective.

Future treatment solutions should be sought that are less invasive, yet still allow normal spine growth and correction of the deformity. Currently, the dual growing rod technique allows surgeons to offer minimal restriction to the normal growth of the spine and maintain deformity correction in the surgical treatment of patients with progressive infantile and early juvenile idiopathic scoliosis. For older patients with progressive juvenile scoliosis, however, definitive spinal fusion may still be the best treatment option available. Surgeons who treat this patient population should be experienced with the techniques available and the potential complications. The surgeon and the family of the patient should understand the level of commitment that is necessary to effectively treat these complex deformities.

## Adolescent Idiopathic Scoliosis

Almost a half-century ago, Cobb stated that "Scoliosis has always been one of the interesting and difficult problems in orthopaedics. André probably had it in mind when he devised his symbol for orthopaedics. It is stimulating and encouraging but can be confusing to those who have to treat scoliosis patients and do not know which new trend to follow." Although the treatment of adolescent idiopathic scoliosis has evolved since that time, Cobb's words still hold true today.

### Epidemiology

Conceptualizing scoliosis as a series of imperfect geometric torsions requires that the three-dimensional nature of the deformity be considered. In general, the prevalence of scoliosis decreases as the magnitude increases. Curves greater than 10° is the minimum accepted to establish a diagnosis of true scoliosis. The prevalence of adolescent idiopathic scoliosis in patients with curves greater than or equal to 10° ranges from 1% to 3%. In patients with larger curves that require treatment (> 30°), the prevalence decreases to 0.15% to 0.3%. In patients with smaller curves, the ratio of females to males is 1.4:1, and this ratio dramatically increases to greater than 5:1 in patients with curves greater than 30° or those that require treatment.

The natural history of adolescent idiopathic scoliosis depends on several factors, including the degree of skeletal maturity, curve magnitude, curve location, and curve pattern. The risk of progression is highly dependent on the amount of growth remaining during adolescence. In females, significant growth occurs 6 to 12 months before the onset of menarche. Peak height velocity in females has been reported to predict the cessation of growth more reliably than other scales of skeletal maturity (Risser sign and chronologic age). Peak height velocity is believed to be a better predictor of spinal growth in patients with delayed menarche. The risk of progression in patients with thoracic curves between 20° to 29° in girls (Risser stages 0 to 1) has been reported to be 68%, and it decreases to 23% in patients with advanced skeletal maturity (Risser stages 2 to 4). Curves with apex above the T12 level have a higher risk of progression compared with lumbar curves. Family history, degree of rotation, and gender do not tend to help predict progression. The determination of cessation of spinal growth is less predictable in males than in females. Closure of the triradiate cartilage on radiographs approximates the timing of peak height or growth velocity in males.

After skeletal maturity is achieved, several factors contribute to the risk of curve progression, which on average progresses 1° per year. Thoracic curves greater than 50°, and thoracolumbar and lumbar curves greater than 30° have been reported in long-term natural history studies to have the highest risk of curve progression.

A recent study reported the health and function of 117 patients with scoliosis who were treated without surgery. At 50-year follow-up, increased chronic back pain was reported in these patients when compared with a matched cohort group (61% and 35%, respectively). The average thoracic curve at skeletal maturity was 60°, and at follow-up it was 85°. However, most patients (68%) reported the pain to be mild. A trend was noted toward increased shortness of breath with activities, although this was not statistically significant. The increased shortness of breath was associated with an increased Cobb angle (> 80°) and having the curve apex in the thoracic region.

### History

A thorough history and physical examination of the patient with adolescent idiopathic scoliosis is important to rule out other known causes of scoliosis, to determine the patient's degree of skeletal maturity and growth remaining, and to determine if other diagnostic studies or consultations are needed. Obtaining an accurate history from the patient and family often will address many of these concerns. Patients may be referred because of a positive school screening result or for back pain. Severe back pain associated with scoliosis may suggest an underlying cause and should be differentiated from a more common fatigue-related pain. Evaluating the severity, duration, and character of a patient's pain may aid in this determination.

Other symptoms suggestive of an underlying neurologic cause such as weakness, balance or coordination concerns, or incontinence may require further diagnostic and imaging studies. Diseases associated with scoliosis, such as Charcot-Marie-Tooth disease, will often be elicited from a family history. A positive family history of idiopathic scoliosis is not predictive for the risk of scoliosis progression.

The distinction between juvenile and adolescent idiopathic scoliosis (before or after age 10 years) can be difficult to discern, and inquiring about age of onset is important. Often, the onset of scoliosis before the age of 10 years by itself may be a manifestation of an underlying neural axis abnormality. Rapid progression of scoliosis may also identify nonidiopathic forms of scoliosis. The age at onset of menarche in females, along with radiographic determinants of skeletal maturity and peak height velocity, provides information to assess the amount of growth remaining and the risk of progression.

### Physical Examination

The physical examination must also be comprehensive and not limited to the evaluation of the spinal deformity alone. A thorough neurologic examination includes the assessment of gait. It should be determined whether the patient is able to walk on the heels and toes, demon-

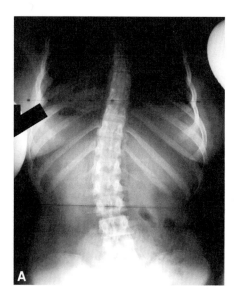
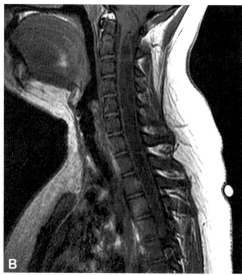

Figure 3 **A,** PA radiograph of a 13-year-old girl with tight hamstrings on physical examination. **B,** MRI demonstrating Arnold-Chiari type I malformation and syringomyelia.

strate a tandem walk, perform a deep knee bend or squat, or do a single-leg hop. Balance can also be tested by performing a Romberg test. Motor strength of all four extremities should be assessed, as well as deep tendon reflexes, clonus, and the presence of hyperreflexia. Charcot-Marie-Tooth disease may present in patients with absent deep tendon reflexes, cavus feet, and a kyphotic deformity in addition to scoliosis. Asymmetry of the superficial cutaneous abdominal reflex has been shown to be sensitive for the presence of syringomyelia.

Observing the patient erect and discretely clothed allows for the assessment of trunk balance, shoulder height, scapula prominence, paraspinal asymmetry or prominence, and flank crease asymmetry. An unequal iliac crest height may indicate an underlying limb-length discrepancy and may contribute to a postural scoliosis. The posterior midline skin must be examined for cutaneous stigmata such as dimples or tufts of hair that may indicate an underlying neural axis abnormality. The Tanner stages of pubertal development provide additional information in assessing growth remaining and risk of progression. Height measurements at each subsequent visit enable the peak height velocity to be determined.

The presence of asymmetric thigh or calf circumference or a unilateral cavovarus foot may be as sensitive as MRI in detecting an underlying spinal cord abnormality. The general physical examination should also include an assessment of joint laxity and possible elongated anatomic proportions to rule out the presence of Marfan syndrome or other connective tissue disorders. The identification of café-au-lait spots and/or axillary freckling is highly suggestive of neurofibromatosis. The forward bend test requires the patient to bend forward at the waist with the knees fully extended and palms together. The spine should also be evaluated from behind the patient, in front of the patient (to identify high thoracic rotational asymmetry), and from the side to iden-

**Table 1 | Classification of Scoliosis**

Idiopathic
Neuropathic
Congenital
Mesenchymal (Marfan syndrome or other connective tissue disorders)
Neurofibromatosis
Neural tube defects
Metabolic
Osteochondrodystrophies
Miscellaneous (tumor, infection, or traumatic)
Thoracogenic
Functional

tify a prominent kyphotic sagittal plane deformity. Range of motion and flexibility of the spine can also be evaluated. Limited range of motion of the spine (caused by hamstring tightness) and deviation of the trunk to one side upon forward bending may represent an underlying pathology such as spondylolisthesis or spinal cord abnormality (Figure 3).

*Differential Diagnosis*

The diagnosis of adolescent idiopathic scoliosis requires the exclusion of known causes of nonidiopathic scoliosis, and a comprehensive examination will often rule these out or suggest the need for further diagnostic studies. Most instances of scoliosis at this time and with the present level of diagnostic sophistication are idiopathic (80% of patients), and the list of causes of scoliosis defined by the Scoliosis Research Society is extensive (Table 1). Patients may present with a reactive scoliosis secondary to an underlying painful condition such as a tumor, infection, or spondylolysis. Scoliosis will often resolve or not progress once the primary process is addressed.

## Diagnostic Testing

The initial or screening radiograph should be a standing PA view on a long 36-inch cassette to include the entire thoracolumbar spine and pelvis. A limb-length discrepancy greater than or equal to 2 cm noted on clinical examination should be corrected using a lift to level the pelvis and eliminate a potential postural component of the scoliosis. Lateral radiographs should be obtained in patients with back pain or in those in whom a sagittal plane deformity is detected clinically. The radiographs should be used to assess for curve pattern, magnitude, location, trunk balance, and skeletal maturity.

Curve magnitudes are quantified by the Cobb angle measurement. Intraobserver and interobserver error has been reported to range from 5° to 10° and is better when the end vertebrae have been preselected, which highlights the importance of consistent end vertebrae selection with serial radiographs. Skeletal maturity is most commonly evaluated by the Risser stage of ossification of the iliac apophyses. Additional radiographic markers include the closure of the triradiate cartilage and the greater trochanteric apophysis to help determine the degree of skeletal maturity.

MRI has been an invaluable diagnostic imaging technique for identifying spinal cord abnormalities that manifest scoliosis, including Arnold-Chiari malformations, tethered cord, split cord malformations, syringomyelia, hydromyelia, and intraspinal lipomas. The role of MRI in diagnosing juvenile scoliosis is firmly established, but the indications for using MRI in diagnosing adolescent idiopathic scoliosis continue to evolve. If obtained, MRI scans should extend from the brain stem to the lumbar spine with proper sequences and orientation.

Several retrospective studies have assessed clinical and radiographic criteria or variables that may be associated with an underlying neural axis abnormality. In a multicenter study of 41 patients with Arnold-Chiari type I malformation and/or syringomyelia, a high prevalence (51%) of typical radiographic curve patterns (left thoracic, double thoracic, triple, and a long right thoracic curve with end vertebrae distal to T12) and high or low apex and/or end vertebrae were noted. Sagittal plane deformities (in particular the lack of apical thoracic lordosis) may be highly suggestive of the presence of an underlying syringomyelia. A high index of suspicion should also be maintained for male patients with these atypical scoliosis curve patterns. Identification and, when possible, treatment of these neural axis abnormalities may improve or prevent progression of the spinal deformity. Preoperative identification may decrease the risk of intraoperative neurologic complications and mandate the use of titanium spinal instrumentation to allow for future diagnostic imaging.

Patients with pain associated with a spinal deformity may require other diagnostic imaging modalities, depending on and directed by their clinical examination findings. Neoplasms, infection, or spondylolysis should always be considered in these patients. Bone scanning is a sensitive screening diagnostic modality and should be considered before MRI or CT.

Bending films are obtained preoperatively to assess flexibility of the primary and compensatory curves, disk space mobility, and to select levels of spinal instrumentation. The Lenke classification uses bending films to differentiate structural versus nonstructural curves. Supine lateral bending films have been the gold standard, but several other techniques, including fulcrum bending, traction, and push-prone radiographs have been reported. Maximum coronal flexibility using the fulcrum bend technique has been reported to be best for patients with primary thoracic curves, and side bending views have been reported to be best for those with upper thoracic and thoracolumbar curves. The push-prone technique has been advocated to most accurately reflect the effect that correction of the primary curve has on the compensatory curves above and below the fused structural curve; it also best predicts the translation correction and rotation of the lowest instrumented vertebrae.

## Nonsurgical Treatment

The short- and long-term natural history of a disease such as scoliosis should be fully understood to ensure that the treatment affects its natural history in a positive manner. Many types of nonsurgical treatment, including exercise, manipulation, and electrical stimulation have been shown to be no more effective than the natural history of scoliosis. Bracing has been shown to be the only form of nonsurgical treatment that is more effective than the natural history of scoliosis, and its use is widely accepted despite healthy skepticism regarding its efficacy. In a nonrandomized prospective study, bracing was successful (defined as < 5° of progression) in 74% of patients compared with 34% of patients without bracing and 33% of patients who underwent electrical stimulation.

The goal of bracing is to prevent progression of scoliosis until skeletal maturity is reached. The indications for brace treatment include spine curves greater than 25° to 45° on initial presentation, spine curves greater than 20° with documented progression, patients with significant growth remaining (Risser stages 0 to 2), and patients with significant spinal decompensation. Relative contraindications for orthotic device treatment include patients with thoracic lordosis. Orthotic device decisions must be individualized for each patient. Higher rates of failure are noted with younger patients, male patients, and in patients with pretreatment curves greater than 40°. Success with brace treatment is defined as 5° or less of progression.

Criteria for successful brace treatment include the amount of correction achieved while the patient is in the brace and the amount of time the brace is worn each day. Part-time bracing (16 hours per day) was formerly advocated to be as effective as full-time bracing. A recent meta-analysis study demonstrated a dose-dependent correlation with the amount of time the brace is worn and preventing progression of scoliosis. Compliance with brace treatment calls into question its effectiveness. A recent study analyzed compliance with brace wear using a skin-brace temperature gauge. The authors found that the average compliance with brace wear was 65% (range, 8% to 90%) and that patients overestimated compliance by 150%.

Monitoring patients and the frequency of follow-up during orthotic device treatment primarily depends on the age and growth of the patient. A dedicated team approach involving the orthotist, nursing staff, physical therapists, and the patient's family are critical to improving the compliance and success of brace treatment.

## Surgical Treatment

The degree of skeletal maturity, curve magnitude, and location or pattern of scoliosis determines the risk of progression and natural history of adolescent scoliosis. In a skeletally immature patient, curves greater than 40° meet the indications for surgical intervention. Because the presence of an open triradiate cartilage indicates an increased risk for the crankshaft phenomenon, surgery may be delayed in such patients. In children who have reached skeletal maturity, the indications for surgery include thoracic curves greater than 50°, thoracolumbar or lumbar curves greater than 40° with increased apical rotation or translation, double major curves greater than 50°, and curves creating severe imbalance.

The goals of surgical treatment have remained constant despite evolving concepts, techniques, and approaches for scoliosis. Treatment must achieve a solid arthrodesis and prevent progression of the spinal deformity. Attention to the time-honored concepts of thorough facetectomies, decortication, and bone grafting are important to achieve a fusion. Preserving distal motion segments, maintaining balance and alignment in both the coronal and sagittal planes, and achieving correction of the deformity in all three planes are the other key objectives of surgical management.

## Classification

The King-Moe classification for thoracic adolescent idiopathic scoliosis describes five curve patterns based on coronal radiographs. This classification scheme was developed in part to identify specific curve patterns (type II) that were amenable to selective thoracic fusion using Harrington distraction instrumentation and to thereby preserve distal motion segments. This classification system remains the gold standard for adolescent idiopathic scoliosis.

Limitations of the King-Moe classification scheme were noted in part when derotational and multiplanar corrective techniques were used. The problem of coronal decompensation or imbalance was frequently reported after selective fusion of patients with King-Moe type II curve patterns. Other limitations of the King-Moe classification scheme include its inability to account for many of the curve patterns observed in patients with adolescent idiopathic scoliosis and poor intraobserver and interobserver reliability.

The Lenke classification system (Figure 4), now commonly used, was developed in response to these concerns. The intended goals of this classification system are to be comprehensive, two-dimensional, treatment based, able to recommend selective fusions when appropriate, and have better intraobserver and interobserver reliability. This triad classification system comprises six curve patterns, three lumbar modifiers, and a sagittal alignment modifier. The system uses curve magnitude and flexibility based on bending radiographs, deviation of the lumbar curve from the center sacral vertical line, and the sagittal alignment to provide a framework to determine fusion levels.

### Preoperative Evaluation and Planning

The comprehensive framework of the Lenke classification system refocuses attention on preserving motion of the spine and helps identify scoliosis patterns that are amenable for selective thoracic fusion within the context of newer approaches and techniques, such as anterior instrumentation and thoracic pedicle screw instrumentation. Many of the previously published guidelines for the selection of instrumented end vertebrae and the application of corrective forces were primarily used for posterior segmental instrumentation. The guidelines for anterior instrumentation and thoracic pedicle screw instrumentation continue to evolve.

In general, the patient evaluation should evaluate shoulder balance, flank crease asymmetry, paraspinal asymmetry or rotation, and sagittal contour. The end vertebrae, neutral vertebrae, and the apical vertebrae for each curve are determined from the weight-bearing PA radiograph. Cobb angle measurements are made of the primary and compensatory or nonstructural curves. The ratios of each of these measures help in deciding which curves are appropriate for selective fusions (those > 25%), particularly false double major curves (King-Moe type II or Lenke type 1). The Lenke classification differentiates primary curves from minor compensatory curves depending on the bending radiographs (< 25°). The lateral radiograph helps determine whether a junctional kyphosis is present in the proximal thoracic region

## Curve Type

| Type | Proximal Thoracic | Main Thoracic | Thoracolumbar/ Lumbar | Curve Type |
|---|---|---|---|---|
| 1 | Nonstructural | Structural (Major*) | Nonstructural | Main Thoracic (MT) |
| 2 | Structural | Structural (Major*) | Nonstructural | Double Thoracic (DT) |
| 3 | Nonstructural | Structural (Major*) | Structural | Double Major (DM) |
| 4 | Structural | Structural (Major*) | Structural | Triple Major (TM) |
| 5 | Nonstructural | Nonstructural | Structural (Major*) | Thoracolumbar/Lumbar (TL/L) |
| 6 | Nonstructural | Structural | Structural (Major*) | Main Thoracic (TL/L - MT) |

**STRUCTURAL CRITERIA**
(Minor Curves)

*Proximal Thoracic:* - Side Bending Cobb ≥ 25°
       - T2 - T5 Kyphosis ≥ +20°

*Main Thoracic:* - Side Bending Cobb ≥ 25°
       - T10 - L2 Kyphosis ≥ +20°

*Thoracolumbar/Lumbar:* - Side Bending Cobb ≥ 25°
       - T10 - L2 Kyphosis ≥ +20°

*Major = Largest Cobb Measurement, always structural
Minor = all other curvs with structural criteria applied

**LOCATION OF APEX**
(SRS definition)

| CURVE | APEX |
|---|---|
| Thoracic | T2 - T11-12 disk |
| Thoracolumbar | T12 - I1 |
| Lumbar | L1-2 disk - L4 |

## Modifiers

| Lumbar Spine Modifier | CSVL to Lumbar Apex | | | | Thoracic Sagittal Profile T5 - T12 | | |
|---|---|---|---|---|---|---|---|
| A | CSVL Between Pedicles | | | | — | (Hypo) | (< 10° |
| B | CSVL Touches Apical Body(ies) | 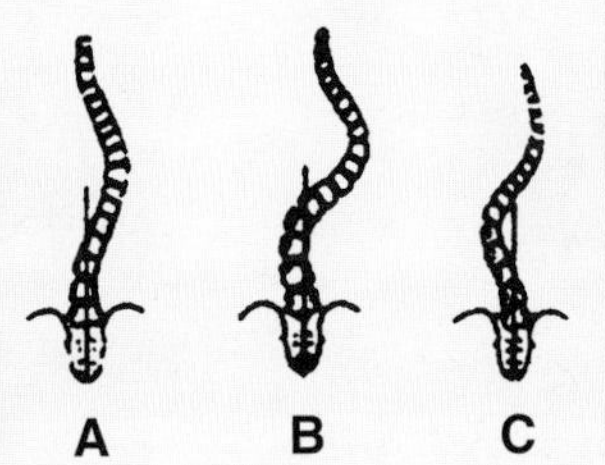 A | B | C | N | (Normal) | 10° - 40° |
| C | CSVL Completely Medial | | | | + | (Hyper) | > 40° |

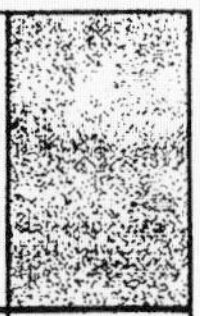

Curve Type (1-6) + Lumbar Spine Modifier (A, B, or C) + Thoracic Sagittal Modifier (–, N, or +)

**Classification (eg, 1B+):** _____

**Figure 4** The Lenke classification for adolescent idiopathic scoliosis. SRS = Scoliosis Research Society, CSVL = central sacral vertical line. *(Reproduced with permission from Lenke LG, Betz RR, Harms J, et al: Adolescent idiopathic scoliosis: A new classification to determine extent of spinal arthrodesis.* J Bone Joint Surg Am *2001;83:1169-1181.)*

or at the thoracolumbar junction. All primary curves and minor structural curves, as well as sagittal plane junctional deformities should be included in the fusion. The lower instrumented vertebrae has generated considerable controversy, in particular for patients with King-Moe type II or Lenke type 1 curve patterns. It can be quite difficult to determine whether to preserve motion and accept a considerable degree of residual deformity of both curves to maintain coronal balance in a selective thoracic fusion or improve correction of both curves with a longer distal fusion at the expense of motion.

### Posterior Instrumentation
Pedicle screw fixation, initially used in the lumbar spine to treat scoliosis, demonstrated significant advantages in the correction of deformity, rotation, and the ability to save motion segments compared with hook fixation. Pedicle screw instrumentation in the thoracic spine using translation correction or direct vertebral rotation

techniques is being used with increasing frequency in North America (Figure 5). Proponents of thoracic pedicle screw instrumentation cite several advantages for its use. It is a significantly more rigid instrumentation system in that it addresses all three columns of the spine. Preliminary anterior release was formerly advocated for patients with severe rigid thoracic curves greater than 75° that did not correct to less than 50° on bending radiographs. The power of the instrumentation may decrease the need for concomitant anterior release in skeletally immature patients who are at risk for the crankshaft phenomenon and for those with severe deformities (up to 90°); it may also decrease the number of motion segments fused. Apical vertebral rotation with thoracic pedicle screws may decrease the need for convex thoracoplasty and may improve the three-dimensional correction of the spinal deformity. Avoiding the chest cavity with either an anterior approach or thoracoplasty may optimize pulmonary function.

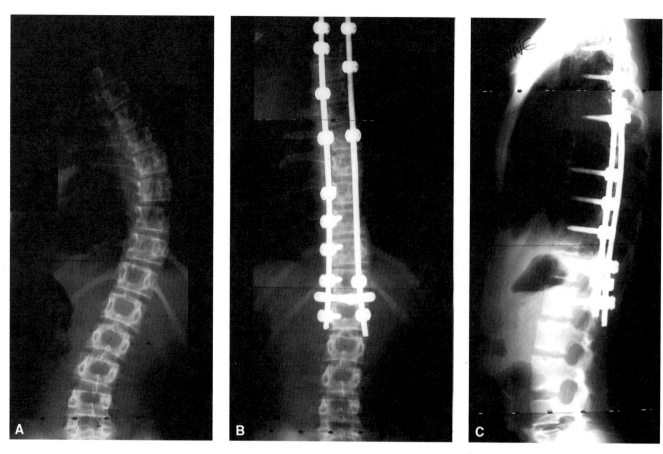

Figure 5 **A,** Preoperative PA radiograph of an 11-year-old girl with double thoracic scoliosis or Lenke type 2 curve pattern. Postoperative PA **(B)** and lateral **(C)** radiographs of the same patient with pedicle screw instrumentation and lowest instrumented vertebrae at L1.

Critics of thoracic pedicle screw fixation to treat spinal deformity point out the potential neurologic, vascular, and visceral risks of improperly placed pedicle screws. The small size and orientation of the thoracic pedicles, in particular on the concave side of the scoliosis deformity, can make screw placement technically challenging and requires precise placement to avoid penetration and potential complications. Lateral penetration of the pedicle screw places the tip in close proximity to the aorta, and medial penetration places the tip within the spinal canal. The freehand technique has been shown to be quite safe at one major spine center. The use of C-arm fluoroscopy and triggered electromyographic monitoring of the rectus abdominis muscle for T6-T12 pedicle screw insertion have been advocated to identify and minimize these risks. The cost-benefit ratio of pedicle screw instrumentation (compared with hook/wire anchors) also has not been demonstrated to date. The expense of thoracic pedicle screws at multiple levels was noted to be almost double the cost of hook implants for a standard scoliosis construct. Despite showing improvement in the degree of spinal deformity correction, it is still unclear whether this correlates with a measurable improvement in clinical outcomes. Despite the cost and safety concerns of thoracic pedicle screw fixation, this powerful technique of spinal deformity correction offers many potential advantages in the hands of experienced spinal surgeons. Long-term studies may provide answers regarding the efficacy of this technique.

### Anterior Instrumentation

Anterior instrumentation is indicated for patients with primary thoracic curves and thoracolumbar curves, with the goal to save two or more levels compared with that predicted using posterior instrumentation (Figure 6). Fusion levels tend to extend from the proximal to the distal end vertebrae as measured by the Cobb angle. Potential advantages of the anterior approach include avoiding disruption of the posterior extensor musculature, decreased risk of junctional problems, superior long-term correction of the compensatory noninstrumented curves with less postoperative coronal decompensation, and better correction of thoracic hypokyphosis. The anterior approach is also indicated for skeletally immature patients (those with open triradiate cartilage) at risk for the crankshaft phenomenon. The contraindications for this anterior approach include significant

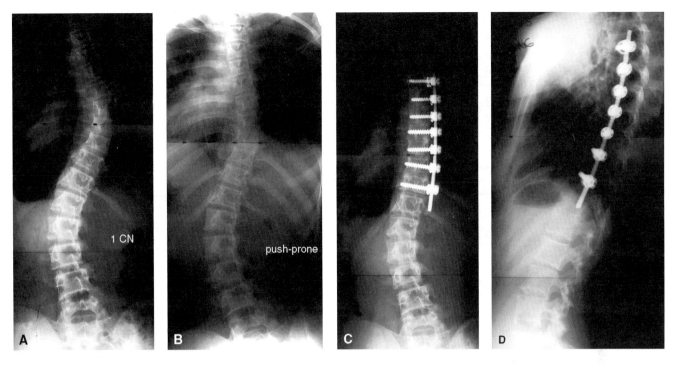

**Figure 6** Preoperative PA **(A)** and push-prone **(B)** radiographs of a 12-year-old girl with Lenke 1CN curve pattern. **C,** Postoperative PA **(C)** and lateral **(D)** radiographs demonstrating selective thoracic fusion with anterior thoracic instrumentation.

preoperative kyphosis (> 40°), curves greater than 75° to 80°, impaired respiratory function (vital capacity < 50%), and double or triple structural curves. Historical complications with anterior instrumentation included rod breakage, pull-out of the proximal screw, pseudarthrosis, and kyphosis. These complications have been addressed with the use of larger rods and structural grafts and spacers to provide anterior column reconstruction and maintain lordosis for thoracolumbar curves. Stability of the proximal screw is achieved with eccentric insertion in the superior one third of the vertebral body, use of one to two washers, and bicortical purchase. Newer trends in anterior instrumentation also include the use of dual rod instrumentation.

The role of minimally invasive video-assisted thoracoscopic surgery for anterior release and instrumentation of single thoracic curves continues to progress. The technique is technically challenging, has a steep learning curve, but is believed to result in decreased chest wall and pulmonary function morbidity. Patients traditionally are positioned in the lateral position for thoracoscopic procedures. Prone positioning is gaining favor because it eliminates the need to change patient positioning if an anterior release is performed before a posterior instrumentation; moreover, the prone position avoids the potential problems of single-lung ventilation. Recent studies evaluating the results of open versus thoracoscopic anterior instrumentation have demonstrated comparable rates of correction. A trend toward more rapid re-

turn of shoulder girdle function in the video-assisted thoracoscopic surgery group has been cited.

A potential concern with anterior thoracic instrumentation is the close proximity of the vertebral screws to vital structures such as the aorta. Postoperative CT scans were evaluated in one study to evaluate the location of the screws to the spinal canal and the aorta. The screws were believed to create a contour deformity of the aorta with 12% of the screws, and an additional 14% were adjacent to the aorta. In a related study from the same institution, the position of the aorta relative to the spine was compared in patients with a right thoracic scoliosis to normal patients using MRI and plain radiography. The aorta was found to be positioned more lateral and posterior relative to the vertebral body at the T5-T12 levels in patients with scoliosis compared with normal patients. This was more distinct near the apical regions of the curve, with increasing coronal Cobb angles, and with increased apical vertebral rotation. These findings highlight the need for careful placement of anterior vertebral screws or concave posterior pedicle screws in patients with a right thoracic idiopathic scoliosis to minimize the risk of vascular, neurologic, or visceral complications.

## Acknowledgment

Dr. Akbarnia would like to acknowledge Sarah Canale, BS, for her assistance with manuscript preparation.

## Annotated Bibliography
### Infantile and Juvenile Idiopathic Scoliosis

Akbarnia BA, Marks DS, Boachie-Adjei O, Thompson AG, Asher MA: Dual growing rod technique for the treatment of progressive early-onset scoliosis: A multicenter study. *Spine* 2005;30(17S):S46-S57.

The authors present the initial results of the dual growing rod technique in the treatment of 23 patients with progressive early onset scoliosis. The technique is shown to preserve the initial scoliosis correction throughout treatment and permit continued growth of the spine.

Betz RR, Kim J, D'Andrea LP, Mulcahey MJ, Balsara RK, Clements DH: An innovative technique of vertebral body stapling for the treatment of patients with adolescent idiopathic scoliosis: A feasibility, safety, and utility study. *Spine* 2003;28:S255-S265.

The efficacy and safety of vertebral body stapling in stabilizing curves was demonstrated in 21 patients with adolescent idiopathic scoliosis. Initial critiques call for better staple design, placement near the end plates, and control of all curves.

Blakemore LC, Scoles PV, Poe-Kochert C, Thompson GH: Submuscular Isola rod with or without limited apical fusion in the management of severe spinal deformities in young children: Preliminary report. *Spine* 2001;26:2044-2048.

In this study, 29 children with progressive scoliosis and kyphoscoliosis were treated with submuscular single rod instrumentation with and without apical fusion. Although balance improved, spinal growth was minimal, and no additional deformity correction was observed after initial surgery and with subsequent distractions.

Campbell RM, Smith MD, Mayes TC, et al: The characteristics of thoracic insufficiency syndrome associated with fused ribs and congenital scoliosis. *J Bone Joint Surg Am* 2003;85-A:399-408.

The clinical indications, space available for the lungs, radiography, and three-dimensional CT to diagnose thoracic insufficiency syndrome are discussed. Evaluation of pulmonary compromise associated with thoracic deformity is important in the treatment of congenital scoliosis with fused ribs.

Dobbs MB, Lenke LG, Szymanski DA, et al: Prevalence of neural axis abnormalities in patients with infantile idiopathic scoliosis. *J Bone Joint Surg Am* 2002;84-A:2230-2234.

The authors of this study reported that the incidence of neural axis abnormalities in infantile idiopathic scoliosis was 21.7%, which is similar to the prevalence in juvenile idiopathic scoliosis in previous reports. Total spine MRI is recommended for all patients with infantile idiopathic scoliosis who have a curve that is 20° or greater.

Thompson GH, Akbarnia BA, Kostial P, et al: Comparison of single and dual growing rod techniques followed through definitive surgery: A preliminary study. *Spine* 2005;30:2039-2044.

Submuscular single and subcutaneous dual growing rods with and without apical fusion were compared in the treatment of patients with progressive scoliosis. Dual rods were shown to be more effective in maintaining correction and encouraging growth. The authors advised against using apical fusions with growing rod instrumentation.

### Adolescent Idiopathic Scoliosis

Lee SM, Suk SI, Chung ER: Direct vertebral rotation: A new technique of three-dimensional deformity correction with segmental pedicle screw fixation in adolescent idiopathic scoliosis. *Spine* 2004;29:343-349.

This prospective study was conducted to compare the new technique of direct vertebral rotation and simple rod rotation. Statistically significant differences were noted in coronal curve correction, lowest instrumented vertebra tilt, and rotational correction with the direct vertebral rotation technique.

Lenke LG, Betz RR, Harms J, et al: Adolescent idiopathic scoliosis: A new classification to determine extent of spinal arthrodesis. *J Bone Joint Surg Am* 2001;83:1169-1181.

The authors presented a comprehensive classification of adolescent idiopathic scoliosis based on three components, six curve patterns, three lumbar modifiers, and a sagittal thoracic modifier. The intraobserver and interobserver reliability of this new two-dimensional classification scheme was found to be more reliable than those of the King-Moe classification system for adolescent idiopathic scoliosis.

Lenke LG, Edwards CC II, Bridwell KH: The Lenke classification of adolescent idiopathic scoliosis: How it organizes curve patterns as a template to perform selective fusions of the spine. *Spine* 2003;28:S199-S207.

This retrospective study evaluated the results of using the Lenke classification for adolescent idiopathic scoliosis, specifically for its utility of determining selective fusions. Clinical and radiographic criteria are outlined for selective patterns of thoracic and thoracolumbar scoliosis. Instrumentation techniques are discussed to obtain major curve correction and allow for minor curve correction and coronal balance.

Lowe TG, Betz R, Lenke L: Anterior single-rod instrumentation of the thoracic and lumbar spine: Saving levels. *Spine* 2003;28:S208-S216.

The authors of this review article discuss the utility of anterior single-rod instrumentation in the treatment of specific curve patterns described by the Lenke classification system. The authors noted that one to three distal fusion levels will often be saved when treating isolated thoracic, thoracolumbar, or lumbar curves. They also reported that anterior single-rod instrumentation predictably corrects hypokyphosis of the thoracic spine.

Newton PO, Marks M, Faro F, et al: Use of video-assisted thorascopic surgery to reduce perioperative morbidity in scoliosis surgery. *Spine* 2003;28:S249-S254.

The authors of this retrospective case study compared video-assisted thorascopic surgery and open anterior instrumentation for the treatment of adolescent idiopathic scoliosis. Perioperative and early postoperative outcomes were compared. The authors reported that the radiographic outcomes were similar for the two groups. The minimally invasive approach was noted to have reduced chest wall morbidity, but the authors found that it took longer to perform compared with the open approach.

Ouellet JA, LaPlaza J, Erickson MA, et al: Sagittal plane deformity in the thoracic spine: A clue to the presence of syringomyelia as a cause of scoliosis. *Spine* 2003;28: 2147-2151.

In this retrospective review of 93 patients with idiopathic or syringomyelia-associated scoliosis, the authors assessed radiographs for the presence or absence of thoracic apical lordosis. They noted that thoracic apical lordosis was present in 97% of patients with adolescent idiopathic scoliosis, but absent in 75% of patients with syringomyelia-related scoliosis.

Spiegel DA, Flynn JM, Stasikelis PJ: Scoliotic curve pattern in patients with Chiari I malformations and/or syringomyelia. *Spine* 2003;28:2139-2146.

The authors of this retrospective review of scoliosis curve patterns in 41 patients with Arnold-Chiari I malformations and/or syringomyelia reported that 50% of patients had atypical curve patterns or abnormal features (shift of apical vertebral or upper/lower end vertebrae) in normal curve patterns. They concluded that MRI should be considered in patients with these atypical curve patterns, in male patients, or patients with normal or hyperkyphotic thoracic spines.

Sucato DJ, Duchene C: The position of the aorta relative to the spine: A comparison of patients with and without idiopathic scoliosis. *J Bone Joint Surg Am* 2003; 85:1461-1469.

The authors of this MRI study of patients with adolescent idiopathic scoliosis noted an increased lateral and posterior position of the descending aorta compared with patients without spinal deformity. These findings highlight the need for careful placement of anterior vertebral or concave posterior pedicle screws in patients with a right thoracic idiopathic scoliosis to minimize the risk of vascular, neurologic, or visceral complications.

Weinstein SL, Dolan LA, Spratt KF, et al: Health and function of patients with untreated idiopathic scoliosis: A 50-year natural history study. *JAMA* 2003;289:559-567.

The authors updated their prospective report of 117 patients with adolescent idiopathic scoliosis who were treated without surgery at 50-year follow-up. Compared with a matched cohort, these patients were noted to have a higher incidence of chronic back pain. The average thoracic curve at skeletal maturity was 60°, and at follow-up it was 85°. The authors noted an increased trend toward shortness of breath with activities.

## Classic Bibliography

Akbarnia BA, Marks DS: Instrumentation with limited arthrodesis for the treatment of progressive early-onset scoliosis. *Spine* 2000;14:181-189.

Cobb JR: Scoliosis: Quo vadis? *J Bone Joint Surg Am* 1958;40:507-510.

Dubousset J, Herring JA, Shufflebarger H: The crankshaft phenomenon. *J Pediatr Orthop* 1989;9:541-550.

Gupta P, Lenke LG, Bridwell KH: Incidence of neural axis abnormalities in infantile and juvenile patients with spinal deformity: Is a magnetic resonance image screening necessary? *Spine* 1998;23:206-210.

King HA, Moe JH, Bradford DS, et al: The selection of fusion levels in thoracic idiopathic scoliosis. *J Bone Joint Surg Am* 1983;65:1302-1313.

Klemme WR, Denis F, Winter RB, Lonstein JW, Koop SE: Spinal instrumentation without fusion for progressive scoliosis in young children. *J Pediatr Orthop* 1997; 17:734-742.

Lenke LG, Bridwell KH, Baldus C, et al: Preventing decompensation in King type II curves treated with Cotrel-Dubousset instrumentation: Strict guidelines for selective thoracic fusion. *Spine* 1992;17:S274-S281.

Little DG, Song KM, Katz D, et al: Relationship of peak height velocity to other maturity indicators in idiopathic scoliosis in girls. *J Bone Joint Surg Am* 2000;82:685-693.

Lonstein JE, Carlson JM: The prediction of curve progression in untreated idiopathic scoliosis during growth. *J Bone Joint Surg Am* 1984;66:1061-1071.

Luque ER, Cardosa A: Segmental spinal instrumentation in growing children. *Orthop Trans* 1977;1:37.

Mardjetko SM, Hammerberg KW, Lubicky JP, Fister JS: The Luque trolley revisited: Review of nine cases requiring revision. *Spine* 1992;17:582-589.

Marks DS, Iqbal MJ, Thompson AG, Piggott H: Convex spinal epiphysiodesis in the management of progressive infantile idiopathic scoliosis. *Spine* 1996;21:1884-1888.

Mehta MH: The rib-vertebra angle in the early diagnosis between resolving and progressive infantile scoliosis. *J Bone Joint Surg Br* 1972;54:230-243.

Moe JH, Kharrat K, Winter RB, Cummine JL: Harrington instrumentation without fusion plus external orthotic support for the treatment of difficult curvature problems in young children. *Clin Orthop Relat Res* 1984; 185:35-45.

Nachemson AL, Peterson LE: Effectiveness of treatment with a brace in girls who have adolescent idiopathic scoliosis: A prospective, controlled study based on data from The Brace Study of the Scoliosis Research Society. *J Bone Joint Surg Am* 1995;77:815-822.

Rogala EJ, Drummond DS, Gurr J: Scoliosis: Incidence and natural history: A prospective epidemiological study. *J Bone Joint Surg Am* 1978;60:173-176.

Vedantam R, Lenke LG, Bridwell KH, et al: Comparison of push-prone and lateral bending radiographs for predicting postoperative coronal alignment in thoracolumbar and lumbar scoliotic curves. *Spine* 2000;25:76-81.

Weinstein SL, Ponseti IV: Curve progression in idiopathic scoliosis. *J Bone Joint Surg Am* 1983;65:447-455.

Wynne-Davies R: Infantile idiopathic scoliosis: Causative factors, particularly in the first six months of life. *J Bone Joint Surg Br* 1975;57:138-141.

# Chapter 47

# Neuromuscular Scoliosis

Freeman Miller, MD

Kirk W. Dabney, MD

## Introduction

Spinal deformity occurs as a result of an abnormality in the neuromuscular system in childhood. The pathologic abnormalities of the neuromuscular system present in different patterns, including conditions related to muscle tone and motor control, muscle weakness, or paralysis.

Children with problems related to motor control and muscle tone most commonly have cerebral palsy. The most common pattern of cerebral palsy that develops into spinal deformity is severe quadriplegic pattern involvement in children with no ability for independent seating. Spinal deformity is relatively uncommon in children who are able to ambulate. The most common spinal deformity that develops in these children is a typical neuromuscular scoliosis; however, many different patterns of spinal deformity may develop. These nonambulatory children often have several comorbidities including seizures, gastroesophageal reflux, chronic aspiration, poor nutrition, and delayed growth.

Conditions causing muscle weakness (with pathology primarily involving the muscles) include Duchenne muscular dystrophy and spinal muscular atrophy. Spinal curves in patients with Duchenne muscular dystrophy typically develop during adolescence, starting with mild hyperlordosis that later results in a general kyphosis and scoliosis with varying degrees of pelvic obliquity. The major comorbid condition related to Duchenne muscular dystrophy is a restrictive type of pulmonary involvement, with a dramatic drop in forced vital capacity. Forced vital capacity should be monitored along with the radiographs of the spine. Children with spinal muscular atrophy also experience a decrease in respiratory function, but this condition is usually more specifically related to weakness and less to a restrictive component. The second comorbid condition in the myopathies that has to be monitored is the possibility of cardiomyopathy or cardioconduction defects.

The paralytic syndromes include childhood spinal cord injury; however, this category also includes poliomyelitis. Children who develop paralysis after the adolescent growth spurt are at very low risk for developing spinal deformity. However, the development of scoliosis is almost universal in those children who develop a high thoracic or cervical spinal cord injury before the age of 8 years. The major comorbid conditions to monitor in children with paralysis are the possibility of hyperreflexia and chronic urinary conditions, especially chronic urinary infections.

## Natural History

The natural history of neuromuscular scoliosis for most conditions includes the slow development of flexible scoliosis in middle childhood with the rapid development of more severe fixed scoliotic deformities during the adolescent growth spurt. Often the scoliosis includes a significant component of kyphosis and lordosis, and some children have a primary sagittal plane deformity. The natural history of these sagittal plane deformities is less well defined and less predictable. Progression of the scoliosis is common in both cerebral palsy and Duchenne muscular dystrophy. The rate of progression is 1° to 2° per month starting at age 8 to 10 years; however, progression of more than 4° per month often occurs during the year of most rapid adolescent growth. Some children with cerebral palsy or a congenital type of cerebral palsy may develop curves very early (before age 8 years) and need to be treated between the ages of 4 and 6 years. Also, children with severe spinal muscular atrophy may develop severe spinal deformities that start to become fixed deformities between the ages of 6 and 8 years. Almost all paralytic curves remain flexible and do not develop a large magnitude (greater than 90°) until the adolescent growth spurt. Data on progression of neuromuscular scoliosis in adulthood are limited but evidence exists that there is a significant incidence of progression if the scoliosis is more than 30° at the end of growth. There are no data on change of kyphosis or lordosis in adulthood.

## Treatment

The nonsurgical treatment of neuromuscular scoliosis has involved multiple attempts at orthotic management

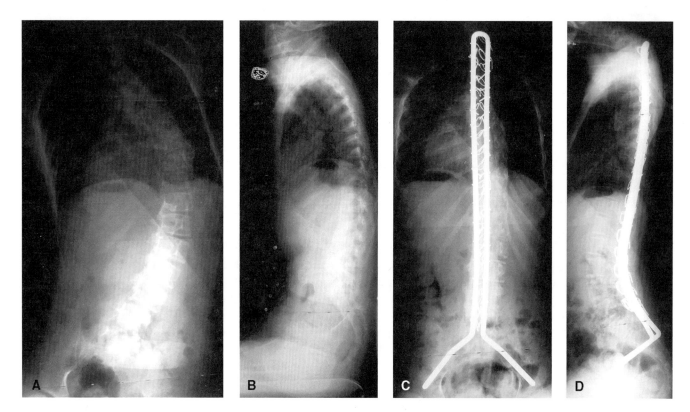

**Figure 1** **A,** Neuromuscular scoliosis in cerebral palsy usually is a long, single curve with a thoracolumber apex and pelvic obliquity. **B,** The lateral position varies with kyphosis and is often increased with an increased lumbar lordosis. **C,** Instrumentation should focus on correction of the pelvic obliquity and trunk alignment, which is most consistently done using the precontoured unit rod. **D,** The instrumentation also needs to correct the kyphosis and lordosis with the cranial extension of the fusion going to T1 or T2.

of these deformities. Currently, a well-padded corset type of thoracolumbosacral orthoses (TLSO) is useful to assist with seating during childhood. However, these devices do not impact the rate of development or the time at which the fixed spinal deformity develops. Other treatment modalities such as seating adjustments, physical therapy, electrical stimulation, or manipulative treatments have not demonstrated any impact on the development of the fixed scoliosis. The only treatment that has demonstrated a definitive impact upon the spinal deformity is surgical correction and fusion.

During middle childhood (to age 10 years) the use of a soft TLSO or seating adjustments is recommended to maintain optimal seating comfort. Usually, the TLSO or seating adaptations can be used in the child with cerebral palsy until the scoliotic curve is approximately 90° or is developing substantial stiffness, typically occurring near the middle to end of the adolescent growth spurt. If the child has completed growth and has a scoliotic curve of more than 40°, it is recommended to proceed with arthrodesis because there is a high risk of slow progression during early adulthood. In children with muscle weakness, specifically Duchenne muscular dystrophy, the scoliosis progression and forced vital capacity should be monitored during the adolescent growth spurt. When the scoliotic curve becomes larger than 30° to 40° or the forced vital capacity drops below 35%, sur-

gical correction is indicated. Surgical correction for spinal muscular atrophy is typically indicated when the child is not tolerating seating with the combination of either soft TLSO or seating adjustments. The same approach is used for children with paralytic curves. Typically, during the middle part of the adolescent growth period the scoliotic curve becomes much larger and causes stiffness, making seating very difficult. Fusion is recommended in these patients.

The primary surgical procedure for instrumentation of patients with neuromuscular scoliosis is a posterior spinal fusion, typically from T1 to the sacrum with the most predominant instrumentation using the unit rod instrumentation with sublaminar wires (Figure 1). Individually bent rods with sublaminar wires that are cross-connected is another option; multiple pedicle screws are being used as a third option. The unit rod is especially powerful to correct severe pelvic obliquity but is more difficult to use if significant lordosis is present. Except for some children with Duchenne muscular dystrophy who are near the end of growth and have no evidence of pelvic obliquity, in all other patients it is strongly recommended that fusion should extend to the pelvis to prevent the later development of pelvic obliquity. Patients with Duchenne muscular dystrophy who have no pelvic obliquity do not develop severe obliquity after a fusion ending at L5.

Anterior release is required for a scoliotic curve of a large magnitude, usually over 90°, that has caused significant curve stiffness. Also, for patients with severe kyphosis or severe lordosis, anterior release and diskectomy are recommended to allow flexibility. If the unit rod is used, there is no need to be concerned about the crankshaft phenomenon, and therefore anterior release is not required in children who have not achieved skeletal maturity.

The surgical procedure should be planned with the possibility of substantial blood loss, especially in some children with cerebral palsy who are on seizure medications and have rather poor nutrition. Two blood volumes of transfusion sometimes are required. Good vascular access is necessary. Large volumes of bank bone graft should also be available for good bone grafting with decortication of the transverse processes and fasciectomies so that good fusions are obtained. Good fusion is especially important in children with spasticity and movement disorders and is less important in children with conditions such as Duchenne muscular dystrophy and spinal muscular atrophy who put less stress on their instrumentation.

The usefulness of spinal cord monitoring for neuromuscular scoliosis remains unclear. Most children with neuropathies and myopathies can be monitored; however, reliable monitoring often cannot be performed in children with severe cerebral palsy (those children with severe mental retardation, no ambulatory function, and poor oral motor function). It is also not clear that the results of the monitoring would provide much useful information in this patient group because there is little motor function to preserve. Removal of implanted hardware cannot be justified because the risk of death in this patient population is so great that a second operation to reimplant instrumentation to preserve nonessential motor function does not seem to be reasonable. In a child with any functional standing or ambulatory ability, monitoring of somatosensory-evoked potentials with cervical leads and motor-evoked potential monitoring can be done and the response to monitoring changes should be similar to those of patients with idiopathic scoliosis.

The postoperative care of these children usually involves managing several comorbidities. For that reason, it is important to have a high level intensive care unit with good intensive care follow-up available to manage the ventilatory support that is often needed. Nutritional needs should also be aggressively managed with the initiation of early feeding. If the gastrointestinal system is not functioning to properly absorb nutrients by the third or fourth postoperative day, the use of central venous hyperalimentation is recommended. Mobilization of these patients should begin as soon as respiratory status is stable. The instrumentation used for neuromuscular fusions allow mobilization without any external casts or orthotic devices. Early mobilization is important to manage the respiratory system and stimulate the gastrointestinal system. Wheelchairs should be adjusted to the child's new body shape to prevent the development of postoperative decubiti.

## Complications

Complications of postoperative management of scoliosis include the requirement for prolonged ventilatory support. Some children may develop pneumothorax or a hemothorax as a result of ventilatory support or fluid from the posterior wound may leak into the chest. Gastrointestinal conditions including gastritis, cholelithiasis, and pancreatitis are also relatively common and should be expected if there is a prolonged period of ileus or abdominal discomfort. Aggressive treatment of postoperative constipation is also required. Wound infections occur in 3% to 5% of patients and can almost always be treated with local wound débridement without the removal of hardware, and a good long-term outcome is possible. Pseudarthrosis is rare, especially with the use of the unit rod and exuberant grafting with fasciectomies and decortications.

## Outcomes

In ambulating children who develop scoliosis, the spine can be fused to the pelvis with no risk of loss of ambulatory ability. Nonambulatory children generally are better able to sit, and caretakers tend to report that these children are also much more comfortable while sitting. Recurrent deformity seldom occurs. Long-term outcome after the acute surgical complications is excellent with very few late complications. Life expectancy after spinal fusion for a child with cerebral palsy is shorter than that for an age-matched child; however, there are no data to confirm whether correction of the spinal deformity has a positive or negative impact on the patient's life expectancy.

## Summary

Neuromuscular scoliosis is common in children with significant neurologic motor disability. Surgical correction and spinal fusion is the only treatment that has a documented beneficial impact on the deformity. Parents and caretakers report excellent improvement in the child's quality of life after deformity correction.

## Annotated Bibliography

### Natural History

Chuah SL, Kareem BA, Selvakumar K, Oh KS, Borhan Tan A, Harwant S: The natural history of scoliosis: Curve progression of untreated curves of different aetiology, with early (mean 2 year) follow up in surgically treated curves. *Med J Malaysia* 2001;56(suppl C):37-40.

A comparison of idiopathic scoliosis to neuromuscular scoliosis showed an annual progression rate of 7° for idiopathic adolescent scoliosis and 17° for neuromuscular scoliosis over a 2-year period before spinal fusion.

## Treatment

Lipton GE, Letonoff EJ, Dabney KW, Miller F, McCarthy HC: Correction of sagittal plane spinal deformities with unit rod instrumentation in children with cerebral palsy. *J Bone Joint Surg Am* 2003;85-A:2349-2357.

The purpose of the present study was to identify the indications for and the results of treatment of patients with cerebral palsy who have a spinal curve deformity solely in the sagittal plane. Patients with cerebral palsy and a severe sagittal plane deformity (> or =70°) can be treated successfully with posterior spinal fusion with use of unit rod instrumentation. Indications for treatment include loss of sitting ability or balance, back pain, loss of bowel or bladder function, and superior mesenteric artery syndrome that is unresponsive to medical management.

Shoham Y, Meyer S, Katz-Leurer M, Tamar Weiss PL: The influence of seat adjustment and a thoraco-lumbar-sacral orthosis on the distribution of body-seat pressure in children with scoliosis and pelvic obliquity. *Disabil Rehabil* 2004;26:21-26.

Application of a TLSO in a child with scoliosis and contralateral pelvic obliquity significantly reduced the spinal curvature and interface sitting pressure. Manipulation of sitting by use of wedges under the pelvis had no significant effect on pressure distribution; therefore, the TLSO seems better at improving seating than seating adjustments only.

## Complications

Brenn BR, Theroux MC, Dabney KW, Miller F: Clotting parameters and thromboelastography in children with neuromuscular and idiopathic scoliosis undergoing posterior spinal fusion. *Spine* 2004;29:E310-E314.

This study compared standard tests of coagulation and thromboelastography parameters between idiopathic scoliosis and cerebral palsy patients undergoing posterior spinal fusion. Children with cerebral palsy demonstrated a much more significant change in thromboelastography after 15% blood volume loss than children with idiopathic scoliosis although all clotting tests were normal preoperatively. Therefore, there is some physiologic reason for greater blood loss in some children with cerebral palsy and this expectation needs to be considered in planning surgical management.

DiCindio S, Theroux M, Shah S, et al: Multimodality monitoring of transcranial electric motor and somatosensory-evoked potentials during surgical correction of spinal deformity in patients with cerebral palsy and other neuromuscular disorders. *Spine* 2003;28:1851-1855.

This prospective study determined the reliability of transcranial electric motor and posterior tibial nerve somatosensory-evoked potentials in children with neuromuscular scoliosis. Both transcranial electric motor and posterior

tibial nerve somatosensory-evoked potentials can be monitored reliably in many patients with neuromuscular scoliosis. Those with severe cerebral palsy and severe mental retardation with no ambulatory function could be monitored in 39% of cases. Because it is difficult to obtain reliable monitoring in children with severe cerebral palsy and because there is limited motor function to preserve, electrically monitoring this population is less clinically useful.

Edler A, Murray DJ, Forbes RB: Blood loss during posterior spinal fusion surgery in patients with neuromuscular disease: Is there an increased risk? *Paediatr Anaesth* 2003;13:818-822.

This study examined the risk of extensive blood loss (> 50% of total blood volume) in patients with neuromuscular disease compared with patients who did not have neuromuscular disease when the extent of the surgery (number of segments fused), age, and preoperative coagulation profile were taken into consideration. Patients with neuromuscular disease did not vary significantly in age, weight, or preoperative hematocrit and platelet count from patients without neuromuscular disease. When the number of vertebral segments fused was controlled statistically, neuromuscular patients had an almost sevenfold higher risk of losing > 50% of their estimated total blood volume during scoliosis surgery. Recognizing this situation may help anesthesiologists and surgeons more accurately prepare for and treat intraoperative blood loss during scoliosis surgery in patients with neuromuscular disease.

Smucker JD, Miller F: Crankshaft effect after posterior spinal fusion and unit rod instrumentation in children with cerebral palsy. *J Pediatr Orthop* 2001;21:108-112.

Fifty patients were found to have an open triradiate cartilage at the time of posterior spine fusion. None of the 43 patients with at least 2 years of clinical follow-up had any radiographic change that was clinically significant on chart review. Therefore, posterior spinal fusion alone with unit rod instrumentation is adequate treatment to control crankshaft deformity in skeletally immature children with neuromuscular scoliosis caused by cerebral palsy.

Tsirikos AI, Chang WN, Dabney KW, Miller F: Comparison of one-stage versus two-stage anteroposterior spinal fusion in pediatric patients with cerebral palsy and neuromuscular scoliosis. *Spine* 2003;28:1300-1305.

Sequentially performed spinal procedures on one day were associated with increased intraoperative blood loss, prolonged surgical time, and a considerably higher incidence of medical and technical complications, including two perioperative deaths, compared with staged procedures 1 week apart. Two-stage anteroposterior spinal fusion provides safer and more consistent outcome.

Westerlund LE, Gill SS, Jarosz TS, Abel MF, Blanco JS: Posterior-only unit rod instrumentation and fusion for neuromuscular scoliosis. *Spine* 2001;26:1984-1989.

Results from this study indicate that even in the very young patient with neuromuscular scoliosis, acceptable amounts of curve correction can be achieved and maintained with posterior-only unit rod instrumentation and fusion. The biomechanical stiffness of this construct seemed to be able to prevent the crankshaft phenomenon in most patients at risk.

## Outcomes

Jones KB, Sponseller PD, Shindle MK, McCarthy ML: Longitudinal parental perceptions of spinal fusion for neuromuscular spine deformity in patients with totally involved cerebral palsy. *J Pediatr Orthop* 2003;23:143-149.

Retrospective surveys of caregivers of patients with totally involved cerebral palsy who are undergoing arthrodesis for spine deformity have demonstrated satisfaction with results but are subject to retrospective bias. There were no significant changes between preoperative and postoperative assessments of physical function, school absence, comorbidities, and parental health. Patient pain, happiness, frequency of feeling sick and tired, and parental satisfaction improved significantly by 1 year postoperatively. The presence of complications did not significantly affect questionnaire results. This prospective study substantiates the subjective gains noted in previous retrospective studies of spinal fusion for neuromuscular spine deformity in cerebral palsy.

Tsirikos AI, Chang WN, Dabney KW, Miller F: Comparison of parents' and caregivers' satisfaction after spinal fusion in children with cerebral palsy. *J Pediatr Orthop* 2004;24:54-58.

A questionnaire assessing patients' functional improvement after spinal arthrodesis for correcting scoliosis was addressed to 190 parents. An expanded questionnaire was also addressed to 122 educators and therapists working in the care of children with cerebral palsy. Considering that the benefits from scoliosis correction clearly outweigh the increased risk of surgical complications, most parents (95.8%) and caretakers (84.3%) would recommend spine surgery.

Tsirikos AI, Chang WN, Dabney KW, Miller F, Glutting J: Life expectancy in pediatric patients with cerebral palsy and neuromuscular scoliosis who underwent spinal fusion. *Dev Med Child Neurol* 2003;45:677-682.

The goal of this study was to document the rate of survival among 288 severely affected pediatric patients (154 females, 134 males) with spasticity and neuromuscular scoliosis who underwent spinal fusion (mean age at surgery 13 years) and to identify exposure variables that could significantly predict survival times. The number of days in the intensive care unit after surgery and the presence of severe preoperative thoracic hyperkyphosis were the only factors affecting survival rates. This study demonstrated statistically significant predictability for decreased life expectancy after spinal fusion in children with cerebral palsy; however, there was no control group with untreated scoliosis used for comparison.

Tsirikos AI, Chang WN, Shah SA, Dabney KW, Miller F: Preserving ambulatory potential in pediatric patients with cerebral palsy who undergo spinal fusion using unit rod instrumentation. *Spine* 2003;28:480-483.

Spine surgery with fusion extending to the pelvis in ambulatory patients with cerebral palsy provided excellent deformity correction and preserved their ambulatory function. These results refute the widespread dogma that fusion to the pelvis will cause children with cerebral palsy to stop walking.

## Classic Bibliography

Dias RC, Miller F, Dabney K, Lipton G, Temple T: Surgical correction of spinal deformity using a unit rod in children with cerebral palsy. *J Pediatr Orthop* 1996;16:734-740.

Ferguson RL, Hansen MM, Nicholas DA, Allen BL Jr: Same-day versus staged anterior-posterior spinal surgery in a neuromuscular scoliosis population: The evaluation of medical complications. *J Pediatr Orthop* 1996;16:293-303.

Lipton GE, Miller F, Dabney KW, Altiok H, Bachrach SJ: Factors predicting postoperative complications following spinal fusions in children with cerebral palsy. *J Spinal Disord* 1999;12:197-205.

Madigan RR, Wallace SL: Scoliosis in the institutionalized cerebral palsy population. *Spine* 1981;6:583-590.

Miller A, Temple T, Miller F: Impact of orthoses on the rate of scoliosis progression in children with cerebral palsy. *J Pediatr Orthop* 1996;16:332-335.

Noordeen MH, Lee J, Gibbons CE, Taylor BA, Bentley G: Spinal cord monitoring in operations for neuromuscular scoliosis. *J Bone Joint Surg Br* 1997;79:53-57.

Olafsson Y, Saraste H, Al-Dabbagh Z: Brace treatment in neuromuscular spine deformity. *J Pediatr Orthop* 1999;19:376-379.

Sponseller PD, LaPorte DM, Hungerford MW, Eck K, Bridwell KH, Lenke LG: Deep wound infections after neuromuscular scoliosis surgery: A multicenter study of risk factors and treatment outcomes. *Spine* 2000;25:2461-2466.

Szoke G, Lipton G, Miller F, Dabney K: Wound infection after spinal fusion in children with cerebral palsy. *J Pediatr Orthop* 1998;18:727-733.

Sussman MD, Little D, Alley RM, McCoig JA: Posterior instrumentation and fusion of the thoracolumbar spine for treatment of neuromuscular scoliosis. *J Pediatr Orthop* 1996;16:304-313.

# Chapter 48

# Scheuermann's Disease

David A. Spiegel, MD

## Etiology/Epidemiology

Scheuermann's disease may be described as a hyperkyphosis in the thoracic or thoracolumbar spine associated with apical vertebral wedging, end-plate irregularities, and often Schmorl's nodes. The etiology remains unknown, but most likely involves the influence of mechanical forces in a genetically susceptible individual. The reported incidence has varied from 0.4% to 10%, and is most likely in the range of 1%. The disease is most commonly observed in males.

Both biologic and mechanical theories have been proposed to explain the characteristic histologic and radiographic findings in Scheuermann's disease. Biologic theories suggest a primary impairment in anterior vertebral growth because of either a genetic predisposition or hormonal/metabolic abnormality (juvenile osteoporosis, growth hormone deficiency, vitamin A deficiency). Although evidence to support a hormonal/metabolic etiology is lacking, there is considerable evidence to support a genetic etiology; however, the responsible gene has yet to be identified. The disease has been reported in monozygotic twins, and previous studies have supported an autosomal dominant mode of inheritance, most likely with an incomplete, gender-dependent penetrance. Alternatively, it has been suggested that mechanical loading of the immature vertebral column results in a secondary impairment of vertebral growth.

Although the available evidence suggests that a primary mechanical etiology is unlikely, mechanical forces may play a role in the progression of deformity. Normal growth of immature musculoskeletal tissues is influenced by mechanical forces, and stresses outside a normal range or "window" would be expected to either stimulate or retard growth. With respect to the thoracic spine, the anterior column is normally loaded in compression, and the posterior column in tension. Increases in either the frequency or magnitude of anterior compressive forces may potentially impair anterior vertebral growth, resulting in an increase in kyphosis. Increased tensile forces along the posterior column of the spine might be expected to stimulate growth, also increasing kyphosis. The importance of mechanical forces is supported by the response to bracing in a subset of skeletally immature patients, in whom a permanent reconstitution of vertebral height has been documented.

Studies of pathologic specimens have revealed a disturbance in endochondral ossification at the vertebral end plate; however, histologic analysis is unable to determine whether such changes are primary or secondary. Abnormalities in both collagen and proteoglycans in the extracellular matrix have been documented, along with irregular mineralization and ossification of the end plates.

## History/Physical Examination

The physical signs and symptoms usually become apparent during the prepubertal growth spurt, when patients present with either cosmetic concerns relating to an accentuation of thoracic kyphosis, back pain, or both. Any discomfort is usually dull in character, and is more pronounced following activities. Pain is most commonly experienced at the apex of the deformity, but may also occur at the cervicothoracic junction or in the lumbar spine. Although the origin of pain remains unclear, potential sources include the disks, the facet joints (either at the apex or in the adjacent, more mobile segments), or the paraspinal muscles. The presence of symptoms does not correlate with either the magnitude of kyphosis or with progression of the deformity. Lumbar pain may be caused by a coexisting spondylolysis or spondylolisthesis.

A standing examination of the spine reveals excessive thoracic kyphosis, which may be accompanied by an increase in cervical and/or lumbar lordosis. The Adams forward bending test may help to identify both the apex of the deformity and the presence of a coexisting scoliosis. Flexibility may be assessed by voluntary hyperextension of the spine, or by placing a bolster at or just below the apex of the deformity while the patient is supine. As the hamstring muscles are frequently contracted, the femoral-popliteal angle should be measured. A thorough neurologic examination also should be performed.

Neurologic abnormalities are infrequent, and are more likely to be encountered in adults.

## Differential Diagnosis

The list of conditions that may be associated with thoracic hyperkyphosis is extensive. Categories include posttraumatic, postinfectious (bacterial, tuberculous, fungal), metabolic (osteogenesis imperfecta, osteoporosis), iatrogenic (postlaminectomy, postradiation), neuromuscular, neoplastic, and congenital/developmental. Examples of the last category might include disorders of collagen (Marfan's), and several dysplasias (neurofibromatosis, achondroplasia, mucopolysaccharidosis). The condition most likely to be confused with Scheuermann's disease is postural hyperkyphosis. On occasion, the radiographic features in a congenital kyphosis (failure of segmentation) or a progressive noninfectious anterior vertebral fusion may be similar to those seen in Scheuermann's disease. Patients with postural hyperkyphosis are typically asymptomatic, and their hyperkyphosis can be voluntarily corrected. The deformity is distributed evenly throughout the thoracic spine. Progressive noninfectious vertebral fusion is very rare, and involves a partial or complete ankylosis of one or more vertebral bodies. The fusion is usually anterior, and may represent a variant of congenital kyphosis. The radiographic findings during childhood include narrowing of the disk space, with approximation of the anterior corners of the vertebral bodies. Older patients will demonstrate bony ankylosis anteriorly; the kyphotic deformity progresses as a result of tethering of anterior vertebral growth.

## Diagnostic Testing

The diagnosis of Scheuermann's disease is based on plain radiographic findings; other imaging studies may be helpful to further evaluate atypical features identified in the patient's history or physical examination. A standing lateral radiograph of the thoracic and lumbar spine demonstrates thoracic hyperkyphosis with vertebral wedging at the apex, which is usually between T7 and T9. It has been proposed that anterior wedging of more than 5° in three adjacent vertebrae is required to establish the diagnosis, a criterion that has gained wide acceptance. The normal range of thoracic kyphosis in children is 20° to 50°, as measured using the Cobb technique from the superior end plate of T3 to the inferior end plate of T12. Ideally, when following patients over time, a similar radiographic technique will be used for all films, and the measurements will be completed by the same observer with previous radiographs available for comparison.

Associated findings, which may also be encountered with some frequency in asymptomatic adolescents, include disk space narrowing, end-plate irregularities, and Schmorl's nodes. These findings are most commonly observed in the apical region, but may also be identified at other levels. The lumbosacral region should be evaluated for the presence of spondylolisthesis, and a standing posteroanterior radiograph should be routinely obtained because mild scoliosis is common. A hyperextension film of the thoracic spine is required to assess the degree of flexibility, especially when contemplating treatment. The patient is placed supine, and a bolster is placed as a fulcrum at or just below the apex of the kyphosis.

Maintenance of sagittal spinal balance is also important because a balanced state implies that little or no muscular action is required to maintain normal upright posture. On the standing lateral radiograph, a plumb line dropped from C7 should fall within 2 cm of the posterosuperior corner of the S1 vertebral body. In addition to the primary thoracic deformity, compensatory changes in the cervical spine, the lumbar spine, and the pelvis may occur to maintain sagittal spinal balance.

Other diagnostic studies, most commonly MRI, may be indicated when neurologic abnormalities are identified on physical examination, or when the symptoms are atypical or unresponsive to conservative care. Atypical symptoms may include night pain, pain in another region of the spine, and/or radicular complaints. Abnormal findings on advanced imaging studies have included epidural cysts, thoracic spinal stenosis, thoracic disk herniation, and degenerative disk disease.

## Natural History and Nonsurgical Treatment

An appreciation for the natural history of a condition helps to educate the patient/family, and to make recommendations for treatment. There has been some difference of opinion in the literature with respect to the natural history of Scheuermann's disease. Although some studies have suggested that significant degenerative changes and pain are common at long-term follow-up, usually with curves in excess of 75°, others have reported a more benign outcome. In a study of 67 patients with a mean kyphosis of 71° who were followed for 32 years, the patients with Scheuermann's disease were found to have more intense back pain, decreased trunk range of motion and strength, and more sedentary occupations than the patients in the control group. However, there were no significant differences in self consciousness, self esteem, participation in recreational activities or activities of daily living, level of education, use of medications for back pain, or absence from work because of back pain. Restrictive lung disease was associated with those kyphotic deformities with an apex above T8 with curve progression that was in excess of 100°. A more recent investigation found no significant difference in functional outcome between those patients who were observed and those who were treated (nonsurgically and surgically);

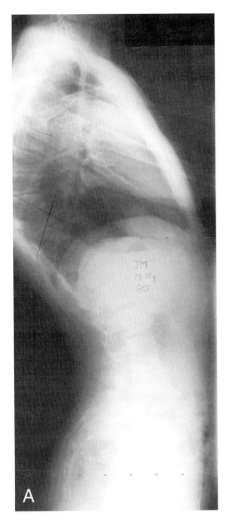 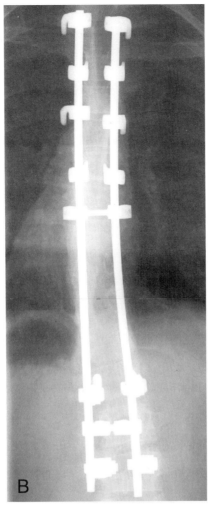 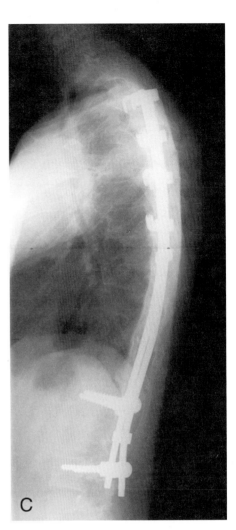

Figure 1  **A,** Preoperative lateral radiograph in a patient with Scheuermann's disease. **B** and **C,** An instrumented posterior spinal fusion was performed, using the cantilever technique. Fixation included two claws proximally and distally. The deformity was corrected to within the upper range of normal values, and sagittal balance was maintained.

however, the outcome was worse in patients with residual curves of greater than 70°.

Alternatives for nonsurgical treatment include observation, stretching and strengthening exercises, or use of an orthotic device. Observation is generally recommended for the asymptomatic patient with a nonprogressive deformity that lies within the accepted range of values. Although thoracic back pain may respond to a combined regimen of activity modification and an exercise program, a permanent reduction in thoracic hyperkyphosis in unlikely. The program should focus on thoracic hyperextension exercises, strengthening of the abdominal muscles and spinal extensors, and stretching of the hamstrings.

A bracing program may be offered for a progressive kyphosis (> 50° to 60°) associated with an unacceptable cosmetic appearance and/or pain. The goals are not only to arrest progression and/or relieve pain, but also to affect a permanent improvement in spinal alignment through the reconstitution of vertebral height. The fail-

ure to correct vertebral wedging will necessarily result in a return to the pretreatment alignment when the brace is discontinued.

Prerequisites for a successful bracing program include adequate curve flexibility (ideally less than 40° on a hyperextension radiograph), sufficient growth remaining (more than 18 months is generally required to correct vertebral wedging), a mechanically sound orthotic device, and adequate patient compliance. Bracing is less effective for larger curves, and is not recommended for curves in excess of 75°.

As the "in brace" correction correlates with the success of a bracing program, efforts to improve curve flexibility are often required. Options include sequential orthotic modifications as the patient is weaned into the brace, or a period of serial casting before the initiation of bracing. Deformities of greater magnitude and rigidity may respond better to serial casting. An underarm cast is applied on the Risser table, and may be changed every few weeks until sufficient correction is achieved.

Alternatively, an approach popularized in Europe uses two to three casts over a 9-month period. Once an acceptable "in brace" correction is achieved, the orthotic device serves to maintain the correction.

The type of spinal orthosis depends on the apex of the curvature. A Milwaukee brace will be required for most patients in whom the apex lies at or above the eight thoracic vertebra. An underarm thoracolumbosacral orthosis may suffice when the apex is below this level. Recommendations in the literature have varied with respect to both the number of hours that the brace should be worn, and the degree of skeletal maturity at which it is appropriate to discontinue treatment. Although a minimum of 16 hours has been recommended in some studies, other studies indicate that 20 to 22 hours of brace use per day offers the greatest chance of success.

Compliance may be a challenge in the asymptomatic adolescent in whom physical appearance is not a concern. Furthermore, compliance may be poor should discomfort be experienced during the course of treatment, for example, when trying to control a rigid curve or when attempting to increase curve flexibility through sequential orthotic adjustments.

## Surgical Treatment

Surgical management is indicated for chronic back pain that is unresponsive to nonsurgical measures, and/or a progressive deformity that is unacceptable to the patient. Although some authors have offered spinal fusion for progressive deformities greater than 60°, most have suggested a lower limit of 70° to 75°. The goals of surgery are to reduce the thoracic hyperkyphosis to a cosmetically acceptable range while maintaining sagittal balance and relieving pain.

A posterior spinal fusion with instrumentation is required in all patients, and the current trend has been to reserve anterior release/fusion for larger, stiffer curvatures. The arthrodesis should extend from the upper end vertebra (highest vertebra that is tilted into the curve) to the vertebra distal to the first lordotic disk space. Correction may be achieved by applying cantilever forces (Figure 1), or by sequential compression following segmental shortening of the posterior column by multiple osteotomies. Complications include neurologic deficit, excessive blood loss, infection, pseudarthrosis, sagittal imbalance, and implant-related problems including loss of fixation, fracture or prominence of the implant, and bursitis. Sagittal imbalance may be avoided by choosing the correct fusion levels, and by correcting the deformity to less than 50% of the original magnitude.

Overall, the reported outcomes following the surgical treatment of Scheuermann's disease have been variable. Although cosmesis can be reliably improved with-

out complications in most patients, it remains unclear whether surgical intervention alters the natural history. Patients should be counseled in detail regarding the natural history of Scheuermann's disease and the goals, complications, and expected outcome following an instrumented spinal arthrodesis.

## Annotated Bibliography

### Etiology/Epidemiology

Axenovich TI, Zaidman AM, Zorkoltseva IV, Kalashnikova EV, Borodin PM: Segregation analysis of Scheuermann disease in ninety families from Siberia. *Am J Med Genet* 2001;100:275-279.

Scheuermann's disease may fit into an autosomal dominant model with incomplete, gender-dependent penetrance.

### History/Physical Examination

Loder RT: The sagittal profile of the cervical and the lumbosacral spine in Scheuermann thoracic kyphosis. *J Spinal Disord* 2001;14:226-231.

Cervical lordosis was correlated with both lumbar lordosis and the sagittal difference (thoracic kyphosis minus lumbar lordosis). Flexible cervical and lumbar segments are linked by a rigid intermediate thoracic segment. The cervical spine compensates for an increase in sagittal difference to maintain forward gaze.

### Diagnostic Testing

Stotts AK, Smith JT, Santora SD, Roach JW, D'Astous JL: Measurement of spinal kyphosis: Implications for the management of Scheuermann's kyphosis. *Spine* 2002;27:2143-2146.

The 95% confidence limit for intraobserver variance was +/- 9.6°, and for interobserver variance was +/- 8.7°. This range of variability should be kept in mind when reviewing the indications for treatment, and in reporting the outcome following treatment.

### Natural History and Nonsurgical Treatment

Riddle EC, Bowen JR, Shah SA, et al: The duPont kyphosis brace for the treatment of adolescent Scheuermann kyphosis. *J South Orthop Assoc* 2003;12:135-140.

Thirty-four adolescents with a mean kyphosis of 63° (apex T7-T9 in 50%) were treated with an underarm thoracolumbosacral orthosis for 15 hours per day. Of the 22 (64%) who were compliant, 16 demonstrated no progression (mean improvement 9°). Flexible curves had a better outcome.

Soo CL, Noble PC, Esses SI: Scheuermann kyphosis: Long term followup. *Spine J* 2002;2:49-56.

Sixty-three patients were treated by observation, bracing, or surgery. At 14-year follow-up, there were no differences in functional outcome between these groups with respect to marital status, educational level, general health, occupation, and level of pain. However, the outcome was inferior in patients with a residual kyphosis greater than 70°.

## Surgical Treatment

Hosman AJ, de Kleuver M, Anderson PG, et al: Scheuermann kyphosis: The importance of tight hamstrings in the surgical correction. *Spine* 2003;28:2252-2259.

Patients with hamstring contracture may be at increased risk for postoperative sagittal imbalance, especially if the arthrodesis extends into the lumbar spine, as they rely on lumbar flexibility for compensation.

Hosman AJ, Langeloo DD, de Kleuver M, et al: Analysis of the sagitttal plane after surgical management for Scheuermann's disease: A view on overcorrection and the use of an anterior release. *Spine* 2002;27:167-175.

Thirty-three patients treated by posterior (76.6° preoperative, 55.8° follow-up, 1.3° correction loss) or anterior/posterior fusion (80.8° preoperative, 52.6° follow-up, 1.5° correction loss) were compared. All patients had a significant improvement in both pain and cosmesis. Posterior spinal fusion (correction to 40° to 50°) is recommended in the absence of anterior bony bridging.

Papagelopoulos PJ, Klassen RA, Peterson HA, et al: Surgical treatment of Scheuermann's kyphosis with segmental compression instrumentation. *Clin Orthop Relat Res* 2001;386:139-149.

Twenty-one adolescents/adults underwent an instrumented posterior fusion (68.5° preoperative, 40° at follow-up, 5.8° correction loss) or an anterior/posterior fusion (86.3° preoperative, 46.4° at follow-up, 4.4° correction loss). Cosmesis was restored, and complications included one perioperative death (superior mesenteric artery syndrome), rod fracture (2), junctional kyphosis (2), and symptomatic bursae (3). Eleven patients had mild low back pain at follow-up.

Poolman RW, Been HD, Ubags LH: Clinical outcome and radiographic results after operative treatment in Scheuermann's disease. *Eur Spine J* 2002;11:561-569.

A "fair" outcome was observed following anterior/posterior fusion in this prospective study of 23 patients. Removal of implants (for localized pain) resulted in a loss of correction despite a solid fusion mass. The authors question the value of surgical intervention in patients with Scheuermann's disease.

## Classic Bibliography

Boseker EH, Moe JH, Winter RB, Koop SE: Determination of "normal" thoracic kyphosis: A roentgenographic study of 121 "normal" children. *J Pediatr Orthop* 2000; 20:796-798.

Bradford DS, Ahmed KB, Moe JH, et al: The surgical management of patients with Scheuermann's disease: A review of twenty-four cases treated by combined anterior and posterior spinal fusion. *J Bone Joint Surg Am* 1980;62:705-712.

Ippolito E, Bellocci M, Montanaro A, Ascani E, Ponseti IV: Juvenile kyphosis: An ultrastructural study. *J Pediatr Orthop* 1985;5:315-322.

Lowe TG, Kasten MD: An analysis of sagittal curves and balance after Cotrel-Dubousset instrumentation for kyphosis secondary to Scheuermann's disease: A review of 32 patients. *Spine* 1994;19:1680-1685.

McKenzie L, Sillence D: Familial Scheuermann disease: A genetic and linkage study. *J Med Genet* 1992;29:41-45.

Murray PM, Weinstein SL, Spratt KF: The natural history and long-term follow-up of Scheuermann's kyphosis. *J Bone Joint Surg Am* 1993;75:236-248.

Sachs B, Bradford D, Winter RB, Lonstein JE, Moe J, Willson S: Scheuermann kyphosis: Followup of Milwaukee-brace treatment. *J Bone Joint Surg Am* 1987; 69:50-57.

Sorenson KH: Scheuermann's juvenile kyphosis: Clinical appearances, radiography, etiology, and prognosis. Copenhagen, Denmark, Munksgaard, 1964.

Sturm PF, Dobson JC, Armstrong GW: The surgical management of Scheuermann's disease. *Spine* 1993;18: 685-691.

# Section 5

# Future Developments

Section Editor:
Jeffrey C. Wang, MD

# Chapter 49

# Biologic Enhancement of Spinal Arthrodesis

Arya Nick Shamie, MD

Jeffrey C. Wang, MD

## Introduction

Spinal arthrodesis is the mainstay of all spinal surgeries; more than 250,000 procedures are performed annually, with fusion as the ultimate goal. Prior to the use of spinal instrumentation, the rate of success of spinal fusion surgery was 65% to 95%. With the advent of rigid fixation methods such as pedicle screws, cervical plates, and lateral mass screws, the fusion rates reported in recent studies are in the 90th percentile. Until recently, the best results of fusion have been reported with the use of autogenous iliac crest bone graft. The use of iliac crest bone graft has an overall 15% risk of minor complications such as wound infections and up to an 8% risk of major complications such as pelvic fractures. Alternatives to autogenous bone have been desirable for fusion surgeries but until recently were not considered by surgeons because of the suboptimal results achieved in comparison with iliac crest autograft. With the use of rigid spinal instrumentation, the results of fusion with allograft bone have been promising.

Many substitutes for iliac crest bone graft have been used in spinal fusion surgeries, with mixed results. The two main categories for enhancement of spinal fusion are electromagnetic stimulation, both transcutaneous and implantable, and biologic implants that have one or more of the properties of autograft bone: osteoconduction, osteoinduction, and osteogenic potential. Any product that has living cells is by definition a graft material; an implant has no living cells present. The focus of this chapter will be on biologically active grafts or implants.

## Patient Factors Affecting Biology

The patient's own biologic makeup, along with other factors, plays an important role in outcome after surgery. Proper nutrition has been shown to affect wound healing and fusion rates. One indicator is the serum total protein and hematocrit, which in subnormal levels can predict poor healing rates. Severe vitamin D deficiency has also been associated with poor spinal fusion rates. Patients who have recently received local radia-

tion treatment should also be considered at risk for poor fusion. Gamma radiation and x-ray exposure cause a zone of stasis, in which local blood supply is impaired by coagulative necrosis because of thrombotic occlusion of smaller arteries. Gamma and x-ray radiation also increase free radicals in the tissues, which adversely affects DNA. The result is inhibition of regeneration of tissues and dividing cells.

Elderly patients are also at a higher risk for nonunion or pseudarthrosis, possibly because of poor fixation in osteoporotic bone and poor nutritional status. Another factor influencing union rates in these patients may be deficient amounts of endogenous bone induction material. Studies have shown a significant decrease in the amount of endogenous bone morphogenetic proteins (BMPs) extracted from bone harvested from elderly patients. This decrease in endogenous BMPs can be responsible for poor healing potential in these patients. Higher levels of circulating anti-BMP antibodies have also been shown in age-matched elderly women with osteoporosis compared with elderly women without osteoporosis. This difference in the circulating antibodies may also affect the healing potentials of exogenous BMPs implanted in these patients.

To understand the efficacy of various products used for enhancement of fusion in spine surgery, it is important to define the three key characteristics that independently play a role in the de novo bone formation process: osteoinduction, osteoconduction, and osteogenic properties.

## Biologic Properties
### Osteoinduction

Osteoinduction is the process resulting in nascent bone formation by the induction of local pluripotential mesenchymal cells. The classic bioassay for this osteoinductive property is the implantation of a product in the hindquarter of mice and radiographic detection of bone by 21 days. Recent in vitro bioassays measure the alkaline phosphatase and osteocalcin production of rat skeletal muscle myoblasts in response to osteoinductive protein exposure.

BMPs are the only clinically available proteins with proven osteoinductive potential. BMP is normally found in minute quantities of 0.001% of cortical bone weight and plays an important role in normal morphogenesis of bone. It is also found in various tissues in the developing embryo. BMPs are members of the transforming growth factor-beta (TGF-β) superfamily. BMPs have also been identified in T lymphocytes of patients with fibrodysplasia ossificans progressiva and may be responsible for heterotopic ossification of the connective tissue of these patients. More than 15 isoforms of BMP have been identified to date; BMP-1 has no morphogenetic activity and is a procollagenase.

In bone, BMPs, in their various isoforms, are bound to noncollagenous proteins. Noncollagenous proteins include osteopontin, osteonectin, and gla proteins. Upon completion of isolation of BMP from bone matrix, it remains complexed with noncollagenous proteins, which function as a carrier for BMP. Further separation of BMP from noncollagenous proteins requires a very low pH, which will denature BMP. Noncollagenous proteins alone have no osteoinductive properties. BMPs derived from human bone (hBMPs) were the first BMP to be implanted clinically. Based on more than 20 years of follow-up of over 100 patients implanted with hBMP, no adverse effects of infection, allergic reaction, or tumorigenesis have been noted.

The first isoform of BMP-2 was produced in 1996 using recombinant technology. For approval by the United States Food and Drug Administration (FDA), extensive laboratory and clinical studies had to be performed. BMP-2 gained FDA approval in July 2002 for use in anterior interbody fusions with a metallic cage. Fusion rates of 100% have been reported in patients in whom a metallic cage and BMP-2 were used. Since the publication of these early studies, the use of metallic cages as fusion devices has somewhat fallen out of favor. It is difficult to observe the fusion mass through these cages, even with an axial CT scan, and therefore some surgeons are favoring allograft interbody devices or radiolucent devices such as the poly-ethyl-ether-ketone (PEEK) implants. Fusion results with BMP-2 and these other interbody implant devices are forthcoming.

When used in posterolateral fusion surgery, BMP-2 has had mixed results. One explanation for the suboptimal fusion in this scenario is the pressure the overlying muscles exert on the collagen sponge that acts as a carrier for the BMP. It has been observed that the induced bone formation either occurs in the surrounding muscles or not at all. BMP that escapes from the carrier and is released into the blood stream or the surrounding tissues is degraded or diluted to inactivity. Modified compression-resistant carriers that resist the muscular compression in the lateral gutter are under investigation and may offer improved fusion results in this location.

BMP-7 (osteogenic protein-1) was approved by the FDA under humanitarian exemption in 2004 for use in treating resistant posterolateral nonunions of the lumbar spine. This isoform with the accompanying carrier has been shown to have similar results in posterolateral fusion in comparison with iliac crest bone grafts.

Current studies on recombinant human growth/differentiation factor-S (rhGDF-S) are ongoing. This member of the TGF-β superfamily is undergoing clinical investigation as a promoter of fusion in the posterolateral spine. In the experimental animal model, rhGDF-S increases the adhesion proliferation of cartilage cells during endochondral bone formation.

## Osteoconduction

Osteoconduction is defined by the biologic scaffolding provided for the endogenous (host) or exogenous (graft) pluripotential cells to move across a gap between two bony surfaces. If the cells do not have a scaffolding to move across the gap between two bony surfaces, bony union will not occur. Critical size defect is a gap between two bony surfaces that will not heal without a bone graft or implant material. An osteoconductive material decreases this defect size to allow for bony union.

The osteoconductive material can range in density with varied mechanical properties. The more dense the material (for example, cortical bone or ceramics) the more structural support it can provide. Hence, a dense implant can be effectively used in defects under axial compression, such as a corpectomy defect. However, the more dense the material, the longer it takes for its resorption and integration with the host bone. Therefore, the best material for a posterolateral instrumented fusion, where no axial compression is present, is a more porous cancellous bone to encourage more rapid resorption and replacement with the de novo bone.

Osteoconductive materials are often used as carriers for bioactive proteins such as BMP. BMPs are known to be bound to the collagen matrix of bone in their natural state. It is this affinity of BMPs to the collagen matrix that makes a collagen-based osteoconductive material superior to other synthetic carriers. BMP is thought to have a hydrogen link to the collagen, as reducing agents are known to release the BMPs into the solution in laboratory experiments. The carrier plays an important role in the actions of BMP. The BMP that escapes the carrier attachments and gathers into the surrounding tissues or the bloodstream will form heterotopic bone or may be degraded by the serum enzymatic activity, respectively. Autolyzed antigen extracted allogeneic bone was used as a carrier for hBMP for more than 20 years before the synthesis of recombinant forms of BMP (rhBMP). This autolized antigen extracted allogenic bone/hBMP combination was effective in treating more than 100 patients with resistant nonunions and failed spinal arthrodeses;

there were no adverse effects. However, the limited supply of donor bone led to the development of various synthetic and bone derived implants to aid in spinal fusion surgeries.

## Osteogenesis

The osteogenic potential of a graft is dependent on its cellular content. If a graft has pluripotential cells that can be induced to become osteoblasts, the graft is by definition osteogenic. Although the presence of osteoconductive material and stimulus of osteoinductive material in a fusion site is important, the absence of pluripotential cells will result in failure of the fusion surgery. The pluripotential cells are present in autogenous bone derived from the spinous processes or lamina, and the harvested iliac crest bone. These pluripotential cells are more abundant in cancellous bone than in cortical bone; therefore, cancellous bone graft possesses better fusion characteristics. These mesenchymal pluripotential cells can also migrate to the fusion site from the decorticated host bony surfaces or the surrounding vascular tissues and pericytes.

The most commonly used graft with osteogenic potential is autogenous iliac crest bone graft. Because open harvest of iliac crest autograft is associated with increased morbidity, alternative methods of minimally invasive iliac crest bone marrow harvesting have been studied. The bone marrow cells can be harvested by inserting a hollow point Jamshidi needle into the crest and then aspirating the pluripotential cells. The cellular composition of this bone marrow aspirate is more than 80% red blood cells with less than 5% pluripotential cells. Various techniques for separating and concentrating this subset of pluripotential cells have been used. In animal studies, allograft and synthetic osteoconductive material mixed with concentrated bone marrow aspirate has shown promise. The technique is currently under clinical evaluation in randomized clinical trials.

## Bone Graft Extenders

Many options are available for autogenous bone graft augmentation or substitution, mixed clinical results. Two general categories are bone derivatives and synthetic material. Bone derivatives can be either allogeneic or xenogeneic (mostly bovine or porcine). In addition to patient variability in their biologic response, there may be some inherent variability in the efficacy of these products. This variability is especially true for bone-derived products such as demineralized bone matrices or allograft bone; synthetic materials are inherently more consistent in their composition. This variability is especially apparent in the product's inductive potential. Biodegradation time is defined as the time elapsed from the death of the donor to the time the harvested bone is processed or frozen to -70°C. During the lag time, be-

fore the freezing of bone or its processing, endogenous anti-BMPases continue to degrade the osteoinductive potential of the bone. Lyophilization of the bone will ultimately halt the BMP degradation process and maintain the bone's osteoinductive potential. Therefore, each batch of bone processed in the bone bank may have varied osteoinductive potential depending on the age of the donor patient, the initial amount of BMP present in the bone, and the biodegradation time. Most allogeneic bone used in surgery has minimal osteoinductive potential and is mostly osteoconductive.

## Gene Therapy

Gene therapy is the transfer of a gene (DNA) for a specific protein or cytokine into a cell so that the cell transcribes the messenger RNA (mRNA) of that protein. The cell's internal mechanism then translates the mRNA into the index protein (cytokine) using its ribosomes. The gene is produced in the laboratory using the reverse transcriptase, which uses the mRNA of a protein to produce a complementary DNA (cDNA). Because the cDNA is produced directly from the mRNA, it lacks the noncoding nucleotides of the DNA (introns). Only the coding nucleotides (extrons) are present in the cDNA.

The cDNA is then inserted into a plasmid, a self-replicating DNA found naturally in bacteria and yeast. The cDNA plasmid is then cleaved with restriction enzymes and then inserted into a larger plasmid with a promoter sequence. The promoter sequence is necessary for the transcription of the cDNA once the gene is transferred into a cell. This plasmid is then termed an expression plasmid because it now has the potential to become a template for protein expression. There are two types of promoters available: constitutive (always on) and regulated (can be turned on and off with external stimuli).

Once an expression plasmid is produced, an effective transfer into a cell needs to be planned. A vector is the tool that facilitates the transfer of a gene into a cell. Vectors can be viral or nonviral. The most commonly used nonviral vectors are liposomes, which are phospholipid vacuoles capable of integrating with a cell membrane, as the cell membranes are also made up of phospholipids. Through this fusion, the contents of the liposomes can be delivered into the cell's cytoplasm. Other forms of nonviral vectors are gene gun (DNA loaded on an element injected into the cell using a helium gun), DNA conjugates (DNA bound to polycations to help DNA binding to cell membranes), and gene-activated matrices (matrices with attached expression plasmids). The efficiency of nonviral vectors is far inferior to viral vectors in accomplishing this gene transfer into the cell. Successful gene transfer using nonviral vec-

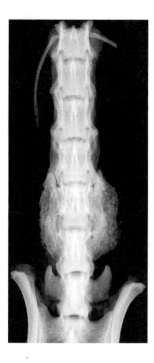

**Figure 1** AP radiograph of the lumbar spine of a rat that had a complete fusion of the intertransverse processes at 4 weeks after treatment with BMP-2-producing transduced marrow cells; solid fusion on manual palpation was noted.

tors is called transfection; gene transfer using viral vectors is called transduction.

The viral vectors most commonly used are adenoviruses, followed by retroviruses, and herpes simplex viruses. Adenoviruses have been successfully used in the transduction of hamster ovary cells to produce the rhBMP-2 that is now commercially available. The adenovirus gene is inserted into the cell as an episome and is not integrated with the cell genome. Furthermore, adenoviruses can cause transduction of dividing and nondividing cells. Retroviral vectors cause transduction of actively dividing cells only. Viruses are used in gene therapy applications and clinically to produce a protein in vitro. This protein is then implanted to produce its effects. Alternatively, a patient's cells can be used to produce the index protein after transduction either ex vivo or in vivo. Causes for concern with introduction of a virus into a patient are possible increased risk of infection from the virus, or uncontrolled viral transduction. If the transduction is accomplished in the laboratory, although the risk of infection for the patient will be decreased, the cells may cease production of the index protein before the index protein has reached full effectiveness. Another concern with using retroviral vectors is that the index gene can randomly be spliced into the cellular genome and can theoretically alter oncogene expression. Despite these concerns, studies have shown successful results with ex vivo transduction of allogeneic marrow cells of rats with the rhBMP-2 gene followed by bone formation after grafting of these cells in the posterolateral spine.

After introduction of a DNA sequence into the cell, the cell is manipulated to produce the therapeutic pro-

teins. More than a decade of research has been devoted to gene therapy, mainly to supplement a genetic deficiency causing a specific disease. Research on gene therapy for the treatment of systemic disease has thus far been largely disappointing, and the clinical utility of this type of therapy has not been realized. However, local gene therapy for spinal fusion has shown great promise in the laboratory.

BMP is a potent osteoinductive agent. It is present in minute amounts in bone tissue, and more recently has been produced using recombinant technology. Regardless of the mode of BMP production, either through extraction from bone or using recombinant technology, both methods require a large dose of the BMP implantation for successful fusion. There has also been some concern regarding the potential of infection from extracted BMP products. Although hBMP has been used clinically without any incidence of infection or immunogenicity with over 10 years of follow-up, the potential of prion or viral transmission may theoretically exist. The risk of disease transmission has been eliminated by using the recombinant forms of BMP; however, immunogenic reaction has been shown in a small percentage of patients. The significance of this immunogenicity in repeat recipients of rhBMP is not known. Using genetic engineering technology, a viable alternative to the extracted or recombinant forms of BMP will be available. Using this technology, the need for large doses of BMP implantation can be eliminated. The gene transfer can be performed either in vivo or ex vivo. With ex vivo gene transfer, the BMP gene is introduced in the autogeneic or allogeneic cells; after confirmation of the gene transfer, the cells are introduced in the fusion site.

In genetic engineering experiments, viral vectors are used to introduce rhBMP-2 cDNA intracellularly using ex vivo methods. In animal studies, adenoviral vectors carrying rhBMP-2 DNA have been used for transduction of allogeneic rat bone marrow cells. These cells can then secrete BMP-2 in the transplanted sites of the posterolateral spine. When compared with autograft and rhBMP-2 implantation (when transduced bone marrow cells were implanted), bone formation was abundant. When tested both manually and histologically (Figures 1 and 2), the implanted areas were solidly fused. These experiments show promise in the future usefulness of this technology for patients undergoing spinal fusion.

## Stem Cells

Stem cells are the key component of de novo bone formation and determine the osteogenic potential of a graft or implant. For bone formation to take place, osteoconductivity, osteoinductivity, and osteogenicity need to be present. Without living cells from either the graft or the host site, bone formation will not occur. One source for the stem cells is the host mesenchymal stem cells, which arrive into the fusion site when the marrow of the bone is exposed by decortication.

Mesenchymal stem cells are most responsive to growth factors and osteoinductive proteins. Mesenchymal stem cells are the resting stem cells capable of producing various connective tissue and skeletal tissues including muscles, tendons, bone, and cartilage. These cells are ideal for tissue engineering with various growth factors, and are abundant in the stroma of the bone marrow, muscle tissue, and in soft tissues and organs such as the brain, kidney, and urinary bladder. Mesenchymal stem cells can be obtained from the bone marrow by biopsy. Various ongoing clinical studies using bone marrow aspirate plus osteoconductive material have shown promise in enhancing spinal fusion. Pericytes of vessels found in a muscle pouch are also capable of producing bone when exposed to osteoinductive material. Mesenchymal stem cell transplants have also been used clinically to treat neonates with osteogenesis imperfecta.

Isolation of fully differentiated cells such as osteoblasts and chondroblasts is not feasible because of donor availability and is associated with significant morbidity in the donor site. Therefore, tissue engineering is theoretically ideal for replacement of tissue defects and establishing bony fusions. The stem cells can either be induced in vivo or ex vivo. The autogeneic cells can also be replicated and induced in vitro before implantation back into the patient.

## Future Directions

The future of spinal surgery is changing rapidly. With the recent FDA approval of spinal arthroplasty devices, the rate of fusion surgery, compared with motion preservation surgery, may decrease. However, based on strict qualification criteria for spinal arthroplasty, only 5% to 10% of all patients currently having spine surgery qualify for spinal arthroplasty according to a recent study. This group of patients is currently being treated with diskectomy and not fusion. Osteoinductive protein stimulation of spine arthroplasty implants may improve the surface of these implants. Revision surgery following spinal arthroplasty may also require biologic materials to help fill in large defects created by these implants.

Although genetic engineering technology is currently focused on producing osteoinductive proteins, intracellular upregulatory proteins of osteoinductive proteins may be used in genetic engineering. One such protein is the LIM mineralization protein-1 (LMP-1) which has been shown to induce spinal fusion in rats after ex vivo transduction of allogeneic bone marrow cells and implantation in the posterolateral spine.

An in vivo strategy for gene therapy in a rat model has also been described. In this experiment an adenoviral vector containing the rhBMP-9 was injected in the posterolateral muscles creating a solid arthrodesis. This

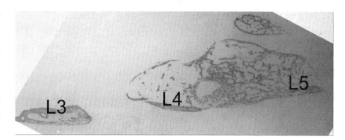

Figure 2 Histologic section obtained 4 weeks after arthrodesis with transduced bone marrow cells producing BMP-2 showed new trabecular bone formation bridging the transverse processes of L4 and L5.

technique demonstrates an alternative strategy for gene therapy and uses a different isoform of recombinant BMP.

Although rhBMP-2 and rhBMP-7 have shown excellent results in animal models in establishing spinal fusion, the optimal carrier for these proteins for clinical use has not yet been determined. The rhBMP-2 is usually packaged with a collagen sponge carrier that is not resistant to compression. Although the BMP is bound to the collagen at implantation, the muscle compression of the implant in the posterolateral spine has been shown to cause BMP to escape into the surrounding muscle, resulting in either no fusion or heterotopic ossification. Other carriers currently under clinical investigation may be more appropriate for lumbar posterolateral fusion surgery. The optimal carrier for the BMP is one that time-releases the protein into the surrounding tissue, is resorbed as new bone is laid, is immune neutral, has easy handling characteristics, and does not dilute the action of the protein.

As diagnostic tools improve, genetic and phenotypic deletions that cause certain degenerative conditions currently treated with fusion surgery may be diagnosed early. Patients will then be treated with prophylactic gene therapy and surgery prior to advanced disease states.

## Annotated Bibliography

### Biologic Properties

Muschler GF, Nitto H, Matsukura Y, et al: Spine fusion using cell matrix composites enriched in bone marrow-derived cells. *Clin Orthop Relat Res* 2003;407:102-118.

Bone matrix alone was compared with bone matrix and bone marrow clot. In this animal model, fusion rates were significantly better using the addition of bone marrow clot based on union score, quantitative CT, and mechanical testing.

Takikawa S, Bauer TW, Kambic H, Togawa D: Comparative evaluation of the osteoinductivity of two formulations of human demineralized bone matrix. *J Biomed Mater Res A* 2003;65:37-42.

Using the athymic rat muscle pouch bioassay, various commercially available allografts prepared using various techniques were compared. A significant difference was observed between the tested demineralized bone matrix.

### Bone Graft Extenders

Boden SD: Overview of the biology of lumbar spine fusion and principles for selecting a bone graft substitute. *Spine* 2002;27(16 suppl 1)S26-S31.

This review article presents a discussion of various bone graft options. A literature review is offered with a focus on finding suitable substitutes for autogenous iliac crest bone graft to promote spine fusion.

Sandhu HS: Bone morphogenetic proteins and spinal surgery. *Spine* 2003;28(suppl 15):S64-S73.

The role of BMP in spinal fusion surgery is discussed. Preclinical experiments that enabled regulated human clinical trials of rBMPs for spinal fusion are also discussed.

Vaccaro AR, Chiba K, Heller JG, et al: Bone grafting alternatives in spinal surgery. *Spine J* 2002;2:206-215.

Autogenous bone graft alternatives are discussed, with a focus on BMPs. Clinical and animal studies of each alternative implant were reviewed.

### Gene Therapy

Dumont RJ, Dayoub H, Li JZ, et al: Ex vivo bone morphogenetic protein-9 gene therapy using human mesenchymal stem cells induces spinal fusion in rodents. *Neurosurgery* 2002;51:1239-1244.

Human mesenchymal stem cells were transduced with recombinant, replication-defective type 5 adenovirus containing the cytomegalovirus promoter *BMP-9* gene to show large volumes of ectopic bone, resulting in successful spinal fusion in an animal model.

Laurent JJ, Webb KM, Beres EJ, et al: The use of bone morphogenetic protein-6 gene therapy for percutaneous spinal fusion in rabbits. *J Neurosurg Spine* 2004;1:90-94.

Percutaneous injection of adenoviral vectors containing the *BMP-6* gene was shown to induce bone formation in a rodent model. This study offers a novel method for gene therapy in experimental spinal fusion surgery.

Pola E, Gao W, Zhou Y, et al: Efficient bone formation by gene transfer of human LIM mineralization protein-3. *Gene Ther* 2004;11:683-693.

Human LMP-3 was used to induce bone mineralization and the expression of the bone-specific genes and BMP-2 in human mesenchymal stem cells in a dose-dependent manner.

Both in vitro experiments and animal experiments with human LMP-3 showing ectopic bone formation are discussed.

Viggeswarapu M, Boden SD, Liu Y, et al: Adenoviral delivery of LIM mineralization protein-1 induces new-bone formation in vitro and in vivo. *J Bone Joint Surg Am* 2001;83-A:364-376.

The novel BMP upregulator gene *LMP-1* was used with successful ex vivo gene transfer and spinal fusions in a rabbit model. A theoretic clinical application of this technique is discussed.

Wang JC, Kanim LE, Yoo S, Campbell PA, Berk AJ, Lieberman JR: Effect of regional gene therapy with bone morphogenetic protein-2-producing bone marrow cells on spinal fusion in rats. *J Bone Joint Surg Am* 2003;85-A:905-911.

Ex vivo transduction of bone marrow cells successfully formed a solid fusion mass in the rat posterolateral fusion model. Histologic analysis of the specimens revealed that the fusion masses formed by the BMP-2-producing autogenous bone marrow cells were of higher density bone compared with bone formed by the implantation of rhBMP-2 protein alone.

### Future Directions

Huang RC, Girardi FP, Lim MR, Cammisa FR Jr: Advantages and disadvantages of nonfusion technology in spine surgery. *Orthop Clin North Am* 2005;36:263-269.

Current evidence on the potential benefits and risks of nonfusion technology in spine surgery is presented in this article.

## Classic Bibliography

Boden SD, Schimandle JH, Hutton WC: The use of an osteoinductive growth factor for lumbar spinal fusion: Part II. Study of dose, carrier, and species. *Spine* 1995;20: 2633-2644.

Lovell TP, Dawson EG, Nilsson OS, Urist MR: Augmentation of spinal fusion with bone morphogenetic protein in dogs. *Clin Orthop Relat Res* 1989;243:266-274.

Urist MR: Bone: Formation by autoinduction. *Science* 1965;150:893-899.

Urist MR, Budy AM, McLean FC: Endosteal-bone formation in estrogen-treated mice. *J. Bone Joint Surg Am* 1950;32:143-162.

Wang EA, Rosen V, D'Alessandro JS, et al: Recombinant human bone morphogenetic protein induces bone formation. *Proc Natl Acad Sci USA* 1990;87:2220-2224.

# Chapter 50

# Intervertebral Disk Repair

Eric A. Levicoff, MD

James W. Larson III, MD

Lars G. Gilbertson, PhD

James D. Kang, MD

## Introduction

Back pain is a common condition that has enormous personal, social, and economic ramifications. Most instances of chronic back pain are caused by disorders of the spine, particularly degeneration of the intervertebral disk, which can occur in many different clinical conditions including disk herniation, spinal stenosis, instability, radiculopathy, myelopathy, and arthritis. Current treatments of back pain, including bed rest, administration of nonsteroidal anti-inflammatory drugs, diskectomy, and fusion remain somewhat limited in efficacy. Most of these treatments do not produce reliable outcomes, nor do they result in a complete return to preinjury levels of function, because they are directed mostly toward symptom reduction.

However, recent advances in biotechnology and in understanding the process of degeneration make possible the development of novel treatments aimed at disk preservation during the multiple stages of degeneration. Certain genes have a significant impact on matrix synthesis and catabolism within the disk and have provided targets for scientists seeking to alter the balance between these two processes. In parallel to the biologic approach to disk repair, many physicians have been working toward a better understanding of how the mechanical changes in the process of degeneration originate, and how they interact with the biologic changes. An improved understanding of the mechanical pathology at the early and later stages of disk degeneration would allow for a better attempt at the restoration of normal disk biomechanics, and therefore prevention of any effect these altered forces have in the process of degeneration. As a result, much attention over the past several years has centered on both mechanical and biologic disk repair. The early results of these efforts have been promising, and have formed the basis for a new approach to the treatment of intervertebral disk disease.

## The Degenerative Cascade

Degeneration of the intervertebral disk is a multifactorial process involving mechanical, genetic, and biologic factors. The structural and functional changes in the disk during degeneration have been well described, although the exact pathophysiologic pathway has yet to be fully understood. Normal disks consist of a gelatinous nucleus pulposus surrounded by a tough peripheral structure called the anulus fibrosus. Proper biomechanical and biologic interaction between these two distinct structures enables the disk to perform various functions including bending, load distribution, and shock absorption. This entire mechanism is highly dependent on the ability of normal disk tissue to imbibe and release water; as the water content of the disk decreases, abnormalities of function increase.

Disk hydration is maintained mainly via the extracellular matrix (ECM) produced by the chondroid cells of the disk. Chondrocytic cells within the normal nucleus produce and maintain a matrix consisting largely of a type II collagen scaffold supporting a network of proteoglycans, which attract and hold water within the disk by means of multiple negatively charged glycosaminoglycan side chains (Figure 1). This makeup is fairly similar to articular cartilage, and the ability of the matrix to imbibe and release water in relation to the stresses placed on it allows the disk to cushion compressive loads. During disk degeneration, there is a net loss of proteoglycans and water from the nucleus. This reduction in proteoglycan content and water is hypothesized to lead to the clinical evidence of degeneration including decreased disk height, decreased fluid content on T2-weighted MRI (the "black disk" phenomenon), and increased load on the surrounding structures of the spine. Abnormal distribution of forces across the disk results in cracking and fissuring of the anulus fibrosus, loss of normal nucleus matrix, herniation of the nucleus, and vertebral body pathology including subchondral sclerosis, end-plate ossification, and osteophyte formation.

Further studies have investigated the alterations in the biochemical makeup of the degenerating disk. Although the complete mechanism has yet to be determined, research suggests that degenerating disks display an imbalance between degradation and anabolism of this matrix. Biochemical investigations of degenerated

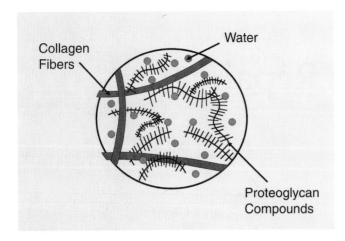

Figure 1 The major components of the ECM produced by the chondrocytes in the nucleus pulposus are shown. Type II collagen fibers support the major structure of the tissue. Proteoglycans consisting mainly of aggrecan and hyaluronic acid provide the highly charged environment that allows for strong attraction of water molecules into the ECM. This matrix is regularly degraded by the production of the enzymes in the MMP and ADAMTS families, which consist of aggrecanases, collagenases, and other degradative enzymes.

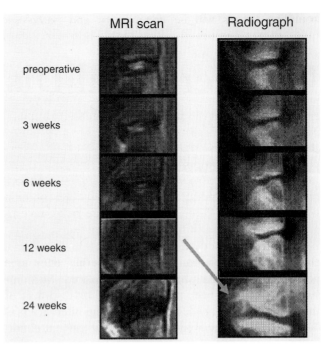

Figure 2 The degeneration induced in a rabbit lumbar spine after a stab incision through the anulus fibrosus with a 16-gauge hypodermic needle. In the serial T2-weighted MRI scans there is the steady loss of disk height and signal intensity, corresponding to degeneration of the nucleus and loss of water from this structure. Radiographs taken at the same points in time also illustrate the progressive degeneration, with loss of disk height and the formation of osteophytes (arrow).

disk cells taken from patients with herniated disks reveal increased production of catabolic proteins and inflammatory cytokines. Degradative enzymes, collectively known as matrix metalloproteinases (MMPs), are produced at levels that begin to outstrip production of their negative regulators, the tissue inhibitors of metalloproteinases (TIMPs). Upregulation of MMPs, nitric oxide, interleukin-6, and prostaglandin E2 seem to correlate with disk degeneration in humans. Although the entire family of MMPs is known to metabolize ECM in many tissues, results from recent studies of disk degeneration have revealed an imbalance with both MMP-3 (stromelysin) and its natural inhibitor TIMP-1, as well as with another catabolic protein, aggrecanase (ADAMTS-4), and its inhibitor TIMP-3.

This overabundance of catabolism is the proposed biologic mechanism, although currently there is still debate as to whether it is the altered biologic milieu or the altered biomechanical forces that set into motion the cascade of degeneration. It is quite possible that either or both may be the case. Some patients are able to trace their spinal problems back to a specific mechanical injury, whereas others have no report of such an incident, reporting merely the slowly progressing symptoms associated with the onset of disk degeneration. Models of disk degeneration support both hypotheses as well; some models rely on discrete damage to the disk, whereas others rely on chronic mechanical compression of the spine, without any traumatic damage to the disk. Although the presence or absence of acute inflammation represents a considerable difference between the two types of degenerative models, both models have been successful in creating reproducible changes consistent with chronic disk degeneration (Figure 2).

The importance of proteoglycans in maintaining disk health, together with advances in the understanding of the molecular, biochemical, and biomechanical changes that occur during the process of degeneration, has formed the basis for new research focusing on the clinical potential of novel therapeutic strategies. Although none of these strategies have attained widespread clinical application, there have been notable advances in both mechanical and biologic methods of disk repair.

## Mechanical Repair

Just as some scientists are researching the exact relationship between altered mechanical forces and disk degeneration, others are trying to show that correction of these forces can produce clinical benefit. In repairs of this nature, implanting what amounts to a prosthesis only for the nucleus pulposus is emphasized, in contrast to the larger and more invasive procedure of total disk replacement. One way these procedures differ is in the timing of the intervention. The nucleus replacement is intended for an earlier time point in degeneration, usually when the pathology at first becomes evident, such as with a herniated nucleus. In this instance, only the nucleus would be removed, then replaced with one of a variety of artificial matrices that replicates the normal biomechanics of the disk, allowing for normal compression, height, and mobility characteristics. With normal function of the disk restored, the hope is that further compensation by the surrounding tissues will be unnecessary, and pathologic outcomes such as loss of motion, osteophyte production, and spinal stenosis will be prevented.

Several different polymers are being investigated for mechanical repair, as well as different methods of delivery. There are many important aspects of these constructs. The most basic requirement is biocompatibility. The constructs also must have the ability to withstand the compression and repetitive loading that they will encounter in vivo. Prostheses should be easily handled and implanted, and they should be stable following implantation to avoid extrusion. These are indeed the common goals, but many different innovations are being investigated and refined to fit into those guidelines.

The first device designed to replace a nucleus was a steel ball, developed in 1966, which merely acted as a space holder, fulfilling few of the goals previously outlined. The nuclear prostheses currently under investigation often are grouped into one of three categories: in situ curable polymers, preformed implants, and implants that are preformed but can be altered in size during the process of implantation. Hydrogels that are being investigated as both preformed and curable implants include poly (vinyl alcohol), poly (vinyl pyrrolidone), and polyurethane as well as other proprietary hydrogels. Complications that can be encountered with in situ cured hydrogels include the prepolymerization toxicity of the monomers from which the gels are formed. Implant wear is also an issue, and one of the preformed implants now in development actually is encased in a polyethylene jacket so that frictional wear on the implant itself may be reduced. Unfortunately, although this prosthesis does help to restore normal disk function, results from preclinical studies have shown implant extrusion rates of up to 33%. Extrusions can result in catastrophic failure because many extrusions do not simply enter the implant site, but often enter the spinal canal itself. The third design technique involves preformed implants that can be sized after placement into the nuclear space, such as a polycarbonate urethane, which has a strong coiling memory and curls up on itself on implantation, much like a pigtail catheter. With this device, the delivery system is designed to stop inserting the prosthesis once the space is full, solving the problem of device sizing. A review of studies on this implant found that it fulfilled many of the biomechanical and safety goals of nuclear prostheses. In all, these prostheses appear to have some potential for clinical application, but whether they will ultimately prevent end-stage spinal degeneration and prove to have long-term durability is currently unknown.

## Biologic Repair
### Growth Factors for Disk Regeneration

In an effort to avoid the need for major surgeries such as nuclear replacement, methods for biologic repair of

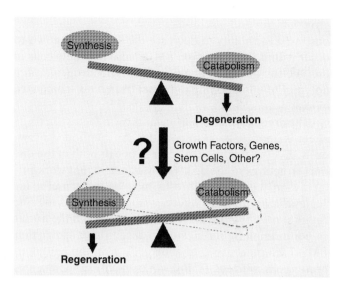

**Figure 3** Schematic representation of the general philosophy regarding the biologic strategy for disk repair. As disk degeneration is believed to occur secondary to an overall shift in the disk to a catabolic state, any alteration causing a return to an anabolic state is potentially therapeutic.

disks are being investigated. In recent years, much research regarding the intervertebral disk has centered on different growth factors now known to influence its biochemical makeup. Growth factors are molecules that bind to cells via autocrine, paracrine, or endocrine pathways to effect some change in cellular growth or differentiation. Although hundreds of growth factors are known to exist throughout the body, a select few have beneficial effects on the intervertebral disk, and studies have focused on these as forming the basis for future biologic therapies. Although there have been many exciting advances regarding the basic science of disk biochemistry, many of the potential effects of growth factors, as well as the mechanisms through which they work, remain poorly understood. Although it is currently impractical to examine each growth factor and determine its independent effect on the disk, there are certain concepts regarding the eventual clinical application of these biologic agents that deserve attention.

One issue to be considered is the type of effect a particular molecule exerts on the disk. Disk pathology is related to many factors, including decreased cellularity and decreased ECM. Although the exact mechanisms of degeneration remain unknown, it has become clear that in disk degeneration the rate of catabolism is greater than the rate of ECM synthesis; therefore, the administration of proteins that push the disk cell toward an anabolic state theoretically may improve disk health (Figure 3). Some growth factors such as transforming growth factor-beta (TGF-β) and bone morphogenetic proteins-2 and -7 (BMP-2 and BMP-7) have been shown not only to increase the production of ECM, but also to enhance cellular proliferation. Others such as platelet-derived growth factor and insulin-like growth factor-1 have demonstrated the ability to decrease the apoptosis known to occur within the aging disk. BMP-2 also may help cells in the nucleus pulposus to retain their chondrogenic phenotype, thereby delaying the onset of fibrosis, a hallmark of disk degeneration.

The area in which a particular growth factor exerts its effect is another issue to consider. As mentioned previously, disk breakdown can occur in one or both of the distinct structures of the disk. Growth factors that work primarily on the anulus fibrosus may be most useful for acute disk herniations, whereas other conditions may be better served by proteins that work on cells of the nucleus. For example, in recent studies, results have shown that BMP-7 exerts a strong anabolic effect on the anulus fibrosus cells, whereas TGF-β works mainly in the nucleus and has very little effect on the anulus fibrosus. With continued study, growth factor technology may advance to the point that therapy can be tailored to fit specific needs of the disk depending on the site of pathology.

A third issue to consider, and one that is perhaps most important, is protein delivery. Because access to the intervertebral disk would most likely require surgical dissection, therapies using growth factor injections would come with a definite level of risk to the patient. Although these procedures would be minor compared with those involving diskectomy and fusion and would result in less associated tissue loss, the need for multiple injections could dramatically increase the risk to patients. Disk degeneration and its associated pathology are usually the result of chronic processes. Even acute annular tears often are caused by a progression of damage over several years, and therapies aimed at delaying or preventing this type of insult must be capable of sustaining their effect for extended periods of time. The short half-life of an injected protein limits its ultimate clinical usefulness. Studies in which multiple injections were given in series over longer periods of time have demonstrated success, but such strategies are somewhat impractical for application to humans because of the increasing morbidity associated with each surgical procedure. Work is being done to develop a method of sustained release capable of implantation, but no such system presently exists.

## Gene Therapy

In contrast to growth factor injection therapy, the goal of gene therapy is the prolonged expression of genes, leading to a sustained, high level of protein production within the intervertebral disk. With gene therapy, actual genetic material is transferred to target cells, which then become virtual biologic factories, synthesizing and exporting proteins of interest. Although the location of the disk is somewhat of a hindrance to repeated injections of growth factors, its physical properties and biologic envi-

ronment may confer some significant advantages with regard to gene therapy. For example, the immunogenicity of foreign DNA remains a considerable obstacle to sustained protein delivery via gene transduction, as the immune response mounted by host organisms against the foreign material largely prohibits long-term gene expression. However, although this is certainly true of most tissues, there are some sites within the body that sequester injected genes from a systemic response, theoretically allowing for longer-term expression. Because of its encapsulated, virtually avascular environment, the disk is considered to be largely "immune-privileged," with cells in the nucleus sometimes up to 1 cm away from the nearest point of access to the systemic circulation. Although studies have demonstrated a mild immune response to DNA placed within the nucleus pulposus, gene expression there has lasted far longer than in other tissues. Documentation shows some expression as being only slightly diminished at 1 year following transduction.

As with treatments involving the use of growth factors, the study of gene therapy must include an examination of the pertinent issues to arrive at a coherent strategy for eventual clinical application. All gene therapy can be broken down into two general categories. Ex vivo gene therapy involves the genetic alteration of explanted host cells, followed by reimplantation into the target tissue. Advantages of this approach include transduction of cells in a more controlled environment and the ability to enhance efficacy of reinserted cells by deselecting those that are not transduced. Disadvantages include increased procedural complexity and the dedifferentiation of explanted cells while being handled in vitro. The second category is called in vivo gene therapy, during which targeted cells are transduced in their natural habitat without being removed from the host organism. Although this process is much less cumbersome than its counterpart, it cannot guarantee total transduction of cells in the target tissue, and transduced cells cannot be processed following transduction. As attempts to harvest cells from within the intervertebral disk would cause significant annular disruption, the ex vivo approach to gene therapy is less feasible for disk repair. Because cells of the nucleus depend on unique phenotypic traits that may be lost when they are cultured out of their natural environment, these cells are unable to survive reimplantation. For these reasons, most of the work done thus far regarding gene therapy in the intervertebral disk has used the in vivo model; it is this approach that seems to have the most promise for future clinical application.

A third consideration in the development of a strategy for gene therapy is the route, or vector, by which foreign DNA is transferred to target cells. Vectors can be classified as viral or nonviral, depending on the type of carrier used for the genetic material of interest. As cellular invasion and gene transfer are part of the natu-

**Table 1 | Common Viral Vectors Currently in Use in Gene Therapy Research**

| Viral Vector | Advantages | Disadvantages | Intervertebral Disk-Related Comments |
|---|---|---|---|
| Adenovirus | Highly efficient transduction<br>Cell division not necessary<br>Transduces cells of many different species and tissues | Nonincorporating<br>Safety issues: associated with a human death in clinical trials<br>Highly immunogenic | Much historical research value<br>Shown to transduce intervertebral disk cells efficiently<br>Cell division not required<br>Safety near vital structures? |
| Adeno-Associated Virus | Regarded as safest viral vector to date<br>Cell division not necessary | Less efficient transduction<br>Nonincorporating | Has been shown to transduce cells of the intervertebral disk<br>Little associated inflammation |
| Herpes Simplex Virus | Cell division not required<br>Very efficient transduction<br>Can encode large genes | Nonincorporating<br>Potentially damaging to host cells | Few data regarding use in intervertebral disk<br>Host cell damage in disk may be limiting |
| Retrovirus (such as oncoretrovirus) | Incorporating<br>Large virus capable of encoding large genes | May increase risk of leukemia<br>Some serotypes require cell division | Mitotic requirements may limit in vivo potential in disk<br>Few data regarding use in intervertebral disk |

ral life cycle of viruses, most of the successes in gene therapy research to date have been achieved using viral vectors. In these constructs, genes of interest are spliced into the viral genome, taking the place of removed pathologic DNA. Nonviral vectors, such as electroporation, gene gun, and DNA-liposome or DNA-polymer complexes, are becoming more advanced and avoid some of the risks associated with viral transduction, but they are still beset by problems of inefficiency and short-term gene expression. Within the class of viral vectors are several different types of viruses that all have particular advantages and disadvantages with respect to gene transfer in different tissues (Table 1). Safety, ability of the virus to infect nondividing cells, and length of expression of transferred genes are some of the properties associated with viral vectors that are particularly important with regard to the intervertebral disk. Because most of the disk is composed of nondividing cells, in vivo viral transduction must use viral vectors capable of invading cells that are mitotically quiescent. Viruses that incorporate into the host genome, rather than simply remaining as free plasmids, generally confer longer-term expression because the transferred genes are passed on to progeny. However, most incorporating viral vectors are able to infect only dividing cells and carry the risk of insertional mutagenesis, which rarely occurs but can cause potentially harmful side effects.

To date, successful transduction of cells of the anulus fibrosus and nucleus has been achieved, and intradiskal transgene expression has lasted longer in these structures than in other tissues. In addition, animal models of disk degeneration have been developed, and studies using these models have shown that cells of degenerated disks not only are amenable to gene transfer, but also that they are able to upregulate production of ECM in response to transduction with therapeutic genes. Adenoviral vector technology has been used for much of this gene therapy work on the intervertebral disk. Adenovirus has shown exceptional efficiency of transduction along with reasonable safety profiles in animal models. However, concerns over the safety of using the adenovirus in humans have grown in recent years, and the eventual clinical application of gene therapy will most likely depend on the continued development of safer vectors, such as adeno-associated virus, and improvements in the regulation of transgenes following transduction.

### Stem Cell Therapy

In addition to growth factor treatments and gene therapy, repopulation of the nucleus pulposus using stem cell technology is gaining rapid acceptance as another potential approach to preventing complications associated with disk degeneration. Because cells of the nucleus pulposus do not actively divide, one popular theory regarding the decline in matrix production is that these cells grow old and die, decreasing the total cell population within the nucleus. As the cellularity slowly declines, the remaining cells become unable to produce enough matrix to keep up with ongoing degradative processes. Although the success of gene therapy and growth factor injection depends on a critical mass of cells within the disk, cell-based therapy does not share this requirement, and may therefore be appropriate for a wide range of disease states, including severe degenerative disease in which the fibrotic nucleus is largely acellular. Stem cell research is still in its very early stages, but mesenchymal stem cells have been made to phenotypically resemble cells of the nucleus pulposus when placed under certain environmental conditions. Repopulation of the nucleus with these differentiated stem cells may some day be used to assist not only in the treatment of early disk disease, but also to regenerate, or "rescue" disks from a severely degenerated state. Although there is much to be learned about stem cells, and future research will have to address many medical-legal issues, cell-based therapy, used alone or in combination with growth factor injection and gene therapy, has shown promise in biologic disk repair.

## Future Directions

The understanding of disk degeneration and its associated pathologic conditions has grown in recent years. This expansion in knowledge has been accompanied by advances in mechanical and biologic strategies for disk repair. Although newer strategies for disk repair are promising, much work needs to be done before these strategies can be used regularly. Synthetic nucleus pulposus implants currently are in existence, yet safer, more biocompatible constructs must be developed. In addition, less toxic, injectable polymers are necessary, and surgical techniques used for implantation of these materials must be refined to avoid nucleus extrusion.

Biologic approaches to disk repair have also shown great potential to aid in the treatment of pathology associated with disk degeneration. The study of growth factors will continue, and more research must be done regarding not only which growth factors work in the disk, but also the mechanisms by which they exert their proanabolic influence. Advances in gene therapy are dependent on a more complete understanding of these mechanisms, as well as the continued development of safer, more efficient vectors for gene transfer. Although the study of transgene regulation is in its infancy, the ability to modulate foreign genes once they gain access to target cells will be critical to the ultimate success of this treatment strategy. Cell-based therapy using differentiated mesenchymal stem cells also has inspired great optimism in those studying disk repair. Stem cell repopulation may allow the rescue of previously degenerated disks. Although stem cell research may become more logistically difficult because of political, social, and religious concerns, the mechanisms by which differentiation occurs, and the length of stem cell survival within the disk require additional study. The explosion of knowledge related to disk degeneration has led to increased interest in the development of multiple new approaches to the degenerating intervertebral disk. Continued work is necessary to ultimately add these strategies to the therapeutic arsenal.

## Annotated Bibliography

### The Degenerative Cascade

Le Maitre CL, Freemont AJ, Hoyland JA: Localization of degradative enzymes and their inhibitors in the degenerate human intervertebral disc. *J Pathol* 2004;204: 47-54.

This study reported on a survey of degenerative and non-degenerative disks from surgical samples and postmortem samples. Immunohistochemistry was used to quantify the production of anabolic enzymes and their inhibitors. Results showed increases in all catabolic enzymes, but with proportional increases in their inhibitors except in the case of ADAMTS-4 (a disintegrin and metalloproteinase domain with thrombospondin). Its inhibitor, tissue inhibitor of MMP-3, was upregulated but not to the same degree.

### Mechanical Repair

Allen MJ, Schoonmaker JE, Bauer TW, Williams PF, Higham PA, Yuan HA: Preclinical evaluation of a poly (vinyl alcohol) hydrogel implant as a replacement for the nucleus pulposus. *Spine* 2004;29:515-523.

This study focused on an animal model of diskectomy. In baboons, the nucleus was removed from lumbar spine segments and replaced with a jacketed poly (vinyl alcohol) insert. Study results showed good restoration of height and prevention of degeneration, although there was a high rate of complications, including migration of the implant into the spinal canal and surrounding soft tissues.

Husson JL, Korge A, Polard JL, Nydegger T, Kneubuhler S, Mayer HM: A memory coiling spiral as nucleus pulposus prosthesis: Concept, specifications, bench testing, and first clinical results. *J Spinal Disord Tech* 2003; 16:405-411.

This article summarizes the creation, delivery system, preclinical, and early clinical testing of a coiled nuclear replacement. The prosthesis is implanted through a small anulotomy and can be sized at the time of surgery. The delivery and retention of the device appeared to have very favorable results. It also performed well with biomechanical and biocompatibility testing.

Kroeber MW, Unglaub F, Wang H, et al: New in vivo animal model to create intervertebral disc degeneration and to investigate the effects of therapeutic strategies to stimulate disc regeneration. *Spine* 2002;27:2684-2690.

This study outlines a model for creating degenerate disks in a rabbit. The method involves the application of a device for compressing the spine, which leads to slow and progressive degeneration of the lumbar disks.

Thomas J, Lowman A, Marcolongo M: Novel associated hydrogels for nucleus pulposus replacement. *J Biomed Mater Res A* 2003;67:1329-1337.

This article presents the data for the design of a hydrogel nuclear replacement. Various levels of poly (vinyl alcohol) and poly (vinyl pyrrolidone) are mixed and evaluated for their biomechanical properties. It concludes that low poly (vinyl pyrrolidone) ratios (1%) provide a proper amount of crosslinking, preventing the dissolution of the polymer into the surrounding fluid over 120 days.

## Biologic Repair

Li J, Yoon ST, Hutton WC: Effect of bone morphogenetic protein-2 (BMP-2) on matrix production, other BMPs, and BMP receptors in rat intervertebral disc cells. *J Spinal Disord Tech* 2004;17:423-428.

An in vitro experiment study using rat disk cells was performed to determine the effect of BMP-2 on extracellular matrix production, other BMPs, and BMP receptors.

Nishida K, Kang JD, Gilbertson LG, et al: Modulation of the biologic activity of the rabbit intervertebral disc by gene therapy: An in vivo study of adenovirus-mediated transfer of the human transforming growth factor beta 1 encoding gene. *Spine* 1999;24:2419-2425.

In vivo studies were performed using a rabbit model to determine the biologic effects of adenovirus-mediated transfer of a therapeutic gene to the intervertebral disk. Disks injected with the therapeutic viral vector exhibited a 100% increase in proteoglycan synthesis compared with intact control tissue.

Paul R, Haydon RC, Cheng H, et al: Potential use of Sox9 gene therapy for intervertebral degenerative disc disease. *Spine* 2003;28:755-763.

Adenoviral vector containing the *Sox9* gene efficiently transduced HTB-94 cells and degenerated human disk cells. After transduction, cells with the newly acquired gene demonstrated significant increases in type II collagen production.

Risbud MV, Albert TJ, Guttapalli A, et al: Differentiation of mesenchymal stem cells towards a nucleus pulposus-like phenotype in vitro: Implications for cell-based transplantation therapy. *Spine* 2004;29:2627-2632.

Hypoxic conditions and addition of TGF-β drive mesenchymal stem cell differentiation toward a phenotype consistent with that of the nucleus pulposus, with mechanisms seeming to involve a mitogen-activated protein kinase signaling pathway.

Sobajima S, Nishida K, Moon SH, Kim JS, Gilbertson LG, Kang JD: Gene therapy for degenerative disc disease. *Gene Ther* 2004;11:390-401.

This review article summarizes much of the research to date on gene therapy for the degenerating disk, and list work done on a rabbit model of degeneration. It also reviews research done showing the feasibility of transducing disks in vivo with adenovirus.

Wallach CJ, Sobajima S, Watanabe Y, et al: Gene transfer of the catabolic inhibitor TIMP-1 increases measured proteoglycans in cells from degenerated human intervertebral discs. *Spine* 2003;28:2331-2337.

Cells from degenerated intervertebral disks were transduced with an adenoviral vector delivering tissue inhibitor of metalloproteinase-1, a known inhibitor of the catabolism of extracellular matrix. Successful delivery of the gene resulted in significantly increased proteoglycan synthesis compared with control cells.

Yoon ST, Park JS, Kim KS, et al: LMP-1 upregulates intervertebral disc cell production of proteoglycans and BMPS in vitro and in vivo. *Spine* 2004;29:2603-2611.

Both in vitro and in vivo methods were used to study the effect of LIM mineralization protein-1 on intervertebral disk cell production of proteoglycans and BMPs following adenoviral transduction of the therapeutic gene. The possible mechanism of LIM mineralization protein-1 is also addressed.

## Classic Bibliography

Bao Q, Yuan HA: New technologies in spine: Nucleus replacement. *Spine* 2002;27:1245-1247.

Buckwalter JA: Aging and degeneration of the human intervertebral disc. *Spine* 1995;20:1307-1314.

Handa T, Ishihara H, Ohshima H, Osada R, Tsuji H, Obata K: Effects of hydrostatic pressure on matrix synthesis and matrix metalloproteinase production in the human lumbar intervertebral disc. *Spine* 1997;22:1085-1091.

Kanemoto M, Hukuda S, Komiya Y, et al: Immunohistochemical study of matrix metalloproteinase-3 and tissue inhibitor of metalloproteinase-1 human intervertebral discs. *Spine* 1996;21:1-8.

Kang JD, Georgescu HI, McIntyre-Larkin L, Stefanovic-Racic M, Donaldson WF III, Evans CH: Herniated lumber intervertebral discs spontaneously produce matrix metalloproteinases, nitric oxide, interleukin-6, and prostaglandin E2. *Spine* 1996;21:271-277.

Tal J: Adeno-associated virus-based vectors in gene therapy. *J Biomed Sci* 2000;7:279-291.

Thompson JP, Oegema TR Jr, Bradford DS: Stimulation of mature canine intervertebral disc by growth factors. *Spine* 1991;16:253-260.

Vernon-Roberts B: Disc pathology and disease states, in Ghosh P (ed): *The Biology of the Intervertebral Disc.* Boca Raton, FL, CRC Press, 1988, pp 73-119.

Wehling P, Schulitz KP, Robbins PD, Evans CH, Reinecke JA: Transfer of genes to chondrocytic cells of the lumbar spine: Proposal for a treatment strategy of spinal disorders by local gene therapy. *Spine* 1997;22:1092-1097.

Winn SR, Uludag H, Hollinger JO: Carrier systems for bone morphogenetic proteins. *Clin Orthop* 1999;367(suppl):S95-106.

# Chapter 51

# Minimally Invasive Spinal Surgery

D. Greg Anderson, MD

Chadi Tannoury, MD

## Introduction

The concept of minimally invasive spinal surgery embodies the goal of achieving clinical outcomes comparable to those of conventional open surgery, while minimizing the iatrogenic soft-tissue damage inherent with traditional spinal exposures. The theoretic benefits of the minimally invasive approach to spinal surgery include limited tissue disruption, less injury to the nerve and blood supply to the paraspinous muscles, less postoperative pain, shorter hospital stays, less blood loss, and faster recovery from the surgical procedure. The small incisions used for minimally invasive procedures heal with minimal scarring and therefore are appealing to many patients. Over the past few decades, minimally invasive approaches have been described for all areas of the spinal axis. Beginning with the treatment of lumbar disk disease in the 1960s and 1970s, the early pioneers of less invasive spinal surgery realized that the goals of surgery could be achieved with less exposure and thus less injury to the surrounding tissues.

Modern minimally invasive surgery of the spine has borrowed technologies from many fields to achieve its current level of sophistication. Examples of technological innovations that have led to the current state-of-the-art include advance spinal imaging, fiberoptic endoscopes, microscopes, cannulated screw technology, tubular retraction systems, illumination systems, and image guidance technology.

## Principles of Minimally Invasive Spinal Surgery

Although several techniques fall under the descriptive umbrella of minimally invasive spinal surgery, all existing procedures have certain features in common. Because the goals are to achieve the surgical treatment with minimal injury to the soft tissues, the incision size is generally limited. Rather than cutting and stripping soft tissues and paraspinous muscles, the surgeon performing minimally invasive surgery uses soft-tissue dilation or internervous planes to access the spine. In the posterior spinal region, serial dilation of the soft tissues is often used to open a space between muscle fascicles. In the anterior region of the spine, an attempt is made to limit the amount of disruption to major body cavities such as the chest or abdomen.

Because a limited amount of the spine is exposed, skin incisions must be carefully localized directly over the pathologic segment. The exact location of the spinal pathology must be determined with preoperative imaging studies to allow the surgeon to plan the approach. In most instances, high-powered illumination and magnification are used to provide the surgeon with adequate visualization of the spinal anatomy; fluoroscopy and/or image guidance technology are used to assist with positioning of instruments. Despite the limited exposure of the spine, the surgeon must ensure that the goals of surgery are achieved.

## Specialized Retractors and Instruments

Although many instrument systems have been described for minimally invasive spinal surgical procedures, a theme common to many transmuscular approaches is the concept of serial dilation. In its simplest form, this approach involves a series of enlarging tubes that are introduced sequentially through the skin incision down to the spine. As the tubes are placed, the soft tissues are dilated, ultimately allowing the distance from the skin to the spine to be determined and a final tubular retractor of appropriate length to be placed. The tubular retractor is often attached to the operating table by a rigid "arm" that secures the position of the retractor during the procedure. The tubular retractor is used as a viewing portal to visualize and to operate on the spine.

Optimal visualization generally requires some form of illumination and magnification. To access different regions of the spine, the position and angulation of the tubular retractor can be adjusted or "wanded" over a fairly wide area that often encompasses two lumbar vertebral levels (Figure 1). Wanding also can be used to access the contralateral side of the spinal canal. More complex retractor systems, based on the same concept of serial dilation, are available that expand or open to create a wider

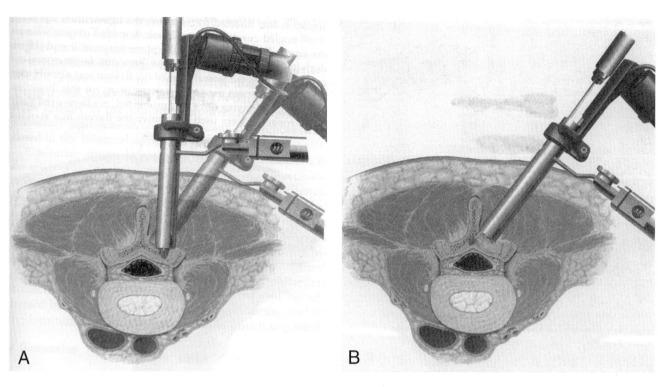

Figure 1 **A** and **B,** A wanding maneuver is used to change the position of the tubular retractor and reach different areas of the spine.

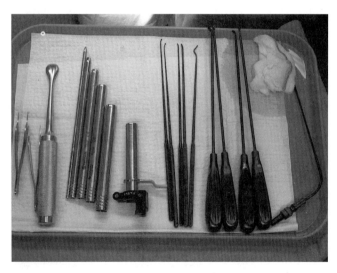

Figure 2 Instruments used for tubular microdiskectomy.

viewing area. These retractors are useful for more complex procedures such as spinal fusions. Some retractors provide a wide view of the anatomy without wanding, and thus can be thought of as a "mini-open" system, allowing the direct placement of spinal implants based on visualization of topographic landmarks.

Minimally invasive surgery requires the use of specialized surgical instrumentation so that surgery will proceed safely, with results comparable with the open techniques. In some instances, the instruments used are simply longer or bayoneted for use through a tubular

retractor system (Figure 2). Other more specialized instruments are available for soft-tissue ablation, interbody fusion, and hemostasis.

## Viewing Technologies

The development of microscopy, endoscopy, fiberoptics, video systems, and high-powered illumination sources all have impacted modern minimally invasive spinal surgery. These technologies allow the surgeon to view and magnify regions of anatomy located well below the skin, providing three-dimensional viewing of the surgical field in some instances (Figure 3).

Each viewing technology has certain advantages and disadvantages. Loupe magnification is simple and useful when working through the larger portals, but simultaneous visualization by the surgeon and assistant is limited. Endoscopy provides excellent lighting, magnification, and allows visualization into tight spaces but limits three-dimensional viewing and may cause smudging or fogging. The microscope provides the best lighting and magnification and allows the surgeon a three-dimensional view of the surgical site. When using the microscope, however, large instruments, such as those required for an interbody fusion, may block visualization through the tubular access channel.

## Minimally Invasive Spinal Implants

The first minimally invasive spinal surgical procedures to be widely adopted have been diskectomies and de-

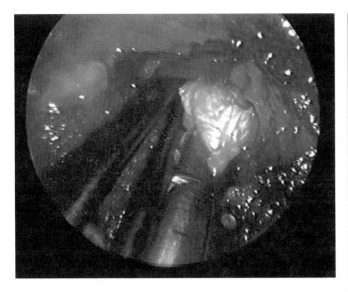

Figure 3 Endoscopic diskectomy. A large extruded disk fragment is being pulled from the spinal canal with a pituitary rongeur. This procedure is done under direct visualization using an endoscopic camera.

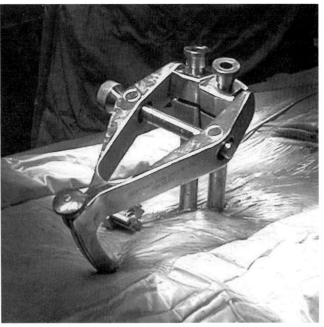

Figure 4 The percutaneous pedicle screw system allows a rod to be passed through pedicle screws using a special jig that guides the rod into the crowns of the pedicle screws.

compressions of the lumbar spine. However, with surgeon experience, it became clear that fusions and instrumentation were feasible using this approach. Initially, spinal implants used for fusion procedures were adopted from traditional open lumbar fusion. Over the past few years, however, specialized implants specifically designed for minimal access spinal fusion have become available. Two types of implants are currently available; one type is cannulated, with the screw placed percutaneously over a guide wire, and others are designed to be placed under direct visualization through a retractor system used for minimally invasive surgery.

The technique for the placement of percutaneous cannulated screws differs somewhat from the placement of traditional pedicle screws and relies on accurate placement of a guide wire down the pedicle. First, a large cannulated needle and obturator are placed through the pedicle under fluoroscopic guidance. The obturator is then removed allowing the placement of a guide wire. Using cannulated instruments, the pedicle is prepared and a cannulated pedicle screw is placed. Finally, a rod is attached and secured to the screws (Figure 4).

## Image Guidance/Computer-Assisted Spinal Surgery

Image guidance involves a system of sensors and a computer that allows the real-time tracking of "virtual" surgical instruments relative to previously acquired imaging studies (Figure 5). Currently, most image guidance systems display the "virtual" position of instruments relative to fluoroscopic and/or CT images on a computer monitor. With image guidance, the surgeon can determine the position of surgical instruments relative to an-

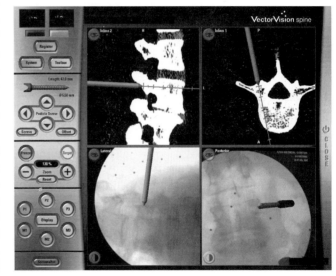

Figure 5 Image guidance can be used to show the position of surgical instruments relative to previously acquired imaging studies. In this figure, the surgeon is using the software to navigate the position of a lumbar pedicle simultaneously using fluoroscopic and CT images.

atomic landmarks on the imaging studies. Because the spine anatomy is complex and the margin of error is low, spinal surgery has been viewed as an ideal application of image guidance technology.

The most important theoretic benefit to the use of image guidance during spinal surgery is the potential for increased safety and accuracy when performing surgery adjacent to vital structures or delicate neural elements.

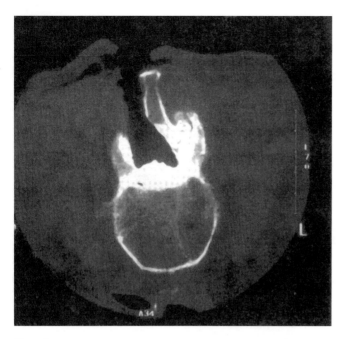

Figure 6   The lamina has been undercut from a unilateral approach to provide bilateral decompression of the spinal canal.

Other important benefits are reduced exposure of the patient and surgical team to ionizing radiation, the ability to perform less invasive procedures, and the ability to follow the position of instruments in multiple planes (images) without using intraoperative fluoroscopy. Certain highly technical instrumentation techniques, such as the placement of C1-C2 transarticular screws, are ideal for use in image guidance because the implants must be placed in a small corridor between critical structures. Image guidance can be used to place instrumentation during revision procedures; normal anatomic landmarks may be absent or difficult to see. Many different spinal procedures have been performed with the assistance of image guidance and some have been systematically studied and compared with traditional techniques.

Image guidance can be a useful adjuvant to many minimally invasive spinal techniques because it allows "virtual" visualization of anatomic landmarks that cannot be directly visualized because of the limited surgical exposure.

## Spinal Decompression

The goal of spinal decompression is to remove mechanical pressure from the neural elements either by excising a herniated disk fragment or by expanding the spinal canal with a laminectomy, medial facetectomy and/or foraminotomy. Lumbar diskectomies are undoubtedly the most commonly performed minimally invasive spinal surgery. The benefits of a less invasive approach have been known since at least the mid 1970s, when most surgeons adopted the use of hemilaminotomy

rather than laminectomy as the mainstay for this procedure. At the current time, microdiskectomy is considered the "gold standard" for treatment of most instances of posterolateral herniated disk with sciatica. Many studies have documented good results using this approach.

In recent years, microdiskectomy has been performed through tubular retractor systems. The benefits of this approach include soft-tissue dilation as opposed to muscle cutting and stripping, and the small incision size. Obese patients, although somewhat more difficult to treat, seem to benefit even more than thin patients because the use of traditional exposure techniques requires a large incision to allow visualization of the spine. The visualization of the spinal canal, dura, and herniated disk using a microscope are excellent. This procedure is technically simpler than other minimally invasive spinal procedures and should be the starting point for those surgeons adopting minimally invasive surgery in their practice. Although rigorous published outcome studies comparing diskectomy using tubular retractors with microdiskectomy using standard retractors are lacking, it appears that results are good with the tubular systems.

Lumbar canal stenosis also has been successfully treated using tubular retractor systems. Using a unilateral or bilateral technique, or partial or complete laminectomy, medial facet resection and foraminotomy can be achieved. In the unilateral technique, the retractor system can be "wanded" to undercut the lamina and reach the contralateral foramen and lateral recess (Figure 6). Similar muscle-splitting approaches with tubular retractors have been successfully used in the posterior cervical spine.

A different approach to lumbar decompression using an endoscope to access the posterolateral disk and lateral portion of the neural foramen outside of the spinal canal has been described (Figure 7). The theoretic advantages of this approach include the avoidance of scarring to the spinal canal and the ability to directly access the lateral disk and lateral neural foramen. Disadvantages of accessing the spine with the endoscopic technique include the steep learning curve for the surgeon and the increased surgical time associated with the approach.

## Spinal Fusion

Both interbody and posterolateral (intertransverse) fusions have been achieved through minimally invasive surgical techniques. In the lumbar spine, the interbody space can be approached through an anterior, lateral, transforaminal, and posterior approach. The transforaminal approach has become popular in recent years because it provides access to the disk space without the need to reposition the patient intraoperatively (in contrast to the anterolateral approach) and requires minimal retraction of the neural elements (unlike the posterolateral approach). Using a tubular retractor system, the facet complex on one side can be removed, providing exposure to the posterolateral disk space. An interbody fusion is then achieved by thoroughly excising all of the disk and cartilaginous end plate and placing an appropriately sized interbody fusion device with bone graft into the interbody space. The segment is then stabilized by placing pedicle screw instrumentation. This relatively technical procedure should be used only after a surgeon has gained significant experience in tubular access lumbar surgery.

Another procedure that has grown in popularity in recent years is the mini-anterolateral interbody fusion. Using a retroperitoneal approach, the anterior aspect of the lower lumbar spine is exposed through a small incision (about 5 cm in a thin patient). This approach provides wide access to the anterior aspect of the disk space, allowing interbody fusion to be performed. In most instances, only minimal postoperative discomfort is experienced by the patient as a result of this approach. Often, a general or vascular surgeon will assist with exposure of the spine because the great vessels must be mobilized for exposures above the L5-S1 disk space.

Fusion of the posterior cervical spine using tubular retractor systems has also been reported. In one report, the authors were able to reduce cervical facet dislocations, place lateral mass screws, and perform a posterior arthrodesis in two patients following cervical trauma.

## Thoracoscopic/Laparoscopic Spinal Surgery

Endoscopic procedures have made a major impact in the fields of general and chest surgery, where they have become the preferred method for addressing many types of pathology. Not surprisingly, these same technologies have been used to approach anterior spinal pathologies including infections, burst fractures, tumors, degenerative disk disease, and spinal deformity.

Laparoscopic and open anterolateral interbody fusion were compared in one study; it was concluded that the laparoscopic approach was associated with a shorter hospital stay and reduced blood loss but required a longer surgical time in many instances. Other studies have compared laparoscopic anterolateral interbody fusion with mini-open anterolateral interbody fusion and it was concluded that the risk of complications, including vein laceration and retrograde ejaculation in males, was high with the laparoscopic approach. For this reason, the popularity of laparoscopic anterolateral interbody fusion above the L5-S1 disk space has diminished in recent years in favor of mini-anterolateral interbody fusion, which also provides many of the benefits of a minimally invasive approach.

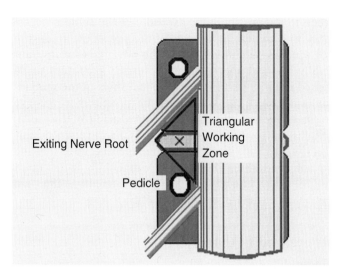

Figure 7 The extraforaminal approach to the lumbar disk is shown. The endoscope is docked against the disk (x) in the triangular working zone below the exiting nerve root. This positioning allows access to the disk and intervertebral foramen.

In one study, decreased blood loss, less postoperative pain, and a shorter hospital stay were reported using video-assisted thoracoscopic anterior diskectomy in the thoracic region compared with thoracotomy for the same diagnosis. Unlike the lumbar spine, deflation of the lung provides good access to the lateral thoracic spine without the need to mobilize the great vessels. This approach also has been used for performing biopsies, thoracic sympathectomies, and thoracic corpectomies. In selected patients with spinal deformities, anterior releases, interbody fusions, and anterior instrumented fusions have been successfully performed. In a 2004 study, a thoracoscopic transdiaphragmatic approach was used to address pathology at the thoracolumbar junction, allowing decompression and instrumentation down to the L2 level.

## Future of Minimally Invasive Surgery

Minimally invasive surgery is a rapidly evolving field with new instruments and techniques being described on a regular basis. Although this approach holds much promise, minimally invasive techniques have not yet been subjected to rigorous scientific scrutiny, comparing the new techniques with the traditional techniques in a prospective fashion. Prospective studies are needed to truly define the role, benefits, and risks of this developing field of spinal surgery. It is important to realize that minimally invasive surgical techniques have a significant learning curve. Therefore, it is prudent that the approach to minimally invasive spinal surgery be progressive, beginning with cadaver training and gaining experience on simple cases before applying these techniques to complex conditions. The real benefits of a minimally invasive surgical approach can only be achieved when the surgeon is able to fully attain the goals of the surgery. Therefore, the surgeon should be prepared to proceed to a more generous exposure of the spine if necessary to complete all aspects of the procedure to ensure an optimal outcome. Despite the advantages of a minimally invasive approach, spine surgery continues to be based in large part on the technical skills of the individual surgeon; these skills must be practiced to achieve mastery. It is likely that with time, many of the techniques and principles of minimally invasive spinal surgery will replace some traditional approaches to treating spinal conditions. Therefore, learned skills in this area will help the surgeon adapt to advancements in the field as outcome data prove the benefits of less invasive surgical techniques.

## Annotated Bibliography

### General

Jaikumar S, Kim DH, Kam AC: History of minimally invasive spine surgery. *Neurosurgery* 2002;51(suppl 5):S1-14.

Minimally invasive spine surgery is designed for conventional surgery involving extensive anatomic dissections performed via small incisions. Advances in lasers, endoscopy, and image-guidance systems have helped to reduce recovery time, decrease postoperative morbidity, and provide cosmetic benefits to patients undergoing minimally invasive spine surgery.

Tong HC, Williams JC, Haig AJ, Geisser ME, Chiodo A: Predicting outcomes of transforaminal epidural injections for sciatica. *Spine J* 2003;3:430-434.

This cross-sectional study attempts to determine which patient factors are associated with the outcomes of epidural injections for patients with sciatica. The poorest outcomes were primarily associated with patients who received Social Security Disability Insurance or Workers' Compensation. For patients with jobs requiring heavy lifting and who receive Social Security Disability Insurance or Workers' Compensation, treatment with epidural injection is questioned.

### Viewing Technologies

Egol KA: Minimally invasive orthopaedic trauma surgery: A review of the latest techniques. *Bull Hosp Jt Dis* 2004;62:6-12.

Malalignment is the main complication with first generation orthopaedic implants. Computer-assisted minimally invasive fluoroscopic surgery and other advanced technologies can provide the surgeon with three-dimensional views and biplanar imaging for placement of orthopaedic implants in difficult to reach areas. The current literature regarding these techniques is limited and poorly defined.

Thongtrangan I, Le H, Park J, Kim DH: Minimally invasive spinal surgery: A historical perspective. *Neurosurg Focus* 2004;16:E13.

The development of microscopy, laser technology, thoracoscopy, endoscopy, and video- and image-guidance systems provided the foundation for minimally invasive spinal surgery. Further improvements in optical devices and imaging re-

sources, the development of biologic agents, and the introduction of instrumentation systems designed for minimally invasive procedures will lead to further applications for minimally invasive spine surgery.

### Image Guidance/Computer-Assisted Spinal Surgery

Austin MS, Vaccaro AR, Brislin B, Nachwalter R, Hilibrand AS, Albert TJ: Image-guided spine surgery: A cadaver study comparing conventional open laminoforaminotomy and two image-guided techniques for pedicle screw placement in posterolateral fusion and nonfusion models. *Spine* 2002;27:2503-2508.

A randomized comparison of conventional and image-guided techniques for pedicle screw placement showed that the use of image-guided methods, particularly CT, increases the accuracy of pedicle screw placement in the thoracolumbosacral spine. Improved accuracy is especially relevant clinically when the anatomy is obscured as a result of inflammatory disorders or when used postoperatively in the setting of posterolateral fusion.

Foley KT, Simon DA, Rampersaud YR: Virtual fluoroscopy: Computer-assisted fluoroscopic navigation. *Spine* 2001;26:347-351.

A novel virtual fluoroscopy system offers several advantages over conventional fluoroscopy while providing acceptable targeting accuracy. A single C-arm can provide real-time, multiplanar procedural guidance. Virtual fluoroscopy dramatically reduces radiation exposure to the patient and surgical team by eliminating the need for repetitive fluoroscopic imaging for tool placement.

Holly LT, Bloch O, Obasi C, Johnson JP: Frameless stereotaxy for anterior spinal procedures. *J Neurosurg* 2001; 95(suppl 2):196-201.

Intraoperative image guidance provides real-time three-dimensional visualization and has been successfully used in many posterior spinal procedures. This study showed that applying these stereotaxic techniques to anterior spinal surgery in a human cadaveric model was successful and practical. The accuracy of the findings in this study indicates that anterior stereotaxy should be applicable in clinical practice.

Holly LT, Foley KT: Three-dimensional fluoroscopy-guided percutaneous thoracolumbar pedicle screw placement: Technical note. *J Neurosurg* 2003;99(suppl 3):324-329.

The feasibility and accuracy of three-dimensional fluoroscopic guidance for percutaneous placement of thoracic and lumbar pedicle screws were evaluated in three cadaveric specimens. This study reported a 95% rate of accurate screw placement. This study found that a highly accurate spinal navigation system will facilitate the application of minimally invasive techniques to the field of spine surgery.

Mirza SK, Wiggins GC, Kuntz C IV, et al: Accuracy of thoracic vertebral body screw placement using standard fluoroscopy, fluoroscopic image guidance, and computed tomographic image guidance: A cadaver study. *Spine* 2003;28:402-413.

A surgical simulation study in human cadaver spine specimens was conducted to evaluate the accuracy, procedure duration, and radiation exposure to the specimen and the surgeon of thoracic vertebral body screw placement using four different intraoperative imaging techniques. Fluoroscopy-based image guidance using a single reference marker for the entire thoracic spine is highly inaccurate and unsafe. Systems using registration based on the instrumented vertebrae provide more accurate placement of thoracic vertebral body screws than standard fluoroscopy, but expose the patient to more radiation and require more time for screw insertion.

Resnick DK: Prospective comparison of virtual fluoroscopy to fluoroscopy and plain radiographs for placement of lumbar pedicle screws. *J Spinal Disord Tech* 2003;16:254-260.

Fluoroscopy-based frameless stereotactic systems provide feedback to the surgeon using virtual fluoroscopic images. The accuracy of pedicle screw placement using these virtual images was studied prospectively in 23 consecutive patients and compared with traditional fluoroscopy. The positive predictive value was 99%.

Wigfield C, Bolger C: A technique for frameless stereotaxy and placement of transarticular screws for atlanto-axial instability in rheumatoid arthritis. *Eur Spine J* 2001;10:264-268.

In this study, 46 patients with atlantoaxial instability resulting from rheumatoid arthritis had minimally invasive posterior stabilization with percutaneous transarticular screws using the StealthStation (Medtronic Sofamor Danek, Memphis, TN) for image guidance to navigate safely through C2. There were no neurovascular injuries.

## Spinal Decompression

Guiot BH, Khoo LT, Fessler RG: A minimally invasive technique for decompression of the lumbar spine. *Spine* 2002;27:432-438.

The purpose of this study was to determine the feasibility of percutaneous microendoscopic bilateral decompression of lumbar stenosis via a unilateral approach in a human cadaver model using a microendoscopic laminotomy technique.

Williams RW: Lumbar disc disease: Microdiscectomy. *Neurosurg Clin N Am* 1993;4:101-108.

This article discusses a rationale for the use of the microsurgical technique when treating lumbar disk herniations. The rigid surgical discipline of microlumbar diskectomy is presented along with a suggested means to best preserve the future competence of the anulus fibrosus.

Yeung AT: The evolution of percutaneous spinal endoscopy and discectomy: State of the art. *Mt Sinai J Med* 2000;67:327-332.

The author relates his 7 years' experience with endoscopic spine surgery for lumbar disk herniations and conditions. These spinal pathologies were treated using the Yeung endoscopic spine system, which features an endoscope with a 2.8 mm operating channel.

Yuguchi T, Nishio M, Akiyama C, Ito M, Yoshimine T: Posterior microendoscopic surgical approach for the degenerative cervical spine. *Neurol Res* 2003;25:17-21.

The authors studied the microendoscopic posterior approach in both cadaver models and in clinical cases. This technique needs only a small surgical route, thus reducing damage to the paraspinous muscles. It also provides a clear view of the operating points.

## Spinal Fusion

Wang MY, Prusmack CJ, Green BA, Gruen JP, Levi AD: Minimally invasive lateral mass screws in the treatment of cervical facet dislocations: Technical note. *Neurosurgery* 2003;52:444-447.

This technical note describes the successful placement of lateral mass screw and rod constructs with the use of a tubular dilator retractor system, preserving the integrity of the muscles and ligaments that maintain the posterior tension band of the cervical spine.

## Thoracoscopic/Laparoscopic Spinal Surgery

Han PP, Kenny K, Dickman CA: Thoracoscopic approaches to the thoracic spine: Experience with 241 surgical procedures. *Neurosurgery* 2002;51(suppl 5):S88-S95.

Microsurgical thoracoscopic approaches to the thoracic spine allow access to the spinal cord, spinal nerves, disk spaces, vertebral bodies, paravertebral soft tissues, and sympathic chain with minimal invasion, lower morbidity rates, and better cosmesis when compared with open thoracotomy. This approach does not replace the open approach for thoracic carpectomies and spinal reconstruction procedures.

Kaiser MG, Haid RW Jr, Subach BR, Miller JS, Smith CD, Rodts GE Jr: Comparison of the mini-open versus laparoscopic approach for anterior lumbar interbody fusion: A retrospective review. *Neurosurgery* 2002;51:97-103.

The anterior lumbar interbody fusion procedure can be done laparoscopically as well as a new "mini-open" approach. In this retrospective review, a comparison of these two anterior lumbar interbody fusion approaches showed that the laparoscopic approach does not seem to have a definitive advantage over the mini-open exposure.

Kim DH, Jahng TA, Balabhadra RS, Potulski M, Beisse R: Thoracoscopic transdiaphragmatic approach to thoracolumbar junction fractures. *Spine J* 2004;4:317-328.

The thoracoscopic transdiaphragmatic approach provides excellent access to the entire thoracolumbar junction, permitting satisfactory spinal decompression, reconstruction, and instrumentation. Diaphragmatic opening and repair can be accomplished safely and effectively without special endoscopic instrumentation and precluding the need for retroperitoneoscopic or open thoracoabdominal approaches and related morbidities.

Krasna MJ, Jiao X, Eslami A, Rutter CM, Levine AM: Thoracoscopic approach for spine deformities. *J Am Coll Surg* 2003;197:777-779.

Minimally invasive thoracoscopic anterior procedures can be used safely and effectively in the treatment of idiopathic scoliosis and kyphotic deformity. These approaches decrease procedure-related trauma, surgical time, blood loss, and length of hospitalization, and may also alleviate postthoracotomy pain.

## Classic Bibliography

Capanna AH, Williams RW, Austin DC, Darmody WR, Thomas LM: Lumbar discectomy: Percentage of disc removal and detection of anterior annulus perforation. *Spine* 1981;6:610-614.

Chiu JC, Clifford TJ, Greenspan M, Richley RC, Lohman G, Sison RB: Percutaneous microdecompressive endoscopic cervical discectomy with laser thermodiskoplasty. *Mt Sinai J Med* 2000;67:278-282.

Connelly CS, Manges PA: Video-assisted thoracoscopic discectomy and fusion. *AORN J* 1998;67:940-956.

Heniford BT, Matthews BD, Lieberman IH: Laparoscopic lumbar interbody spinal fusion. *Surg Clin North Am* 2000;80:1487-1500.

Kambin P, Savitz MH: Arthroscopic microdiscectomy: An alternative to open disc surgery. *Mt Sinai J Med* 2000;67:283-287.

Onik GM, Helms C: Nuances in percutaneous discectomy. *Radiol Clin North Am* 1998;36:523-532.

Reasoner DK, Warner DS, Todd MM, Hunt SW, Kirchner J: A comparison of anesthetic techniques for awake intubation in neurosurgical patients. *J Neurosurg Anesthesiol* 1995;7:94-99.

Regan JJ, Yuan H, McAfee PC: Laparoscopic fusion of the lumbar spine: Minimally invasive spine surgery: A prospective multicenter study evaluating open and laparoscopic lumbar fusion. *Spine* 1999;24:402-411.

Visocchi M, Masferrer R, Sonntag VK, Dickman CA: Thoracoscopic approaches to the thoracic spine. *Acta Neurochir (Wien)* 1998;140:737-743.

Williams RW: Lumbar disc disease: Microdiscectomy. *Neurosurg Clin N Am* 1993;4:101-108.

Wolf O, Meier U: First experiences using microsurgical techniques for minimally invasive ventral interbody fusion of the lumbar spine (MINI-ALIF). *Z Arztl Fortbild Qualitatssich* 1999;93:267-271.

Yeung AT: The evolution of percutaneous spinal endoscopy and discectomy: State of the art. *Mt Sinai J Med* 2000;67:327-332.

# Chapter 52

# Motion-Sparing Technologies

Alan S. Hilibrand, MD

John S. Kirkpatrick, MD

## Introduction

The term "motion-sparing technology" has been used to describe newer surgical techniques designed to preserve spinal motion while eliminating spinal pathology. Currently, the greatest amount of attention in this field has been given to total disk arthroplasty, although many other technologies are being developed for motion preservation, especially in the posterior lumbar spine. The principle behind motion-sparing technology is to allow the surgeon to treat the patient's spinal condition that usually arises from the consequences of aging and disk degeneration, by a means that does not require spinal fusion or alteration of normal spinal biomechanics. This concept is not new.

This chapter summarizes the current knowledge regarding available technology in the field of motion preservation. Although the materials and designs of cervical and lumbar disk prostheses are similar, their indications and rationale differ. Cervical disk arthroplasty has been promoted as an alternative to the fusion that accompanies almost all anterior cervical decompressive procedures. Ideally, these implants would be indicated for many patients undergoing anterior cervical fusion for the treatment of radiculopathy and/or myelopathy. On the other hand, most decompressive procedures for lumbar radiculopathy are performed through a posterior approach, which does not provide adequate access to the anterior disk space to allow placement of any of the current lumbar disk arthroplasty designs. Consequently, the indications for lumbar disk arthroplasty in current Investigational Device Exemption (IDE) trials have focused on symptoms of axial back pain caused by primary lumbar disk degeneration. Other forms of motion-sparing technologies are being developed to preserve motion after posterior lumbar decompressive procedures.

Many of the products and technologies discussed in this chapter are currently undergoing IDE trials conducted by the United States Food and Drug Administration (FDA). Outcomes data are being reported from centers involved in these trials, and comprehensive data

from multicenter trials are likely to be presented within the next year and published within 18 to 24 months.

## Lumbar Spine

Devices are being developed for the lumbar spine to replace or augment the function of all or part of the disk, the posterior ligaments, or other portions of the spinal motion segment. Devices also are being developed to aid in decompression of lumbar stenosis. The rationale for these devices is reviewed with each specific device. These devices are at various stages of availability in the United States, from recent FDA approval to preclinical development. Many of these devices are using proprietary technology with data not yet published, which prevents detailed description at this time.

### Disk Arthroplasty

The general philosophy of disk replacement is similar to that of lumbar fusion for low back pain, but is considered the next generation in the surgical care of degenerative disk disease. This concept is similar to the progression of treatments for arthritis of diarthrodial joints, with historical surgical management consisting of arthrodesis being superseded by total joint arthroplasty more than 25 years ago. Disk arthroplasty aims to replace the "pain generator" degenerative disk with a mobile implant instead of performing an arthrodesis, thus allowing continued motion and in theory preventing adjacent segment degeneration, which is presumed to be the cause of long-term failure of fusions. As the principle of fusion for low back pain remains somewhat controversial, so should the concept of disk arthroplasty. The multidirectional nature of spinal motion and stability, including the contribution of the facet joints and posterior structures, complicates the replication of anatomic motion with simple devices. The complex nature and poorly understood causes of spinal pain also introduce challenges to improving clinical outcomes using disk arthroplasty.

The restoration of the mechanical integrity of the lumbar spinal motion segment involves consideration of

American Academy of Orthopaedic Surgeons

495

kinematics, geometry, and mechanics of the disk prosthesis. Normal kinematics of the disk involves motion in flexion/extension, lateral bending, axial rotation, and translation with a variable instantaneous axis of rotation. With current disk prosthesis designs, the trend is to use mobile bearings to reproduce such complex motions. The use of such mobile bearings leads to some concern over the production of wear debris and the longevity of the prostheses. Disk prosthesis geometry must approximate the geometry of the disk height and axial plane dimensions to provide appropriate stability, fit within the intended level, and preserve normal motion and load on the facet joints. The mechanics of the disk prosthesis must allow for normal load transmission through the disk without failure, load transfer, or shifting to other structures such as the facets. Ideally, the key goal of disk arthroplasty, the prevention of adjacent segment degeneration, must be achieved without producing abnormal motion or stress on adjacent segments. In vitro test methods are being used in an attempt to predict the in vivo mechanical behavior wear properties of disk prostheses. Although preclinical in vitro testing for wear properties failed to predict the catastrophic failures resulting from delamination of the polyurethane that occurred in vivo using the AcroFlex disk (DePuy Spine, Raynham, MA), improved standards for testing are being developed through the American Society for Testing and Materials International and the International Organization for Standardization.

The first lumbar disk prosthesis to gain FDA approval (2004) is the Charite prosthesis (DePuy Spine). Clinical results of the disk replacement (n = 182) were compared with those of anterior lumbar fusion with a cage implant (n = 85) for the treatment of single level degenerative disk disease at L4-5 (approximately 30% of patients) or L5-S1 (approximately 70% of patients). Success was defined as 25% improvement in the Oswestry Disability Index, absence of device failure, absence of major complications, and maintenance of or improvement in neurologic status. Follow-up was maintained at 24 months in 86% of patients who received disk replacement and 79% of patients who underwent fusion. The percentage of patients who had successful results at 6, 12, and 24 months were 44%, 51%, and 63%, respectively, for the Charite group and 35%, 41%, and 53%, respectively, for the fusion group.

The review panel raised the issue that 2 years of follow-up was inadequate to demonstrate proof that disk replacement prevented adjacent segment degeneration. There were also concerns regarding the potential for altered stresses on the facets that could lead to degeneration of the articulation and persistent pain. A postapproval study generating longer-term follow-up data is in progress. Other designs are currently undergoing

clinical trials in the United States with the expectation that regulatory applications will be filed in the next few years.

Although the formal complete clinical trials are not yet published, some data are available from individual centers and from the FDA website. A patient satisfaction measure of those who received the lumbar disk arthroplasty device showed 74% were satisfied and 14% were "somewhat satisfied." Satisfaction among patients in the fusion group was 53% and 26%, respectively.

Other total disk prostheses remain at various stages of development and clinical use. Other metal-on-polyethylene or metal-on-metal designs include the ProDisc Artificial Total Lumbar Disk Replacement (Synthes, Inc, Paoli, PA), the MPD Motion Preservation Devices (Vertebron, Inc, Stratford, CT), Maverick (Medtronic Sofamor Danek, Memphis, TN) and the FlexiCore Lumbar Prosthesis (Stryker, Allendale, NJ), which are in clinical trials under IDE in the United States. Clinical results from one center of the IDE trial for ProDisc showed improved Oswestry scores for disk replacement compared with fusion at 6-month follow-up. Longer-term follow-up results and results from other designs are expected in the near future. A design using an elastomeric core between titanium plates has been the focus of two pilot studies, with clinical results showing an average improvement in the Oswestry index of 15 points. Unfortunately, thin cut CT scans have shown mechanical failure using this design. One novel design approach for a total disk replacement is use of a three-dimensional polyethylene fabric with a bioactive ceramic coating. Biomechanical testing of this design noted similarity to natural intervertebral disk. Preliminary animal studies noted short-term success, but temporary internal fixation was required and later removed.

### Partial Disk Replacement

Several approaches are under development for nucleus pulposus replacement. A mechanical spring design intended for use with annular preservation has been investigated in vitro; motion segment stiffness was similar to that of the intact disk. This device is intended to be inserted through cavities made in the adjacent vertebral bodies, sparing the anulus fibrosus. A hydrogel nuclear replacement (PDN; Raymedica, Bloomington, MN) has been developed and has undergone preliminary clinical trials in China. It is intended for insertion via a laminotomy performed during disk excision for treatment of a herniated disk. This device has been studied in a longitudinal cohort with no concurrent control studies, providing an initial clinical experience demonstrating its initial safety and effectiveness. The PDN device has also been studied in patients with back pain caused by degenerative disk disease, with the device implanted using an anterolateral approach. There were few complications related to the approach used, but the device was noted to have moved postoperatively in four of eight patients, with one requiring revision to a fusion. Six of the eight patients had successful outcomes, with preoperative Oswestry scores (mean, 31.43) improving to 8.0 at 12 months after surgery. An alternative design of a hydrogel implant, made of poly vinyl alcohol, has been implanted in a baboon model with no evidence of local or systemic toxicity. There were six extrusions postoperatively in 20 animals, two of which were into the spinal canal even though the method of insertion was anterolateral or posterolateral.

A memory-coiling spiral of a polycarbonate urethane has also been developed to maintain the intervertebral space after diskectomy. This device is intended to be inserted through the annulotomy after disk excision for radiculopathy. Initial clinical results in five patients have been deemed successful, with no device-related complications. Follow-up flexion and extension radiographs have shown maintenance of disk height and preservation of motion. Long-term performance remains unknown. Injectable polymers are being investigated as a means to replace the turgor and load-carrying capacity of the degenerated nucleus pulposus. Polymer gels contained in a mesh are also being developed as a way to maintain the distraction and mobility of the disk. A polymer material that coils into a spiral when inserted through the anulus fibrosus to then restore the distraction of the disk space is also being developed. Hydrophilic implants that swell when hydrated, allowing a small insertion site through the anulus fibrosus, are under development. These nuclear replacements require variable amounts of integrity of the anulus fibrosus depending on their design and indications.

## Biologic "Devices" for Disk Replacement

Tissue engineering techniques are being developed to provide more biologic solutions to address disk replacement and degeneration. The capability to engineer a composite disk using a scaffold made of polyglycolic and polylactic acid was described in a recent study. Annular cells from sheep were seeded on the device and incubated for 1 day, with nucleus pulposus cells (also from sheep) in alginate gel suspension added 1 day later. The implants were then placed subcutaneously into athymic mice and harvested at 4, 8, and 12 weeks. Gross morphology, histology, collagen typing and proteoglycan, hydroxyproline, and DNA analysis all showed a strong similarity to native disk. Although challenges remain in optimizing scaffolds, cell sources, implantation techniques, fixation, and long-term function, tissue engineering may offer viable solutions in the future.

Biologic regeneration and gene therapy techniques are also being applied to address disk degeneration. Initial findings in vitro and in limited in vivo studies sug-

gest the potential of growth factors to help regenerate or repair degenerated disk. The effects of various growth factors on cells derived from the nucleus pulposus and anulus fibrosus in both animals and humans are being identified. Animal models are being used to determine the effects of the administration of growth factors on the normal disk and some injury models. Although the complexity of growth factor effects has slowed progress in this area of study, the potential remains that administration of one or more growth factors can promote regeneration or repair of disk tissues. The continuing development of gene therapy techniques has led to the application of these techniques to disk degeneration. Efficient transduction of genes into the cells of the nucleus can be done using adenovirus vectors, and several promising transduction factors have been identified. It has been suggested that gene therapy may have the potential to favorably alter the course of the disk degeneration process. Growth factors for disk degeneration and gene therapy are discussed in detail in chapter 50.

## Motion-Sparing Posterior Devices

Posterior nonfusion devices are being developed to address instability and spinal stenosis. The Dynesys spinal system (Centerpulse Orthopaedics, Switzerland; now Zimmer, Warsaw, IN) is being developed to provide spinal alignment and dynamic stabilization while preserving the facets and disk. This system is a combination of polyethylene-terephthalate cords with polycarbonate urethane spacers as load-sharing members between metallic pedicle screws. In a biomechanical study, the Dynesys device restored stability to a destabilized spine to a level between that of the intact spine and fixation with an internal fixator. The device is believed to improve back pain by reducing the painful motion resulting from degenerative disk disease while retaining some motion to minimize adjacent segment problems. One recent clinical study reported that back and leg pain remain moderately high at 2 years after implantation of the Dynesys device. In addition, only half of the patients noted improved quality of life and less than half had improved functional capacity. Using comparisons with historical control subjects, the authors concluded that the Dynesys device had no advantage over fusion for treating degenerative disk disease. In another study that investigated the use of the Dynesys device after nucleotomy for herniated disk, deterioration of the Oswestry index was greater in patients without the stabilization.

Some devices are being developed to provide some stabilizing support to the posterior elements by being applied to the spinous processes of the degenerative segments. These devices are believed to improve back pain caused by degenerative instability, to preserve mobility, and to be reversible. The concept behind these devices is to provide an intermediate step between the degenerative unstable spine and a fused motion segment in hopes of reducing back pain. The Wallis device (SpineNext, Bordeaux, France), the Interspinous U (Fixan, Peronnas, France), and the DIAM (Medtronic, Memphis, TN) are examples of devices being developed with this philosophy.

## Device for Spinal Stenosis "Postural Decompression"

The X Stop interspinous process distraction device was developed as a minimally invasive approach to the relief of claudication from spinal stenosis. This device attempts to prevent the canal and foraminal narrowing that occurs with extension in patients with spinal stenosis, while not limiting flexion of the spine. In a recent FDA submission, clinical results were noted to benefit 45.7% of the study group compared with 4.9% of the nonsurgical control group. Although the concept seems sound and few safety issues were noted, questions were raised by the FDA advisory panel. As proof of concept for the design, the panel requested demonstration that narrowing of the canal and foraminal dimensions is prevented clinically. The panel also believed that the specific population that benefits from the device could be better defined.

## Cervical Spine
### Rationale for Motion-Sparing Technologies
In the cervical spine, the primary rationale for motion-sparing technology (cervical disk arthroplasty) is to avoid any adverse biomechanical effects on adjacent motion segments that may result from current procedures. By doing so, it is hoped that the subsequent radiographic degeneration of those adjacent segments and the development of new clinical disease related to degeneration of those segments might be minimized or avoided. However, when the degeneration of adjacent motion segments is attributed to a prior surgical procedure, the natural history of degenerative disease at motion segments adjacent to unoperated cervical spondylosis is unknown. For example, it is unknown how frequently a patient with a C6-7 spondylosis causing C7 radiculopathy who does not undergo surgical treatment will experience progression of spondylosis at C5-6 that causes C6 radiculopathy. It has been hypothesized that the elimination of segmental motion after anterior interbody fusion of the cervical spine may have deleterious effects on adjacent motion segments over time, possibly accelerating the degenerative process at these levels. Biomechanical studies have shown in vitro that interbody fusion constructs can increase adjacent segment motion and adjacent disk strain, although computerized assessments of motion in vivo up to 2 years after anterior cervical fusion have failed to correlate these results.

The degenerative process at adjacent levels as seen radiographically may be best described as adjacent segment degeneration. This phenomenon has been observed among many patients undergoing anterior cervical decompression and fusion procedures who are assessed many years after surgical treatment. One study reported a higher incidence of degeneration after posterior foraminotomy than after anterior cervical fusion. It should be remembered that the presence of these radiographic changes has not been found to correlate with the development of new clinical symptoms referable to changes at these levels. It has also been shown that among patients undergoing anterior cervical fusion, these changes are much more likely with the application of an anterior cervical plate.

When patients develop new symptoms of cervical radiculopathy and/or myelopathy that correlate with the development of degenerative changes at adjacent levels, the process is called adjacent segment disease. It has been reported that approximately 3% of patients undergoing anterior cervical decompression and fusion for radiculopathy and/or myelopathy will develop adjacent segment disease each year after the index operation, and the likelihood that a patient undergoing such a procedure will develop adjacent segment disease within 10 years is greater than 25%. The motion segments of C5-6 and C6-7 were found to be at highest risk of developing adjacent segment disease when not incorporated into the surgical procedure. In addition, the authors reported a significantly higher rate of adjacent segment disease following single-level procedures when compared with fusions of multiple levels.

Although there are fewer studies in the literature on the likelihood of adjacent segment disease after nonfusion procedures, similar percentages have been identified in studies of patients undergoing posterior foraminotomy without a fusion. Although these patients did not undergo a stabilization procedure, they did undergo an operation that may affect motion segment kinematics at the level of the decompression because of the resection of a portion of the facet joint in the area of the foraminal decompression. Nevertheless, the similarities in rates of adjacent segment disease between anterior cervical fusion and posterior foraminotomy procedures, as well as the finding that adjacent segment disease was more common following single rather than multiple level fusions, continue to fuel the controversy over whether adjacent segment disease is the consequence of the patient's spinal fusion procedure or of the natural history of the patient's cervical spondylosis.

The primary method of motion preservation proposed for the cervical spine has been total disk arthroplasty. One of the benefits of this procedure in the cervical spine is that it allows the same interbody decompressive procedure through an anterior approach that is already routinely performed for cervical radiculopathy and myelopathy caused by either a herniated disk or spondylosis. In patients undergoing cervical disk arthroplasty, an articulating prosthesis is placed into the decompressed disk space instead of a bone graft and anterior cervical plate. Theoretically, such a procedure would not only allow decompression of the neural elements but also potentially decreases or even eliminates the deleterious effects of fusion on adjacent levels by preserving motion at the decompressed level.

Fundamental to the benefits of a cervical disk replacement is its ability to "spare" motion at the segment undergoing surgery. Range of motion is diminished as a result of advancing age in most patients undergoing anterior cervical decompression; therefore, whether these devices can restore native motion at the operated level or preserve the motion that existed before the anterior cervical decompressive procedure is unclear.

## Biomechanics of Cervical Disk Arthroplasty

The biomechanics and biomaterial considerations associated with cervical disk arthroplasty are complex. Biomechanical factors include the number and shape of the articulating surfaces, their centers of rotation, any constraints on motion caused by the design, and the subsequent effect these factors may have on other parts of the motion segment, including the facet joints. Material considerations include the composition of the end plates of the prosthesis, method of implant fixation to the native bone stock, and the materials used to form the articulating surfaces.

Perhaps one of the most important aspects of cervical disk arthroplasty design is an understanding of the bony anatomy where the prosthesis will reside. A series of studies were performed to evaluate this anatomy, including evaluation of end-plate mineralization, trabecular structure of the cervical vertebrae, and the bone density of cervical vertebrae. The results of these studies demonstrated that the most dense bone mineralization in the cervical vertebrae was located in the lateral portions of the end plate. This density in bone mineralization is in part caused by the higher bending loads and increased lateral mobility seen in the cervical spine. Bone density was found to be higher in the cervical spine than in the lumbar spine. The trabeculae were thicker and the space between trabeculae was smaller in the cervical spine than in the lumbar spine. As a result of these findings, certain design properties were recommended: (1) the implant should have a large surface area to maximize contact area with the vertebral body, especially in the areas of highest mineralization; (2) the implant should have a profile that would obviate the need for removal of the highly mineralized bone in the uncovertebral areas; and (3) any porous coating on the implant should account for the dense bone structure of the cervical spine. These principles were suggested as a

way to avoid subsidence of a cervical disk prosthesis, a devastating complication that may lead to focal deformity and loss of local bone stock. These complications could hamper any attempts at salvage and revision.

Implant materials currently being used in cervical disk replacement include titanium alloys, cobalt-chromium alloys, and stainless steel. In addition to metal-on-metal, bearing surfaces also include ultra-high molecular weight polyethylene (UHMWPE) and polyurethane. All of these biomaterials have been used and tested extensively in adult reconstruction. The data regarding strength, biocompatibility, resistance to wear, and generation of debris particles have significantly influenced decisions about the components used in cervical disk prostheses. The physiologic loads placed across the cervical disk space are far less than in the knee or hip, and thus any of these metals/alloys would provide a solid platform. One benefit of using a titanium alloy rather than stainless steel in the cervical spine is that it would result in less artifact on CT and MRI studies.

The choice of bearing surfaces has been a source of controversy in the field of adult reconstruction, and these concerns have affected the development of cervical disk replacements. Hard bearing surfaces such as ceramic-on-ceramic or metal-on-metal have been used to minimize the generation of wear debris that might result in periprosthetic osteolysis. Currently, both hard-on-hard bearing surfaces and hard-on-soft bearing surfaces are being used in cervical disk prosthesis. The intervertebral space is devoid of synovial tissue, which is considered a primary source of macrophages believed to be responsible for the development of osteolysis. In addition, the production of wear debris in the cervical spine will most likely not be as significant as in total knee or total hip arthroplasty because much smaller loads are encountered. The other factor that may cause particulate wear is the sliding distance, which is relatively small in the cervical spine.

Three primary modes of fixation are used in cervical disk replacement. The first method is via a press-fit approach similar to that performed with cementless total hip and total knee arthroplasty. Short-term fixation is achieved through the press-fit with bony ingrowth along the prosthesis providing long-term fixation. A minimal amount of bone resection is typically required, and cutting jigs are not used in this process. The second method of fixation involves the use of screws in the adjacent vertebral bodies in a process similar to that used in anterior cervical plating. A third mode of fixation involves the use of porous ingrowth combined with a prosthetic "fin" to provide immediate stability in all planes.

## Current Cervical Disk Replacements

Five cervical disk replacements are currently in use: the Bryan disk (Medtronic, Minneapolis, MN), Prestige

(Medtronic), Prodisc-C (Synthes), Porous Coated Motion (PCM Cervitech, Rockaway, NJ), and the Cervi-Core (Stryker). In the United States three of these disks (Bryan, Prodisc-C, Prestige) have been placed in humans as part of the FDA's IDE studies. These devices also are discussed in chapter 25.

### Bryan Disk

The Bryan cervical disk replacement is a one-piece prosthesis made of titanium alloy and polyurethane. The titanium end plates articulate with a polyurethane nucleus creating two articulating surfaces. The device is unconstrained in nature and allows for a variable center of rotation. The end plates are porous-coated titanium and the device is implanted in a press-fit fashion, requiring no supplemental fixation. The articulating surfaces are contained within a polyurethane sheath that attaches to the titanium end plates, forming a barrier that can contain any potential wear debris. The prosthesis is configured to five different diameters and one height.

### Prestige

The Prestige cervical disk replacement is a two-piece prosthesis made of stainless steel. The prosthesis has one articulating surface that is titanium (metal-on-metal). The inferior end-plate portion contains a ball configuration that articulates with the superior end plate, which has a trough configuration. The device is a semiconstrained device with a mobile center of rotation. The prosthesis is fixed to the adjacent vertebra via a constrained locking screw mechanism. The prosthesis is available in 6- to 9-mm heights, a constant width of 17.8 mm, and depths of 12 and 14 mm.

### Prodisc-C

The Prodisc-C is a three-piece prosthesis. The end plates are made of cobalt-chromium alloy. The device contains one articulation that is made of UHMWPE. The polymer insert is fixed on the caudal end plate and articulates via a concavity formed in the superior end plate. The prosthesis is semiconstrained and has a fixed center of rotation. The end plates contain sagittal keels that are plasma sprayed. The implantation of this device requires use of a chisel to make slots in the vertebral bodies for the keels. The prosthesis is fixed using a press-fit technique.

### Porous Coated Motion

The Porous Coated Motion has a rectangular footprint to reduce the incidence of subsidence. The end plates are manufactured from cobalt-chromium alloy. The prosthesis is made of two components that are affixed to the respective end plates. An UHMWPE core is affixed to the caudal component. Thus, the bearing surface is cobalt-chromium on polyethylene. The device is provisionally fixed using a press-fit method. The outside of

each component is covered with titanium/calcium phosphate to promote long-term bony ingrowth. This device has a large radius of curvature, allowing near-physiologic unconstrained anterior-posterior translation with flexion and extension.

### CerviCore

The CerviCore is a two-piece, uniarticulating, metal-on-metal device made of a cobalt-chromium composite. The articulation between the pieces is saddle-shaped, which reportedly allows a flexion-extension moving center of rotation in the vertebral body below the prosthesis but allows the center of rotation for lateral bending to be in the vertebral body above the prosthesis. The goal of the saddle design is to allow couple motions characteristic of cervical spine kinematics, such as the lateral bending that occurs with axial rotation. Fixation of the device is via screw placement through anterior flanges.

Currently, there are few published clinical studies evaluating the success of cervical disk arthroplasty. There are, however, a few reports detailing the early clinical experiences associated with this form of treatment. The Porous Coated Motion was studied in 52 patients undergoing 81 disk replacements. After 1 year of follow-up the patients underwent postoperative radiographic and clinical evaluation. The most common condition treated in this group of patients was radiculopathy. Exclusion criteria included infection, tumor, trauma, or any biomechanical instability. Visual analog scale scores at 1 year after surgery had decreased from an average preoperative value of 85 (range, 100 to 50) to an average postoperative value of 20 (range, 50 to 0). The patients were also evaluated using Odom's criteria; 56% reported excellent results, 37% good, 7% fair, and 0% poor at 1 year.

The Bryan cervical disk was placed in 97 patients being treated for either radiculopathy or myelopathy. Patients were evaluated radiographically and the Short Form-36 was used postoperatively. Seventy-three patients underwent a single-level disk replacement and were reviewed at 2 years. Results were excellent in 45 patients, good in 7, fair in 13, and poor in 8 patients. Postoperative radiographs did not show any evidence of subsidence. One early episode of anterior migration (3 mm) was reported. Thirty patients underwent a two-level disk replacement and were reviewed at 1 year. Results were excellent in 21 patients, good in 3, fair in 5, and poor in 1 patient. No evidence of subsidence was reported. Average motion occurring in each disk was 8°.

Additional clinical studies evaluating cervical disk arthroplasty are needed before definitive recommendations can be made regarding their implantation. Some of the variables that need to be critically evaluated include the overall sagittal alignment obtained after cervical disk replacement, pain scores, subsidence, preservation, and the effect on adjacent segment disease.

## Summary

Motion-sparing devices are being developed for both cervical and lumbar indications. As these devices are evaluated, several issues should be considered. The indication for the device should be clear. The theoretical benefits of the device and the mechanism by which it is effective should be demonstrated in both preclinical and clinical testing. Clinical trials should demonstrate safety in that the risks of the device and its insertion should be outweighed by the benefits experienced by the patient. The effectiveness of the device should be demonstrated by improved validated outcome scores compared with those of control populations undergoing surgical procedures that represent the current standard of care. Studies should also establish an individual effectiveness threshold of patient success and show that a significant portion of the study population benefits from the device. New devices are held to the standard of equal or greater effectiveness when compared with existing treatment controls, but clinical studies are typically limited to 2 years of follow-up, limiting evaluation of long-term risks and benefits.

## Annotated Bibliography

### General

Bridwell KH: Introduction for scoliosis research society focus issue on motion preservation. *Spine* 2003;28:S101-S102.

Articles reviewing the considerations involved with motion-sparing technologies, including design and clinical applications, are presented. Disk replacement, minimization of fusion for scoliosis, and fusionless correction of scoliosis are discussed.

Disc arthroplasty: Focus issue. *J Spinal Disord* 2003;16:all.

This supplement to the *Journal of Spinal Disorders* presents 16 articles covering preclinical design and testing through preliminary clinical results of cervical and lumbar disk replacements.

Disc replacement: Special issue. *Spine J* 2004;4(suppl 6): all.

This supplemental issue of *The Spine Journal* presents papers reviewing the history, philosophy, and indications for disk replacement, the biomechanics and clinical results to date, and potential future developments. It is the most recent of these three focus issues of journals and is the most comprehensive coverage of the topic to date.

### Lumbar Spine

Allen MJ, Schoonmaker JE, Bauer TW, Williams PF, Higham PA, Yuan HA: Preclinical evaluation of a poly (vinyl alcohol) Hydrogel implant as a replacement for the nucleus pulposus. *Spine* 2004;29:515-523.

This article describes the rationale and preclinical evaluation of a hydrogel nucleus replacement.

Bertagnoli R, Vazquez RJ: The Anterolateral Trans Psoatic Approach: A new technique for implanting prosthetic disc-nucleus devices. *J Spinal Disord Tech* 2003;16: 398-404.

Technique and early clinical results from nucleus replacement introduced into the anterolateral aspect of the disk are discussed.

Buttermann GR, Beaubien BP: Stiffness of prosthetic nucleus determines stiffness of reconstructed lumbar calf disc. *Spine J* 2004;4:265-274.

An animal model of nuclear replacement and motion segment stiffness is described.

Husson JL, Korge A, Polard JL, Nydegger T, Kneubuhler S, Mayer HM: A memory coiling spiral as nucleus pulposus prosthesis: Concept, specifications, bench testing and first clinical rsults. *J Spinal Disord Tech* 2003;16: 405-411.

The rationale, design, preclinical and initial clinical results of a memory coiling prosthesis for nucleus replacement are discussed.

Jin D, Qu D, Zhao L, Chen J, Jiang J: Prosthetic disc nucleus replacement for lumbar disc herniation: Preliminary report with six month's follow-up. *J Spinal Disord Tech* 2003;16:331-337.

This article describes early (6 months) clinical results from a human trial of nucleus pulposus replacement.

Kotani Y, Abumi K, Shikinami Y, et al: Artificial intervertebral replacement using bioactive three-dimensional fabric: Design, development, and preliminary animal study. *Spine* 2002;27:929-936.

This article describes an alternative disk replacement design using a three-dimensional fabric.

Takahata M, Kotani Y, Abumi K, et al: Bone ingrowth fixation of artificial intervertebral disc consisting of bioceramic coated three-dimensional fabric. *Spine* 2003;28: 637-644.

This article discusses bone ingrowth as fixation for a three-dimensional fabric design.

US Food and Drug Administration Website. In depth statistical review for expedited PMA (P040006) Charite Artificial Disc, DePuy Spine Inc (dated Feb. 23, 2004). Available at: http://www.fda.gov/ohrms/dockets/ac/04/ briefing/4049b1_04_Statistical%20Review%20Memo% 20JCC.pdf. Accessed September, 2005.

This website provides the FDA statistical review of results from the Charite disk replacement premarket approval application.

US Food and Drug Administration Website. Department of Health and Human Services: PMA Memorandum. Available at: http://www.fda.gov/ohrms/dockets/ac/04/briefing/4049b1_03_Clinical%20Review%20Memo%20MAY.pdf. Accessed September, 2005.

This website provides the clinical review of results by the FDA from the Charite disk replacement premarket approval application.

Zigler E, Burd TA, Vialle EN, Sachs BL, Rashbaum RF, Ohnmeiss DD: Lumbar spine arthroplasty: Early results using the ProDisc II: A Prospective radomized trial of arthorplasty versus fusion. *J Spinal Disord* 2003;16:352-361.

Clinical results from an alternative disk replacement design, the ProDisc II, are described.

## Biologic "Devices" for Disk Replacement

Mizuno H, Roy AK, Vacanti CA, Kojima K, Ueda M, Bonassar LJ: Tissue-engineered composites of anulus fibrosus and nucleus pulposus for intervertebral disc replacement. *Spine* 2004;29:1290-1298.

This article describes details about the tissue-engineered composite described in the chapter. Techniques of tissue engineering, scaffold description, and morphology of disk resulting from these techniques are reviewed.

## Motion-Sparing Posterior Devices

Grob D, Benini A, Junge A, Mannion A: Clinical experience with the dynesys semirigid fixation system for the lumbar spine. *Spine* 2005;30:324-331.

This article presents a clinical study of patients undergoing dynamic stabilization of the lumbar spine.

Schmoelz W, Huber JF, Nydegger T, Claes L, Wilke HJ: Dynamic stabilization of the lumbar spine and its effects on adjacent segments: An in vitro experiment. *J Spinal Disord Tech* 2003;16:418-423.

The biomechanical effects of dynamic posterior stabilization of the lumbar spine including the adjacent segment are reviewed.

## Device for Spinal Stenosis "Postural Decompression"

http://www.fda.gov/ohrms/dockets/ac/04/briefing/2004-4064b1_02_clinical%20memo.doc

An FDA review of a premarket application for an interspinous process distraction device for lumbar stenosis is presented.

## Cervical Spine

Link HD, McAfee PC, Pimenta L: Choosing a cervical disc replacement. *Spine J* 2004;4(suppl 6):294S-302S.

This article discusses cervical disk replacement designs and rationale for use.

# Chapter 53

# Restoration of Spinal Cord Function

Jack Chen, MD

Frank Eismont, MD

## Introduction

The incidence of spinal cord injury (SCI) is more than 10,000 instances per year in the United States. Over 200,000 Americans live with a disability related to a SCI. The cost of caring for patients with SCI in the United States has been estimated to be $10 billion per year. Despite extensive research efforts, no treatment currently exists to reliably restore neurologic function below the level of injury. Instead, the current primary treatment of a patient with SCI begins with limiting the effects of the acute injury and minimizing secondary neurologic damage caused by the inflammatory processes. Second, as the patient transitions into the later stages of injury, treatment must evolve to address the multiple issues associated with chronic injury. The third major component of the treatment of SCI is still in an experimental phase and involves the enhancement of axonal regeneration. The management of acute SCI has been covered in chapter 21. It is important to discuss the epidemiology and unique complications seen with chronic SCI and to characterize possible future treatments.

## Epidemiology

In the 1970s, the model SCI care system program was initiated. In this system, the federally funded centers for SCI care were required to contribute patient data to a national database. This database is known as the National Spinal Cord Injury Statistical Center (NSCISC). In the 1980s, the Centers for Disease Control and Prevention (CDC) began funding SCI surveillance systems in various states. The NSCISC and CDC databases were combined to provide a relatively thorough description of the epidemiology of SCI in the United States.

The incidence of SCI ranges from 59 new patients per million per year in Mississippi to 25 new patients per million per year in West Virginia. The average incidence in the United States is approximately 40 new patients per million per year, translating to more than 10,000 new patients per year in the United States. These figures do not include fatal SCIs that occur before hospitalization. Using mathematical models that take into account the incidence of SCI and the life expectancy of patients with SCI, the prevalence of SCI has been estimated to be just under 250,000 patients in 2004. This estimate predicts the prevalence of SCI to be more than 275,000 patients in 2014, because of the improved life expectancies resulting from current standards of care.

Almost 50% of new patients with SCI are between the ages of 15 and 29 years. The NSCISC database reports the most common age of injury is 19 years, and the mean age of injury is 31.8 years. There is a 4:1 gender ratio, with an incidence of 65 injuries per million per year for men versus 16 for women. Women have a higher survival rate. This increase is reflected by a difference in the percentage of men in the estimates of incidence compared with their percentage in the estimates of prevalence. Although 80% of new patients with SCI are men, the percentage of male patients living with SCI is approximately 70%.

In the 1990s, 58.9% of new patients enrolled in the NSCISC database were white, 28.1% were African American, 10.3% were Hispanic, 2.2% were Asian, and 0.5% were Native American. The etiologies of the SCIs were: 38.6% caused by motor vehicle crashes, 23.2% caused by falls, 22.5% resulting from violence, 6.7% were sports related, and 9% were the result of other unknown causes. A closer analysis of ethnicity and etiology reveals a disturbing trend. Among African American and Hispanic males age 16 to 21 years at the time of injury, the percentage of SCI resulting from an act of violence was approximately 35% in the 1970s; this percentage had increased to approximately 70% in the 1990s.

Approximately 50% of patients have cervical injuries, 35% have thoracic and thoracolumbar injuries, 11% have lumbar and lumbosacral injuries, and the remaining injuries are unknown or unreported. In terms of a specific injury level, C5 is the most common, accounting for about 15% of all injuries. Fifty percent of all patients have complete injuries, and thoracic level injuries are the most likely to be complete injuries.

The mortality rate has been estimated to be approximately 6% during the first year after injury. The rate drops to approximately 2% during the second year, declining to about 1% every year thereafter. The latest life expectancy estimates from the NSCISC database can be found online at *www.spinalcord.uab.edu.* The most common cause of death is respiratory disease, with pneumonia accounting for about 70% of deaths from pulmonary causes. Compared with the general population, deaths as a result of septicemia in patients with SCI are more than 60 times the normal rate, deaths caused by pulmonary embolism are almost 50 times normal, and deaths resulting from pneumonia and influenza are about 35 times normal.

Costs for caring for patients with SCI differ for those with complete and incomplete injury. In the first year, the costs of care for a patient with a complete cervical level injury have been estimated to be about $550,000. In contrast, the costs of care are about $160,000 for a patient with incomplete motor function. After the first year, the average annual expenditures are about $98,000 for patients with complete injuries and $11,000 for patients with incomplete injuries. These costs are higher in patients who are ventilator dependent and are almost $750,000 during the first year, dropping to annual costs of over $290,000 thereafter.

## Patient Issues
### Autonomic Dysreflexia
Autonomic dysreflexia (AD) is a syndrome of severe and sudden hypertension in response to a noxious stimulus below the level of SCI in patients with injuries above T6 (above the sympathetic outflow levels). AD has been estimated to occur in up to 85% of all patients with SCI with injuries at or above T6. The exaggerated hypertension, if left untreated, may result in retinal hemorrhage, subarachnoid hemorrhage, intracerebral hemorrhage, myocardial infarction, seizure, and even death. The mechanism causing the syndrome begins with a strong, usually noxious stimulus entering the spinal cord via intact peripheral nerves. This stimulus ascends the spinal cord and incites a reflex release of sympathetic activities, mediated by the release of norepinephrine and dopamine. The increase in blood pressure can lead to a compensatory reflex bradycardia caused by the brainstem vasomotor center.

AD most often occurs between 6 months and 1 year after injury. Symptoms include headache, sweating, and flushing; however, patients may experience no symptoms. To avert the sequelae of the syndrome, early recognition is important and the inciting stimulus must be removed. To prevent worsening of the hypertension while potential causes are being investigated, it is recommended that the patient sit upright and constrictive devices and clothing be removed. Antihypertensive agents with rapid onset and a short half-life, such as nitroglycerine paste, can be used as a temporizing mea-

sure. The most common stimulus causing AD is blockage of the urinary system. The patient should receive a catheter if an indwelling urinary catheter is not in place. If the patient has an indwelling catheter, it needs to be changed or at least checked for kinking of the tube or other obstructions. The second most common cause of AD is fecal impaction. Lidocaine gel should be used before rectal examination. If the cause of AD has not been identified or if the hypertension persists, the patient should be sent to the emergency department for monitoring and further pharmacologic control of blood pressure while other causes of AD are investigated.

### Urologic Issues
Voiding dysfunction may result in an increase in urinary tract infection (UTI), bladder stones, and can potentially lead to renal complications. Bladder storage and emptying are controlled by an interaction between the parasympathetic, sympathetic, and somatic innervation of the lower urinary tract. Sympathetic efferent nerves originate from T11 to L2 and provide inhibitory effects to the bladder, facilitating storage. Parasympathetic efferent nerves begin in the sacral cord (S2 to S4) and provide excitatory input to facilitate bladder contraction and emptying. Most commonly, patients with SCI have injuries above the sacral level. These patients have spastic bladders with uninhibited bladder contractions, resulting in episodes of incontinence. However, the contractions are uncoordinated, leading to high intravesical pressures. These high pressures can result in hydronephrosis and renal deterioration. In contrast, patients with sacral spinal cord and cauda equina injuries have acontractile or flaccid bladders. However, overdistention of the bladder, combined with decreased bladder wall compliance, can also lead to high intravesical pressures, resulting in renal complications similar to those experienced by patients with suprasacral level injuries.

Initially, many patients with acute SCI are in spinal shock, at which time there is no bladder contraction. This condition, combined with posttraumatic fluid shifts, may necessitate the use of an indwelling catheter. Once the patient's fluid status has stabilized, a program of intermittent catheterization should be started. Compared with an indwelling catheter, intermittent catheterization results in less chance of UTI, bladder stones, urethral erosions, and penile scrotal fistulas. Catheterization is performed every 4 hours, with the goal of keeping catheterization volumes below 400 mL. Additionally, a 2 L daily fluid restriction is often encouraged to help meet this goal. Other options of urinary management include indwelling catheterization, suprapubic catheterization, and reflex voiding, which describes the action of spontaneous reflexive voiding once the bladder reaches a certain volume. To collect urine, the patient must wear a condom catheter; therefore, this method is not used in women.

To further avoid high bladder pressures and renal complications, pharmacologic and surgical treatments also are used. Because parasympathetic stimulation of bladder contraction is mediated by cholinergic receptors, the primary pharmacologic agents used are anticholinergics. Oxybutynin is a frequently used oral anticholinergic medication. Adverse effects of anticholinergics include a dry mouth, tachycardia, blurred vision, and constipation. Surgical procedures can be used if conservative treatment and medications have failed to decrease bladder pressures. Bladder augmentation can be performed in patients with poor bladder compliance to increase bladder capacity. Transurethral sphincterotomy is another well-established procedure that can be performed in patients with urine retention caused by sphincter overactivity.

UTIs can result in complications such as pyelonephritis, renal scarring, renal calculi, retroperitoneal abscess, and sepsis. Symptoms of UTI in an insensate patient with SCI include cloudy, foul-smelling urine, increased abdominal or lower extremity spasticity, new onset urinary incontinence, and autonomic dysreflexia. Patients with upper UTI also may have fever and chills. Patients with lower UTI should be treated with a 3- to 7-day course of antibiotics with the use of shorter courses of treatment whenever possible. In patients with pyelonephritis, high fevers, dehydration, or autonomic dysreflexia, treatment should consist of hospitalization, hydration, indwelling Foley catheterization to decompress the bladder, a catheter change for those patients who already have a catheter in place, anticholinergic medication, and a longer course of antibiotics. In addition, patients with pyelonephritis should have a urologic evaluation for stones and reflux.

The treatment of asymptomatic bacteriuria (< 100,000 colony-forming organisms) and asymptomatic UTI (> 100,000 colony-forming organisms) depends on the presence of vesicoureteral reflux. Patients with high grade reflux are more likely to develop pyelonephritis and therefore should be treated with antibiotics. Otherwise, it is generally believed that symptomatic bacteriuria in a patient with an indwelling catheter does not warrant antimicrobial treatment.

Up to 8% of patients with SCI develop renal calculi, the most notorious cause of renal deterioration. It was reported that a patient with a staghorn calculus has a 50% chance of losing the involved kidney. Renal calculi are often associated with UTIs, particularly with *Protease mirabilis* infections. Eradication of the infection, along with procedures such as percutaneous nephrolithotomy and extracorporeal shock wave lithotripsy, are the treatments of choice for renal calculi.

Bladder cancer occurs more frequently in patients with SCI than in the general population. Squamous cell bladder cancer is frequently associated with the use of an indwelling catheter, recurrent UTIs, and bladder stones. In patients who have had indwelling catheters in place for more than 10 years, cystoscopy should be performed each year to rule out the presence of bladder stones and to screen for bladder cancer.

Previously, renal failure was the leading cause of death after SCI. Since the widespread use of intermittent catheterization and sphincterotomy, the rate of death from renal causes has markedly decreased. Avoidance of renal failure in patients with SCI requires an increased index of suspicion for these disorders, lowering bladder pressure, and preventing recurrent infections.

## Psychosocial Issues

Depression is evidenced by persistent loss of interest in people and activities, accompanied by an overall depressed mood. In contrast to the transient states of dysphoria often experienced by patients adapting to SCI, persistent depression is a disabling condition. Depressive disorders have been estimated to occur in 20% to 45% of patients with SCI, and is considered to be the most common form of psychological pathology in these patients. Symptoms include loss of interest in activities, changes in appetite or sleep, and decreased attention to self-care.

Suicidal ideation should be assessed when depression is suspected. Suicide is the leading cause of death in patients with SCI who are younger than 55 years; therefore, depression may be linked to mortality after SCI. Pharmacologic intervention should be considered for patients with mood disturbances. Many antidepressant medications are available. The signs and symptoms of the patient as well as the side-effect profile of the medication should guide the selection of a particular medication. For example, tricyclic antidepressants, because of the risk of overdose, should be avoided in patients with suicidal ideation. Because medications cannot address the cognitive aspects of depression or the social, environmental, and interpersonal concerns of the patient, other psychotherapeutic modalities, such as cognitive therapy, can be offered.

Social support has a direct relationship with adjustment and an inverse relationship with psychological distress. For recently injured patients, social support often begins in the rehabilitation center, where these patients befriend others with SCI. However, as new relationships develop, existing social relationships can be strained. The patient often needs to reestablish their relationships with preexisting friends and with family. Patient apathy or embarrassment, together with their friends' discomfort, contributes to the development of social isolation. Furthermore, family members must adjust to new roles. For example, a spouse has to become both spouse and attendant. To promote communication and foster relationships, counseling should be made available to the patient and family members during medical follow-up visits. Family members can be reminded to maintain their own physical, emotional, and social health.

Overcoming the psychological challenges of SCI often requires the aid of psychologists, the rehabilitation team, and appropriate social support from friends and family. Promoting the mental well-being of the patient with SCI includes maintaining motivation and hopefulness, encouraging self-directed behavior, and improving sense of control. Mental health contributes greatly to regaining as much independence as possible and improving the quality of life. For some, learning to cope with SCI and its psychological impact becomes a lifelong process. For others, adaptation and acceptance are evident when disability is no longer the dominant concern in life.

## Regeneration of Spinal Cord Function
### Nerve Regeneration and Repair
#### The Early Stages of Injury
In SCI, the primary mechanisms of neurologic injury occur from mechanical deformation and ischemia. This primary injury is then followed by the initiation of the inflammatory cascade, leading to further tissue damage (Figure 1). A loss of neurotrophic and growth-promoting factors occurs, coupled with the release of inhibitory factors. Programmed cell death (apoptosis) occurs, and the formation of an astrocytic glial scar creates a barrier for attempts at axonal regeneration. In consideration of the stages of acute injury, there are three steps in the strategy of neural repair: neuroprotection to support neuron survival; modulation of the inhibitory environment present after the injury, including suppression of the astrocytic response; and stimulation of axonal regrowth.

#### Neuroprotection
The administration of steroids is the only current treatment that is believed to be beneficial in the treatment of acute SCI, based on the results of prospective randomized studies. The beneficial effects of methylprednisolone are theorized to be attributable to membrane stabilization and to the suppression of the inflammatory response following acute SCI. However, more recent publications have questioned the risk-benefit ratio of using steroids for acute SCI because steroids increase the risks of infection and gastrointestinal bleeding in these patients. Therefore, steroid use should be carefully considered on an individual basis.

A possible alternative for neuroprotection includes the inhibition of apoptosis. Bcl-2 is a protooncogene that may block the intracellular triggers of apoptosis. Bcl-2 inhibits the release of cytochrome c. Cytochrome c is essential in the activation of caspase, the enzyme that triggers the execution phase of apoptosis. It has been

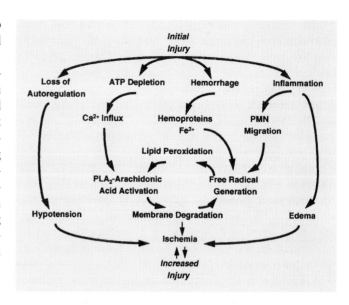

**Figure 1** Biochemical cascade effect following primary SCI. ATP = adenosine triphosphate, PMN = polymorphonuclear leukocytes, PLA$_2$ = phospholipase A$_2$.

shown that overexpression of Bcl-2 increases the survival of axontomized neurons. Consequently, peptides similar to Bcl-2 may serve as effective agents in neuroprotection. Because caspases are essential enzymes in the execution of apoptosis, they have been targeted in other strategies aimed at inhibiting apoptosis. Peptides that inhibit caspases have been shown to block apoptosis of motor neurons.

#### Reversal of Inhibitory Environment
Astrocytes contribute to the formation of a glial scar. This scar poses both a physical and chemical barrier to regenerating axons. (Overcoming the physical barrier posed by the scar will be discussed in the section pertaining to promoting axonal regrowth.) The milieu of the glial scar contains proteoglycans that inhibit axonal regeneration. The major inhibitory mechanism seems to be the interference with growth-promoting cell adhesion molecules such as laminin, which provide guidance cues for axonal growth. To combat this inhibitory effect, researchers have used proteases. In vitro experiments show that proteases can degrade proteoglycans. Furthermore, an in vivo study using rats showed that administration of chondroitinase resulted in regrowth of axons across transected regions.

Other inhibitory molecules have been found in patients with SCI. Some membrane proteins associated with rat oligodendrocytes and central nervous system myelin have been shown to inhibit neurite growth. Inhibitory myelin molecules that have been identified include NI-35, NI-250, Nogo-A, and myelin-associated glycoprotein. When antibodies to these membrane proteins were administered, regrowth of axons in adult rats with transected spinal cords were observed. Other research-

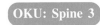

ers have shown that brain- and glial-derived neurotrophic factors can protect neurons from the inhibitory effects of these myelin molecules.

### Promotion of Axonal Regrowth

A much-studied strategy for promoting neuronal regeneration is nerve grafting. Previous studies have shown the ability of axons to enter and grow within peripheral nerve grafts, but these axons were not able to penetrate the distal graft-host interface to continue growing. To overcome the inhibitory environment at the graft-host interface, fibrin glue with fibroblast growth factor (FGF-1) was used to stabilize the graft to the host spinal cord. FGF-1 has been previously found to stimulate axonal outgrowth, and in this study, successful growth of axons past the graft-host interface was demonstrated. Hind limb function in the adult rats in the study exhibited progressive improvement during the 6 months after the nerve grafting procedure.

An alternative to using whole nerve grafts is to use Schwann cell grafts. Studies have shown that Schwann cells express neurotrophic factors and provide guidance cues to regenerating axons via cell adhesion molecules. Schwann cells transplanted with a matrix containing adhesion molecules into an area of spinal cord transection supported the regrowth of ascending and descending axons. Recently, olfactory ensheathing glial (OEG) cells have also been tested in cell transplantation models. Olfactory axons can regenerate and reestablish synaptic contacts within the olfactory bulb. OEG cells normally support olfactory axons, producing trophic factors (platelet-derived growth factor, nerve growth factor, brain-derived neurotrophic factor, neurotrophin-3 [NT-3]) and cell adhesion molecules (laminin, L1, N-CAM). After transplantation of OEG cells into rhizotomies that were anastomosed microsurgically, axonal regrowth was seen across the root-cord junction and into the spinal cord gray matter. In other studies, OEG cells also have been shown to aid in remyelinating dorsal column axons.

Neurotrophic factors, when delivered into an injured region of rat spinal cord, have been shown to promote some axonal regeneration and to be neuroprotective. Different cell populations have different and specific receptors for different neurotrophic factors. Brain-derived neurotrophic factor and NT-3 are two neurotrophic factors that have been shown to have preferential effects on the rubrospinal tract and corticospinal tract, respectively.

Exogenous delivery of neurotrophic factors, however, is a difficult task, limited by pharmacokinetics, systemic antibodies, and the blood-brain barrier. Transplantation of cells that can supply neurotrophic factors can potentially overcome these limitations. Gene therapy has the potential of modifying the cells to produce neurotrophic factors at the site of injury. The accomplishment of gene therapy requires a target cell, a gene encoding for the protein of interest, and a vector to carry the gene into the target cell. Research is still evolving regarding the efficacy and safety of the various vectors used for gene delivery. The theoretic possibility exists of using viral vectors to transplant target genes directly into cells surrounding the injury site. Current work focuses on ex vivo transfection of cells with the intended genes and then implanting the modified cells into the area of injury.

Gene therapy using ex vivo modified fibroblasts and Schwann cells has been reported. Fibroblasts modified to secrete NT-3 showed neuroprotective functions, preventing cell death in the corticospinal tract of injured spinal cords. In another study, fibroblasts that were modified to secrete brain-derived neurotrophic factor induced axonal regeneration in hemitransected rat spinal cords. The animals also had partial recovery of forelimb function. Schwann cells that were modified to deliver brain-derived neurotrophic factor, when injected into spinal cord tissue distal to a transection, resulted in axonal growth across the transection. The new axons were found within guidance tracts established by the injected Schwann cells.

### Recovering Function Through Supported Ambulation and Electrical Stimulation

The plasticity of the central nervous system allows for the possibility that a small biologic bridge can produce dramatic impacts on distal function. After intensive physical therapy such as supported ambulation, adaptable circuitry may be trained to interpret complex sensory information associated with load bearing. It is hoped that this sensory input could "reawaken" spinal circuits, activating central pattern generators in the spinal cord to initiate stepping. Programs studying supported ambulation are ongoing at various institutions, including The Miami Project, Washington University, and at the University of California at Los Angeles. Current obstacles to intensive physical therapy for patients with SCI are budgetary considerations and the need for personnel trained in this type of work.

Functional electrical stimulation (FES) describes the application of an electrical stimulus to paralyzed nerves or muscles to activate their function. FES is used in other medical specialties in the form of cardiac pacemakers and cochlear implants. In the field of SCI, FES has been available for phrenic nerve pacing for more than two decades. Cost, surgical risk, and the need to retain a tracheostomy are some of the limiting factors against widespread use of implanted phrenic nerve pacing. FES technology has also been used for restoration of bladder and bowel function. The system consists of an implantable FES device controlled by radiofrequency signaling. The device activates electrodes placed on the sacral spinal roots (S2-S4), causing contraction of the bladder, urethra, large bowel, and anal sphincter. To prevent unwanted reflex bladder incontinence, detrusor-sphincter dysinergia, and hydronephrosis, implantation of the device must also be combined with sensory (dorsal) rhizotomies at S2 to S5. This results in loss of perineal sensation, reflex erection, and ejaculation. For many patients, the need for major surgery and additional "damage" in the form of rhizotomies are contraindications to this elective procedure. However, in Europe, similar systems have been implanted in more than 1,500 patients. Outcome studies show that by preventing urinary tract complications, the long-term cost savings help the system to pay for itself and net savings begin to accrue within 5 years.

FES has also been applied to the upper extremities. The Freehand system is an implantable FES system approved for use by the Food and Drug Administration. It improves hand function for tetraplegic patients with C5/C6 American Spinal Injury Association motor level. Eligible patients should have intact lower motor neuron function, adequate proximal muscle strength, and good motivation with realistic expectations. More recently, researchers have reported on the use of FES to improve triceps function. Compared with patients who underwent a posterior deltoid to triceps tendon transfer, patients who had FES-activated triceps demonstrated stronger elbow extension moments. This system allowed patients to improve their ability to reach and move objects as well as decrease the amount of time required to acquire an object.

In the lower extremities, FES has been applied for cardiovascular conditioning and strength training. Electrical activation of muscles occurs in a sequentially alternating pattern, via surface electrodes applied to hip extensors, knee extensors, and knee flexors. In studies of patients using FES coupled to a stationary bike, improvements in muscle mass and blood flow were seen. Other potential benefits of FES-assisted exercise are reduction in the risks of venous thrombosis and osteoporosis. FES of the lower extremities has been applied to restoration of standing and stepping, but patients require extensive bracing and assistive walking devices. Furthermore, intensive training and high metabolic energy consumption required for standing and stepping limit the use of FES for these purposes.

## Summary

A few decades ago, patients with SCI had a significantly shorter lifespan and multiple morbidities, with little hope for treatment and recovery. More information is now available about the epidemiology and treatment of the various morbidities associated with SCI. The length and the quality of life have been improved for patients with SCI because the specific issues of SCI patients are better addressed. Because of the advances being made

in cell transplantation and molecular biology, the goal of restoring spinal cord function is closer to being achieved.

## Annotated Bibliography

*Patient Issues*

Elfstrom M, Ryden A, Kreuter M, Taft C, Sullivan M: Relations between coping strategies and health-related quality of life in patients with spinal cord lesion. *J Rehabil Med* 2005;37:9-16.

This study showed that patients with better coping strategies in terms of greater self-acceptance and fewer tendencies towards dependent behavior scored higher in quality of life outcome measures.

Karlsson AK: Autonomic dysreflexia. *Spinal Cord* 1999; 37:383-391.

This article presents a review of the clinical aspects of autonomic dysreflexia. Pathogenesis, prevalence, symptoms, and treatments are discussed.

Weld KJ, Dmochowski RR: Effect of bladder management on urological complications in spinal cord injured patients. *J Urol* 2000;163:768-772.

The authors retrospectively reviewed patients with various methods of bladder management after SCI. Patients treated with clean intermittent catheterization had statistically significant lower complication rates compared with patients treated with chronic urethral catheterization.

*Regeneration of Spinal Cord Function*

Cao L, Liu L, Chen ZY, et al: Olfactory ensheathing cells genetically modified to secrete GDNF to promote spinal cord repair. *Brain* 2004;127:535-549.

In this study, a retroviral vector was used to transduce the *GDNF* gene into olfactory ensheathing cells. The modified olfactory ensheathing cells were then implanted into adult rats with complete cord transection. Both locomotor function recovery and axon regeneration were demonstrated.

Creasey GH, Dahlberg JE: Economic consequences of an implanted neuroprosthesis for bladder and bowel management. *Arch Phys Med Rehabil* 2001;82:1520-1525.

In a study of 12 patients in whom a neuroprosthesis was implanted for stimulation of the sacral nerves, the authors noted cost reductions in bowel and bladder care in comparison to treatment with conventional methods.

Hendriks WT, Ruitenberg MJ, Blits B, Boer GJ, Verhaagen J: Viral vector-mediated gene transfer of neurotrophins to promote regeneration of the injured spinal cord. *Prog Brain Res* 2004;146:451-478.

This article presents a review of gene therapy strategies for spinal cord regeneration. The authors discuss viral vectors, neurotrophic factors, and cell types that have been tested in experimental models of SCI.

Memberg WD, Crago PE, Keith MW: Restoration of elbow extension via functional electrical stimulation in individuals with tetraplegia. *J Rehabil Res Dev* 2003;40: 477-486.

Patients with tricep stimulators were evaluated for elbow extension force and performance in workspace environments. Compared with tendon transfer, tricep stimulation provided a stronger elbow extension moment and significantly increased the ability to move objects.

Ruitenberg MJ, Plant GW, Hamers FP, et al: Ex vivo adenoviral vector-mediated neurotrophin gene transfer to olfactory ensheathing glia: Effects on rubrospinal tract regeneration, lesion size, and functional recovery after implantation in the injured rat spinal cord. *J Neurosci* 2003;23:7045-7058.

This study describes the use of gene therapy to enhance the outgrowth-promoting properties of olfactory ensheathing cells. Adenoviral vectors encoding BDNF, NT-3, or control marker gene LacZ were used to transduce olfactory ensheathing cells. The olfactory ensheathing cells were implanted into rat spinal cords with unilateral transactions. Compared with control subjects without olfactory ensheathing cell implantations, all rats implanted with olfactory ensheathing cells showed smaller injury lesion size. Furthermore, rats with olfactory ensheathing cells transduced to express neurotrophins showed additional improvement in recovery of hindlimb function.

## Classic Bibliography

Alberi S, Reggenbass M, de Bilbao F, et al: Axotomized neonatal motoneurons overexpressing the Bcl-2 proto-oncogene retain functional electrophysiological properties. *Proc Natl Acad Sci USA* 1996;93:3978-3983.

Bracken MB, Shepard MJ, Holford TR, et al: Administration of methylprednisolone for 24 or 48 hours or tirilazad mesylate for 48 hours in the treatment of acute spinal cord injury. *JAMA* 1997;277:1597-1604.

Bregman BS, Kunkel-Bagden E, Schnell L, et al: Recovery from spinal cord injury mediated by antibodies to neurite growth inhibitors. *Nature* 1995;378:498-501.

Cai D, Shen Y, DeBellard ME, et al: Prior exposure to neurotrophins blocks inhibition of axonal regeneration by MAG and myelin via a cAMP-dependent mechanism. *Neuron* 1999;22:89-101.

Cheng H, Cao Y, Olson L: Spinal cord repair in adult paraplegic rats: Partial restoration of hind limb function. *Science* 1996;273:510-513.

Consortium for Spinal Cord: Acute management of autonomic dysreflexia: Adults with spinal cord injury presenting to health-care facilities. *J Spinal Cord Med* 1997; 20:284-318.

Edgerton VR, De Leon RD, Tillakaratne N, et al: Use-dependent plasticity in spinal stepping and standing. *Adv Neurol* 1997;72:233-247.

Farlie PG, Dringen R, Rees SM, et al: Bcl-2 transgene expression can protect neurons against developmental and induced cell death. *Proc Natl Acad Sci USA* 1995; 92:4397-4401.

Grill R, Murai K, Blesch A, et al: Cellular delivery of neurotrophin-3 promotes corticospinal axonal regrowth and partial functional recovery after spinal cord injury. *J Neurosci* 1997;17:5560-5572.

Guest JD, Hesse D, Schnell L, et al: Influence of IN-1 antibody and acidic FGF-fibrin glue on the response of injured corticospinal tract axons to human Schwann cell grafts. *J Neurosci Res* 1997;50:888-905.

Guttmann L, Frankel H: The value of intermittent catheterization in the early management of traumatic paraplegia and tetraplegia. *Paraplegia* 1966;4:63-84.

Harkema SJ, Hurley SL, Patel UK, et al: Human lumbosacral spinal cord interprets loading during stepping. *J Neurophysiol* 1997;77:797-811.

Hayashi T, Sakurai M, Abe K, et al: Apoptosis of motor neurons with induction of caspases in the spinal cord after ischemia. *Stroke* 1998;29:1007-1012.

Himes BT, Solowska-Baird J, Boyne L, et al: Grafting of genetically modified cells that produce neurotrophins in order to rescue axotomized neurons in rat spinal cord. *Soc Neuro Sci Abstr* 1995;21:537.

Lapides J, Diokno AC, Silber SJ, et al: Clean, intermittent self catheterization in the treatment of urinary tract disease. *J Urol* 1972;107:458-461.

Lasfargues JE, Custis DE, Morrone F, et al: A model for estimating spinal core injury prevalence in the United States. *Paraplegia* 1995;33:62-68.

Liu Y, Kim D, Himes BT, et al: Transplants of fibroblasts genetically modified to express BDNF to promote regeneration of adult rat rubrospinal axons. *J Neurosci* 1999;19:4370-4387.

Menei P, Montero-Menei C, Whittemore SR, et al: Schwann cells genetically modified to secrete BDNS promote enhanced axonal regrowth across transected adult rat spinal cord. *Eur J Neurosci* 1998;10:607-621.

Mukhopadhyay G, Doherty P, Walsh FS, et al: A novel role for myelin-associated glycoprotein as an inhibitor of axonal regeneration. *Neuron* 1994;13:757-767.

Ramon-Cueto A, Avila J: Olfactory ensheathing glia: properties and function. *Brain Res Bull* 1998;46:175-187.

Ramon-Cueto A, Plant GW, Avila J, et al: Long distance axonal regeneration in the transected adult rat spinal cord is promoted by olfactory ensheathing glia transplants. *J Neurosci* 1998;18:3803-3815.

Vaidyananthan S, Soni BM, Brown E, et al: Effect of intermittent urethral catheterization and oxybutinin bladder instillation on urinary continence status and quality of life in a selected group of spinal cord injured patients with neuropathic bladder dysfunction. *Spinal Cord* 1998; 36:409-414.

Villa T, Kaufmann SH, Earnshaw WC: Caspases and caspase inhibitors. *Trends Biochem Sci* 1997;22:388-393.

Wyndaele JJ: Pharmacotherapy for urinary bladder dysfunction in spinal cord injury patients. *Paraplegia* 1990; 28:146-150.

Xu XM, Chen A, Guenard V, et al: Bridging Schwann cell transplants promote axonal regeneration from both the rostral and caudal stumps of transected adult rat spinal cord. *J Neurocytol* 1997;26:1-16.

Zuo J, Ferguson TA, Hernandez YJ, et al: Neuronal matrix metalloproteinase-2 degraded and inactivated a neurite inhibiting chondroitin sulfate proteoglycan. *J Neurosci* 1998;18:5203-5211.

# Index